D1605491

HIGH
RISK
OBSTETRICS

The Requisites in Obstetrics and Gynecology

Series Editor:

Mark I. Evans, MD

President, Fetal Medicine Foundation of America
Director, Comprehensive Genetics
Professor of Obstetrics and Gynecology
Mt. Sinai School of Medicine
New York, New York

Other titles in

The Requisites in Obstetrics and Gynecology Series

GENERAL GYNECOLOGY
REPRODUCTIVE ENDOCRINOLOGY AND GYNECOLOGY
GYNECOLOGIC ONCOLOGY   (Coming Soon)

HIGH RISK OBSTETRICS

The Requisites in Obstetrics and Gynecology

Edmund F. Funai, MD

Associate Chair for Clinical Affairs; Co-Chief, Maternal-Fetal Medicine; Associate Professor, Department of Obstetrics, Gynecology, & Reproductive Sciences, Yale University School of Medicine, New Haven, Connecticut

Mark I. Evans, MD

President, Fetal Medicine Foundation of America; Director, Comprehensive Genetics; Professor of Obstetrics and Gynecology, Mt. Sinai School of Medicine, New York, New York

Charles J. Lockwood, MD

Anita O'Keefe Young Professor and Chair, Department of Obstetrics, Gynecology, & Reproductive Sciences, Yale University School of Medicine, New Haven, Connecticut

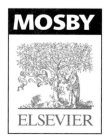

MOSBY

ELSEVIER

1600 John F. Kennedy Blvd.
Ste 1800
Philadelphia, PA 19103-2899

HIGH RISK OBSTETRICS: THE REQUISITES IN OBSTETRICS
AND GYNECOLOGY

ISBN: 978-0-323-03322-0

Library of Congress Cataloging-in-Publication Data

High risk obstetrics : the requisites in obstetrics and gynecology /
[edited by] Edmund Funai, Mark Evans, Charles Lockwood. — 1st ed.
  p. ; cm.
    Includes bibliographical references.
    ISBN 978-0-323-03322-0
  1. Pregnancy—Complications. I. Funai, Edmund. II. Evans, Mark I.
  III. Lockwood, Charles J.
    [DNLM: 1. Pregnancy Complications. 2. Pregnancy, High-Risk. WQ 240
  H6372 2008]
  RG571.H43 2008
  618.3—dc22

2007034987

Acquisitions Editor: Laurie Hee
Developmental Editor: Elizabeth Hart
Project Manager: Bryan Hayward
Design Direction: Steve Stave

Printed in the United States of America

Last digit is the print number: 9 8 7 6 5 4 3 2 1

Dedication

To Maryanne, Peter, and Phoebe for their love and patience.
Edmund F. Funai

To my daughters, Kiera and Shara.
Mark I. Evans

To Nancy, Sarah, and John: their patience, good humor, and encouragement make it all possible.
Charles J. Lockwood

CONTRIBUTORS

Yale S. Arkel, MD
Medical Director, Hemostasis and Thrombosis Laboratory, Bio-Reference Laboratories, Elmwood Park, New Jersey

Mert Ozan Bahtiyar, MD
Assistant Professor, Department of Obstetrics and Gynecology, Section of Maternal-Fetal Medicine, Yale University School of Medicine, New Haven, Connecticut

Yoni Barnhard, MD
Vice Chair, Department of Obstetrics and Gynecology, Lenox Hill Hospital, New York, New York

Jill P. Buyon, MD
Professor and Associate Director, Division of Rheumatology, New York University School of Medicine, New York, New York

Joshua Copel, MD
Professor and Vice Chair of Obstetrics, Department of Obstetrics and Gynecology, Yale University School of Medicine, New Haven, Connecticut

Michael Y. Divon, MD
Chair, Department of Obstetrics and Gynecology, Lenox Hill Hospital, New York, New York

Arie Drugan, MD
Director, Labor and Delivery, Department of Obstetrics & Gynecology, Rambam Medical Center, Haifa, Israel

Mark I. Evans, MD
President, Fetal Medicine Foundation of America; Director, Comprehensive Genetics; Professor, Department of Obstetrics and Gynecology, Mt. Sinai School of Medicine, New York, New York

Michael R. Foley, MD
Medical Director, Phoenix Perinatal Associates, Scottsdale, Arizona

Nastaran Foyouzi, MD
Resident, Department of Obstetrics and Gynecology, Barnes-Jewish Hospital, Washington University, St. Louis, Missouri

Edmund F. Funai, MD
Associate Chair for Clinical Affairs; Co-Chief, Maternal-Fetal Medicine; Associate Professor, Department of Obstetrics, Gynecology, & Reproductive Sciences, Yale University School of Medicine, New Haven, Connecticut

Robert Gagnon, MD, FRCS(c)
Professor, Department of Obstetrics, Gynecology, and Physiology, University of Western Ontario, St. Joseph's Health Care London, London, Ontario, Canada

Benjamin D. Hamar, MD
Instructor, Department of Obstetrics, Gynecology, and Reproductive Biology, Beth Israel Deaconess Medical Center, Boston, Massachussetts

John Paul Hayslett, MD
Professor, Nephrology, Department of Internal Medicine; Medical Director, Physician Associate Program and Obstetrics and Gynecology, Yale University School of Medicine, New Haven, Connecticut

Jon Hyett, MD
Consultant in Obstetrics, Maternal and Fetal Medicine, King's College School of Medicine and Dentistry, London, United Kingdom

Svena Julien, MD
Assistant Professor, Maternal-Fetal Medicine, Department of Obstetrics and Gynecology, Northwestern University, Feinberg School of Medicine, Chicago, Illinois

Nikki Koklanaris, MD
Department of Obstetrics and Gynecology, Carolinas Medical Center, Charlotte, North Carolina

Olympia Kovich, MD
Assistant Professor, Department of Dermatology, New York University School of Medicine, New York, New York

De-Hui W. Ku, PhD
Technical Director, Hemostasis and Thrombosis Laboratory, Bio-Reference Laboratories, Elmwood Park, New Jersey

D. Yvette LaCoursiere, MD, MPH
Assistant Professor, Department of Obstetrics and Gynecology, University of Utah School of Medicine, Salt Lake City, Utah

Hee Joong Lee, MD
Associate Professor, Department of Obstetrics & Gynecology, College of Medicine, The Catholic University of Korea, Seoul, Korea

Men-Jean Lee, MD
Associate Professor, Department of Obstetrics and Gynecology, Mt. Sinai School of Medicine, New York, New York

Charles J. Lockwood, MD
Anita O'Keefe Young Professor and Chair, Department of Obstetrics, Gynecology, & Reproductive Sciences, Yale University School of Medicine, New Haven, Connecticut

Urania Magriples, MD
Associate Professor, Department of Obstetrics and Gynecology, Yale University School of Medicine, New Haven, Connecticut

Stephanie R. Martin, DO
Assistant Medical Director, Pike's Peak Maternal Fetal Medicine, Memorial Health System, Colorado Springs, Colorado

Despina Mavridou, MD
Resident, Department of Obstetrics and Gynecology, St. John's Mercy Medical Center, St. Louis, Missouri

Thomas F. McElrath, MD, PhD
Assistant Professor, Department of Obstetrics, Gynecology, and Reproductive Biology, Brigham and Women's Hospital, Boston, Massachussetts

Ana Monteagudo, MD
Professor, Department of Obstetrics and Gynecology, New York University School of Medicine, New York, New York

Kypros Nickolaides, MD
Professor and Chairman of Obstetrics and Gynecology, Director, Harris Birthright Center, King's College Hospital, London, England

Errol R. Norwitz, MD, PhD
Associate Professor, Yale University School of Medicine; Co-Director, Division of Maternal-Fetal Medicine; Director, Maternal-Fetal Medicine Fellowship Program; Director, Obstetrics & Gynecology Residency Program, Department of Obstetrics, Gynecology, & Reproductive Sciences, Yale-New Haven Hospital, New Haven, Connecticut

Michael J. Paidas, MD
Associate Professor and Director, Yale Center for Thrombosis and Hemostasis in Women's and Children's Health; Department of Obstetrics and Gynecology, Yale University School of Medicine, New Haven, Connecticut

Miriam Keltz Pomeranz, MD
Assistant Professor, Department of Dermatology, New York University School of Medicine, New York, New York

Julian N. Robinson, MD
Medical Director of Maternal-Fetal Medicine, Newton-Wellesley Hospital, Newton, Massachusetts

Michael G. Ross, MD, MPH
Professor and Chairman, Department of Obstetrics and Gynecology, UCLA Harbor Medical Center, Torrance, California

Anna K. Sfakianaki, MD
Assistant Professor, Department of Obstetrics and Gynecology, Yale University School of Medicine, New Haven, Connecticut

Maria J. Small, MD
Assistant Professor, Department of Obstetrics and Gynecology, Duke University School of Medicine, Durham, North Carolina

Stephen F. Thung, MD
Assistant Professor, Department of Obstetrics and Gynecology, Yale University School of Medicine, New Haven, Connecticut

Ilan E. Timor-Tritsch, MD
Professor and Director of OB/GYN Ultrasound, Department of Obstetrics and Gynecology, New York University School of Medicine, New York, New York

Michael Varner, MD
Professor, Department of Obstetrics and Gynecology, University of Utah Medical Center, Salt Lake City, Utah

Karlijn Woensdregt, MD
Faculty of Medicine, Maastricht University, The Netherlands

The Requisites in Obstetrics and Gynecology

FOREWORD

We are living in an era of rapidly changing technologies, in which technical and now many medical services can be performed remotely and often impersonally. At the same time, the cultures of medical practice and training have been radically transformed, as resident work rules, the use of new procedures and equipment, and changing perspectives on the practice of medicine have evolved quite significantly over the past two decades. Consequently, the overall approach to medical education, the slower rate of increasing responsibilities given to residents during their training, and the tolerance for non-standardized approaches to patient care have likewise changed, for both the better and the worse. Thus, the basics—the "requisites"—needed to operate in the current environment likewise have evolved. In this series, the editors and chapter authors crystallize the foundations needed for independent practitioners to survive and thrive in the current medical climate. We hope readers will view the materials as the basis for evolving sophistication in the practice of obstetrics and gynecology.

Mark I. Evans, MD

PREFACE

It has been both a challenge and a privilege to create the first volume of *High Risk Obstetrics: The Requisites in Obstetrics and Gynecology.* Our main aim in this endeavor has been to create a resource that is valuable to the busy generalist obstetrician/gynecologist, and as such, we have strived to provide clear, succinct, and precise guidance for the management of complex obstetric patients. We also crafted this volume as a quick reference for the Maternal-Fetal Medicine specialist who is looking for forthright answers, not a voluminous review of the literature detailing the pros and cons of each management controversy, as many other traditional books have done.

We believe the very best place to begin is the beginning (of course!) and as such, the first chapters are an overview of the genetic basis of human development, with an emphasis on areas in which nature is imperfect. Because screening and diagnosis of aneuploidy are a growing aspect of many OB practices, we cover these topics in detail. Chapters 3-7 then move on to the most common means by which fetal anomalies are now diagnosed: ultrasound. Each of the major organ systems have their own chapter for easy reference.

Chapters 8-16 then cover common complications of pregnancy, such as recurrent pregnancy loss, preterm labor, and preeclampsia. We are fortunate to have some of the leading experts in the world serve as authors for many of these chapters.

Finally, beginning with Chapter 17, we cover many of the more common medical complications of pregnancy, such as diabetes and hypertension, which are diagnoses that have been vexing clinicians for decades.

We hope that this book becomes a trusted old friend to you, and quickly develops dog-ears and a cracked spine. With apologies to our orthopedic colleagues, we wrote it to be abused, not simply to be admired.

Edmund F. Funai, MD

Mark I. Evans, MD

Charles J. Lockwood, MD

CONTENTS

Contents

1

OVERVIEW
OF GENETICS

Arie Drugan and Mark I. Evans

Congenital anomalies are observed in only 2% to 3% of liveborns but have a major effect on the risk of pregnancy loss as well as on perinatal mortality and morbidity.[1] The pioneer work of Mendel with garden peas defined in 1865 "inheritance units" (later called genes) that pass separately and randomly into the egg or sperm, allowing parental traits to appear unchanged in subsequent generations. In the first half of the 20th century, two other major milestones were recorded: Garrod's definition of enzymatic defects as "inborn errors of metabolism" and the identification of the 46 human chromosomes in 1956. Chromosomal DNA is the vehicle that carries the "inheritance units" described by Mendel in his early experiments. During cell division, condensation of the DNA allows the chromosomes to be stained and analyzed. Evaluation of the number and gross structure of the chromosomes enabled the correlation of specific chromosome aberrations with severe syndromes of congenital anomalies described many years before.[2,3]

Laboratory techniques to cut and analyze DNA sequences were developed in the early 1970s.[4,5] First, restriction enzymes were used to recognize specific base pair sequences and to cut the DNA molecule whenever that sequence appears, thus resulting in DNA strands of differing lengths and velocity on gel electrophoresis. These were called "restriction fragment length polymorphisms" (RFLPs). The DNA strands were then sorted out by coupling with molecular probes on the gel.[5] When the actual molecular structure of the gene in investigation is unknown, known RFLPs in close vicinity to the gene can be used as gene markers, enabling us to follow the segregation of the gene within a given family. Direct gene analysis with complementary DNA probes can be used when the sequence of base pairs within the gene is already known. In some families, these techniques enable identification of carrier or affected individuals before they are clinically symptomatic or even before they are born (prenatal diagnosis).

Thus within a relatively short period, the science of genetics evolved from anatomic descriptions of malformation patterns (without an identifiable cause), through the correlation of phenotypic abnormalities with pathology at the microscopic cellular level (i.e., abnormal number or gross structure of the chromosomes), and now to the molecular level—an abnormal gene structure causing an abnormal gene product resulting in phenotypic changes.

The etiology of genetic disease includes chromosome anomalies, single gene disorders, and multifactorial defects. In chromosome disorders, the number or the gross structure of the chromosomes is aberrant, resulting in added or missing genetic material. As a group, they are quite common, affecting about 0.7% of live births.[6] The abnormal dose of thousands of genes causes severe malformations in most organ systems, severe growth and mental retardation, and, in some cases, fetal or neonatal death. Some errors in embryogenesis may result in embryonic loss before implantation, causing the low fecundity rate (25%) per cycle observed in fertile couples trying to conceive.[1] Others may cause loss of pregnancy after it was clinically recognized.

Single gene disorders are caused by *mutations,* changes in the structure of an active gene, causing abnormal transmission of genetic information and resulting in an altered or absent gene product. Single gene disorders are inherited following strict mendelian rules. Knowing the family pedigree and the mode of inheritance of a specific disorder, we can calculate with relative accuracy what the risk is that other family members will be affected.

Multifactorial disorders are the relatively common result of the interaction between genetic predisposition and exogenous factors (i.e., teratogens) to produce a birth defect. Although the risk of multifactorial disorders is higher in families that have been affected before, the risk of recurrence is significantly lower than in single gene disorders and pedigrees are not characteristic. Overall, multifactorial disorders affect approximately 1% of live births.

CLINICAL ASPECTS OF CHROMOSOMAL ANOMALIES

Chromosome aberrations are a frequent cause of congenital malformations, affecting about 1:165 live births.[6] The frequency of chromosome anomalies is much higher in patients with severe mental retardation and in pregnancies affected by congenital anomalies or fetal loss (Table 1-1). About half of all spontaneous abortions in the first trimester are caused by chromosomal problems.[7] Chromosome aberrations have been found in 30% to 35% of amniocenteses performed following the diagnosis of fetal malformations on ultrasound.[8]

Chromosome abnormalities can be classified as numerical or structural. Numerical chromosome anomalies, either additional sets of chromosomes *(polyploidy)* or additional or missing single chromosomes *(aneuploidy)* are by far more common than structural anomalies, representing more than 95% of recognized chromosomal aberrations.[7] Two totally different mechanisms are active in the etiology of these disorders. Polyploidy may be caused by

Table 1-1

Frequency of Chromosome Anomalies

Live births	0.6%
Mentally retarded, institutionalized	12%
Mentally retarded with congenital anomalies	23%
First trimester pregnancy losses	50%
Second trimester pregnancy losses	15%-20%
Third trimester losses (stillbirths)	6%
Major fetal malformations (ultrasound)	35%
Prenatal diagnosis for maternal age >35 yr	1%-3%

failure of cleavage of the fertilized egg at the first mitotic division or, more commonly, by fertilization of the normal oocyte with more than one normal sperm (polyspermy). This is a relatively frequent problem, affecting 1% to 3% of recognized conceptions and approximately 5% of oocytes fertilized in vitro.[9] In contrast, aneuploidy is mainly the result of meiotic nondisjunction and shows a definite association with advanced maternal age (Figure 1-1). The complexity of the female meiosis is the most likely explanation for the strong association between advanced maternal age and an increased risk of aneuploid gestations.[10] In about 80% of trisomic pregnancies, nondisjunction (the failure of homologous chromosomes to separate and segregate into different daughter cells during cell division) is of maternal origin, in most cases occurring during maternal meiosis I.[11] An association between abnormal ovulation patterns and an increased risk of chromosome anomalies has also been documented.[10] Increased paternal age, however, does not increase the risk of aneuploid offspring.

The vast majority of triploid conceptions are caused by fertilization of a haploid egg by two haploid sperm. Thus triploid conceptions may have the karyotype 69,XXX; 69,XXY; or 69,XYY. Most triploid conceptions will be

3

Figure 1-1

Mitosis and meiosis chromosomal division.

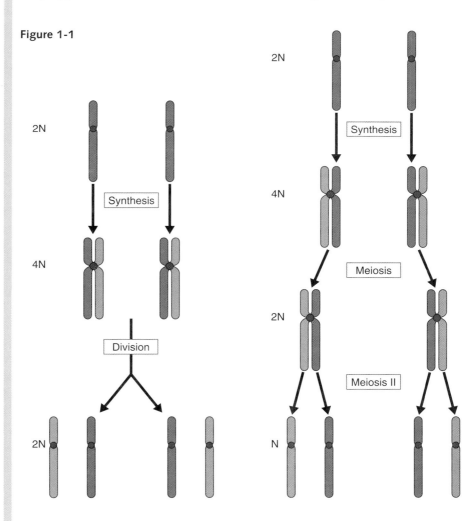

aborted in the first or early second trimester. Triploidy is the cause of about 7% of clinically recognized spontaneous abortions.[12] In those cases surviving into the second or third trimester, the placenta undergoes cystic degeneration typical of partial hydatidiform mole. When the fetus survives into the second or third trimester, generally by virtue of fetal mosaicism, it is severely growth retarded and has omphalocele or other associated congenital anomalies. Maternal serum alpha-fetoprotein (MSAFP) is often elevated in pregnancies affected by triploidy.[12]

The abnormal development of the fetus and placenta in triploid conceptions demonstrates a new and revolutionary concept in medical genetics, termed *genomic imprinting.* Mendel's theory states that allelic genes have equal effects when transmitted from either parent. However, human triploids have twice the normal genetic contribution from one parent and show differential development dependent on the origin of the double genetic dose (paternal or maternal). Most cases of triploidy are the result of dispermy (two paternal and one maternal chromosomal complements) and the abnormalities observed are a large placenta with cystic molar changes and a growth-retarded malformed fetus. However, when two maternal complements and one paternal complement are present, only a small underdeveloped placenta is seen. If a fetus exists, it is not malformed but is markedly underdeveloped, probably related to placental failure. Thus it appears that paternal genetic information is critical to the development of the placenta and fetal membranes, whereas maternal genetic information is essential for early embryonic development. This has also been substantiated by experiments in pronuclear transplantation and parthenogenetic activation in mice. With only paternally derived chromosomes (androgenetic), only placenta and membranes develop, as seen also in complete hydatidiform moles. Conversely, with two sets of only maternally derived chromosomes there is relatively good embryonic development but poor development of the placenta and membranes.[13]

Tetraploidy (92,XXXX or 92,XXYY) arises almost always from failure of the first mitotic division of a normal diploid zygote, so that four copies of each chromosome exist in the multiplying cell. Most of these pregnancies will be miscarried in the first trimester; tetraploidy is observed in about 2% of spontaneous abortions, commonly diagnosed on ultrasonography as an empty sac ("blighted ovum") without embryonic remnants. Isolated cases of liveborn tetraploid fetuses with multiple congenital anomalies have also been reported.[14] Mosaic tetraploidy of amniotic cell cultures is also a relatively common laboratory artifact and is almost always associated with good outcome. The type of cell and the culture medium (i.e., Chang medium) may affect the percentage of tetraploid cells growing in culture. True tetraploidy should be suspected only if a significant percentage of tetraploid cells are discovered in multiple culture flasks. In these cases, confirmation of cytogenetic results by repeat amniocentesis or percutaneous umbilical blood sampling (PUBS) should be sought before operative decisions are taken.[15]

Aneuploidy refers to the addition or absence of single chromosomes (either autosomes or sex chromosomes), causing trisomy or monosomy, respectively. Most autosomal trisomies and some of the X-chromosome trisomies are caused by maternal nondisjunction and increase in frequency with advanced maternal age.[11] For 47,XXY (Klinefelter syndrome) the frequency of maternal and paternal nondisjunction events is almost equal, with a slight excess (57%) of paternal nondisjunction. The age effect appears to be limited to cases of maternal nondisjunction. Unlike the autosomal trisomies, the diagnosis of monosomy X is observed more often in young women. In most cases, the origin of monosomy X is mitotic loss of a paternal sex chromosome post fertilization and during cell division, an event influenced neither by paternal nor by maternal age.[16] Because monosomy X is most commonly the result of a post zygotic event, it is usually observed in mosaic state, with both normal and abnormal cell lines in culture.

Aneuploidy is the most common type of chromosome anomaly in live births as well as in abortion material.[7] The most commonly observed karyotypes in aneuploid infants born alive are trisomy of the autosomes 13, 18, or 21 or of the sex chromosomes and monosomy X. Trisomy 21 is the most common chromosome anomaly in liveborns, being diagnosed in about half of all chromosomally abnormal neonates. Rare case reports of trisomy 8, 9, or 22 or partial trisomies for other chromosomes have also been reported. It is assumed that fetuses with full autosomal trisomies surviving to term have a component of mosaicism with a normal cell line in their placenta, facilitating their intrauterine survival.[17] That is true in particular for unusual trisomies such as trisomy 8 or trisomy 9, which are usually diagnosed in neonates only in mosaic form.

Autosomal trisomies occur in about 3% of recognized conceptions and cause about 25% of all pregnancy losses. The most common autosomal trisomy in first trimester miscarriages is trisomy 16, which has never been reported at term. Monosomy X is the most common single chromosome anomaly found in abortion material—about 18% of all spontaneous miscarriages. It is estimated that 95% to 99% of all conceptions with monosomy X are miscarried, most commonly in the first trimester.[7]

All autosomal trisomies (except for chromosome 1) have been observed in abortion material, but only monosomy X has been described. Because trisomy and monosomy are reciprocal events—the results of meiotic nondisjunction—these data imply that autosomal monosomy and trisomy (of chromosome) 1 have a stronger negative impact on affected conceptions, causing their loss even before pregnancy is clinically recognized. Thus, whether the aneuploid fetus is destined to be miscarried before or after pregnancy is recognized or is allowed to be delivered, malformed, at term, is determined by the chromosome involved in aneuploidy, meaning the amount and type of added or missing genetic material.[18] Chromosome 21 is the smallest chromosome (only 56,000 kilobase of DNA), and most conceptions affected by trisomy 21 will be delivered as liveborns. Chromosomes 13 and 18 are larger than chromosome 21. About 70% of pregnancies affected by trisomy 13 or 18 are miscarried—the rest are born alive with malformations and severe growth and mental retardation and die soon after birth.[19] Chromosome 1 is the largest human chromosome, and pregnancies affected by trisomy 1 are miscarried very early, probably before implantation. Most autosomal monosomies are also miscarried very early, probably because of the effect of uniparental transmission of some genetic information on the developing pregnancy.

Chromosomal mosaicism affects 0.2% to 0.7% of amniotic cell cultures.[20] Because fetal blood sampling confirmed the abnormal karyotype in less than 50% of cases, these results suggest that all cases of mosaic aneuploidy diagnosed at amniocentesis should be reevaluated by fetal blood sampling.[15]

The incidence of mosaicism in chorionic villi specimens is higher than in amniotic fluid, about 1% to 2%.[21] In 90% of cases chromosomal mosaicism is confined to the placenta (confined placental mosaicism [CPM]), and fetal karyotype is normal.[22] Moreover, it appears that the ratio of normal to abnormal cells may change with time, in favor of the normal cell line. Thus the prognosis in pregnancies diagnosed on chorionic villus sampling (CVS) to be affected by chromosome mosaicism is commonly favorable. However, unexplained intrauterine fetal death or intrauterine growth retardation may occur in some cases.[23]

True mosaicism with a normal cell line is found in 1% to 2% of Down syndrome conceptions and up to 20% of liveborns affected by trisomy 13. In general, the phenotype of mosaics should be milder than those of individuals with full aneuploidy. The more severe the effect of aneuploidy, the more likely it is to be mosaic if discovered in a liveborn. Likewise, there are definite differences between potentially viable autosomal and sex chromosome trisomy:

1. Mental retardation in sex chromosome aneuploidy is generally mild and some affected individuals may have normal or above normal intelligence. Profound mental retardation is the rule with autosomal trisomies.
2. The phenotypic expression of sex chromosome aneuploidy affects mainly the development and function of sex organs and sex hormones; reproductive failure is common in these cases and may be the presenting symptom. With autosomal trisomies, somatic expression is common and multiple organ systems are often affected.

Structural chromosome anomalies affect approximately 0.2% of newborns and are most commonly caused by breakage with abnormal repair of the chromosomes. Chromosome damage can occur spontaneously but is more common after exposure to radiation or to mutagenic agents or in specific genetic disorders such as Bloom syndrome, ataxia telangiectasia, or Fanconi anemia. Breaks involving only one chromosome may lead to loss of the broken part *(deletion)* or *inversion* of the repaired chromosomal segment. If the breaks involve two chromosomes, exchange of the broken segments between the two may lead to a *translocation*. The translocation may be balanced (when genetic material was not added or lost in the process) or unbalanced (when added or missing chromosomal segments result in partial trisomy or monosomy, respectively). The phenotypic abnormalities depend on the chromosomes involved in the process and whether the rearrangement is balanced or not. Deletions and duplications are always unbalanced and are always associated with abnormal phenotype and mental retardation. Because deletions or duplications in the offspring may be the product of a balanced structural anomaly in the parents, parental blood karyotypes should be pursued in these cases.

Inversions are the result of two breaks in the chromosome with repair of the broken segment in reversed direction. Because genetic material should not be lost in the process, the phenotype is most commonly normal. The population frequency of pericentric inversions is 0.01%[24] and those involving chromosomes 9, 10, or 11 are so common that they are considered normal population variants. The pericentric inversion of chromosome 9 (p11q13) is particularly common in Africans.

When one of the parents carries a balanced inversion, the risk of unbalanced offspring at the time of amniocentesis is about 6%.[25] This risk seems to differ with the sex of the carrier. The rate of unbalanced offspring is 4% when the father carries the inversion and 7.5% when the mother is the carrier of the balanced inversion. Thus inversion carriers should receive genetic counseling and should be offered prenatal diagnosis by amniocentesis or CVS, regardless of maternal age. Conversely, when an inversion is diagnosed in an amniocentesis or CVS specimen performed for other indications, parental karyotypes should be obtained. If the inversion is also carried by one of the parents (inherited), a normal phenotype should be expected. However, if the inversion appears de novo in the conceptus and parental karyotypes are normal, mental retardation or abnormal phenotype may occur because of positional effects on gene activity (moving the coding part of one gene next to regulatory sequences of another gene), breaks within a gene, or minute deletions at the break lines.

The incidence of balanced inversion or translocation carriers among couples affected by two or more pregnancy losses is 2% to 4%, 10 times higher than the prevalence of translocation carriers in the general population.[24] Among individuals with unbalanced translocations, about one third to one half are inherited from a carrier (balanced) parent—most of the rest arise de novo, commonly in the father's sperm. The pattern of segregation in familial cases exhibits multiple affected siblings and/or multiple miscarriages concentrated on one side of the family. In inherited cases, blood karyotypes of other family members are often necessary to identify additional individuals at risk for unbalanced offspring.

Two main types of translocations are identified—reciprocal and Robertsonian. A reciprocal translocation means that breaks were formed on two different chromosomes and that the segments between the breaks were exchanged between the two. In the balanced carrier, the nomenclature of such a karyotype will be 46, XX or XY, t(a:b), where "a" and "b" represent the numbers of the chromosomes involved in the translocation. Unless minute deletions occurred at the breaking points, the phenotype of carriers of reciprocal translocations is normal. The mathematical risk of unbalanced offspring in these cases is 50%. However, the actual risk of unbalanced offspring when one of the parents is the carrier of a balanced reciprocal translocation is 12% to 14% and is even lower when the father is the carrier.[26]

Robertsonian translocations can take place only between acrocentric chromosomes—13, 14, 15, 21, and 22. In this translocation, the "p" arms of the translocated chromosomes are lost and the "q" arms unite at the centromere. Thus a Robertsonian translocation carrier has *only 45 chromosomes*, but the genetic material is balanced and the phenotype is normal because the p arm of acrocentric chromosomes does not contain euchromatin. The nomenclature of this type of karyotype will be 45, XX or XY, t (a;b). Theoretically, one third of the offspring of a Robertsonian translocation carrier will have an unbalanced karyotype and will possess an abnormal phenotype, one third will carry the balanced translocation like the parent and will have a normal phenotype, and another one third will have normal chromosomes.[24] The actual risk of unbalanced viable offspring is, however, negligible, unless the translocation involves chromosomes 13 or 21. A significant sex difference in the segregation of Robertsonian translocations is also observed. For a female carrier of a Robertsonian translocation involving chromosome 21, the risk of having a viable trisomic 21 offspring is 10% to 20%. The exception are carriers of 21;21 translocations, in which all conceptions will be abnormal—either monosomic (and therefore nonviable and aborted) or trisomic and potentially viable with Down syndrome. The risk for a liveborn unbalanced offspring for female carriers of other Robertsonian translocations or for male carriers is low—1% to 2%. Because all conceptions involving trisomy 14, 15, or 22 and most trisomy 13 pregnancies will be miscarried, the rate of spontaneous abortions is increased in carriers of Robertsonian translocations.[25,26]

Structural chromosome rearrangements are sometime diagnosed incidentally when prenatal diagnosis is performed for unrelated indications (i.e., advanced maternal age). If the rearrangement is unbalanced, the partial monosomy or trisomy implies a serious risk of mental retardation or abnormal phenotype. Available evidence suggests that chromosomal deletions or duplications large enough to be observed by regular cytogenetic techniques usually have serious phenotypic consequences.[27] When the structural rearrangement is seemingly balanced, it is important to determine whether the same rearrangement is carried by one of the parents. The diagnosis of the same chromosome rearrangement in parental karyotype reassures that a normal phenotype is expected in the tested fetus but may prompt chromosome studies of other family membranes and, obviously, in subsequent pregnancies.

When a balanced chromosome rearrangement is not inherited but appears de novo in the index pregnancy, fetal prognosis is guarded. The incidence of de novo, seemingly balanced, translocations or inversions observed at amniocentesis is 0.06%, higher than the 0.04% incidence of these abnormalities reported at term.[27] Thus it appears that about a third of these pregnancies are miscarried between amniocentesis and term. The incidence of dysmorphic features in newborns with de novo rearrangements is 7.6%, two to three times higher than the incidence of congenital anomalies reported in newborns.[27] Moreover, cases of mental retardation or developmental delay that are not associated with dysmorphism may not be reported at birth. In surveys of the mentally retarded, apparently balanced, de novo chromosome rearrangements were seven times more frequent than among newborns surveyed at random. Thus patients that are diagnosed to carry a fetus with de novo chromosome rearrangement should be counseled that the risk of congenital anomalies for that pregnancy is probably in the range of 10% to 15%. The risk is probably higher with reciprocal translocations or with inversions; with de novo Robertsonian translocations, the risk for congenital anomalies is probably small.

MENDELIAN INHERITANCE IN MAN

The Structure and Function of Human Genes

Human chromosomes are made of DNA, double-helix polynucleotide chains formed of two purine and two pyrimidine bases. In the double helix, adenine always pairs with thymine and guanine with cytosine (Figure 1-2). Along the polynucleotide chain, each three-base sequence *(codon)* can code for a specific amino acid. Because there are 64 possible arrangements of nucleotide base triplets but only 20 amino acids, the genetic code is said to be redundant, each amino acid being coded by one to six codons. Overall, the diploid set of chromosomes contains about 7 billion base pairs (bp). However, not all of it is translated into protein. It is estimated that about half of the DNA is formed by "informative" sequences, that being interspaced with DNA stretches that are not translated and whose function is not exactly defined.

9

DNA base pairing.

Figure 1-2   DNA BASE PAIRING

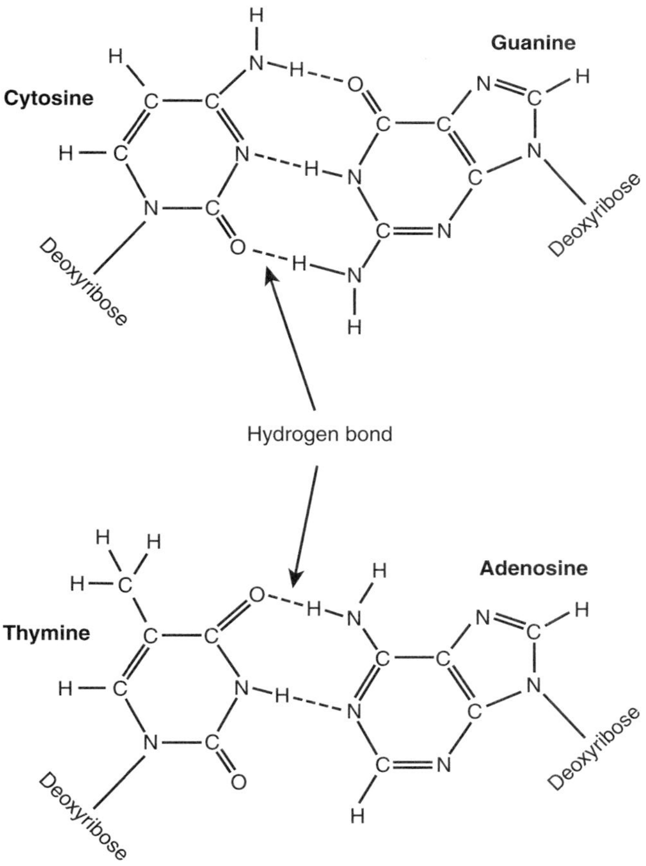

Cytosine — Guanine

Hydrogen bond

Thymine — Adenosine

Three chief classes of DNA are recognized:

1. *Unique sequences*: Approximately 50% to 60% of human DNA is formed of single copy stretches about 2000 bases long. The number of protein coding, unique sequences is probably around 100,000 per haploid genome. They are interspaced with repetitive DNA sequences about 0.3 kb long. The repetitive noncoding DNA sequences probably serve structural or regulatory functions.

2. *Highly repetitive sequences* are found in specific areas such as the heterochromatic region of chromosomes 1, 9, 16, and the Y-chromosome and are usually located near the centromere. These million-fold repetitions of oligonucleotides form about 10% of the human genome. They are highly polymorphic in quantity but without any effect on the phenotype. Because highly repetitive sequences are transmitted from generation to generation in an extremely conserved form, they can be used as markers in population studies.

3. *Moderately repetitive sequences* (about 30% of the human genome) contain some gene families that are necessary in all cells and in each phase of individual development. Genes for ribosomal RNA, generally located in the nucleolus-organizing region (NOR) of human acrocentric chromosomes, immunoglobulins, histones, and transfer RNA are included in this group.

Chromatin structure is the packaging of genomic DNA through association with histone proteins. The nucleosome is the basic repeating unit of chromatin and consists of 146 bp of DNA wrapped around an octameric histone core.[28] Nucleosomal DNA can be further compacted by association with histone 1 as well as by higher order looping and folding of the chromatin fiber. The special organization of chromatin as well as post-translational modifications of histone proteins plays direct regulatory roles on gene expression.[29] They also define genomic landmarks such as heterochromatin and euchromatin. Heterochromatin is the name of functionally inactive regions of the genome, and euchromatin is where actual gene activity occurs.

Protein coding genes are formed from *exons,* the translated sequences of nucleotide bases, interspersed with nontranslated sequences termed *introns* (Figure 1-3). Upstream to the exon-intron complex (toward the 5′ end of the molecule) there are regulatory sequences that control gene expression and

Figure 1-3

Exon to protein.

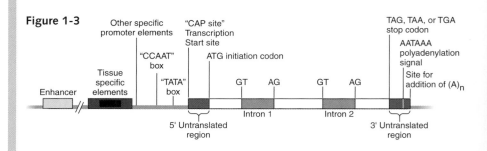

initiate transcription. These are called promoter regions and appear to be similar in all genes. They include signals for initiation of transcription (the TATA box, about 30 bases upstream the gene) and the recognition site for RNA transcriptase (CAT box), about 80 bp upstream the transcribed sequence. The signal to stop transcription is given by a regulatory sequence flanking the transcribed complex downstream (toward the 3′ end of the molecule).

Transcription, the transfer of the genetic code from DNA to messenger RNA (mRNA) is always in the same direction, from the 5′ to the 3′ end of the DNA molecule. The mRNA molecule created is complementary to the DNA sequence copied, meaning that it is the exact copy of the DNA strand that was not transcribed (with the exception that uracil is substituted for thymine). After transcription, a poly adenyl tail is added to the mRNA molecule and the introns are excised (spliced) to form a "mature" form of mRNA that exits the nucleus. In the cytoplasm, the mature mRNA serves as a skeleton along which transfer RNA (tRNA) builds the specific protein by sequentially adding amino acids as encoded by mRNA.

Promoter elements modify gene activity by controlling the rate of transcription. Specific mediator proteins (i.e., steroid hormones) may interact with promoter elements to increase their activity. Gene inactivation is also affected by DNA methylation of the promoter region, the addition of a methyl group to C-G pairs—an increase in methylation inhibits gene expression, whereas a decrease in DNA methylation is associated with an increase in gene expression or with reactivation of expression of suppressed genes. DNA and histone methylation may also be one of the mechanisms to explain parental genomic imprinting[13,30] and X inactivation.[31] Histones are now recognized as active effectors of gene expression and as providers of additional levels of regulation to the standard DNA blueprint.

Mutations—The Pathogenesis of Single Gene Disorders

Mutation is a change in the normal DNA sequence of nucleotides, caused by absence, addition, or substitution of one or more base pairs. If the mutated DNA strand is part of the sequence of base pairs forming a gene, the mutation will result in a different pattern of codons that may cause the formation of an abnormal mRNA template and an abnormal gene product. A single base substitution—"point" mutation—may or may not alter the amino acid sequence coded by the gene because, as previously mentioned, some amino acids are coded by more than one codon. For example, the amino acid leucine is coded by six different codons. Sometimes, however, a single base substitution can cause severe disorders. A common example is sickle cell disease. In this disorder, a single base substitution in codon 6 of the β globin chain causes the replacement of glutamic acid by valine. Glutamic acid has two COOH groups and one NH_2 group, whereas valine has only one COOH group. The charge difference between hemoglobin A and hemoglobin S explains the instability of the latter under specific conditions, causing the sickling phenomenon.

"Frameshift" mutations are caused by insertions or deletions of one or more nucleotide bases in the gene sequence, altering the whole coding system of the gene caudal to the mutation locus. Because the amino acid sequence coded downstream to the mutation will be entirely different than that coded by the original gene, the gene product in these cases will be grossly abnormal, with obvious phenotypic consequences. Such mutations are observed in part of the β thalassemia genotypes or in the Duchenne muscular dystrophy (DMD) locus. Mutations can affect gene activity also by changing the code for termination of transcription (chain termination mutations) or by changing the recognition code for splicing sites. The latter will result in acceptance of part or the whole intron as exon, thus changing significantly the mRNA template. In addition, mutations in regulatory sequences can lead to reduced, abnormal or absent transcription by changing the recognition site of RNA polymerase.

Thus the pathogenesis of genetic disease is, in most cases, an alteration of DNA structure (a mutation) causing abnormal gene function and resulting in an abnormal gene product. The abnormal rate of production or the production of abnormal protein may interfere with enzymatic or metabolic pathways or cause structural anomalies or cell membrane dysfunction. Malfunction of regulatory genes can be even more detrimental because cell differentiation and morphologic development may be altered.

In some cases, the gene-specific DNA sequence is not altered but the space orientation is changed so that the DNA is not accessible for transcription and is targeted for silencing. Active regions of chromatin have unmethylated DNA and have high level of acetylated histones, whereas inactive regions of chromatin contain methylated DNA and diacetylated histones.[32] Thus changes in methylation result in abnormal expression of the specific gene. *Epigenetics* refers to the study of heritable changes in gene expression without a change in DNA sequence. Many deviations from strict mendelian inheritance (i.e., effects of parental genomic imprinting, anticipation, or variability of expression in dominant disorders) as well as multifactorial traits can be explained by epigenetic effects, which have a major impact on embryonic development as well as on the germline and derivatives.[33,34]

Patterns of Single Gene Inheritance

Genetic disorders caused by malfunction of a single gene are inherited following strict mendelian rules. The risk for other family members to be affected is calculated based on the diagnosis, on the pattern of inheritance of the specific disorder, and on the pedigree.

Genes located at the same locus on homologous chromosomes are called *alleles.* According to Mendel, alleles always segregate during meiosis, each mature sex cell (spermatocyte or oocyte) containing only one of each homologous chromosome (and one of each allele). Because the allocation of chromosomes during meiosis is totally random and independent of segregation of other chromosomes, each fertilized oocyte contains a random assortment of alleles contributed by both parents. Thus each genetic locus can be either concordant or discordant in respect to the function of a specific allele pair, this being termed *homozygous* and *heterozygous,* respectively. Moreover, there is a "gene dosage" effect, each allele contributing half the normal gene product. A trait that is expressed in the heterozygous state is considered *dominant.* In dominant disorders, 50% reduction of the activity or the quantity of the normal protein coded by the specific gene will cause phenotypic abnormalities. Dominant disorders will be caused mainly by malfunction of genes coding for structural proteins (i.e., collagen) or for proteins regulating complex metabolic pathways, such as membrane receptors. A trait that is expressed clinically only in the homozygous state is called *recessive*. In recessive conditions, a normal phenotype is maintained with 50% or less of the normal gene function. Disorders associated with enzyme deficiencies (inborn errors of metabolism) are the main group of diseases in this class. Single gene disorders are described and classified by Victor McKusick and the team at John Hopkins in a catalog available on-line at www.ncbi.nlm.nih.gov. The site is named OMIM (Online Mendelian Inheritance in Man), is updated periodically, and is accessible free of charge.

The pattern of inheritance of a disorder is determined by the location of the abnormal allele (on an autosome or on the sex chromosome) and by the dominance of the trait. Building a pedigree helps to identify how a specific disease runs in the family and thus to determine the inheritance pattern and the risk of recurrence in other family members. It should be emphasized that dominance and recessiveness are attributes of the phenotype, not of the presence of the abnormal gene. Because a gene dosage effect always exists (although it may not be fully expressed in the phenotype), we can state that dominance and recessiveness are *quantitative rather than qualitative* and are determined by the sensitivity of the methods used to assay one's phenotype.

Autosomal Dominant Inheritance

Autosomal dominant disorders are inherited from one parent carrying and, in most cases, showing phenotypic expression of the abnormal gene. For practical purposes, most individuals with a dominant disorder are heterozygotes. Only when both parents have the same autosomal dominant disorder, 25% of their offspring could be affected with the homozygous form of the disease, which will always be more severe than that of the parents because of double dosage of the deleterious gene. In many cases, homozygous autosomal dominant disorders will be lethal in utero or in early infancy. For example, offspring of achondroplastic individuals, a disease in which marriage between affected individuals is not uncommon, will be either affected (as the parents) or normal; the homozygous form of achondroplasia is always lethal during pregnancy.

Characteristic criteria of autosomal dominant inheritance include the following:

1. Vertical pattern in a pedigree—the trait appears in every generation without skipping.
2. Inheritance from only one heterozygote parent, with 1 in 2 risk for offspring of either sex to be affected. Father to son transmission is observed almost exclusively in transmission of autosomal dominant traits.
3. Male and female offspring are affected with equal frequency and equal severity. With some exceptions, the sex of affected individuals does not modify the expression of a dominant trait.
4. The frequency of sporadic cases is in negative correlation with the reproductive fitness of affected individuals. In other words, the proportion of cases caused by new mutations (the first case in the family, not inherited from an affected parent) is highest in disorders that are lethal in utero or in early infancy (i.e., thanatophoric dwarfism). Advanced paternal age has also been associated with a higher risk of autosomal dominant

disorders (i.e., achondroplasia or neurofibromatosis), caused by new mutations in offspring. When an autosomal dominant disorder is caused by a new mutation, the risk for other affected offspring (siblings of the affected individual) is very low and probably similar to the frequency of the disorder in the general population.

5. Unaffected family members do not transmit the disorder to their offspring; identification of heterozygotes may be confounded, however, by late or variable age of onset of clinical symptoms and by lack of penetrance or variability in expression of the trait.

Late age of onset is characteristic of Huntington's disease (HD), formerly known as Huntington's chorea. The mean age of onset of this severe degenerative disorder of the nervous system is 38 years, with some heterozygote carriers not being clinically affected until 70 years of age. Thus most patients are asymptomatic in the reproductive years and do not know whether they carry the deleterious gene, a fact that may have significant implications on the health of both parent and offspring. Although the gene for HD has been mapped to human chromosome 4p16.3 and prenatal diagnosis of heterozygote fetuses is feasible,[35] ethical and psychological implications obviate the routine use of gene probes for the diagnosis of asymptomatic carriers of HD.

Lack of penetrance is defined as absence of the dominant phenotype in a heterozygous individual known to carry the abnormal gene by means of an affected parent and an affected child. Some autosomal dominant disorders with reduced penetrance are otosclerosis (40%), retinoblastoma (80%), hereditary pancreatitis (80%), and Gardner's syndrome (84%). In some disorders, penetrance may be influenced by age (see HD). In disorders with reduced penetrance, the risk for offspring of an apparently normal individual almost never exceeds 10%.

Expression of autosomal dominant traits may vary between heterozygotes. Even within the same family some affected individuals may express severe phenotypic changes while others may manifest only minimal, difficult to detect, symptoms. Variability of expression is evident in neurofibromatosis, tuberous sclerosis, and myotonic dystrophy (MD). In such disorders, detailed clinical examination and sometimes special tests may be needed before pronouncing an individual as nonaffected (and therefore not carrying the gene for the disease). That may have obvious implications in terms of genetic risk for affected siblings or offspring. It is important to bear in mind that expression of some disorders may vary between transmitting generations. Thus the severity of the disorder in the parent does not indicate what the expression will be in the affected offspring. Such examples are disorders of late onset, such as HD and MD. Approximately 10% of cases of HD and 10% to 20% of cases of MD are characterized by juvenile onset and a very severe course. In more than 90% of juvenile cases, the gene for the disease is transmitted from a specific parent—in juvenile HD by the father, in congenital MD by the mother. It appears that epigenetic mechanisms resulting in parental genomic imprinting play a major role in determining the variation of expression as well as the appearance of juvenile, severe forms of some dominant disorders.[13,32]

In summary, autosomal dominant phenotypes are commonly associated with malformations, are clinically variable and, in most cases, are less severe than recessive phenotypes. Variability of expression and incomplete penetrance may confound the vertical pattern of autosomal dominant inheritance. As a rule of thumb, individuals affected by autosomal dominant disorders are heterozygous for the disease gene; in the homozygous form, these disorders are almost always lethal in early life.

Autosomal Recessive Inheritance

Disorders inherited in an autosomal recessive pattern are expressed only in the homozygote that has inherited the diseased gene from two heterozygous, phenotypically healthy, parents. Thus the inheritance pattern is horizontal, with only one generation in the pedigree showing clinical manifestations of the disease. Commonly, these disorders are caused by rare enzymatic defects and are termed inborn errors of metabolism. Because the genotype is homozygous, the phenotype of these disorders is less variable and more severe than in dominant conditions.

15

Consanguinity or inbreeding in an isolated (ethnic) group has a significant impact on the frequency of recessive disorders in a specific population. A common example is Tay Sachs. This lysosomal storage disease is characterized by accumulation of ganglioside GM2 in the nervous system, causing mental retardation, blindness, a cherry red spot in the retina, and muscular weakness leading to death in early childhood. The enzymatic defect is absence of hexosaminidase A, and carrier detection is available by determination of Hex A serum levels.[36] The gene for Tay Sachs, mapped to human chromosome 15q22, is carried with a frequency of 1:27 among Ashkenazi Jews and 1:300 among the rest of the North American population. The chance of random mating between two Jewish Tay Sachs carriers can be calculated as 1:729, as compared with 1:90,000 among non-Jews. Thus among Ashkenazi Jews, parents of affected children are usually non-related, whereas in other populations the consanguinity rate among parents of affected cases is high. Tay Sachs carrier determination should be offered routinely to Jewish couples and should be considered even when only one of the parents is Jewish.

The most common autosomal recessive disorder in the white Caucasian population is cystic fibrosis, with a carrier frequency of 1:22. The gene for cystic fibrosis has been mapped to human chromosome 7p; mutations specific to different ethnic groups have been identified and molecular screening to identify carriers of cystic fibrosis or prenatal diagnosis of affected fetuses is increasingly used in clinical setup.[37,38] A panel of 25 mutations has been proposed as pan-ethnic mutation screening by the American College of Medical genetics.[39] Other autosomal recessive disorders in which screening of carriers is used in clinical practice include Canavan, Gaucher (type A), Bloom, Fanconi anemia, glycogen storage disease type 1, mucolipidosis type IV, Niemann Pick type A, familial dysautonomia, maple syrup urine disease, and α1-antitrypsin deficiency (Table 1-2). When available, determination of the carrier status for diseases specific to ethnic groups should be offered as standard of care in pregnancy.

Table 1-2

Disease	Ethnic Group	Carrier Frequency	Disease Frequency
Sickle cell	Blacks	1 in 12	1 in 600
Cystic fibrosis	N. Europeans	1 in 22	1 in 1936
α thalassemia	Asians, Chinese	1 in 25	1 in 2500
β thalassemia	Mediterranean	1 in 30	1 in 3600
Tay Sachs	Ashkenazi Jews	1 in 27	1 in 2916
Familial dysautonomia	Ashkenazi Jews	1 in 36	1 in 5000
Canavan	Ashkenazi Jews	1 in 37	1 in 5476
Nieman Pick	Ashkenazi Jews	1 in 45	1 in 8100
Fanconi anemia	Ashkenazi Jews	1 in 50	1 in 10,000
Mucolipidosis IV	Ashkenazi Jews	1 in 50	1 in 10,000
Bloom syndrome	Ashkenazi Jews	1 in 60	1 in 14,400
Phenylketonuria	E. Europeans	1 in 60	1 in 14,400

16

The following criteria are characteristic of autosomal recessive inheritance:

1. The disorder usually appears only in siblings of an affected case (horizontal pattern of the pedigree). Both parents and offspring (if any) are obligatory carriers but clinically unaffected (Figure 1-4).
2. With mating of two carriers, offspring of either sex has a 1 in 4 chance to be affected. Half the siblings of an affected individual will be carriers like the parents and one fourth will not carry the trait. Thus two thirds of healthy siblings of an affected person are phenotypically normal but carry the trait.
3. Transmission in consecutive generations is rare and is confined to mating between two affected individuals or between affected and carrier. In the former situation, all offspring will be affected.
4. Consanguinity and inbreeding increase the frequency of rare autosomal recessive traits.

Figure 1-4

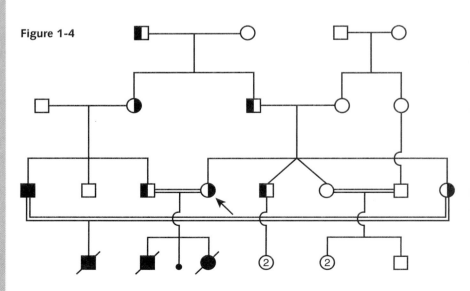

Autosomal recessive
pedigree.

5. All human are heterozygous for three to five lethal equivalents—disorders that would have been lethal if appearing in the homozygous state. This may account for the increase in perinatal mortality and morbidity associated with consanguineous marriages or mating within inbred populations or genetic isolates. The risk of congenital malformations quoted for offspring of first cousins is considered as 6%, about twice the risk in the general population, the difference being attributed to a significantly higher rate of genetic recessive disorders.

Disorders Inherited in Linkage to the Sex Chromosomes

For practical purposes, sex-linked inheritance refers mainly to genetic diseases carried on the X chromosome. The Y chromosome contains only a scarce amount of genetic information, mainly regarding the size of teeth and testes differentiation. For Y-linked inheritance, only male-to-male transmission is observed and only males are affected.

X-linked inheritance patterns are influenced by two major factors:

1. Women have two X chromosomes and can be homozygous or heterozygous to genes on the X. In contrast, males have only one X chromosome. Thus males are said to be *hemizygous* in respect to X-linked genes.
2. Women have only one active X chromosome, the other being inactivated by DNA methylation in the early female embryo. Thus a woman heterozygous for an X-linked gene is an actual mosaic, with the abnormal allele being active in about half of her cells.[40] The inherited allele on the X chromosome will always be active in the hemizygous male.

The characteristic pattern of X-linked inheritance is oblique (Figure 1-5), the disease often affecting a boy and his maternal uncle. The following model is suggestive of X-linked inheritance:

1. Male to male transmission is never observed, because a father does not transmit the X chromosome to his sons.
2. Unaffected males do not transmit the affected phenotype to offspring of either sex.

Figure 1-5

European royal pedigree X-linked transmission.

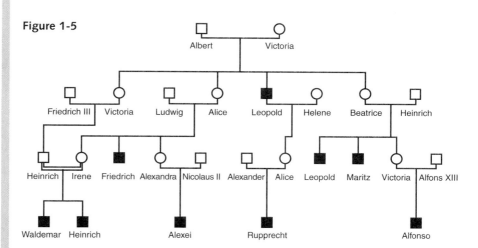

3. Males are usually affected more severely than females. In X-linked dominant disorders, females tend to be affected twice as often (but less severely) than males.
4. All the daughters of an affected male will carry the abnormal gene (and will express it, if dominant).
5. A carrier mother will transmit the mutated gene to half of her offspring of either sex.
6. The proportion of carrier mothers is positively associated with the severity of the condition. Thus for disorders that are always lethal in early childhood (i.e., Duchenne muscular dystrophy), about one third of cases are caused by new mutations.
7. On average, the age of the father of the first heterozygous woman in the pedigree will be advanced.

It appears that the expression of the X-linked phenotype is dependent on a "gene dosage effect." Affected males have only the mutant gene and express its full dosage. Carrier females are mosaic for the abnormal gene and the phenotypic expression will depend on the amount of abnormal gene that was inactivated in early embryonic life. In situations that do not allow inactivation of the specific X chromosome carrying the abnormal gene (i.e., translocation of that X on an autosome), women exhibit the phenotype with the same severity as males. As with autosomal disorders, whether the phenotype is called recessive or dominant depends on the sensitivity of the assay.

Multifactorial Inheritance

Multifactorial disorders appear to result from the additive action of genetic and environmental, non-genetic factors (a threshold effect). Diabetes, congenital heart defects, neural tube defects (NTDs), pyloric stenosis, cleft lip and palate, and epilepsy are all examples of disorders with multifactorial inheritance.

In mendelian (single gene) inheritance, the risk of recurrence in siblings was calculated based on the odds that a specific allele will segregate into the fertilized oocyte. Genetic contribution from both parents was equally important and the risk for proband was not modified by the number of affected individuals in the family or by environmental influences. With multifactorial disorders, the risk of recurrence is based on empirical data obtained from clinical observations and population studies. Moreover, the population frequency of the disorder, the sex of the proband and the affected individual, and the relationship of the proband to the latter may all influence recurrence risk. The population frequency of many of these disorders is 1%, with a risk of recurrence of 3% to 4% in first-degree relatives. Although specific recurrence risks are available for different disorders (Table 1-3), some common rules may apply in many such situations:

1. The risk is highest among closest relatives and decreases rapidly with distance of relationship. The correlation between relatives is proportional to the genes in common—the risk is seldom increased above the risk of the general population in third-degree or more distant relatives. In contrast, the risk to subsequent siblings is higher when parents are consanguineous.

Table 1-3

	Population Incidence (%)	Risk to First-Degree Relatives (%)
Congenital heart defects	1	2-3
VSD	0.5	2-4
ASD	0.1	3.0
Tetralogy of Fallot	0.07	3.0
Pulmonary stenosis	0.08	2.0
Pyloric stenosis* (M:F–5:1)	0.5	3-5
Duodenal ulcer	1.7	10.5
Neural tube defects	0.2	3-4
Cleft lip and/or palate	0.2	2-4
CDH* (F:M–3:1)	0.5	5.0

ASD, Atrial septal defect; CDH, congenital dislocation of hip; VSD, ventricular septal defect.
*Sex predilection–the risk for relatives is higher if disorder is expressed in member of the less commonly affected sex.

2. The risk for affected siblings equals the risk of affected offspring.
3. Recurrence risk depends on the population frequency of the disorder; for first-degree relatives, this risk is approximately the square root of the incidence of the disorder in the population studied. The lower the population risk, the higher the relative risk of recurrence in siblings.
4. When there is unequal sex distribution of a disorder, recurrence risk is higher when a member of the more rarely affected case has the disease. A common example is pyloric stenosis, which is five times more frequent in males than in females. The risk of recurrence is 3.8% for brothers of a male index case but 9.2% for brothers of an affected female.
5. Recurrence risk is higher when more than one family member is affected or when the disease in the index case is more severe.

The common denominator of these rules is a higher genetic liability (lower threshold) associated with increased risk of recurrence in other family members, probably because of genes shared by the affected individuals. Many affected members in one family may reflect a higher genetic liability, as is observed with more severe expression of the disease or with members of the more rarely affected sex being affected. The association of some disorders with specific HLA haplotypes also substantiates the concept of genetic liability.

Environmental factors (i.e., geographic location or diet) are also essential determinants in the occurrence of multifactorial disorders. Common examples are NTDs, a spectrum of disorders of closure of the neural crest that includes anencephaly and spina bifida. The overall incidence before folic acid supplementation was approximately 1 in 500 to 1 in 1000 in the United States. Throughout the world, the prevalence of NTD was highest in Northern Ireland (about 8 per 1000 births) and lowest in Japan. For couples of Irish descent who immigrated to the United States, the risk for NTD was halved. However, the risk for NTD was doubled for Japanese couples living in Hawaii. Overall in the United States, the highest rate of NTD is observed among the white Appalachian population. For any given place, there are marked differences between African and Caucasian populations.[41]

Following the birth of one child with NTD, the risk of recurrent NTD in another offspring is 3% (in the United States) to 5% (in the United Kingdom). The birth of another affected child increases the risk of recurrent NTD in that family to 10% to 15%. However, the risk of recurrence can be lowered significantly by preconceptional administration of folic acid, to be continued until the closure of the neural tube is completed (about 6 to 8 weeks of gestation). In high-risk families, dietary supplementation with folic acid is advocated to reduce the risk of recurrent NTD to less than 1%.[42] On the other hand, some medications (e.g., valproic acid), maternal diabetes, or surgery performed on the mother in the first trimester[43] are reported to be associated with an increased risk for NTD in offspring. This may be mediated through fluctuations in DNA methylation patterns in response to low dietary levels of folate, methionine, and selenium, which can lead to hypomethylation and genetic instability—methyl groups are acquired through the diet and are donated to DNA through the folate and methionine pathways.[32,44]

NONTRADITIONAL INHERITANCE

Not all heritable traits or even all single gene disorders follow the laws of traditional mendelian inheritance. Genetic phenomena that cannot be explained by mendelian rules of genetics include mitochondrial inheritance, genomic imprinting, uniparental disomy (UPD), mosaicism (somatic and germline), and trinucleotides repeat expansion. Many of these problems are mediated through *epigenetic* control—heritable changes in gene expression that are affected by DNA methylation and histone acetylation.[29] Understanding the mechanisms associated with nontraditional modes of inheritance provides the basic principles to evaluate genetic risks and rates of recurrence in these situations.

Mitochondrial Inheritance

Each human cell contains thousands of mitochondria that are the major sites of ATP production. The mitochondrial genome is a circular DNA molecule with 16,569 nucleotides encoding 37 genes. There are 2 to 10 copies of mitochondrial DNA (mtDNA) per mitochondrion, amounting to thousands of copies in every nucleated cell. It has highly conserved sequences in divergent species. It encodes for two rRNAs, 22 tRNAs, and 13 polypeptide chains (Complexes I-V), which are part of the oxidative phosphorylation system and of the respiratory pathway. Complex II is completely encoded by mtDNA, whereas Complexes I, III, IV, and V require the products of nuclear genes as well. The mitochondrial genome replicates asynchronously with the cell cycle, and the mitochondria are then randomly distributed to the daughter cells during cytokinesis.

There are several features that differentiate the mitochondrial genome from the nuclear genome. Nearly every nucleotide appears to be part of a coding sequence, either for a protein or for one of the RNAs. Hence, there are very few introns in the mitochondrial genome. Total noncoding DNA is just a little over 1 kb and is thought to be a control region containing both origins of replication for the heavy (H) strand of mtDNA and promoters for H strand and light (L) strand transcription. Both the H and the L strands contain coding sequences.

Comparison of mitochondrial gene sequences and the amino acid sequences of the corresponding proteins indicates that the genetic code in mtDNA is different from that which is used in the nuclear genome. Four of the 64 codons code for different amino acids in the mitochondrial genome. Although greater than 30 tRNAs specify amino acids in the cytoplasm, mitochondrial protein synthesis requires only 22. Many of the tRNA molecules recognize any one of the four nucleotides in the third position that allows one tRNA to pair with any one of four codons, allowing protein synthesis with fewer tRNAs. In other words, the rules for codon-anticodon pairing appear to be changed in the mitochondrial genome.

The rate of nucleotide substitution in mtDNA is much higher than in nuclear DNA. Comparisons of DNA sequences in different organisms reveal that the rate of nucleotide substitutions during evolution is about 10 times greater in mitochondrial genomes than in nuclear genomes, presumably secondary to reduced fidelity of mtDNA replication, a paucity of DNA repair mechanisms, or both. Deletions also occur more often.

The relative proportion of mutant and normal mtDNA in the affected tissue determines variability of phenotypic expression, which is characteristic of mitochondrial disease. Unlike nuclear DNA that is evenly divided between daughter cells, the cytoplasm and therefore the mtDNA are randomly distributed to daughter cells. The term *heteroplasmy* is used to refer to the presence of both normal and abnormal mitochondria, as opposed to *homoplasmy*, in which all the mitochondria are either normal or abnormal. The proportion of normal genomes determines the phenotype of the cell. Once the proportion of either normal or abnormal mitochondria exceeds a certain tissue-specific threshold, the biologic behavior of the cell will change. This threshold may be influenced by such factors as energy demands of the cell or age.

The ovum is the source of all mitochondria in the embryo because sperm contain only few mitochondria that are located in the tail region. Because only the nucleus of the sperm fuses with the ovum, the mitochondria from the sperm do not persist in the offspring. Hence, mitochondrial inheritance is exclusively maternal (only the mother can inherit the trait to offspring).

Somatic mtDNA Mutations and Aging

The majority of cellular oxidation and most of the cell's ATP is produced in the mitochondria. Free radicals are produced in the mitochondria during oxidative phosphorylation. Free radical production is increased by inhibition of the electron transport pathways and is thus a self-perpetuating process. Oxidative damage to mtDNA, either directly or indirectly by oxidative products such as lipids and proteins, can cause mtDNA mutations, which further impair oxidative phosphorylation efficiency. MtDNA is more susceptible to damage by free radicals because of its close proximity to the site of free radical generation, the lack of protective histones, and the relatively poor repair mechanisms of the mitochondrial genome.

With aging there is a decrease in mitochondrial respiratory function. Accumulation of mtDNA mutations in a tissue is inversely proportional to its potential to replicate and is directly related to its metabolic state, specifically its energy requirements, which are met through oxidative phosphorylation. Hence, such mutations are found to a greater extent in the brain and muscle (skeletal and cardiac) than in other tissues. Certain areas within the brain are at greater risk than others. The basal ganglia are at particularly high risk as they are rich in dopaminergic neurons that generate hydrogen peroxide by deamination of dopamine, a reaction that is catalyzed by monoamine oxidase B (MAO-B). MAO-B levels increase with age concomitantly with the accumulation of mtDNA mutations. By contrast, the cerebellum and myelinated axons, which are not dopaminergic and have a low rate of glucose utilization, have the lowest rate of mtDNA mutations.

Mitochondrial Disease

Leber hereditary optic neuropathy (LHON) is characterized by rapid loss of central vision during early adult life. Eyes may be affected simultaneously or sequentially. LHON patients and their maternal relatives have also been reported to manifest a variety of additional symptoms. Cardiac conduction defects have been noted in some families.[45] Various minor neurologic problems (altered reflexes, ataxia, and sensory neuropathy) have been described, as well as skeletal abnormalities. The penetrance in males who inherit the mutation at bp 11778 is about 50% but only 20% in females. This difference cannot be explained by heteroplasmy and is thought to suggest involvement of an X-linked gene that may be affected by a variety of mutations.[46]

Myoclonus Epilepsy and Ragged-Red Fibers (MERRF Syndrome)

MERRF syndrome consists of myopathy, myoclonus, generalized seizures, hearing loss, intellectual deterioration, and ataxia. The term *ragged red fibers* is derived from histologic characteristics observed with the modified Gomori trichrome staining of fresh frozen muscle, in which accumulated mitochondria appear red, resulting from rearrangements of mtDNA or point mutations affecting tRNA genes.

An A-to-G mutation at nucleotide 8344 accounts for 80% to 90% of cases of MERRF syndrome. The mutation is a missense mutation in the gene for a transfer RNA for lysine, producing multiple deficiencies in the enzyme complexes of the respiratory chain.[47] The clinical phenotype varies greatly within a pedigree, consistent with a heteroplasmic population of mtDNA.

Mitochondrial Myopathy, Encephalopathy, Lactic Acidosis, and Stroke-like Episodes (MELAS)

MELAS is first manifested in childhood as stunted growth; recurrent stroke-like episodes manifest as hemiparesis, hemianopsia, and cortical blindness. Focal or generalized seizures, myoclonic epilepsy, and hearing loss may also be seen. Episodic vomiting may also be present. Death often occurs before the age of 20 years. MELAS is associated with a point mutation in the tRNA for leucine.[48]

Kearns-Sayre and Chronic Progressive External Ophthalmoplegia (KSS/CPEO)

KSS/CPEO is characterized by ophthalmoplegia, atypical retinitis pigmentosa, and mitochondrial myopathy. Cardiac conduction defects may be present. The age of onset is usually before age 20 years. Other features may include ataxia, hearing loss, dementia, short stature, delayed secondary sexual characteristics, hypoparathyroidism, and hypothyroidism. The mtDNA mutations, most commonly deletions, usually occur spontaneously, so this disease is not inherited. Heteroplasmy is usually demonstrable in muscle mtDNA.

Neuropathy, Ataxia, and Retinitis Pigmentosa (NARP)

As the name implies, NARP is characterized by a variable combination of retinitis pigmentosa, ataxia, and sensory neuropathy. Other features include developmental delay, dementia, seizures, and proximal limb weakness. NARP was first described in 1990 by Holt et al.[49] and is associated with an mtDNA point mutation in the gene for subunit 6 of mitochondrial H^+-ATPase. This same mutation has also been seen in families with Leigh disease.

Cytochrome C Oxidase Deficiency (Complex IV Deficiency)

There are three established clinical syndromes of cytochrome C oxidase (COX) deficiency, two of which represent variant forms of infantile myopathy. One is benign, characterized by spontaneous recovery by age two to three. The other form presents in the neonatal period and results in respiratory failure. The fatal form, also associated with a renal tubular defect, is inherited as a recessive trait and is thought to represent a defect in a nuclear-encoded polypeptide in the respiratory chain. The third form of COX deficiency affects the central nervous system and is known as Leigh syndrome. The typical presentation in the neonatal period is one of hypotonia, recurrent vomiting, and retinitis pigmentosa leading to visual loss. Lactic acid levels are increased in blood and cerebrospinal fluid. Several heteroplasmic mtDNA mutations have been demonstrated in Leigh syndrome.

Maternally Inherited Diabetes Mellitus

Several retrospective studies showed that patients with non-insulin-dependent diabetes mellitus (NIDDM) were much more likely to have a mother who was diagnosed with NIDDM than a father.[50] This was also noted to be true for women with gestational diabetes.[51] These studies may be subject to certain biases, however, as all of them used patient recollection to ascertain affected first-degree relatives.

Glucose intolerance or NIDDM has been reported in some subjects with mitochondrial myopathy. Up to 20% of patients with MELAS have been shown to be diabetic. Diabetes in this group of patients has been associated with nerve deafness and a point mutation in a mitochondrial gene for leucine tRNA.[52] It therefore seems probable that mitochondrial mutations may be involved in the pathogenesis of a small, but clinically significant, proportion of cases of NIDDM.

Genomic Imprinting

Genomic imprinting refers to the process whereby specific genes are differentially marked (imprinted) during parental gametogenesis. The result is differential expression of these genes, depending on whether they are inherited either maternally or paternally. The existence of genomic imprinting was first suspected after experiments with pronuclear transplantation. If one of the pronuclei is removed and replaced with a pronucleus of the opposite parental origin, the result is lethal. However, depending on whether the pronuclei are of maternal or paternal origin, the consequences are very different. If both are of maternal origin (a gynogenetic embryo), the embryo initially develops normally but development of the placenta and fetal membranes is deficient. If the pronuclei are male in origin (an androgenetic embryo), the membranes and placenta develop normally while the embryo develops poorly. This latter situation is seen in triploid conceptions with a partial molar pregnancy. These experiments and observations imply that both maternal and paternal genomes are necessary for normal growth and development. Therefore, their contributions cannot be equivalent.

Several theories (avoidance of genetic conflict, prevention of parthenogenesis, optimizing placental function while avoiding the development of gestational trophoblastic disease, dominance modification, and gene regulation) have been proposed to explain the reason for the existence of genomic imprinting. Genomic imprinting is also thought to be operative in X inactivation, a process that results in dosage compensation so that structural genes on the X chromosome are expressed at the same levels in males and females.

Genes that are transcriptionally inactive contain 5-methyl-cytosine residues. Methylation of DNA in mammalian cells occurs in CpG dinucleotides (cytosine-guanine pairs), regions of the genome with an unusually high concentration of the dinucleotide 5'-CG-3'. Typically, unmethylated clusters of CpG pairs in tissue-specific genes and in essential "housekeeping" genes are expressed in most tissues. Proteins that bind to unmethylated CpG areas initiate gene transcription.[32] When methylation occurs in the promoter region, the gene becomes transcriptionally inactive. In addition, changes to histone proteins effect DNA organization and gene expression by ensuring that a receptive DNA region is either accessible for transcription or is targeted for silencing. Active regions of chromatin have unmethylated DNA and have high levels of acetylated histones.[34] These epigenetic changes control tissue-specific gene expression and also play a critical role in the activation of phenomena such as genomic imprinting and X inactivation.

Genomic Imprinting in Human Disease

Prader-Willi and Angelman syndromes are examples of genetic imprinting. Prader-Willi syndrome (PWS) is characterized by short stature, obesity, polyphagia, hypogonadism, and mental retardation. High-resolution chromosome banding reveals small interstitial deletions of the 15q11-q13 regions in a large proportion of these patients.

An identical deletion was reported in 1987 by Magenis et al.[53] in patients with the uncommon Angelman (or "happy puppet") syndrome (AS), characterized by microcephaly, jerky movements, seizures, mental retardation, inappropriate laughter, a large mouth, and protruding tongue. In a rare subset of patients with PWS who did not have detectable cytogenetic deletion, Nicholls et al.[54] reported both copies of chromosome 15 were maternal in origin. It was subsequently discovered in PWS that the deletion always involved the paternally derived chromosome 15, whereas the deletion was present on the maternal copy in AS.[55] These findings strongly suggest a parent-of-origin effect or genomic imprinting in which PWS and AS are caused by two closely linked genes that are oppositely imprinted. Both PWS and AS have been documented to result from UPD in which both copies of chromosome 15 are inherited from one parent. In the case of PWS, both copies are maternal, whereas in AS both copies are paternal in origin.

Beckwith-Wiedemann syndrome (BWS) is characterized by general and regional overgrowth—macroglossia, large kidneys with medullary dysplasia, pancreatic hyperplasia, and cytomegaly within the fetal adrenal cortex. Omphalocele may also be present. Birth weight averages 4 kg, and excessive growth continues in early childhood. There is a significant predisposition toward the development of certain malignancies, most commonly Wilms' tumor, but also adrenocortical carcinoma, hepatoblastoma, and rhabdomyosarcoma. The gene for BWS has been mapped to 11p15. An increased frequency of several 11p15.5 markers in sporadic cases, paternal duplication in trisomic BWS patients, retention of paternal alleles in Wilms' tumor and adrenocortical carcinoma, as well as higher penetrance in individuals who are born to female carriers all suggest that maternal genomic imprinting is operative. The proposed mechanism is failure of methylation to suppress the maternally derived gene, IGF2 (insulin-like growth factor 2).[56]

Uniparental Disomy

Engel first suggested UPD in 1980.[57] UPD refers to the inheritance of two copies of a chromosome (or part of a chromosome) from the same parent. When a chromosome or gene is present in duplicate, it is called isodisomy. If both nonidentical homologs are present, it is designated as heterodisomy. UPD can involve both autosomes and the sex chromosomes. Eight years after Engel advanced his hypothesis, cystic fibrosis and growth deficiency were diagnosed in a patient who had inherited two copies of the same mutation in the CF gene but had only one carrier parent with that mutation.[58] The patient with CF had evidence of intrauterine growth restriction that was thought to be secondary to the effects of UPD, rather than that of CF.

As noted previously, UPD has been recognized as a cause of both PWS and AS. UPD has since been described for chromosomes 5, 6, 7, 9, 11, 13, 14, 15, 16, 21, 22, and the XY pair.[59] Vidaud et al.[60] described a phenotypically normal boy with sex chromosome UPD that was detected because both the boy and his father had hemophilia. Maternal isodisomy for chromosome 16 is associated with pregnancy loss and severe intrauterine growth retardation (IUGR) but can be compatible with a viable pregnancy.[61] The consequences of UPD will depend on the existence of genomic imprinting for a given gene,

25

the presence of recessive mutations in the case of isodisomy, and the extent of mosaicism which may be present in these individuals.

The most common cause of UPD is thought to be "trisomy rescue," which occurs when a trisomic zygote loses the extra chromosome. If the loss happens randomly, two thirds of the cases will not exhibit UPD, and one third will. Isodisomy results when nondisjunction occurs during meiosis I, and heterodisomy results from nondisjunction in meiosis II. The existence of confined placental mosaicism as evidenced on CVS is thought to support the theory of trisomy rescue as the most common cause of UPD. Nondisjunction occurs far more commonly in female gametes than in male gametes and, hence, the significantly higher frequency of PWS compared with AS. The role of nondisjunction in the genesis of UPD is supported by the observation of increased risk for PWS or AS with advanced parental age. There are, however, several other proposed mechanisms that are reviewed by Engel.[62]

Germline Mosaicism

Germline mosaicism is defined as the presence of two or more genetically different populations of germline cells. These result from a somatic mutation in a germline precursor that subsequently persists in all the clonal descendants of that cell. Because only the germline cells are affected, the carrier of this mutation is phenotypically normal. Germline mutations are usually suspected when phenotypically normal parents have more than one child with a disorder that is usually inherited as an autosomal dominant or an X-linked trait.

Somatic Mosaicism

If a mutation within the primordial inner cell mass occurs before differentiation of somatic and germline cells, it will be present in both somatic and germline cells. If this mutation were present in progenitor cells from which the germline cells were derived, then all subsequent germline cells would contain this mutation that would be transmissible to all of the offspring, although the transmitting parent will be mosaic. If the mutation occurs only in the somatic cell line after separation of the somatic and germline cells, it will not be transmissible. The carrier of such a somatic mutation will exhibit a segmental or patchy pattern of expression, depending on the proportion and distribution of cells carrying the mutation.

Trinucleotide Repeat Expansion

About three fourths of the linear length of the genome consists of single-copy or unique DNA, with the remainder consisting of several classes of repetitive DNA. Tandem (head-to-tail) repeated sequences might be transcriptionally active or inactive. Tandem repeats in coding DNA can vary from short to very large repeat sequences that can include whole genes. Sequence exchange between the repeats can result in either a reduction or an increase (expansion) in the number of tandem repeats. Expansion of trinucleotide or triplet repeat sequences is now a recognized cause of human disease and provides an explanation of the phenomenon known as genetic anticipation.

Genetic anticipation is defined as progressively earlier onset and increased severity of a disease with each subsequent generation. Anticipation was originally thought to reflect ascertainment bias; that is, the family was only studied when a severely affected individual was found. It is now known in at least 10 disorders that anticipation occurs as the result of instability of trinucleotide repeats.[63] In certain disorders such as the fragile-X syndrome, the GC-rich triplet repeats can exist in a premutation state in which the number of repeats is greater than that found in alleles of the normal population but insufficient to cause expression of the disease. When the number of repeats exceeds a threshold, which varies with the given disorder, the replication machinery cannot faithfully replicate the sequence with resultant variation in repeat numbers. This can result in amplification of these triplet sequences and is usually thought to occur during meiosis. However, amplification may also occur post-conception, during mitosis. The process of amplification may differ in maternal and paternal meiosis.

The fragile-X syndrome was the first disorder recognized to result from trinucleotide repeat expansion. It was originally diagnosed cytogenetically and identified by a fragile site on Xq27, a folate-dependent area where the chromatin fails to condense during mitosis, and consequently does not stain when cells are grown in folate-deficient media. On examination the chromosome appears broken or distorted in this region. Fragile-X syndrome is now recognized to be the most common inherited form of moderate mental retardation and the second most common chromosomal cause of mental retardation. Current prevalence estimates suggest that 1 in 1200 males and 1 in 2500 females are affected with fragile-X syndrome.[64] Approximately one in 700 females will carry a mutation in the gene for fragile-X syndrome *(FMR-1)*. Males affected with this disorder usually have mental retardation, coarse facial features, and macroorchidism. Affected females are less dysmorphic, but as many as one third will exhibit mild mental retardation.

The expression of the fragile-X mutation depends on the number of CGG repeats within the CpG island in the promoter region of the *FMR-1* gene.[65] Amplification of the CGG repeat is associated with subsequent methylation of the CpG island, effectively silencing expression of the gene so that it resembles the FMR-1 locus on the inactive X chromosome. The *FMR-1* gene has one of the highest mutation rates of any gene in the human genome. The DNA diagnosis for the fragile-X syndrome is based on the size of the CGG expansion as well as the degree of methylation of the *FMR-1* gene.

In fragile-X syndrome, alleles of normal individuals have fewer than 50 copies of the CGG repeat. Small expansions known as premutation involve up to 200 repeats. Males and females carrying the premutation are said to be carriers and are phenotypically normal. The disorder becomes clinically apparent when the triplet is expanded preferentially during maternal meiosis to greater than 200 repeats and the gene is inactivated through methylation with loss of the as yet unknown *FMR-1* gene product. However, there is no sharp delineation between the upper limit of normal and the lower limit of the premutation. Fifty to 60 copies of the CGG are considered a gray area. Expansion of the repeats from generation to generation varies considerably among families but occurs only when the X chromosome is inherited through a female. Expression also requires inheritance of the X chromosome from a female. Expansion occurs during early embryogenesis so there may be considerable variation between cells in the length of the repeat. It has been observed that the greater the size of the premutation, the greater the risk of expansion to a full mutation (the Sherman paradox).

Unaffected males who carry the premutation (normal transmitting males) may pass the mutation on to their daughters, who will also be unaffected. However, their daughters may pass on the expanded allele to their offspring, who are then at risk for expansion to a full mutation and expression of the fragile-X syndrome.

Sutherland and Baker[66] identified a second site of fragility in patients with the cytogenetic changes typical of some patients with fragile-X syndrome but lacking the molecular changes. This site has been designated FRAXE and is 150 to 600 kb distal to FMR-1. FRAXE has since been cloned and patients expressing this site have evidence of amplification of a GCC repeat adjacent to a CpG island in Xq28. Normal individuals have 6 to 25 copies of the repeat, whereas patients with mental retardation have more than 200 copies.[67] As with FMR-1, there is also evidence of methylation of the CpG island in affected individuals. Expansion of the GCC repeat at the FRAXE site generally results in a milder degree of mental retardation than that which is seen in patients with the FMR-1 mutation.

All males and 50% of women carrying far more than 200 CGG copies will be affected. Predicting the phenotype in patients carrying $\approx$ 200 CGG repeats is problematic. Moreover, patients carrying the premutation may be affected in adult life by disorders that are seemingly unrelated to the classic Martin Bell syndrome. A higher rate of premature ovarian failure has been observed in female patients with the FraX premutation.[68] Likewise, male individuals with the premutation are at higher risk of a tremor/ataxia syndrome.[69]

The phenomenon of anticipation and dynamic mutation may explain differences in expression and in penetrance observed in some other X-linked dominant disorders as well as the variability in clinical phenotype noted for certain genetic diseases with autosomal dominant inheritance. In specific autosomal dominant disorders, such as HD, the effect of transmission by either maternal or paternal chromosome on age of onset and severity of symptoms in offspring may be explained by such a dynamic mutation.[70]

HD is a progressive neurologic disorder characterized by chorea, dementia, rigidity, seizures, and often psychiatric symptoms. It has been observed that the offspring of affected males have significantly younger age of onset than the offspring of affected females, which is thought to result from paternal genomic imprinting involving DNA methylation.[71] Late-onset cases are much more likely to be inherited from an affected mother.

HD is inherited as an autosomal dominant trait. The gene is on the short arm of chromosome 4 and is now known as *huntingtin*. It contains an expanded, unstable CAG triplet repeat in HD patients. The risk of expansion is greater during spermatogenesis than in oogenesis. The normal range of CAG repeats is 11 to 34 copies, 30 to 37 copies define the premutation, and the disease is expressed when 38 to 86 copies are present.

Myotonia, muscular dystrophy, cataracts, hypogonadism, cardiac arrhythmias, and frontal balding are the main symptoms of MD. Symptoms usually appear in midlife but age of onset may be considerably earlier. Distal muscles of the extremities are initially affected with later involvement of proximal muscles of the extremities and extraocular and facial muscles.

The gene for MD is located on chromosome 19 and codes for a protein kinase. The defect is caused by amplification of a CTG triplet repeat. Less than 30 copies of the repeat is considered normal, 30 to 50 copies is consistent with the premutation, and overt expression is seen with greater than 50 copies. The severity of the disease is directly correlated with the number of copies. Mildly affected patients will have from 50 to 80 copies, whereas the most severely affected patients may have more than 2000 copies. The expanded repeats affect DNA methylation and chromatin structure and inhibiting expression of adjacent genes. There is no apparent effect on transcription or on the structure of the gene product. Amplification is observed but only when transmission is maternal. The most severe congenital form is seen in offspring of affected women.

Spinocerebellar ataxia type I (SCA1) is a neurodegenerative disease characterized by ataxia, progressive dementia, and spasticity. Symptoms usually begin in the third or fourth decade of life.[72]

The gene for SCA1 has been mapped to chromosome 6. The mutation consists of a CAG repeat expansion. Early onset of disease is associated with a larger number of repeats and paternal transmission. Twenty-five to 36 repeats is considered normal, 35 to 43 constitutes the premutation, and 42 to 81 copies coincides with expression of the disease.

Spinal and Bulbar Muscular Atrophy

Spinal and bulbar muscular atrophy (SBMA; Kennedy disease) was first described by Kennedy et al.,[73] in 1968, in nine males in two unrelated kindreds. Fasciculations followed by muscle weakness and wasting occurs at approximately 40 years of age. Pyramidal, sensory, and cerebellar signs were absent. The disorder is compatible with long life. The main feature of Kennedy disease distinguishing it from the autosomal recessive and autosomal dominant forms of spinal muscular atrophy is the presence of sensory abnormalities. Gynecomastia is often the first clinical sign, suggesting androgen deficiency and estrogen excess.

The gene for SBMA has been mapped to Xq11-q12 and is inherited as an X-linked autosomal disorder. La Spada et al.[74] discovered enlargement of a tandem CAG repeat within the first exon of the androgen receptor *(AR)* gene, in each of 35 unrelated SBMA patients. The AR CAG repeat is normally polymorphic, with an average repeat number of 22 ± 3. In SBMA patients, these investigators found 11 different (CAG) alleles, with repeat numbers ranging from 40 to 52. The *AR* gene abnormality was found to segregate with the disease in 15 SBMA families. The CAG repeat correlates with disease severity such that the mildest clinical manifestations are associated with the smallest CAG repeat. However, other factors seem to contribute to phenotypic variability. As with other diseases resulting from triplet repeat expansion, expansion tends to vary with gender. In the case of Kennedy disease, there is a greater rate of instability and subsequent expansion in male meiosis than in female meiosis.

SUMMARY

Genetic diseases are a heterogeneous group of disorders whose pathophysiology can be viewed as gene malfunction resulting in abnormal quality or quantity of the gene product. When single genes are involved these disorders follow, in most cases, mathematical rules of inheritance. Multifactorial disorders are the result of the interaction between genetic predisposition and external (environmental) factors, and their inheritance is based on empirical observations. Chromosome anomalies can be viewed as a generalized effect of multiple gene dosage abnormalities, resulting in a pattern of mental and growth retardation and developmental defects of some organ systems specific to the chromosome involved. In many cases these defects will be lethal in the perinatal period.

Nonclassical modes of inheritance are recognized with increasing frequency for a diverse and increasing number of single gene disorders. Mitochondrial inheritance, genomic imprinting, UPD, somatic and germline mosaicism, and trinucleotide repeat expansion may explain the unorthodox pattern of inheritance of some genetic disorders. Examples of disorders associated with each of these mechanisms will undoubtedly grow as the molecular basis of genetic disease continues to be elucidated and gene defects linked to medical diseases emerge through the Human Genome Project.

The era of epigenetics is just beginning. These heritable changes in gene function, without the need for changes in primary DNA sequence, will be a source of intense investigation over the next decade. It is undoubtedly through such mechanisms that we see variation between supposedly "identical" twins. Although only the "tip of the iceberg" is currently evident, we do know that such changes are labile, are reversible, and undergo dynamic reprogramming. Such changes are mediated by differential gene expression or other mechanisms involving DNA methylation, chromatin structure, histone modification, and protein changes. Epigenetic programming regulates the combination of genes expressed in each cell and allows tissue-specific genes to be expressed in certain cells and repressed in others. A decade from now, we will certainly see epigenetic changes as truly a second genetic code with almost as much importance to normal functioning as the original one. Thus the quest for a human epigenome project [75] is a necessity for better understanding of human disease as well as for designation of better ways to understand and combat cancer, cell aging, and death.

KEY POINTS

1. Chromosome abnormalities are the cause of only 10% of congenital malformations.
2. Mutations affecting gene function are inherited at random segregation.
3. Mutations causing genetic disease are typical to specific families.
4. Unorthodox patterns of inheritance may explain some cases of multifactorial disease.
5. Epigenetic effects on gene expression are increasingly recognized as a reversible mechanism of inherited disease.

REFERENCES

1. Delhanty JDA, Handyside AH: The origin of genetic defects in the human and their detection in the preimplantation embryo, *Hum Reprod Update* 1:201, 1995.
2. Down JLH: Observations of an ethnic classification of idiots, *Clin Lect Rep Lond Hosp* 3:259, 1866.
3. Lejeune J, Gauthier M, Turpin R: Etude des chromosomes somatiques de neuf enfants mongoliens, *Cr Acad Sci Paris* 248:1721, 1959.
4. Smith HO, Wilcox KW: A restriction enzyme from Hemophilus influenza; I. purification and general properties, *J Mol Biol* 51:393, 1970.
5. Southern EM: Detection of specific sequences among DNA fragments separated by gel electrophoresis, *J Mol Biol* 98:503, 1975.
6. Hsu LYF: Prenatal diagnosis of chromosome anomalies. In Milunski A, editor: *Genetic Disorders and the Fetus*, ed 2, New York, 1986, Plenum Press, pp 115-183.
7. Warburton D: Chromosomal causes of fetal death, *Clin Obstet Gynecol* 30:268, 1987.
8. Williamson RA et al: Abnormal pregnancy sonogram: Selective indication for fetal karyotype, *Obstet Gynecol* 69:15, 1987.
9. Boyers SP et al: The effect of polyploidy on embryo cleavage after in vitro fertilization in humans, *Fertil Steril* 48:624, 1987.
10. Fisher JM et al: Trisomy 18: studies of the parent and cell division of origin and the effect of aberrant recombination on nondisjunction, *Am J Hum Genet* 56:669, 1995.
11. Eggerman T et al: Trisomy of human chromosome 18: molecular studies on parental origin and cell stage of nondisjunction, *Hum Genet* 97:218, 1996.
12. O'Brien WF et al: Elevated maternal serum alpha-fetoprotein in triploidy, *Obstet Gynecol* 71:994, 1988.
13. Hall JG: Genomic imprinting: Review and relevance to human diseases, *Am J Hum Genet* 46:857, 1990.
14. Scarbrough PR et al: Tetraploidy: a report of three liveborn infants, *Am J Med Genet* 19:29, 1984.
15. Godsen C, Rodeck CH, Nicolaides KH: Fetal blood sampling in the investigation of chromosome mosaicism in amniotic fluid cell culture, *Lancet* 1:613, 1988.
16. Hassold T, Benham F, Leppert M: Cytogenetics and molecular analysis of sex chromosome monosomy, *Am J Hum Genet* 42:534, 1988.
17. Kalousek DK, Barrett IJ, McGillivray BC: Placental mosaicism and intrauterine survival of trisomies 13 and 18, *Am J Hum Genet* 44:338, 1989.
18. Drugan A et al: Age of gestation (size) at embryonic demise: Tailoring counseling for lethal versus potentially viable aneuploidy, *Fetal Diagn Ther* 8(2):179-83, 1993.
19. Snijders RJM, Schire NJ, Nicolaides KH: Maternal age and gestational age specific risk for chromosomal defects, *Fetal Diagn Ther* 10:356-67, 1995.
20. Bell JA, Pearn JH, Smith A: Prenatal cytogenetic diagnosis, amniotic cell culture Vs chorionic villus sampling, *Med J Aust* 146:27, 1987.
21. Wright DJ et al: Interpretation of chorionic villus sampling laboratory results is just as reliable as amniocentesis, *Obstet Gynecol* 74:739, 1989.
22. Phillips OP et al: Risk of fetal mosaicism when placental mosaicism is diagnosed by chorionic villus sampling, *Am J Obstet Gynecol* 174:850, 1996.
23. Kalousek D: The role of confined chromosomal mosaicism in placental function and human development, *Growth Genet Horm* 4:1, 1988.
24. DeWald GW, Michels VV: Recurrent miscarriages: Cytogenetic causes and genetic counseling of affected families, *Clin Obstet Gynecol* 29:865, 1986.
25. Boue A, Gallano P: A collaborative study of the segregation of inherited chromosome structural rearrangements in 1356 prenatal diagnoses, *Prenat Diagn* 4:45, 1984.
26. Petrosky DL, Borgaonkar DS: Segregation analysis in reciprocal translocation carriers, *Am J Med Genet* 19:137, 1984.
27. Warburton D: Outcome of cases of de novo structural rearrangements diagnosed at amniocentesis, *Prenat Diagn* 4:69, 1984.
28. Kornberg RD, Lorch Y: Twenty-five years of the nucleosome, fundamental particle of the eukaryote chromosome, *Cell* 98:285, 1999.
29. Cheung P, Lau P: Epigenetic regulation by histone methylation and histone variants, *Mol Endocrinol* 19:563, 2005.
30. Verona RI, Mann MR, Bartolomei MS: Genomic imprinting: intricacies of epigenetic regulation in clusters, *Annu Rev Cell Dev Biol* 19:237, 2003.
31. Avner P, Heard E: X chromosome inactivation: counting, choice and initiation, *Nat Rev Genet* 2:59, 2001.
32. Rodenhiser D, Mann M: Epigenetics and human disease: translating basic biology into clinical applications, *CMAJ* 174:341, 2006.
33. Allegruci C et al: Epigenetics and the germline, *Reproduction* 129:137, 2005.
34. Peterson CL, Laniel MA: Histones and histone modifications, *Curr Biol* 14:R546, 2004.
35. Hayden MR et al: First trimester prenatal diagnosis for Huntington's disease with DNA probes, *Lancet* 1:1284, 1987.
36. Ben Yoseph Y et al: Maternal serum Hexosaminidase A in pregnancy: Effects of gestational age and fetal genotype, *Am J Med Genet* 29:891, 1988.
37. Witt DR et al: Cystic fibrosis heterozygote screening in 5161 pregnant women, *Am J Hum Genet* 58:823, 1996.
38. Bekker H et al: The impact of population based screening for carriers of cystic fibrosis, *J Med Genet* 31:364, 1994.
39. Cystic fibrosis population carrier screening: 2004 revision of American College of Medical Genetics mutation panel, *Genet Med* 6:387, 2004.

40. Heard E: Recent advances in X chromosome inactivation, *Curr Opin Cell Biol* 16:247, 2004.
41. Holmes LB: The health problem: neural tube defects. In Gastel B, Haddow JE, Fletcher JC, editors: *Maternal serum alpha-fetoprotein: Issues in the prenatal screening and diagnosis of neural tube defects,* Washington, DC, 1981, US Government Printing Office, pp 1-4.
42. Olney RS, Mulinare J: Trends in neural tube defects—prevalence, folic acid fortification and vitamins supplement use, *Semin Perinatol* 26:277, 2002.
43. Kallen B, Mazze RI: Neural tube defects and first trimester operations, *Teratology* 41:717, 1990.
44. Ulrey CL et al: The impact of metabolism on DNA methylation, *Hum Mol Genet* 14(suppl 1): R139, 2005.
45. Nikoskelainen E, Wanne O, Dahl M: Pre-excitation syndrome and Leber's hereditary optic neuroretinopathy, *Lancet* 1:696, 1985 (letter).
46. Vikki J et al: Optic atrophy in Leber hereditary optic neuroretinopathy is determined by an X-chromosomal gene closely linked to DXS7, *Am J Hum Genet* 45:206, 1991.
47. Shoffner JM et al: Myoclonic epilepsy and ragged-red fiber disease (MERRF) is associated with a mitochondrial DNA tRNA-lys mutation, *Cell* 61:931, 1990.
48. Goto Y, Nonaka I, Horai S: A mutation in the tRNA leu(vir) gene associated with the MELAS subgroup of mitochondrial encephalomyopathy, *Nature* 348:651, 1990.
49. Holt IJ et al: A new mitochondrial disease associated with mitochondrial DNA heteroplasmy, *Am J Hum Genet* 46:428, 1990.
50. Alcolado JC, Thomas AW: Maternally inherited diabetes mellitus: the role of mitochondrial DNA defects, *Diabetic Med* 12:102, 1995.
51. Martin AO et al: Frequency of diabetes mellitus in mothers of probands with gestational diabetes: possible maternal influence on the predisposition to gestational diabetes, *Am J Obstet Gynecol* 151:471, 1985.
52. Alcolado JC et al: Mitochondrial gene defects in patients with NIDDM, *Diabetologia* 37:372, 1994.
53. Magenis RE et al: Is Angelman syndrome an alternate result of lel(15)(q11q13)? *Am J Med Genet* 28:829, 1987.
54. Nicholls RD et al: Genetic imprinting suggested by maternal heterodisomy in non-deletion Prader-Willi syndrome, *Nature* 342:281, 1989.
55. Magenis RE et al: Comparison of the 15q deletions in Prader-Willi and Angelman syndromes: Specific regions, extent of deletions, parental origin, and clinical consequences, *Am J Med Genet* 35:333, 1990.
56. Weksberg R et al: Disruption of insulin like growth factor 2 imprinting in Beckwith-Wiedemann syndrome, *Nat Genet* 5:143, 1993.
57. Engel E: A new genetic concept: uniparental disomy and its potential effect, isodisomy, *Am J Med Genet* 6:137, 1980.
58. Spence JE et al: Uniparental disomy as a mechanism for human genetic disease, *Am J Hum Genet* 42:217, 1988.
59. Chatkupt S, Antonowicz M, Johnson WG: Parents do matter: genomic imprinting and prenatal sex effects in neurological disorders, *J Neurological Sci* 130:1, 1995.
60. Vidaud D et al: *Father-to-son transmission of hemophilia A due to uniparental disomy,* 40th Annual Meeting of the American Society of Human Genetics, 1989 (Abstract 889).
61. Wolstenholme J: An audit of trisomy 16 in man, *Prenat Diagn* 15:109, 1995.
62. Engel E: Uniparental disomy revisited: the first twelve years, *Am J Med Genet* 46:670, 1993.
63. Erickson RP, Lewis SE: The new human genetics, *Environ Mol Mutagen* 25(suppl 26):7, 1995.
64. Nussbaum RL, Ledbetter DL: The fragile X syndrome. In Scriver CR, Beaudette AL, Sly WS, Valle D, editors: *The metabolic and molecular bases of inherited disease,* ed 7, New York, 1995, McGraw-Hill, pp 795-810.
65. Migeon BR: Role of DNA methylation in X inactivation and the fragile X syndrome, *Am J Med Genet* 47:685, 1993.
66. Sutherland GR, Baker E: Characterization of a new rare fragile site easily confused with the fragile X, *Hum Mol Genet* 1:111, 1993.
67. Knight SJL et al: Triplet repeat expansion at the FRAXE locus and X-linked mild mental handicap, *Am J Hum Genet* 55:81, 1994.
68. Marozzi A et al: Association between idiopathic premature ovarian failure and fragile X premutation, *Hum Reprod* 15:197, 2000.
69. Moore CJ et al: A neuropsychological investigation of male premutation carriers of fragile X syndrome, *Neuropsychologia* 42:1934, 2004.
70. Hayden MR, Kremer B: Huntington disease. In Scriver CR, Beaudette AL, Sly WS, Valle D, editors: *The Metabolic and Molecular Bases of Inherited Disease,* ed 7, New York, 1995, McGraw-Hill, pp 4483-4510.
71. Ridley RM et al: Anticipation in Huntington's disease is inherited through the male line but may originate in the female, *J Med Genet* 25:589, 1988.
72. Orr, HT et al: Expansion of an unstable trinucleotide CAG repeats in spinocerebellar ataxia type 1, *Nat Genet* 4:221, 1993.
73. Kennedy W R, Alter M, Sung JH: Progressive proximal spinal and bulbar muscular atrophy of late onset: a sex-linked recessive trait, *Neurology* 18:671, 1968.
74. La Spada AR et al: Androgen receptor gene mutations in X-linked spinal and bulbar muscular atrophy, *Nature* 352:77, 1991.
75. Esteller M: The necessity of a human epigenome project, *Carcinogenesis* 27:1121, 2006.

2

GENETIC SCREENING AND CLINICAL TESTING

Mark I. Evans, Jon Hyett,
and Kypros Nickolaides

Two areas of nearly universally accepted established screening procedures in obstetrics and gynecology have existed for decades. The first was for cervical cancer via the Papanicolaou smear. The second was obstetrical for fetuses with neural tube defects (NTDs) and later chromosome abnormalities such as Down syndrome; the approach was originally with alpha-fetoprotein (AFP), and later with other biochemical and sometimes biophysical markers.

Identifying individuals with disease usually involves tests or procedures performed on persons who, for whatever reason, were felt to be at increased risk. Investigations come in many fashions. They may be clinical, laboratory testing, and minor invasive procedures, such as obtaining blood, or, in fact, even major surgical ones. Only a small portion of the overall population has enough risk to justify expensive or invasive tests being performed. Particularly for genetic disorders, there are often population subgroups known to be at particularly high risk, whether it be advanced maternal age and Down syndrome, Ashkenazi Jewish heritage and Tay-Sachs disease, African heritage and sickle cell disease, or numerous others.[1] However, for some of these disorders, although the risk for any given individual in the high-risk category is certainly higher than for those in the low-risk category, if the high-risk category is small enough, the majority of affected individuals may actually come from a low-risk group.[1] Particularly with the advent of molecular technologies and the application of knowledge from the Human Genome Project, we will now have the ability to look for literally thousands of potential disorders in any individual who may be totally asymptomatic.[2]

PRINCIPLES OF SCREENING TESTS

The foundation of screening for any disease process requires a fundamental understanding of the differences between diagnostic and screening tests. Diagnostic tests are designed to give a definitive answer to the question: Does the patient have this particular problem? They are generally complex tests and commonly require sophisticated analysis and interpretation. They tend to be expensive, and they are usually only performed on patients felt to be "at risk." Conversely, screening tests are generally performed on healthy patients and are often offered to the entire relevant population. They therefore should be cheap, easy to use, and interpretable by everyone; their function is only to help define who, among the low-risk group, is, in fact, at high risk.

Screening test results are, by definition, not pathognomonic for the disease.[1] All they do is delineate who needs further testing. Fortunately the concept of screening tests is certainly not new to obstetrics and gynecology, having been pioneered decades ago with the development of the Pap smear for cervical cancer screening.

Detailed understanding of all the applications of these principles is beyond the space limitations of this chapter. The interested reader is referred to more extensive explanations, as in Evans et al.[3]

Neural Tube Defects

It is now more than three decades since Brock and Sutcliffe[4] first described the use of AFP in amniotic fluid, and later in maternal serum,[5] for the prenatal detection of NTDs. Since the mid-1970s, routine prenatal screening became accepted in the United Kingdom and since the mid-1980s in the United States. Evaluation of the impact of such screening has clearly shown that the birth rate of children with NTDs has declined from 1.3 per 1000 births in 1970 to 0.6 per 1000 births in 1989.[6] The fall was even more dramatic in some sections of the United States such as the southeast, which had higher than average rates. Since the introduction of folic acid fortification of breads and grains in the United States in 1998, the fall of NTDs as evidenced by birth registry data has been about 20%[7] and by high maternal serum AFP levels more than 30%.[8] The successful application of folic acid has been a dramatic public health success story.[9-19]

Several changes in the epidemiologic characteristics of NTDs have also been observed:

1. The proportion of spina bifida cases has increased.
2. The proportion of NTDs combined with other unrelated defects, that is, syndromes, has increased.
3. The incidence in the white population has decreased relative to the incidence in other races.
4. The incidence of isolated NTDs in females has decreased.[6,7]

It has long been appreciated that there are racial, geographic, and ethnic variations in the incidence of NTDs and that there are patients at increased risk based on other medical conditions. For example, diabetics are known to have an increased risk of NTDs, as are women taking antiepileptic drugs.[20] Patients undergoing ovulation induction do not have higher than background rates of NTDs.[21]

Second-Trimester Screening for Chromosome Abnormalities

In 1984, Merkatz et al.[22] first published the association of low maternal serum AFP with an increased risk of chromosome abnormalities, particularly Down syndrome. In subsequent years, there was also an eventual understanding that Down syndrome is not the only aneuploid condition association with low maternal serum AFP. For example, trisomy 18 usually has even lower AFP values.[23]

The adoption of wide-scale screening with maternal serum AFP effectively doubled the potential detection of chromosome abnormalities in the population. Before the massive explosion of infertility therapies, only about 20% of Down syndrome babies were born to women older than age 35 years. More recent data suggest that the proportion of births to women older than 35 years has gone from about 5% to nearly 15%, and the proportion of Down syndrome cases in women older than 35 years is now more than 30%.[24] The addition of a well-coordinated maternal serum AFP screening program as developed in the late 1980s could detect approximately 30% of the 75% of cases that were born to women younger than age 35 years. The detailed mechanics of biochemical screening, that is, with adjustments for gestational age, race, diabetic status, multiple gestation status, maternal weight, and adjustments via a different database or correction factors for maternal race, have been published previously and are not repeated here.[25]

In 1988, Wald et al.[26] suggested that a combination of parameters including AFP, beta human chorionic gonadotrophin (β-hCG), and unconjugated estriol (uE3) could significantly increase the detection frequency of Down syndrome to approximately 60% of the total. There have been multiple studies that have corroborated the increased efficacy of multiple marker screening as opposed to AFP alone in detecting chromosome abnormalities, particularly Down syndrome.[27-32]

Despite overwhelming data and recommendations of national organizations such as the American College of Obstetricians and Gynecologists that multiple numbers be offered, by the millennium still nearly 20% of patients in the United States who had screening were still just having AFP alone.[33]

Fetal Cells in the Maternal Circulation

Another promising marker has been the search for fetal cells in maternal circulation. Studies throughout the 1990s suggested that isolation and analysis of fetal cells may, in fact, become practical and useful as a screening test.[34-36] The current state follows essentially two decades of various starts and stops that have alternatively looked promising and very frustrating since Hertzenberg et al.[37] first demonstrated detection and enrichment by fluorescent activated cell sorting (FACS). Much of the past two decades has focused on ways to improve the efficacy of detection methods, primarily centered on the need to increase the enrichment of fetal cells from the maternal blood circulation, whose prevalence has been estimated to be approximately 1 in 10,000,000 cells.[38-40]

Three types of fetal cells have been sought extensively in the past several years—trophoblasts, lymphocytes, and nucleated fetal red cells. Trophoblasts, although being the most obvious candidates because they are purely fetal, have proven to be very frustrating because there is huge variability in their passage through the maternal circulation, and most antibodies used to be trophoblast-specific have been disappointing.[34] Lymphoblasts have the advantage of being much more stable; in fact, they are often too stable. There is documentation of lymphocytes persisting in the maternal circulation decades after a woman's last pregnancy. It certainly could persist from pregnancy to pregnancy if there were a recent miscarriage followed by another pregnancy.

The cell type most likely to be successful is felt to be nucleated red blood cells. Bianchi et al.[38] were the first to use slow sorting to isolate nucleated fetal erythrocytes using an antibody to the transfer interceptor. In the late 1990s, studies focused on two general approaches; those using FACS and those using magnetic activated cell sorting (MACS).[34,40] Trisomic concepti subsequently confirmed by invasive testing were found by both methods.[41-43] Analysis of progress through the millennium suggested that the MACS approach appeared to have a better ability than FACS to isolate fetal cells and that the overall sensitivity of fetal cells was not an improvement over current screens but that the specificity of fetal cells might be much better. If so, then a two-step approach might emerge in which a higher percentage of patients—perhaps 10% using double or triple testing—would be called positive to raise the sensitivity to around 80%. Then these 10% would undergo fetal cell testing to reduce that risk group to 2% to 3% but not lose sensitivity.

Another area of potential applicability of fetal cells in maternal blood is for the isolation of molecular diagnosis of mendelian disorders. Lo et al.[44] were able to determine fetal Rh status in women known to be sensitized and married to heterozygous men. By 2004, fetal cell/DNA analysis was already being offered commercially (but not in the United States) for Rh determination and sex selection.

Fetal cell analysis has been met with enthusiasm then despair and now once again some hope; the next several years will ultimately determine how successful fetal cell sorting is as a screening test. It was originally hoped that it could be a diagnostic test and replace the need for invasive testing; however, as of this writing, fetal karyotypes cannot be obtained from cells that are isolated, and therefore only fluorescent in situ hybridization (FISH)-related results are possible. Although this is very good as a screening test for aneuploidy, our experiences show that approximately one third of abnormal karyotypes seen in prenatal diagnosis programs are, in fact, not ones that would be detected by the standard probes for chromosomes 13, 18, 21, X, and Y.[45] Until and unless complete karyotypes can be obtained, fetal cells will not completely replace invasive testing but may potentially be an important addition to the armamentarium of screening technologies.

As reproductive techniques have dramatically increased the proportions of multiple pregnancies, questions arise about the efficacy of screening tests. We and others have debated the data of biochemical screening on twins or more. There have been several papers that have promoted "pseudo risks" for twins by biochemical data. We continue to be concerned about the accuracy of these tests and believe that in multiples biophysical data are more likely to be accurate.[46-51]

Trisomy 18

Although screening has generally focused on trisomy 21, our data and those of others have always shown a varied pattern of anomalies detected by screening.[52] A different pattern of analyte levels has been observed in trisomy 18. The values of AFP, hCG, and uE3 appear to be very low.[53] This suggests a different pathophysiology than for Down syndrome. In Down syndrome, the low AFP and uE3 and high hCG can be explained as reflecting inappropriate immaturity or dysmaturity of the fetus, that is, all values are consistent with a younger gestational age. In trisomy 18, however, that explanation does not work.[54] We have previously shown that there are different patterns of genomically directed intrauterine growth restriction in different aneuploidies,[52] but how this translates into serum markers is unclear. Nevertheless, some reports have shown that a second-trimester algorithm can be used to identify the majority of trisomy 18 cases while adding about 0.75% to the population being offered amniocentesis.[54]

FIRST-TRIMESTER SCREENING

Introduction

The phenotypic features of trisomy 21 were first described by Langdon Down[55] in 1866 and included the observation that "the skin appears to be too large for the body, the nose is small and the face is flat." In the last decade, it has become possible to observe these features by ultrasound examination at 11^{+0} to 13^{+6} weeks' gestation, and there is extensive evidence that effective screening for major chromosomal abnormalities can be provided at this early stage of pregnancy.

Measuring Fetal Nuchal Translucency Thickness

The process of risk assessment, described previously, involves the development of a likelihood ratio as a statistical representation of the test result. Accuracy of measurement is therefore essential to ensure that an accurate likelihood ratio is used in calculating a new level of risk. Although processes of quality assurance are well described in chemical pathology, they have not previously been universally applied to imaging techniques. The Fetal Medicine Foundation (FMF), which is a UK registered charity, has established a process of training and quality assurance for the appropriate introduction of nuchal translucency (NT) screening into clinical practice.[56] Training is based on a theoretical course and practical instruction on how to obtain the appropriate image and make the correct measurement of the NT.

The optimal gestational age for measurement of fetal NT is 11^{+0} weeks to 13^{+6} weeks, which corresponds to a crown-rump length of 45 to 84 mm. The lower gestational limit allows sufficient embryologic development to detect most major anatomical defects. For example, the diagnosis or exclusion of acrania and therefore anencephaly cannot be made before 11 weeks because sonographic assessment of ossification of the fetal skull is not reliable before this gestation.[57] At 8 to 10 weeks all fetuses demonstrate herniation of the midgut that is visualized as a hyperechogenic mass in the base of the umbilical cord, and it is therefore unsafe to diagnose or exclude exomphalos at this gestation.[58-61] In addition, in the early 1990s it was appreciated that chorionic villous sampling before 10 weeks was associated with transverse limb reduction defects, so NT screening between 11^{+0} and 13^{+6} weeks' gestation provides risk assessment at a gestation at which invasive testing can be immediately offered.[62,63]

NT measurement becomes more difficult from 14 weeks onward because the fetus is often in a vertical position.[64,65] The incidence of abnormal accumulation of nuchal fluid in chromosomally abnormal fetuses also decreases beyond 14 weeks.[66-69]

Clear images and accurate NT measurements are best obtained with a high-resolution ultrasound machine that has a video-loop function and calipers that provide measurements to one decimal point. Fetal NT can be

37

measured successfully by transabdominal ultrasound examination in about 95% of cases; in the others, it is necessary to perform transvaginal sonography. The results from transabdominal and transvaginal scanning are similar.[70] A good sagittal section of the fetus, as for measurement of fetal crown-rump length, should be obtained and the NT should be measured with the fetus in the neutral position.[68] The image should be magnified so that only the fetal head and upper thorax are included and so that each slight movement of the calipers produces only a 0.1-mm change in the measurement. Care must be taken to distinguish between fetal skin and amnion because, at this gestation, both structures appear as thin membranes.[68] This is achieved by waiting for spontaneous fetal movement away from the amniotic membrane; alternatively, the fetus is bounced off the amnion by asking the mother to cough and/or by tapping the maternal abdomen.

Precise caliper placement is another key part of the process of measurement standardization. The maximum thickness of the subcutaneous translucency between the skin and the soft tissue overlying the cervical spine should be measured.[68] The calipers should be placed on the lines that define the NT thickness—the crossbar of the caliper should be such that it is hardly visible as it merges with the white line of the border and not in the nuchal fluid. Reducing the gain and removing harmonics prevents the edge of the nuchal space being blurred, which leads to underestimation of the nuchal measurement.[71] During the scan, more than one measurement must be taken and the maximum one should be used for risk assessment.

Other factors that can cause the nuchal measurement to be inaccurate include hyperextension of the fetal neck, which can artificially increase the NT measurement by 0.6 mm, or flexion, which can decrease the measurement by 0.4 mm.[72] The umbilical cord may be around the fetal neck in 5% to 10% of cases, and this finding may produce a falsely increased NT, adding about 0.8 mm to the measurement.[73,74] In such cases, the measurements of NT above and below the cord are different and, in the calculation of risk, it is more appropriate to use the average of the two measurements.[74] Unlike in the second trimester, there are no clinically relevant effects on NT measurements by ethnic origin,[75,76] parity or gravidity,[77] cigarette smoking,[78,79] diabetic control,[80] conception by assisted reproduction techniques,[81-84] bleeding in early pregnancy,[85] or fetal gender.[86-88] The intraobserver and interobserver differences in measurements of fetal NT are less than 0.5 mm in 95% of cases.[89-91]

NT Thickness and Risk for Chromosomal Abnormalities

The largest prospective study examining the association between increased NT and chromosomal abnormalities was coordinated by the FMF. It involved 100,311 singleton pregnancies examined by 306 appropriately trained sonographers in 22 UK centers.[92] Fetal NT and crown-rump length were measured in all cases and individual patient-specific risks, based on maternal age, gestational age, and fetal NT, were calculated. Follow-up was obtained from 96,127 cases, including 326 with trisomy 21 and 325 with other chromosomal abnormalities. The median gestation at the time of screening was 12 weeks (range 10 to 14 weeks) and the median maternal age was 31 years. The estimated risk for trisomy 21 was greater than 1 in 300 in 7907 (8.3%) of the normal pregnancies, in 268 (82.2%) of those with trisomy 21, and in 253 (77.8%) with other chromosomal abnormalities. For a screen-positive rate of 5%, the detection rate was 77% (95% confidence interval 72% to 82%).[92]

The results of this study are supported by other prospective studies that have examined the implementation of NT screening in clinical practice (Tables 2-1 and 2-2).

In some of these studies the screen positive group was defined by a cut-off in fetal NT (Table 2-1), whereas others used a combined risk derived from the maternal age and deviation in fetal NT from the normal median for fetal crown-rump length (Table 2-2). Collectively, these studies demonstrate that fetal NT can be successfully measured in more than 99% of cases and the combined data of more than 200,000 pregnancies, including more than 900 fetuses with trisomy 21, demonstrates that fetal NT screening identifies more than 75% of fetuses with trisomy 21 and other major chromosomal abnormalities for a false-positive rate of 5%. Alternatively, a detection rate of about 60% can be achieved with a false-positive rate of 1%.

Combined First-Trimester Screening

Trisomic pregnancies are associated with altered maternal serum concentrations of various fetoplacental products. At 10^{+3} to 13^{+6} weeks' gestation, the maternal serum concentration of free β-hCG is increased and pregnancy associated plasma protein-A (PAPP-A) is decreased in pregnancies affected by trisomy 21.[117-122] These biochemical markers have no significant association between fetal NT in either trisomy 21 or chromosomally normal pregnancies, and therefore the ultrasononographic and biochemical markers can be combined to provide more effective screening than either method individually.[95-98,123] In a retrospective study of 210 singleton pregnancies with trisomy 21 and 946 chromosomally normal controls, matched for maternal age, gestation, and sample storage time, we estimated that the detection rate for trisomy 21 by a combination of maternal age, fetal NT, and maternal serum PAPP-A and free β-hCG would be about 90% for a screen-positive rate of 5%.[123]

Prospective screening studies have confirmed the feasibility and effectiveness of combining fetal NT and maternal serum free β-hCG and PAPP-A.[124-127,154] The study of Bindra et al.[128] also reported the detection rates for fixed false-positive rates between 1% and 5% and the false-positive rates for fixed detection rates between 60% and 90% of screening for trisomy 21 by maternal age alone; maternal age and fetal NT; maternal age and serum free β-hCG and PAPP-A; and maternal age, fetal NT, and maternal serum biochemistry. Thus for a 5% false-positive rate, the detection rate of trisomy 21 by the first-trimester combined test was 90%, which is superior to the 30% achieved by maternal age and 65% by second-trimester biochemistry. Alternatively, the detection rate of 65% achieved by second-trimester biochemical testing at a 5% false-positive rate can be achieved by first-trimester combined testing with a false-positive rate of only 0.5%.[128] Some authors have suggested that the total hCG can be used instead of free β. However, Evans et al.[129] has shown by analysis that free β substantially outperforms total β-hCG.

Screening Multiple Pregnancies

The prenatal diagnosis of chromosomal abnormalities in multiple pregnancies is potentially complicated by a number of factors. Chorionicity can be determined reliably by ultrasonography in early pregnancy.[130,131] In counseling

Table 2-1

Prospective Screening Studies for Trisomy 21 by Measurement of Fetal Nuchal Translucency (NT) Thickness

Author	Gestation (wk)	N	Successful Measurement (%)	NT Cut-off	FPR (%)	DR Trisomy 21
Pandya et al., 1995[93]	10-13^{+6}	1763	100.0	2.5 mm	3.4	3/4 (75.0%)
Schwarzler et al., 1999[94]	10-13^{+6}	4523	100.0	2.5 mm	2.7	8/12 (66.7%)
Schuchter et al., 2001[95]	10-12^{+6}	9342	100.0	2.5 mm	2.1	11/19 (57.9%)
Wayda et al., 2001[96]	10-13^{+0}	6841	100.0	2.5 mm	4.1	17/17 (100.0%)
Panburana et al., 2001[97]	10-13^{+6}	2067	100.0	2.5 mm	2.9	2/2 (100.0%)
Snijders et al., 1998[98]	10-13^{+6}	96,127	100.0	95th percentile	4.4	234/326 (71.8%)
Theodoropoulos et al., 1998[99]	10-13^{+6}	3550	100.0	95th percentile	2.3	10/11 (90.9%)
Zoppi et al., 2001[100]	10-13^{+6}	10,111	100.0	95th percentile	5.1	52/64 (81.3%)
Gasiorek-Wiens et al., 2001[101]	10-13^{+6}	21,959	100.0	95th percentile	8.0	174/210 (82.9%)
Brizot et al., 2001[102]	10-13^{+6}	2492	100.0	95th percentile	6.4	7/10 (70.0%)
Comas et al., 2002[103]	10-13^{+6}	7345	100.0	95th percentile	4.9	38/38 (100.0%)
Chasen et al., 2003[104]	11-13^{+6}	2248	100.0	95th percentile	3.4	9/12 (75.0%)
Szabo et al., 1995[105]	9-12^{+6}	3380	100.0	3.0 mm	1.6	27/30 (90.0%)
Taipale et al., 1997[106]	10-13^{+6}	6939	98.6	3.0 mm	0.7	4/6 (66.7%)
Pajkrt et al., 1998, 1998[107,108]	10-13^{+6}	3614	100.0	3.0 mm	4.2	32/46 (69.6%)
Audibert et al., 2001[109]	10-13^{+6}	4130	95.5	3.0 mm	1.7	7/12 (58.3%)
Rozenberg et al., 2002[110]	12-14^{+0}	6234	98.6	3.0 mm	2.8	13/21 (61.9%)
Economides et al., 1998[111]	11-14^{+6}	2256	100.0	99th percentile	0.4	6/8 (75.0%)
Whitlow et al., 1999[112]	11-14^{+6}	5947	100.0	99th percentile	0.7	15/23 (65.2%)
Total		200,868	99.8		4.2	669/871 (76.8%)

In some of the studies a cut-off in NT was used to define the screen-positive group and in others the Fetal Medicine Foundation software was used to estimate patient-specific risks based on maternal age, gestational age, and fetal NT.
DR, Detection rate; *FPR*, false-positive rate.

Table 2-2

Author	Mean Maternal Age (yr)	Cut-off	Screen Positive		
			Normal	Chromosomal Abnormalities	
				Trisomy 21	Other
Snijders et al., 1998[98]	31	1 in 300	7,907/95,476 (8.3%)	268/326 (82.2%)*	253/325 (77.8%)
Theodoropoulos et al., 1998[99]	29	1 in 300	151/3528 (4.3%)	10/11 (90.9%)	11/11 (100.0%)
Thilaganathan et al., 1999[113]	29	1 in 300	762/9,753 (7.8%)	17/21 (81.0%)*	25/28 (89.3%)
Schwarzler et al., 1999[94]	29	1 in 270	212/4,500 (4.7%)	10/12 (83.3%)	8/11 (72.7%)
O'Callaghan et al., 2000[114]	32	1 in 300	59/989 (6.0%)	6/8 (75.0%)	3/3 (100.0%
Brizot et al., 2001[102]	28	1 in 300	183/2470 (7.4%)	9/10 (90.0%)	9/12 (75.0%)
Gasiorek-Wiens et al., 2001[101]	33	1 in 300	2800/21,475 (13.0%)	184/210 (87.6%)	239/274 (88.2%)
Sau et al., 2001[115]	28	1 in 100	61/2,600 (2.3%)	8/8 (100%)	5/7 (71.4%)
Zoppi et al., 2001[100]	33	1 in 300	887/10,001 (8.9%)	58/64 (90.6%)	39/46 (84.8%)
Prefumo & Thilaganathan, 2002[116]	31	1 in 300	565/11,820 (4.8%)	22/27 (81.5%)	—
Chasen et al., 2003[104]	33	1 in 300	169/2,216 (7.5%)	10/12 (83.3%)*	15/20 (75.0%)
Total			13,756/164,828 (8.3%)	602/709 (84.9%)	607/737 (82.4%)

*In three studies the detection rate at a fixed 5% false-positive rate was estimated. In the combined data on a total of 359 cases of trisomy 21 it was estimated that 278 (78.4%) would have been detected.

parents it is possible to give more specific estimates of one and/or both fetuses being affected depending on chorionicity. Thus in monochorionic twins the parents can be counseled that both fetuses would be affected and this risk is similar to that in singleton pregnancies. If the pregnancy is dichorionic, then the parents can be counseled that the risk of discordancy for a chromosomal abnormality is about twice that in singleton pregnancies, whereas the risk that both fetuses would be affected can be derived by squaring the singleton risk ratio. This is in reality an oversimplification because, unlike monochorionic pregnancies, which are always monozygotic, only about 90% of dichorionic pregnancies are dizygotic.

Both chorionic villus sampling and amniocentesis can be performed in twin pregnancies, but in some circumstances they may be associated with higher risks of miscarriage and of uncertain diagnosis.[132-135] If twins are discordant for an anomaly, one of the options for the subsequent management may be selective feticide, with risks of spontaneous abortion or severe preterm delivery that has an inverse correlation with the gestation at feticide.[136]

The effectiveness of NT as a means of screening for trisomy 21 was examined in a series of 448 twin pregnancies that found that NT thickness was above the 95th percentile in 7 of 8 (87.5%) fetuses with trisomy 21.[137] Although the false-positive rate was only 5.4% in dichorionic pregnancies, it was increased to 8.4% in monochorionic pregnancies, a finding confirmed in other studies.[138,139] The increase in the false-positive rate in monochorionic twins occurs because increased NT is an early manifestation of twin-to-twin transfusion syndrome.[137-141]

In dichorionic twins, NT can be used as an effective means of screening for chromosomal abnormalities. This allows earlier prenatal diagnosis and therefore safer selective feticide for parents with an affected fetus that choose this option. An important advantage of using fetal NT to assess risk for chromosomal abnormality is that, when there is discordance for a chromosomal abnormality, the presence of a sonographically detectable marker helps ensure the correct identification of the abnormal twin should the parents choose selective termination.

In monochorionic twins, which are almost always of identical chromosomal constitution, the numbers of cases with discordant NT measurements are too small to draw definite conclusions about counseling for the risk of chromosomal abnormalities. The risk of twin-twin transfusion syndrome should also be considered and if there are no other ultrasound features of aneuploidy, one option may be to delay invasive testing until a later stage, once other features of twin-twin transfusion syndrome can also be assessed.

The first-trimester biochemical markers free β-hCG and PAPP-A are also increased in pregnancies affected by trisomy 21 and can be combined with the measurement of NT to screen for chromosomal abnormality.[142] In a study of 159 twin pregnancies, the average free β-hCG was 2.1 and the PAPP-A 1.9 times greater than in 3466 singleton pregnancies. Using statistical modeling techniques, it was predicted that at a 5% false-positive rate screening by a combination of fetal NT and maternal serum biochemistry would identify about 80% of trisomy 21 pregnancies.[143] In a prospective screening study in 206 twin pregnancies, the false-positive rate was 9.0% (19 of 206) of pregnancies and 6.9% of fetuses (28 of 412), and the detection rate of trisomy 21 was 75% (3 of 4).[144]

Absent Nasal Bone and Screening for Chromosomal Abnormality

As the first-trimester scan has become more established, the technique has developed to include sequential examination of fetal systems rather than being restricted to NT measurement. Several other markers for chromosomal abnormality have been noted. In his original description of the phenotypic features of infants affected by trisomy 21, Langdon Down[55] noted that a common characteristic was a small nose. An anthropometric study in 105 patients with Down syndrome at 7 months to 36 years of age reported that the nasal root depth was abnormally short in 49.5% of cases.[145] In the combined data from four postmortem radiologic studies in a total of 105 aborted fetuses with trisomy 21 at 12 to 25 weeks of gestation there was absence of ossification of the nasal bone in 32.4% and nasal hypoplasia in 21.4% of cases.[146-149] Sonographic studies at 15 to 24 weeks of gestation reported that about 65% of trisomy 21 fetuses have absent or short nasal bone.[150-154]

The fetal nasal bone can be visualized by sonography at 11^{+0} to 13^{+6} weeks of gestation.[155] This examination requires that the image is magnified so that the head and the upper thorax only are included in the screen. A mid-sagittal view of the fetal profile is obtained with the ultrasound transducer held in parallel to the longitudinal axis of the nasal bone. The angle of insonation is crucial as the nasal bone will almost invariably not be visible when the longitudinal axis of the bone is perpendicular to the ultrasound transducer. In the correct view there are three distinct lines. The first two, which are proximal to the forehead, are horizontal and parallel to each other, resembling an "equal sign." The top line represents the skin and the bottom line, which is thicker and more echogenic than the overlying skin, represents the nasal bone. A third line, almost in continuity with the skin but at a higher level, represents the tip of the nose. When the nasal bone line appears as a thin line, less echogenic than the overlying skin, it suggests that the nasal bone is not yet ossified, and it is therefore classified as being absent.

A study investigating the necessary training of 15 sonographers with experience in measuring fetal NT to become competent in examining the fetal nasal bone at 11^{+0} to 13^{+6} weeks has demonstrated that the number of supervised scans required is on average 80, with a range of 40 to 120.[156] Another study of 501 consecutively scanned fetuses by experienced sonographers reported that the fetal nasal bone can be successfully examined and measured in all cases without extending the length of time required for scanning.[157]

Several studies have demonstrated a high association between absent nasal bone at 11^{+0} to 13^{+6} weeks and trisomy 21, as well as in other chromosomal abnormalities (Tables 2-3 and 2-4). In the combined data from these studies on a total of 15,822 fetuses the fetal profile was successfully examined in 15,413 (97.4%) cases and the nasal bone was absent in 176 of 12,652 (1.4%) chromosomally normal fetuses and in 274 of 397 (69.0%) fetuses with trisomy 21. An important finding of these studies was that the incidence of absent nasal bone decreased with fetal crown-rump length, increased with NT thickness, and was substantially higher in Afro-Caribbeans than in Caucasians. Consequently, in the calculation of likelihood ratios in screening for trisomy 21, adjustments must be made for these confounding factors.[164,165]

In contrast to the previous studies, Malone et al.[166] reported that they were able to examine the fetal nose in only 75.9% of 6316 fetuses scanned at 10 to 13 weeks and that the nasal bone was apparently present in all nine of their trisomy 21 fetuses. However, the image they published to illustrate their technique reports the nasal bone at the tip rather than the base of the nose.[167] Similarly, De Biasio and Venturini,[168] who examined retrospectively the photographs obtained for measurement of fetal NT, reported that the nasal bone was present in all five fetuses with trisomy 21. However, all five images that they published were inappropriate both for the measurement of fetal NT and for examination of the nasal bone, because they were either too small or the fetus was too vertical or too oblique.

It can be concluded that at 11^{+0} to 13^{+6} weeks the fetal profile can be successfully examined in more than 95% of cases and that the nasal bone is

Table 2-3

Author	Type of Study	Gestation (wk)	N	Successful Examination (%)	FPR (%)	DR Trisomy 21
Cicero et al., 2001[155]	Pre-CVS	11-13^{+6}	701	100	0.5	43/59 (72.9%)
Otano et al., 2002[158]	Pre-CVS	11-13^{+6}	194	94.3	0.6	3/5 (60.0%)
Zoppi et al., 2003[125]	Screening	11-13^{+6}	5532	99.8	0.2	19/27 (70.0%)
Orlandi et al., 2003[126]	Screening	11-13^{+6}	1089	94.3	1.0	10/15 (66.7%)
Viora et al., 2003[127]	Screening	11-13^{+6}	1906	91.9	1.4	8/10 (80.0%)
Senat et al., 2003[159]	Retrospective	11-13^{+6}	1040	91.9	0.4	3/4 (75.0%)
Wong et al., 2003[160]	Pre-CVS	11-13^{+6}	143	83.2	0.9	2/3 (66.7%)
Cicero et al., 2003[161]	Pre-CVS	11-13^{+6}	3829	98.9	2.8	162/242 (67.0%)
Cicero et al., 2004[162]	Pre-CVS	11-13^{+6}	5918	98.9	2.5	229/333 (68.8%)
Total			15,822	97.4	1.4	274/397 (69.0%)

CVS, Chorionic villus sampling; DR, detection rate; FPR, false-positive rate.
*Included in Cicero et al., 2004, xliv.

absent in about 70% of trisomy 21 fetuses and 55% of trisomy 13 fetuses. In chromosomally normal fetuses the incidence of absent nasal bone is less than 1% in Caucasian populations and about 10% in Afro-Caribbeans. Consequently, absence of the nasal bone is an important marker of trisomy 21. However, it is imperative that sonographers undertaking risk assessment by examination of the fetal profile receive appropriate training and certification of their competence in performing such a scan.

The potential performance of combining the ultrasound markers of increased NT and absent nasal bone with the biochemical markers β-hCG and PAPP-A at 11^{+0} to 13^{+6} weeks has been examined in a case-control study of 100 trisomy 21 and 400 chromosomally normal singleton pregnancies. This estimated that the detection rate for trisomy 21 would be 97% for a false-positive rate of 5% or 91% for a false-positive rate of 0.5% (see Table 2-4).[162]

Table 2-4

Chromosomal Abnormality	Absent Nasal Bone (%)
Trisomy 21	229/333 (68.8)
Trisomy 18	68/124 (54.8)
Trisomy 13	13/38 (34.2)
Triploidy	0/19 (0)
Turner's syndrome	5/46 (10.9)
XXY, XXX, XYY	1/20 (5)
Other	8/48 (16.7)

Increased NT in the Chromosomally Normal Fetus

As well as being an effective screening tool for chromosomal abnormalities, increased NT is associated with miscarriage, fetal death, and a wide range of fetal malformations and genetic syndromes.[92,169-171]

In chromosomally normal fetuses, the prevalence of fetal death increases exponentially with NT thickness. In the combined data from two studies on a total of 4540 chromosomally normal fetuses with increased NT but no obvious fetal defects, the prevalence of miscarriage or fetal death increased from 1.3% in those with NT between the 95th and 99th percentiles to about 20% for NT of 6.5 mm or more.[169,170] The majority of fetuses that die do so by 20 weeks and they usually show progression from increased NT to severe hydrops. Another study of 6650 pregnancies undergoing NT screening reported that in chromosomally normal fetuses the prevalence of miscarriage or fetal death was 1.3% in those with NT below the 95th percentile, 1.2% for NT between the 95th and 99th percentiles, and 12.3% for NT above the 99th percentile.[171]

Several studies have reported that increased fetal NT thickness is associated with a high prevalence of major fetal abnormalities (see Table 2-2) [138-176] In the combined data of 28 studies on a total of 6153 chromosomally normal fetuses with increased NT, the prevalence of major defects was 7.3%. However, there were large differences between the studies in the prevalence of major abnormalities, ranging from 3% to 50%, because of differences in their definition of the minimum abnormal NT thickness, which ranged from 2 to 5 mm. The prevalence of major fetal abnormalities in chromosomally normal fetuses increases with NT thickness, from 1.6% in those with NT below the 95th percentile,[140] to 2.5% for NT between the 95th and 99th percentiles, and exponentially thereafter to about 45% for NT of 6.5 mm or more.[169,170]

Although a wide range of fetal abnormalities have been reported in fetuses with increased NT, the prevalence of many of these may not differ from that seen in the general population. However, the prevalence of major cardiac defects, diaphragmatic hernia, exomphalos, body stalk anomaly, skeletal defects, and certain genetic syndromes, such as congenital adrenal hyperplasia, fetal akinesia deformation sequence, Noonan syndrome, Smith-Lemli-Opitz syndrome, and spinal muscular atrophy, appears to be substantially higher than in the general population and it is therefore likely that there is a true association between these abnormalities and increased NT.

The heterogeneity of conditions associated with increased NT suggests that there may not be a single underlying mechanism for this condition. Possible mechanisms include cardiac dysfunction in association with abnormalities of the heart and great arteries, venous congestion in the head and neck, altered composition of the extracellular matrix, failure of lymphatic drainage resulting from abnormal or delayed development of the lymphatic system or impaired fetal movements, fetal anemia or hypoproteinemia, and congenital infection.[177-186] Investigation of these mechanisms has, in part, led to a better understanding of the clinical associations between increased NT and structural abnormalities.

In pathologic studies of both chromosomally abnormal and normal fetuses, there is a high association between increased NT and abnormalities of the heart and great arteries.[187-191] This has also been observed clinically, and in three studies with a combined total of 30 fetuses with major cardiac defects diagnosed by echocardiography at 11 to 14 weeks, 83% had increased NT.[192-194] Similarly, in six studies with a combined total of 3911 fetuses with increased NT, there was a high prevalence of cardiac defects (41.2 per 1000) and this increased with NT thickness from 16.8 per 1000 in those with NT of 2.5 to 3.4 mm to 75.2 per 1000 in those with NT of 3.5 mm or more.

This has led several groups to investigate the screening performance of NT thickness for the detection of cardiac defects.[140,190,195-198]

In total, 67,256 pregnancies were examined and the prevalence of major cardiac defects was 2.4 per 1000. For a false-positive rate of 4.9%, the detection rate of cardiac defects was 37.5%. A meta-analysis of screening studies reported that the detection rates were about 37% and 31% for the respective NT cut-offs of the 95th and 99th percentiles.[195] It was estimated that specialist fetal echocardiography in all chromosomally normal fetuses with NT above the 99th percentile would identify one major cardiac defect in every 16 patients examined. Additionally, this analysis showed that the performance of screening by increased NT does vary with the type of cardiac defect.

The clinical implication of these findings is that increased NT constitutes an indication for specialist fetal echocardiography. Certainly, the overall prevalence of major cardiac defects in such a group of fetuses (1% to 2%) is similar to that found in pregnancies affected by maternal diabetes mellitus or with a history of a previously affected offspring, which are well accepted indications for fetal echocardiography. At present, there may not be sufficient facilities for specialist fetal echocardiography to accommodate the potential increase in demand if the 95th percentile of NT thickness is used as the cut-off for referral. In contrast, a cut-off of the 99th percentile would result in only a small increase in workload and, in this population, the prevalence of major cardiac defects would be very high.

Other structural abnormalities are also associated with increased NT. Increased NT thickness is present in about 40% of fetuses with diaphragmatic hernia, including more than 80% of those that result in neonatal death resulting from pulmonary hypoplasia and in about 20% of the survivors.[196] Increased NT is observed in about 85% of chromosomally abnormal and 40% of chromosomally normal fetuses with exomphalos.[197] Similarly, megacystis, defined as a bladder diameter of 7 mm or more, is associated with increased NT, in particular trisomy 13, which was observed in about 75% of those with chromosomal abnormalities and in about 30% of those with normal karyotype.[198] Body stalk anomaly has also being diagnosed in 25 of 106,727 fetuses screened at 10 to 14 weeks' gestation. The major ultrasonographic features were a major abdominal wall defect, severe kyphoscoliosis, and short umbilical cord with a single artery.[174,175] Although the fetal NT was increased in 84% of the fetuses, the karyotype was normal in all cases.[199,200]

Increased NT has also been associated with a variety of genetic syndromes. As most genetic conditions are relatively rare, it is often difficult to know whether these are true associations, but the prevalence of increased NT in conditions such as congenital adrenal hyperplasia, fetal akinesia deformation sequence, Noonan syndrome, Smith-Lemli-Opitz syndrome, and spinal muscular atrophy suggest that there is a pathologic association. Multiple genetic syndromes have been associated with increased NT.

EVOLVING DIRECTIONS

The evidence that first-trimester screening followed by first-trimester diagnosis by chorionic villus sampling (CVS) can bring about a substantially higher sensitivity and specificity within the same time frame as advanced maternal age (AMA)-indicated CVS is overwhelming. The question thus reduces to how and when to update the accepted "culture" in the United States to be consistent with the current scientific knowledge base.

Cultures and behaviors do evolve with technology, but there has been no simple or predictable timetable for adoption of new ways of thinking. The reality is that asking a patient "How old are you?" is merely a cheap and not very good screening test. Until there is a general perception of age as merely a screening test and not a fixed generator of rights to a test because of risks inherent in age, it will be difficult to gain widespread acceptance from the general population for a shift.

There has to be the understanding that age is not being discarded but will merely become one of a number of variables that can be assessed to give the most accurate assessment of risk possible. With education, the ultrasound portion of the equation will become more standardized to laboratory levels of quality assurance. Nonprofit organizations such as the FMF in London and the FMF in America as well as others will help coordinate the transition and training needed to make such a reality.

It is also not realistic to expect a shift of "standards" and practice to change on a single day. Thus there will have to be a short phase-in period, under which the old and the new approach will be considered acceptable. However, it is also reasonable to expect that the insurance companies who will have to pay for such to vociferously and clearly articulate to their subscribers and physicians that they are not about to vastly increase the numbers of patients having tests. Thus the right will be likely the "right" to pay out of one's own pocket for testing for AMA per se.

DIAGNOSTIC TESTING

The second aspect of prenatal diagnosis involves obtaining fetal specimens for the laboratory to analyze. Traditionally, for more than 40 years, the principal method to obtain such has been through mid-trimester amniocentesis performed with or without ultrasound (US) guidance. Space does not permit a thorough examination of all the relevant issues, but suffice it to say that, although US has made the procedure considerably safer than in previous years, experience, feel, and judgment are still critical components of the equation of risks and benefits for any invasive procedure.

The literature and, even more importantly, patient counseling in practice have been extremely variable, with anecdotal reports quoting risks as low as 1 per 1000 or less on one extreme to the only truly randomized trial—that by Tabor nearly 20 years ago that suggested risks of fetal loss in patients who had amniocentesis by experienced practitioners to be about 1% higher than their corresponding control population.[201,202] Although risks in very experienced hands are certainly now considerably less, it is hard to accept risks as being much lower than 1 in 300.[203]

HISTORICAL PERSPECTIVE

Amniocentesis began in the late 1960s and early 1970s as a tertiary procedure reserved for the highest-risk patients.[204,205] Ultrasound was either nonexistent or virtually useless under any circumstances, and the procedure was essentially blind. By waiting until about 17 weeks, there was usually adequate fluid volume surrounding the fetus that the chances of being able to obtain fluid while avoiding hitting the fetus were felt to be reasonable.[181,206] Early reports suggested complications rates at about 2%, which, although nontrivial, were felt to be a reasonable risk to take in high-risk situations such as for patients at risk for mendelian disorders such as Tay-Sachs disease, previous aneuploidy, or previous NTDs.

Amniocenteses, and later CVS, have followed the traditional paradigm of technology development, that is, going through phases of "development" and "diffusion."[207,208] There is an entire literature with national and international societies devoted to these principles. Space limitations will not permit an entire recitation of the models developed for the multiple technologies that apply here. However, amniocentesis and CVS both moved through a phase in which they were essentially "quaternary" technologies, with patients traveling often across the country to find experienced physicians to perform the procedures.[185] By the late 1970s for amniocentesis and the late 1980s for CVS, the procedures had moved to tertiary technologies; that is, there were commonly one or more centers in large cities with experienced physicians such that at least intercity travel was diminished. For amniocentesis, particularly with increasing utilization of ultrasound guidance, an increasing number of generalist and subspecialist physicians felt qualified to perform the procedure. Although not well documented at the time, it is appreciated that as the phase of diffusion was happening, use rapidly increased and so did complication rates.

For CVS, the diffusion phase was just beginning in the early 1990s. The United States Food and Drug Administration (FDA) and the American Medical Association (AMA) had removed the restrictions on CVS as being an experimental procedure to now a routine one.[185] Use in cities with experienced operators was rising rapidly, and there was a general anticipation of a shift of prenatal diagnosis to the first trimester.[209] Then, in March of 1991, Firth et al.[210] published a letter to the editor of the *Lancet* in which they described their experience in Oxford, England, of their new program. Five patients out of their first 500 procedures, performed transabdominally at 7 to 8 weeks, had babies with limb reduction defects. Four of these patients had oromandibular hypogenesis syndrome. The authors reported these cases and appropriately asked the readership if anyone had comparable experience.

Because the majority of physicians performing CVS in the United States and Europe were doing so transcervically at 10 weeks or more, not surprisingly, no one could confirm their concerns. Then, in October of 1991, Barbara Burton reported results from the new program at Michael Reece Hospital in Chicago, where out of their first 500 procedures, they also had four cases. However, instead of reporting the cases in the literature, they held a press conference in which they stated that everyone should stop doing the procedure. There was widespread lay press attention and considerable patient panic. Use rapidly fell in the United States. When the actual paper was finally published in May 1992, the data showed that their operators had a pregnancy loss rate four times the published averages (8% vs. 2%), and if two passes were required, the loss rate was 20%.[211] The conclusion of most experts in the field was that this report reflected operator inexperience or poor technique and not a systemic problem with CVS when performed at the correct gestational age by physicians with experience.

The risks of having a baby with a limb reduction defect following CVS performed at 10 weeks or more appears to be identical to the background population.[212,213] However, if CVS is performed extremely early (e.g., 6 to 7 weeks), there clearly is an increased risk.[214] Brambati et al.[214] and Wapner and Evans[215] have published a series of "early CVSs" performed at approximately 7 weeks for religious reasons. Brambati, in Milan, has a large Catholic population at high risk for β thalassemia, and Wapner and Evans see Orthodox Jews at high risk for Ashkenazi Jewish disorders such as Tay Sachs disease. In Orthodox Judaism, terminations are considered acceptable up to 40 days post conception, such that for a couple with a 25% risk, taking an increased risk of pregnancy loss and limb reduction defects may be an acceptable choice with appropriate informed consent. Although Catholicism makes no distinction beyond fertilization, many patients at high risk want prenatal diagnosis as early as possible in gestation.

There was a period of time in the mid- to late-1990s in which some programs were touting "early amniocentesis" as a "safer" alternative to CVS.[216] One of the major problems was that there was no standardization of what constituted an early amniocentesis. To some it meant 11 to 13 weeks or earlier, that is, comparable to CVS. Others talked about early amniocentesis meaning at 15 weeks 6 days as opposed to 16 weeks 1 day. It is well established that any invasive procedure, or even wishing the patient a "good day," is associated with a higher rate of pregnancy loss if done at 10 weeks than at 16 weeks. Obviously, the differences are principally related to falling background loss rates, not to the harshness of wishing her a good day. Ironically, it then turned out that patients having an amniocentesis at less than 14 weeks 0 days did not have a lower complication risk than CVS; actually, there was both a higher pregnancy loss rate and increased risks of talipes, approaching 1% of patients.[217] Studies from Europe and North America independently found that about 15% of patients had amniotic fluid leakage, and of those patients, there was approximately 15% risk of talipes.[218,219] The consensus from the literature was that for patients wishing invasive prenatal diagnosis before 13 completed weeks, CVS was the considerably safer choice. At 15 weeks, there are much more data on amniocentesis, and at 14 weeks the data are not definitive in either direction.[181,185]

CURRENT DATA

With the expansion of first-trimester screening seen already worldwide and anticipated to occur in the United States, there will be an increasing number of patients confronting significant changes in their a priori, that is, maternal age risks. As a result of screening data, patients will have to choose among three distinct options, having amniocentesis, CVS, or no procedure.[220] How they are counseled as to the risks and benefits of each option can be expected to profoundly influence the choices made by literally millions of patients every year. Furthermore, even when there is a basic consensus of risk assessment among experienced operators, the reality is that not all operators are created equal; there are often profound differences in actual data among practitioners. A parallel situation was seen previously with success rates quoted of in vitro fertilization programs, with less competent programs often quoting "national" data when in fact in some cases they had never had one successful pregnancy. In response, the Society of Assisted Reproductive Technologies (SART) and the Centers for Disease Control (CDC) created (by law) a database of center-specific results for patients to access before making decisions as to where to go. Although there are always factors that can influence the data among good centers, the database has, to some degree, leveled the playing field of reporting, if not actual successes.[221]

Recent data (<5 years old) have varied markedly in reported risks. The EATA-BUN study showed loss rates up to 20 weeks for early amniocentesis to be 1.5% versus 0.9% for CVS. The incidence of talipes was 0.16% for CVS and 0.66% for early amniocentesis (p = 0.017). Pregnancy loss rate data have varied from the Danish study of Phillip showing 2.3%, the Cochrane database report showing an increase of 0.7% over control, a French study by Muller also showing 0.7%, and unpublished data from the FASTER trial suggesting risks less than 1 per 1000.[222-234] Blessed et al.[235] compared midtrimester amniocentesis loss rates for procedures performed by trained perinatologists versus generalists at their institution. They found a loss rate for perinatologists of 0.3% and 2.5% for the generalists. In a later paper (unpublished), they describe incidence of maternal cell contamination and "bloody taps" to likewise be higher with less trained operators.

Likewise, a number of studies in the past several years have compared rates among mid-trimester amniocentesis, early amniocentesis, and CVS.[236-240] Risks of mid-trimester amniocentesis varied from 0.3% to 5.9% depending on the gestational age at which one begins to follow the pregnancies. Risks of early amniocentesis varied from 0.4% to more than 7%. Transcervical CVS had a slightly higher rate (2.2% vs. 1.7%) versus transabdominal CVS.

In 2006, data from the FASTER trial suggested amniocentesis risks to be only 1/1600.[241] However, multiple analyses of the same data revealed the true procedure risks to be closer to 1/300.[242,243] A meta-analysis of CVS and amniocentesis showed loss rates within two weeks of amniocentesis to be 0.6% and for CVS 0.7%, which was statistically equivalent.[244] We believe that in very experienced hands, the procedure risks are equivalent and therefore CVS, because of its gestational age advantage, should emerge as the predominant procedure.

Patient acceptance of procedures and acceptance of screening is also, in large part, a function of their societal, religious, and cultural backgrounds.[245,246] We have furthermore refined the concept of "framing," that is, through what lens does the patient view the situation to include the following:

"Medical" frame, in which patients are most interested in statistics, data, and likely outcomes.

"Fundamentalist" frame for patients of deeply religious background who view data and risks from the perspective of their religion.

"Lifestyle" frame, in which the impact of a child with serious disabilities controls their decisions on testing and pregnancy management.

These concepts still need further development, but we believe they will be essential in interpreting data as first-trimester screening replaces the decades-old concept of advanced maternal age as the prevailing method to determine who has invasive prenatal diagnosis.

51

CONCLUSIONS

Just as the SART registry for IVF has shown wide variation among centers with differing levels of experience, we believe the data on invasive procedures show the same wide variation in risks. We therefore believe that quoting "national" data to patients can be extremely misleading. Furthermore, the risks of both amniocentesis and CVS have to be stratified by experience, gestational age, the quality of ultrasound visualization, and other maternal factors such as body habitus.

We conclude the following:

1. The procedure risks of mid-trimester amniocentesis in experienced hands are likely to be about 1 in 300.
2. The published data do not support assertions of risks of less than 1 in 1000 even in the most experienced of hands.
3. In less experienced hands, the risks are likely to be considerably higher.
4. The procedure risks of "early amniocentesis" (<13 completed weeks), even with very experienced operators, are probably in the 1 in 50 range or more with a risk of talipes of about 1%.
5. The risks of CVS at 10 weeks' gestation or higher, in the most experienced of hands, are about 1 in 200.
6. In less experienced hands, the risks may be much higher.
7. There is seldom justification for performing amniocentesis at less than 13 completed weeks.
8. For patients desiring invasive prenatal diagnosis at less than 13 completed weeks, CVS is the safer procedure.
9. CVS can be done extremely early (e.g., 7 weeks) for religious reasons but has higher risks as compared with the now common 11-week time frame.
10. In less experienced hands, the risks of all procedures can be considerably higher.
11. Patient decisions are easily influenced by reported risks (of both procedures and screening detection rates), which if inaccurate can cause spurious conclusions.

LABORATORY TESTING

The third component in the triad of screening, procedures, and laboratory testing has had perhaps the most significant advances of the three. Advances in cytogenetics and its ultimate replacement with "molecular" cytogenetics will allow for routine evaluation for disorders not even contemplated at the moment. The increasing use of linear arrays, proteomics, and a fuller understanding of the implications of epigenetic phenomena will overwhelm the clinician and patient with more data than they can possibly absorb. For many of the molecular sequences that will be elucidated, it is likely that we will have abnormalities with considerable uncertainty as to their clinical implications. We are already beginning to see this in patients who request "everything" be tested.

It is likely that there will be even further demarcations between the "fetal" doctors and the "maternal" doctors within maternal-fetal medicine. The role of the geneticist, particularly the obstetrical geneticist, cannot be overemphasized as playing a critical role in coordinating the care of the complex patient at risk for an ever-increasing array of disorders, many of which have until recently been completely a "black box" of confusion and misunderstanding and commonly a tremendous nidus for litigation.

REFERENCES

1. Evans MI, Krivchenia EL, Yaron Y: Screening in Evans MI and Bui: genomic revolution and obstetrics and gynecology, *Ballieres Clin Obstet Gynecol* 16:645, 2002.
2. Evans MI Wapner RJ, Bui TH: Future directions in genomic revolution and obstetrics and gynecology, *Ballieres Obstet Gynecol* 16:757, 2002.
3. Evans MI et al, editors: *Prenatal diagnosis*, New York, 2006, McGraw Hill.
4. Brock DJH, Sutcliffe RG: Alpha-fetoprotein in the antenatal diagnosis of anencephaly and spina bifida, *Lancet* 2:197, 1972.
5. Brock DJH, Bolton AE, Monaghan JM: Prenatal diagnosis of anencephaly through maternal serum alpha-fetoprotein measurements, *Lancet* ii:923, 1973.
6. Yen IH et al The changing epidemiology of neural tube defects: United States, 1968-1989. *AJDC* 146:857, 1992.
7. Honein MA et al: Impact of folic acid fortification of the US food supply on the occurrence of neural tube defects, *JAMA* 285:2981-6, 2001.
8. Evans MI et al: Impact of folic acid supplementation in the United States: markedly diminished high maternal serum AFPs, *Obstet Gynecol* 103:474, 2004.
9. Shane B, Stokstad ELR: Vitamin B12 folate interrelationships, *Ann Rev Nutr* 5:115, 1985.
10. Shoiania AM: Folic acid and vitamin B12 deficiency in pregnancy and the neonatal period, *Clin Perinatol* 11:433, 1984.
11. Smithells RW, Sheppard S, Schorah CJ: Vitamin deficiencies and neural-tube defects, *Arch Dis Child* 51:944, 1976
12. Smithells RW et al: Possible prevention of neural-tube defects by periconceptional vitamin supplementation, *Lancet* 1:339, 1980.
13. Smithells RW et al: Further experience of vitamin supplementation for prevention of neural-tube defect recurrences, *Lancet* 1:1027, 1983.
14. Smithells RW et al: Prevention of neural-tube defect recurrences in Yorkshire: final report, *Lancet* 2:498, 1989.
15. Steegers-Theunissen RPM et al: Neural-tube defects and derangement of homocysteine metabolism, *N Engl J Med* 324:199, 1991.
16. Yates JRW et al: Is disordered folate metabolism the basis for the genetic predisposition to neural-tube defects? *Clin Genet* 31:279, 1987.
17. Wald J et al: Investigation of factors influencing folate status in women who have had a neural tube defect-affected infant, *Br J Obstet Gynaecol* 100:546, 1993.

18. Holmes-Siedle M et al: Long term effects of peri-conceptional multivitamin supplements for prevention of neural tube defects: a seven to 10 year follow up, *Arch Dis Child* 67:1436, 1992.

19. From the Centers for Disease Control and Prevention, Leads from the Morbidity and Mortality Weekly Report, Atlanta, GA: Recommendations for use of folic acid to reduce number of spina bifida cases and other neural tube defects, *JAMA* 69:1233, 1993.

20. Steegers-Theunissen Rdgine PM, Smithells RW, Eskes TKAB: Update of new risk factors and prevention of neural-tube defects, *Obstet Gynecol Surv* 48:287, 1993.

21. Van Loon K, Besseghir K, Eshkol A: Neural tube defects after infertility treatment: a review, *Fertil Steril* 58:875, 1992.

22. Merkatz IR et al: An association between low maternal serum alpha-fetoprotein and fetal chromosome abnormalities, *Am J Obstet Gynecol* 148:886, 1984.

23. Nyberg DA et al: Prenatal monographic findings of trisomy 18: review of 47 cases, *J Ultrasound Med* 2:103, 1993.

24. Martin JA et al: *Births: final data for 2001*, National Vital Statistics Report 51, #2. Hyattsville, MD, 2002, National Center for Health Statistics.

25. Evans MI, Galen RS, Drugan A: Biochemical screening. In Evans MI et al, editors: *Prenatal diagnosis*, New York, 2006, McGraw Hill, pp 227-288.

26. Wald NJ et al: Maternal serum screening for Down syndrome in early pregnancy, *Br Med J* 297:883, 1988.

27. Cheng EY et al: A prospective evaluation of a second-trimester screening test for fetal Down syndrome using maternal serum alpha-fetoprotein, hCG, and unconjugated estriol, *Obstet Gynecol* 81:72, 1993.

28. Aitken DA et al: First-trimester biochemical screening for fetal chromosome abnormalities and neural tube defects, *Prenat Diagn* 13:681, 1993.

29. Rodriguez L et al: Results of 12 years' combined maternal serum alpha-fetoprotein screening and ultrasound fetal monitoring for prenatal detection of fetal malformations in Havana City, Cuba, *Prenat Diagn* 17:301, 1997.

30. Wald N et al: The use of free 1993, β-hCG -in antenatal screening for Down's syndrome, *Br J Obstet Gynaecol* 100:550, 1993.

31. Goodburn SF et al: Second-trimester maternal serum screening using alpha-fetoprotein, human chorionic gonadotrophin, and unconjugated oestriol: experience of a regional programme, *Prenat Diagn* 14:391, 1994.

32. Gardosi J, Mongelli M: Risk assessment adjusted for gestational age in maternal serum screening for Down's syndrome, *Br Med J* 306:1509, 1993.

33. Evans MI: Unpublished data.

34. Elias S, Simpson JL: Prenatal diagnosis. In Rimoin DL, Connor JM, Pyeritz PE, editors: *Emery and Rimoin's principles and practice of medical genetics*, ed 3, New York, 1997, Churchill Livingstone.

35. Elias S, Simpson JL: Prospects for prenatal diagnosis by isolating fetal cells from maternal blood, *Contemp Rev Obstet Gynecol* 7:135, 1995.

36. Lewis DE et al: Rare event selection of fetal nucleated erythrocytes in maternal blood by flow cytometry, *Cytometry* 23:218, 1996.

37. Herzenberg LA, Bianchi DW, Schroder J: Fetal cells in the blood of pregnant women: detection and enrichment by fluorescence-activated cell sorting, *Proc Nat Acad Sci U S A* 76:1453, 1979.

38. Bianchi DW et al: Isolation of fetal DNA from nucleated erythrocytes in maternal blood, *Proc Natl Acad Sci U S A* 87:3279, 1990.

39. Bianchi DW, Klinger KW: Prenatal diagnosis through the analysis of fetal cells in the maternal circulation. In Milunsky A, editor: *Genetic disorders and the fetus*, ed 3, Baltimore, 1992, Johns Hopkins University Press, p 759.

40. Ganshirt-Ahlert D et al: Detection of fetal trisomies 21 and 18 from maternal blood using triple gradient and magnetic cell sorting, *Am J Reprod Immunol* 30:194, 1994.

41. Elias S et al: First trimester prenatal diagnosis of trisomy 21 in fetal cells from maternal blood, *Lancet* 34:1033, 1992.

42. Ganshirt D et al: Noninvasive prenatal diagnosis: isolation of fetal cells from maternal circulation. In Zakuk H, editor: *Seventh International Conference on Early Prenatal Diagnosis*, Bologna, 1994, Monduzzi Editore, p 19.

43. Bianchi DW et al: Fetal gender and aneuploidy detection using fetal cells in maternal blood: analysis of NIFTY I data, *Prenat Diagn* 22:609, 2002.

44. Lo YMD et al: Prenatal determination of fetal RhD status by analysis of peripheral blood f rhesus negative mothers, *Lancet* 341:1147, 1993.

45. Evans MI et al: International, collaborative assessment of 146,000 prenatal karyotypes: expected limitations if only chromosome-specific probes and fluorescent in situ hybridization were used, *Hum Reprod* 14:1213, 1999.

46. Crossley JA et al: Combined ultrasound and biochemical screening for Down's syndrome in the first trimester: a Scottish multicentre study, *BJOG* 109:667, 2002.

47. Drugan A et al: Multiple marker screening in multifetal gestations: prediction of adverse pregnancy outcomes, *Fetal Diagn Ther* 11:16, 1996.

48. O'Brien JE et al: Differential increases in AFP, HCG, and uE3 in twin pregnancies: impact upon attempts to quantify Down syndrome screening calculations, *Am J Med Genet* 73:109, 1997.

49. Wald N et al: Maternal serum unconjugated oestriol and human chorionic gonadotrophin levels in twin pregnancies: implications for screening for Down's syndrome, *Br J Obstet Gynaecol* 98:905, 1991.

50. Cuckle H: Down's syndrome screening in twins, *J Med Screen* 5(1):3, 1998.

51. Wald NJ, Rish S, Hackshaw AK: Combining nuchal translucency and serum markers in prenatal screening for Down syndrome in twin pregnancies, *Prenat Diagn* 23:588, 2003.

53

52. Johnson MP et al: Symmetrical intrauterine growth retardation is not symmetrical: organ specific gravimetric deficits in midtrimester and neonatal trisomy 18, *Fetal Ther* 4(2-3):110-09, 1989.

53. Drugan A et al: Counseling for low maternal serum alpha-fetoprotein should emphasize all chromosome anomalies, not just Down syndrome! *Obstet Gynecol* 73:271, 1989.

54. Palomaki GE et al: Risk-based prenatal screening for trisomy 18 using alpha-fetoprotein, unconjugated estriol, and human chorionic gonadotropin, *Prenat Diagn* 15:713, 1995.

55. Langdon Down J: Observations on an ethnic classification of idiots, *Clin Lect Rep Lond Hosp* 3:259, 1866.

56. Down's screening at 11-14 weeks. Fetal Medicine Foundation www.fetalmedicine.com.

57. acrania paper

58. Green JJ, Hobbins JC: Abdominal ultrasound examination of the first trimester fetus, *Am J Obstet Gynecol* 159:165, 1988.

59. Timor-Tritsch IE et al: First-trimester midgut herniation: a high frequency transvaginal sonographic study, *Am J Obstet Gynecol* 161:831, 1989.

60. van Zalen-Sprock RM, van Vugt JMG, van Geijn HP: First-trimester sonography of physiological midgut herniation and early diagnosis of omphalocele, *Prenat Diagn* 17:511, 1997.

61. Snijders RJ et al: Fetal exomphalos and chromosomal defects: relationship to maternal age and gestation, *Ultrasound Obstet Gynecol* 6:250, 1995.

62. Firth HV et al: Severe limb abnormalities after chorion villous sampling at 56–66 days' gestation, *Lancet* 337:762, 1991.

63. Firth HV et al: Analysis of limb reduction defects in babies exposed to chorion villus sampling, *Lancet* 343:1069, 1994.

64. Whitlow BJ, Economides DL: The optimal gestational age to examine fetal anatomy and measure nuchal translucency in the first trimester, *Ultrasound Obstet Gynecol* 11:258, 1998.

65. Mulvey S et al: Optimising the timing for nuchal translucency measurement, *Prenat Diagn* 22:775, 2002.

66. Benacerraf BR, Gelman R, Frigoletto FD: Sonographic identification of second trimester fetuses with Down's syndrome, *N Engl J Med* 317:1371, 1987.

67. Nicolaides KH et al: Fetal nuchal edema: associated malformations and chromosomal defects, *Fetal Diagn Ther* 7:123, 1992.

68. Nicolaides KH et al: Fetal nuchal translucency: ultrasound screening for chromosomal defects in first trimester of pregnancy, *Br Med J* 304:867, 1992.

69. Comas C et al: Measurement of nuchal translucency as a single strategy in trisomy 21 screening: should we use any other marker? *Obstet Gynecol* 100:648, 2002.

70. Braithwaite JM, Economides DL: The measurement of nuchal translucency with transabdominal and transvaginal sonography—success rates, repeatability and levels of agreement, *Br J Radiol* 68:720, 1995.

71. Edwards A, Mulvey S, Wallace EM: The effect of image size on nuchal translucency measurement, *Prenat Diagn* 23:284, 2003.

72. Whitlow BJ, Chatzipapas IK, Economides DL: The effect of fetal neck position on nuchal translucency measurement, *Br J Obstet Gynaecol* 105:872, 1998.

73. Schaefer M, Laurichesse-Delmas H, Ville Y: The effect of nuchal cord on nuchal translucency measurement at 10-14 weeks, *Ultrasound Obstet Gynecol* 11:271, 1998.

74. Miguelez J et al: Nuchal cord at the 11-14 week scan: effect on nuchal translucency measurement, *Ultrasound Obstet Gynecol* 2004. in press.

75. Thilaganathan B et al: Influence of ethnic origin on nuchal translucency screening for Down's syndrome, *Ultrasound Obstet Gynecol* 12:112, 1998.

76. Chen M et al: The effect of ethnic origin on nuchal translucency at 10-14 weeks of gestation, *Prenat Diagn* 22:576, 2002.

77. Spencer K et al: The influence of parity and gravidity on first trimester markers of chromosomal abnormality, *Prenat Diagn* 20:792, 2000.

78. Spencer K et al: First trimester markers of trisomy 21 and the influence of maternal cigarette smoking status, *Prenat Diagn* 20:852, 2000.

79. Niemimaa M et al: The influence of smoking on the pregnancy-associated plasma protein A, free beta human chorionic gonadotrophin and nuchal translucency, *BJOG* 110:664, 2003.

80. Bartha JL et al: The effect of metabolic control on fetal nuchal translucency in women with insulin-dependent diabetes: a preliminary study, *Ultrasound Obstet Gynecol* 21:451, 2003.

81. Liao AW et al: First-trimester screening for trisomy 21 in singleton pregnancies achieved by assisted reproduction, *Hum Reprod* 16:1501, 2001.

82. Wojdemann KR et al: First trimester screening for Down syndrome and assisted reproduction: no basis for concern, *Prenat Diagn* 21:563, 2001.

83. Maymon R, Shulman A: Serial first- and second-trimester Down's syndrome screening tests among IVF-versus naturally-conceived singletons, *Hum Reprod* 17:1081, 2002.

84. Orlandi F et al: First trimester screening with free beta-hCG, PAPP-A and nuchal translucency in pregnancies conceived with assisted reproduction, *Prenat Diagn* 22:718, 2002.

85. De Biasio P et al: Early vaginal bleeding and first-trimester markers for Down syndrome, *Prenat Diagn* 23:470, 2003.

86. Spencer K et al: The influence of fetal sex in screening for trisomy 21 by fetal nuchal translucency, maternal serum free beta-hCG and PAPP-A at 10-14 weeks of gestation, *Prenat Diagn* 20:673, 2000.

87. Yaron Y et al: Effect of fetal gender on first trimester markers and on Down syndrome screening, *Prenat Diagn* 2001;21:1027, 2001.

88. Larsen SO et al: Gender impact on first trimester markers in Down syndrome screening, *Prenat Diagn* 22:1207, 2002.

89. Pandya PP et al: Repeatability of measurement of fetal nuchal translucency thickness, *Ultrasound Obstet Gynecol* 5:334, 1995.

90. Schuchter K et al: The distribution of nuchal translucency at 10-13 weeks of pregnancy, *Prenat Diagn* 18:281, 1998.

91. Pajkrt E et al: Weekly nuchal translucency measurements in normal fetuses, *Obstet Gynecol* 91:208, 1998.

92. Snijders RJM et al: UK multicentre project on assessment of risk of trisomy 21 by maternal age and fetal nuchal translucency thickness at 10-14 weeks of gestation, *Lancet* 351:343, 1998.

93. Pandya PP et al: The implementation of first-trimester scanning at 10–13 weeks' gestation and the measurement of fetal nuchal translucency thickness in two maternity units, *Ultrasound Obstet Gynecol* 5:20, 1995.

94. Schwarzler P et al: Screening for fetal aneuploidies and fetal cardiac abnormalities by nuchal translucency thickness measurement at 10-14 weeks of gestation as part of routine antenatal care in an unselected population, *Br J Obstet Gynaecol* 106:1029, 1999.

95. Schuchter K et al: Sequential screening for trisomy 21 by nuchal translucency measurement in the first trimester and maternal serum biochemistry in the second trimester in a low-risk population, *Ultrasound Obstet Gynecol* 2001;18:23, 2001.

96. Wayda K et al: Four years experience of first-trimester nuchal translucency screening for fetal aneuploidies with increasing regional availability, *Acta Obstet Gynecol Scand* 80:1104, 2001.

97. Panburana P, Ajjimakorn S, Tungkajiwangoon P: First trimester Down syndrome screening by nuchal translucency in a Thai population, *Int J Gynaecol Obstet* 75:311, 2001.

98. Snijders RJM et al: UK multicentre project on assessment of risk of trisomy 21 by maternal age and fetal nuchal translucency thickness at 10-14 weeks of gestation, *Lancet* 351:343, 1998.

99. Theodoropoulos P et al: Evaluation of first-trimester screening by fetal nuchal translucency and maternal age, *Prenat Diagn* 18:133, 1998.

100. Zoppi MA et al: Fetal nuchal translucency screening in 12,495 pregnancies in Sardinia, *Ultrasound Obstet Gynecol* 18:649, 2001.

101. Gasiorek-Wiens A et al: Screening for trisomy 21 by fetal nuchal translucency and maternal age: a multicenter project in Germany, Austria and Switzerland, *Ultrasound Obstet Gynecol* 18:645, 2001.

102. Brizot ML et al: First-trimester screening for chromosomal abnormalities by fetal nuchal translucency in a Brazilian population, *Ultrasound Obstet Gynecol* 18:652, 2001.

103. Comas C et al: Measurement of nuchal translucency as a single strategy in trisomy 21 screening: should we use any other marker? *Obstet Gynecol* 100:648, 2002.

104. Chasen ST et al: First-trimester screening for aneuploidy with fetal nuchal translucency in a United States population, *Ultrasound Obstet Gynecol* 22:149, 2003.

105. Szabo J, Gellen J, Szemere G: First-trimester ultrasound screening for fetal aneuploidies in women over 35 and under 35 years of age, *Ultrasound Obstet Gynecol* 5:161, 1995.

106. Taipale P et al: Ylostalo P. Increased nuchal translucency as a marker for fetal chromosomal defects, *N Engl J Med* 337:1654, 1997.

107. Pajkrt E et al: Screening for Down's syndrome by fetal nuchal translucency measurement in a general obstetric population, *Ultrasound Obstet Gynecol* 12:163, 1998.

108. Pajkrt E et al: Screening for Down's syndrome by fetal nuchal translucency measurement in a high-risk population, *Ultrasound Obstet Gynecol* 12:156, 1998.

109. Audibert F et al: Screening for Down syndrome using first-trimester ultrasound and second-trimester maternal serum markers in a low-risk population: a prospective longitudinal study, *Ultrasound Obstet Gynecol* 18:26, 2001.

110. Rozenberg P et al: Down's syndrome screening with nuchal translucency at 12(+0)-14(+0) weeks and maternal serum markers at 14(+1)-17(+0) weeks: a prospective study, *Hum Reprod* 17:1093, 2002.

111. Economides DL et al: First trimester sonographic detection of chromosomal abnormalities in an unselected population, *BJOG* 105:58, 1998.

112. Whitlow BJ et al: The value of sonography in early pregnancy for the detection of fetal abnormalities in an unselected population, *BJOG* 106:929, 1999.

113. Thilaganathan B et al: First trimester nuchal translucency: effective routine screening for Down's syndrome, *Br J Radiol* 72:946, 1999.

114. O'Callaghan SP et al: First trimester ultrasound with nuchal translucency measurement for Down syndrome risk estimation using software developed by the Fetal Medicine Foundation, United Kingdom—the first 2000 examinations in Newcastle, New South Wales, Australia, *Aust N Z J Obstet Gynaecol* 40:292, 2000.

115. Sau A et al: Screening for trisomy 21: the significance of a positive second trimester serum screen in women screen negative after nuchal translucency scan, *J Obstet Gynaecol* 21:145, 2001.

116. Prefumo F, Thilaganathan B: Agreement between predicted risk and prevalence of Down syndrome in first trimester nuchal translucency screening, *Prenat Diagn* 22:917, 2002.

117. Macri JN et al: Maternal serum Down syndrome screening: free beta protein is a more effective marker than human chorionic gonadotrophin, *Am J Obstet Gynecol* 163:1248, 1990.

118. Brambati B et al: Low maternal serum level of pregnancy associated plasma protein (PAPP-A) in the first trimester in association with abnormal fetal karyotype. *BJOG* 100:324, 1993.

119. Cuckle HS, van Lith JM: Appropriate biochemical parameters in first-trimester screening for Down syndrome, *Prenat Diagn* 19:505, 1999.

55

120. Brizot ML et al: Maternal serum pregnancy associated placental protein A and fetal nuchal translucency thickness for the prediction of fetal trisomies in early pregnancy, *Obstet Gynecol* 84:918, 1994.

121. Brizot ML et al: Maternal serum hCG and fetal nuchal translucency thickness for the prediction of fetal trisomies in the first trimester of pregnancy, *Br J Obstet Gynaecol* 102:1227, 1995.

122. Noble PL et al: Screening for fetal trisomy 21 in the first trimester of pregnancy: maternal serum free beta-hCG and fetal nuchal translucency thickness, *Ultrasound Obstet Gynecol* 6:390, 1995.

123. Spencer K et al: A screening program for trisomy 21 at 10-14 weeks using fetal nuchal translucency, maternal serum free β-human chorionic gonadotropin and pregnancy-associated plasma protein-A, *Ultrasound Obstet Gynecol* 13:231, 1999.

124. Otano L et al: Association between first trimester absence of fetal nasal bone on ultrasound and Down's syndrome, *Prenat Diagn* 22:930, 2002.

125. Zoppi MA et al: Absence of fetal nasal bone and aneuploidies at first-trimester nuchal translucency screening in unselected pregnancies, *Prenat Diagn* 23:496, 2003.

126. Orlandi F et al: Measurement of nasal bone length at 11-14 weeks of pregnancy and its potential role in Down's syndrome risk assessment, *Ultrasound Obstet Gynecol* 22:36, 2003.

127. Viora E et al: Ultrasound evaluation of fetal nasal bone at 11 to 14 weeks in a consecutive series of 1906 fetuses, *Prenat Diagn* 23:784, 2003.

128. Bindra R et al: One stop clinic for assessment of risk for trisomy 21 at 11-14 weeks: a prospective study of 15,030 pregnancies, *Ultrasound Obstet Gynecol* 20:219, 2002.

129. Evans MI et al, editors: *Prenatal diagnosis*, New York, 2006, McGraw Hill.

130. Monteagudo A, Timor-Tritsch I, Sharma S: Early and simple determination of chorionic and amniotic type in multifetal gestations in the first 14 weeks by high frequency transvaginal ultrasound. *Am J Obstet Gynecol* 170:824-9, 1994.

131. Sepulveda W et al: The lambda sign at 10-14 weeks of gestation as a predictor of chorionicity in twin pregnancies, *Ultrasound Obstet Gynecol* 7:421, 1996.

132. Yukobowich E et al: Risk of fetal loss in twin pregnancies undergoing second trimester amniocentesis, *Obstet Gynecol* 98:231, 2001.

133. Aytoz A et al: Obstetric outcome after prenatal diagnosis in pregnancies obtained after intracytoplasmic sperm injection. *Hum Reprod* 13:2958, 1998.

134. De Catte L, Liebaers I, Foulon W: Outcome of twin gestations after first trimester chorionic villus sampling, *Obstet Gynecol* 96:714, 2000.

135. Brambati B et al: Outcome of first-trimester chorionic villus sampling for genetic investigation in multiple pregnancy, *Ultrasound Obstet Gynecol* 17:209, 2001.

136. Evans MI et al: Efficacy of second-trimester selective termination for fetal abnormalities: international collaborative experience among the world's largest centers, *Am J Obstet Gynecol* 171:90, 1994.

137. Sebire NJ et al: Screening for trisomy 21 in twin pregnancies by maternal age and fetal nuchal translucency thickness at 10-14 weeks of gestation, *BJOG* 103:999, 1996.

138. Monni G et al: Nuchal translucency in multiple pregnancies. *Croat Med J* 41:266, 2000.

139. Sebire NJ et al: Early prediction of severe twin-to-twin transfusion syndrome, *Hum Reprod* 15: 2008, 2000.

140. Sebire NJ et al: Increased fetal nuchal translucency at 10-14 weeks as a predictor of severe twin-to-twin transfusion syndrome, *Ultrasound Obstet Gynecol* 10:86, 1997.

141. Sebire NJ et al: Increased fetal nuchal translucency at 10-14 weeks as a predictor of severe twin-to-twin transfusion syndrome, *Ultrasound Obstet. Gynecol* 10:86, 1997.

142. Noble PL et al: Maternal serum free beta-hCG at 10 to 14 weeks in trisomic twin pregnancies, *BJOG* 104:741, 1997.

143. Spencer K: Screening for trisomy 21 in twin pregnancies in the first trimester using free beta-hCG and PAPP-A, combined with fetal nuchal translucency thickness, *Prenat Diagn* 20:91, 2000.

144. Spencer K, Nicolaides KH: Screening for trisomy 21 in twins using first trimester ultrasound and maternal serum biochemistry in a one-stop clinic: a review of three years experience, *BJOG* 110: 276, 2003.

145. Farkas LG et al: Surface anatomy of the face in Down's syndrome: linear and angular measurements in the craniofacial regions, *J Craniofac Surg* 12:373, 2001.

146. Stempfle N et al: Skeletal abnormalities in fetuses with Down's syndrome: a radiographic postmortem study, *Pediatr Radiol* 29:682, 1999.

147. Keeling JW, Hansen BF, Kjaer I: Pattern of malformations in the axial skeleton in human trisomy 21 fetuses, *Am J Med Genet* 68:466, 1997.

148. Tuxen A et al: A histological and radiological investigation of the nasal bone in fetuses with Down syndrome, *Ultrasound Obstet Gynecol* 22:22, 2003.

149. Larose C et al: Comparison of fetal nasal bone assessment by ultrasound at 11-14 weeks and by postmortem X-ray in trisomy 21: a prospective observational study, *Ultrasound Obstet Gynecol* 22:27, 2003.

150. Sonek J, Nicolaides KH: Prenatal ultrasonographic diagnosis of nasal bone abnormalities in three fetuses with Down syndrome, *Am J Obstet Gynecol* 186:139, 2002.

151. Cicero S et al: Nasal bone hypoplasia in trisomy 21 at 15-22 weeks' gestation, *Ultrasound Obstet Gynecol* 21:15, 2003.

152. Bunduki V et al: Fetal nasal bone length: reference range and clinical application in ultrasound screening for trisomy 21, *Ultrasound Obstet Gynecol* 21:156, 2003.

153. Bromley B et al: Fetal nose bone length: a marker for Down syndrome in the second trimester, *J Ultrasound Med* 21:1387, 2002.

154. Gamez F, Ferreiro P, Salmean JM: Ultrasonographic measurement of fetal nasal bone in a low risk population at 19-22 gestational weeks, *Ultrasound Obstet Gynecol* 23(2):152-53, 2004.

155. Cicero S et al: Absence of nasal bone in fetuses with Trisomy 21 at 11-14 weeks of gestation: an observational study, *Lancet* 358:1665, 2001.

156. Cicero S et al: Learning curve for sonographic examination of the fetal nasal bone at 11-14 weeks, *Ultrasound Obstet Gynecol* 22:135, 2003.

157. Kanellopoulos V, Katsetos C, Economides DL: Examination of fetal nasal bone and repeatability of measurement in early pregnancy, *Ultrasound Obstet Gynecol* 22:131, 2003.

158. Otano L et al: Association between first trimester absence of fetal nasal bone on ultrasound and Down's syndrome, *Prenat Diagn* 22:930, 2002.

159. Senat MV et al: Intra- and interoperator variability in fetal nasal bone assessment at 11-14 weeks of gestation, *Ultrasound Obstet Gynecol* 22:138, 2003.

160. Wong SF, Choi H, Ho LC: Nasal bone hypoplasia: is it a common finding amongst chromosomally normal fetuses of southern Chinese women? *Gynecol Obstet Invest* 56:99, 2003.

161. Cicero S et al: Absent nasal bone at 11-14 weeks of gestation and chromosomal defects, *Ultrasound Obstet Gynecol* 22:31, 2003.

162. Cicero S et al: Likelihood ratio for Trisomy 21 in fetuses with absent nasal bone at the 11-14 weeks scan, *Ultrasound Obstet Gynecol* 2004. in press.

163. Ghi T et al: Incidence of major structural cardiac defects associated with increased nuchal translucency but normal karyotype, *Ultrasound Obstet Gynecol* 18:610, 2001.

164. Cicero S et al: Absent nasal bone at 11-14 weeks of gestation and chromosomal defects, *Ultrasound Obstet Gynecol* 22:31, 2003.

165. Cicero S et al: Likelihood ratio for Trisomy 21 in fetuses with absent nasal bone at the 11-14 weeks scan. *Ultrasound Obstet Gynecol* 2004. in press.

166. Malone FD et al: First trimester nasal bone evaluation for aneuploidy in an unselected general population: results from the FASTER trial, SMFM 2004 (Abstract 58).

167. Welch KK, Malone FD: Nuchal translucency-based screening, *Clin Obstet Gynecol* 46:909, 2003.

168. De Biasio P, Venturini PL: Absence of nasal bone and detection of trisomy 21, *Lancet* 13:1344, 2002.

169. Souka AP et al: Defects and syndromes in chromosomally normal fetuses with increased nuchal translucency at 10-14 weeks of gestation, *Ultrasound Obstet Gynecol* 11:391, 1998.

170. Souka AP et al: Outcome of pregnancy in chromosomally normal fetuses with increased nuchal translucency in the first trimester, *Ultrasound Obstet Gynecol* 18:9, 2001.

171. Michailidis GD, Economides DL: Nuchal translucency measurement and pregnancy outcome in karyotypically normal fetuses, *Ultrasound Obstet Gynecol* 17:102, 2001.

172. Schwarzler P et al: Screening for fetal aneuploidies and fetal cardiac abnormalities by nuchal translucency thickness measurement at 10-14 weeks of gestation as part of routine antenatal care in an unselected population, *Br J Obstet Gynaecol* 106:1029, 1999.

173. Pajkrt E et al: Screening for Down's syndrome by fetal nuchal translucency measurement in a general obstetric population, *Ultrasound Obstet Gynecol* 12:163, 1998.

174. Hiippala A et al: Fetal nuchal translucency and normal chromosomes: a long-term follow-up study, *Ultrasound Obstet Gynecol* 18:18, 2001.

175. Cheng C et al: Pregnancy outcomes with increased nuchal translucency after routine Down syndrome screening, *Int J Gynaecol Obstet* 84:5, 2004.

176. Mangione R et al: Pregnancy outcome and prognosis in fetuses with increased first-trimester nuchal translucency, *Fetal Diagn Ther* 16:360, 2001.

177. Hyett JA et al: Cardiac gene expression of atrial natriuretic peptide and brain natriuretic peptide in trisomic fetuses, *Obstet Gynecol* 87:506, 1996.

178. Matias A et al: Screening for chromosomal abnormalities at 11-14 weeks: the role of ductus venosus blood flow, *Ultrasound Obstet Gynecol* 2:380, 1998.

179. Matias A et al: Cardiac defects in chromosomally normal fetuses with abnormal ductus venosus blood flow at 10-14 weeks, *Ultrasound Obstet Gynecol* 14:307, 1999.

180. von Kaisenberg CS et al: Collagen type VI gene expression in the skin of trisomy 21 fetuses, *Obstet Gynecol* 91:319, 1998.

181. von Kaisenberg CS et al: Morphological classification of nuchal skin in fetuses with trisomy 21, 18 and 13 at 12-18 weeks and in a trisomy 16 mouse, *Anat Embryol* 197:105, 1998.

182. Bohlandt S et al: Hyaluronan in the nuchal skin of chromosomally abnormal fetuses, *Hum Reprod* 15:1155, 2000.

183. Chitayat D, Kalousek DK, Bamforth JS: Lymphatic abnormalities in fetuses with posterior cervical cystic hygroma, *Am J Med Genet* 33:352, 1989.

184. von Kaisenberg CS, Nicolaides KH, Brand-Saberi B: Lymphatic vessel hypoplasia in fetuses with Turner syndrome, *Hum Reprod* 14:823, 1999.

185. von Kaisenberg CS et al: Glycosaminoglycans and proteoglycans in the skin of aneuploid fetuses with increased nuchal translucency, *Hum Reprod* 18:2544, 2003.

186. Sebire NJ et al: Increased fetal nuchal translucency thickness at 10-14 weeks: is screening for maternal-fetal infection necessary? *Br J Obstet Gynaecol* 104:212, 1997.

187. Hyett JA, Moscoso G, Nicolaides KH: First trimester nuchal translucency and cardiac septal defects in fetuses with trisomy 21, *Am J Obstet Gynecol* 172:1411, 1995.

188. Hyett JA, Moscoso G, Nicolaides KH: Increased nuchal translucency in Trisomy 21 fetuses: relation to narrowing of the aortic isthmus, *Hum Reprod* 10:3049, 1995.

189. Hyett JA, Moscoso G, Nicolaides KH: Cardiac defects in first trimester fetuses with trisomy 18, *Fetal Diagn Ther* 10:381, 1995.

190. Hyett JA, Moscoso G, Nicolaides KH: Abnormalities of the heart and great arteries in first trimester chromosomally abnormal fetuses, *Am J Med Genet* 69:207, 1997.

191. Hyett J et al: Abnormalities of the heart and great arteries in chromosomally normal fetuses with increased nuchal translucency thickness at 11-13 weeks of gestation, *Ultrasound Obstet Gynecol* 7:245, 1996.

192. Gembruch U et al: Early diagnosis of fetal congenital heart disease by transvaginal echocardiography, *Ultrasound Obstet Gynecol* 3:310, 1993.

193. Achiron R et al: First-trimester diagnosis of fetal congenital heart disease by transvaginal ultrasonography, *Obstet Gynecol* 84:69, 1994.

194. Smrcek JM et al: The evaluation of cardiac biometry in major cardiac defects detected in early pregnancy, *Arch Gynecol Obstet* 268:94, 2003.

195. Makrydimas G, Sotiriadis A, Ioannidis JP: Screening performance of first-trimester nuchal translucency for major cardiac defects: a meta-analysis, *Am J Obstet Gynecol* 189:1330, 2003.

196. Sebire NJ et al: Fetal nuchal translucency thickness at 10-14 weeks of gestation and congenital diaphragmatic hernia, *Obstet Gynecol* 90:943, 1997.

197. Snijders RJM et al: Fetal exomphalos at 11-14 weeks of gestation, *J Ultrasound Med* 14:569, 1995.

198. Liao AW et al: Megacystis at 10-14 weeks of gestation: chromosomal defects and outcome according to bladder length, *Ultrasound Obstet Gynecol* 21:338, 2003.

199. Daskalakis G et al: Body stalk anomaly at 10-14 weeks of gestation, *Ultrasound Obstet Gynecol* 10:416, 1997.

200. Smrcek JM et al: Prenatal ultrasound diagnosis and management of body stalk anomaly: analysis of nine singleton and two multiple pregnancies, *Ultrasound Obstet Gynecol* 21:322, 2003.

201. Drugan A, Evans MI: Invasive procedures for prenatal diagnosis. In Ransom SB et al., editors: *Contemporary therapy in obstetrics and gynecology*, Philadelphia, 2002, WB Saunders, pp 207-215.

202. Evans MI et al: Parental perception of genetic risk: Correlation with choice of prenatal diagnostic procedures, *Int J Obstet Gynecol* 31:25, 1990.

203. Evans MI, Wapner RJ: Invasive prenatal diagnostic procedures 2005, *Semin Perinatol* 29:215, 2005.

204. Jacobson CB, Barter RH: Intrauterine diagnosis and management of genetic defects, *Am J Obstet Gynecol* 99:795, 1967.

205. Nadler HL, Gerbie AB: Role of amniocentesis in the intrauterine detection of genetic disorders, *N Engl J Med* 282:596, 1970.

206. Evans MI: *Reproductive risks and prenatal diagnosis*, New York, 1992, McGraw Hill.

207. Evans MI, Hanft RS: The introduction of new technologies. *ACOG Clin Semin* 2:1, 1997.

208. Cohen AB, Hanft RS: *Technology in American health care: Policy directions for effective evaluation and management*, Ann Arbor, 2004, University of Michigan Press.

209. Evans MI et al: Genetic diagnosis in the first trimester: the norm for the 90s, *Am J Obstet Gynecol* 160:1332, 1989.

210. Firth HV et al: Severe limb abnormalities after chorion villus sampling at 56-66 days' gestation, *Lancet* 337:726, 1991.

211. Burton BK, Schulz CJ, Burd LI: Limb anomalies associated with chorionic villus sampling, *Obstet Gynecol* 79:726, 1992.

212. Froster UG, Jackson L: Limb defects and chorionic villus sampling: results from an international registry, 1992-94, *Lancet* 347:489, 1996.

213. Kuliev A et al: Chorionic villus sampling safety. Report of World Health Organization/EURO meeting in association with the Seventh International Conference on Early Prenatal Diagnosis of Genetic Diseases, Tel-Aviv, Israel, May 21, 1994, *Am J Obstet Gynecol* 174:807, 1996.

214. Brambati B, Simoni G, Traui M: Genetic diagnosis by chorionic villus sampling before 8 gestational weeks: efficiency, reliability, and risks on 317 completed pregnancies, *Prenat Diagn* 12:784, 1992.

215. Wapner RJ et al: Procedural risks versus theology: chorionic villus sampling for orthodox Jews at less than 8 weeks' gestation, *Am J Obstet Gynecol* 186:1133, 2002.

216. Wilson RD: Early amniocentesis: a clinical review, *Prenat Diagn* 15:1259, 1995.

217. The Canadian Early and Mid-trimester Amniocentesis Trial (CEMAT) Group: Randomized trial to assess safety and fetal outcome of early and mid-trimester amniocentesis, *Lancet* 351:242, 1998.

218. Nagel HTC et al: Amniocentesis before 14 completed weeks as an alternative to transabdominal chorionic villus sampling: a controlled trial with infant follow-up, *Prenat Diagn* 18:465, 1998.

219. Nicolaides K et al: Comparison of chorion villus sampling and early amniocentesis for karyotyping in 1492 singleton pregnancies, *Fetal Diagn Ther* 11:9, 1996.

220. Evans MI, Krivchenia EL, Yaron Y: Screening. In Evans MI, Bui TH, editors: The genome revolution and obstetrics and gynecology, *Ballieres Best Pract Res Clin Obstet Gynecol* 16:645, 2002.

221. Evans MI et al: Selective reduction, *Clin Perinatol* 30:103, 2003.
222. Phillip J et al: Late first-trimester invasive prenatal diagnosis: results of an international randomized trial, *Obstet Gynecol* 103:1164, 2004.
223. Alfirevic Z, Sundberg K, Brigham S: Amniocentesis and chorionic villus sampling for prenatal diagnosis, *Cochrane Database Syst Rev* CD 003252, 2003.
224. Antsaklis A et al: Genetic amniocentesis in women 20-34 years old: associated risks, *Prenat Diagn* 20:247, 2000.
225. Cavollotti D et al: Early complications of prenatal invasive diagnostics: perspective analysis, *Acta Biomed Ateneo Parmense* 75 (Suppl 1):23, 2004.
226. Sangalli M, Langdana F, Thurlow C: Prenancy loss rate following routine genetic amniocentesis at Wellington Hospital, *N Z Med J* 117:U818, 2004.
227. Johnson JM et al: Technical factors in early amniocentesis predict adverse outcome. Results of the Canadian early (EA) versus mid-trimester (MA) amniocentesis trial, *Prenat Diagn* 19:732, 1999.
228. Roper EC et al: Genetic amniocentesis: gestation specific pregnancy outcome and comparison of outcome following early and traditional amniocentesis, *Prenat Diagn* 19:803, 1999.
229. Scott F et al: the loss rates for invasive prenatal testing in a specialized obstetric ultrasound practice, *Aust N Z J Obstet Gynaecol* 42:55, 2002.
230. Muller F et al: Risk of amniocentesis in women screened positive for Down syndrome with second trimester maternal serum markers. *Prenat Diagn* 22:1036, 2002.
231. Centini G et al: A report of early (13 + 0 to 14 +6 weeks) and mid-trimester amniocentesis: 10 years' experience, *J Matern Fetal Neonatal Med* 14:113, 2003.
232. Saltvedt S, Almstrom H: Fetal loss rate after second trimester amniocentesis at different gestational age, *Acta Obstet Gynecol Scand* 78:10, 1999.
233. Wilson RD: Amniocentesis and chorionic villus sampling, *Curr Opin Obstet Gynecol* 12:81, 2000.
234. Toth-Pal E et al: Genetic amniocentesis in multiple pregnancy, *Fetal Diagn Ther* 19:138, 2004.
235. Blessed WB, Lacoste H, Welch RA: Obstetrician-gynecologists performing genetic amniocentesis may be misleading themselves and their patients, *Am J Obstet Gynecol* 184:1340, 2001.
236. Kolibianakis E et al: Prenatal genetic testing by amniocentesis appears to result in lower risk of fetal loss than chorionic villus sampling in pregnancies achieved by intracytoplasmic sperm injection, *Fertil Steril* 79:374, 2003.
237. Cederholm M, Haglund B, Axelsson O: Maternal complications following amniocentesis and chorionic villus sampling for prenatal karyotyping, *BJOG* 110:392, 2003.
238. Alfirevic Z: early amniocentesis versus transabdominal chorion villus sampling for prenatal diagnosis, *Cochrane Database Syst Rev* CD 000077, 2002.
239. Brambati B et al: Outcome of first-trimester chorionic villus sampling for genetic investigation in multiple pregnancy, *Ultrasound Obstet Gynecol* 17:209, 2001.
240. Van den Berg C et al: Amniocentesis or chorionic villus sampling in multiple gestation: experience with 500 cases, *Prenatal Diagn* 19:234, 1999.
241. Edelman KA, Malone F, Sullivan L, et al: Pregnancy loss rates after mid-trimester amniocentesis, *Obstet Gynecol* 108:1067-72, 2006.
242. Wagner RJ, Evans MF, Platt LD: Pregnancy loss rates after amniocentesis, *Obstet Gynecol* 109:780, 2007.
243. Evans MF, Andriole SA: CVS and amniocentesis in 2008, *Curr Opin Obstet Gynecol* (in press).
244. Majezinovic F, Alfirevil Z: Procedure related complications of amniocentesis and chorionic villus sampling, *Obstet Gynecol* 110:687-94, 2007.
245. Britt DW et al: Framing the decision: Determinants of how women considering MFPR as a pregnancy-management strategy frame their moral dilemma, *Fetal Diagn Ther* 19:232, 2004.
246. Britt DW et al: Devastation and relief: conflicting meanings in discovering fetal anomalies, *Ultrasound Obstet Gynecol* 20:1, 2002.

3

GENERAL PRINCIPLES OF OBSTETRIC SONOGRAPHY

Anna K. Sfakianaki and Joshua A. Copel

INTRODUCTION AND BACKGROUND

Ultrasound imaging is used throughout pregnancy and is the most commonly used diagnostic modality in pregnancy. It is used in the estimation of gestational age, in the evaluation of fetal anatomy, and in the assessment of fetal growth. Ultrasound is used as an adjunct to invasive procedures such as chorionic villus sampling, amniocentesis, and cordocentesis. Fetal well-being is assessed though ultrasound. The monitoring of high-risk pregnancies, such as those complicated by growth restriction, is achieved through serial sonography. Doppler ultrasound is used to evaluate the placental circulation, which indirectly is used to assess fetal well-being. Transvaginal assessment of cervical length has become an important tool to predict the risk of preterm delivery. No adverse effects of obstetric ultrasound on the developing fetus have been documented, and ultrasound is considered to be safe in pregnancy.

Ultrasound transducers are composed of crystals of a piezoelectric material to which electrical stimulation is applied. This stimulation induces a mechanical deformation, which creates sound waves. The basis of diagnostic ultrasound is that sound waves generated by the transducer reflect off of a target tissue and, on their return to that transducer, the echoes induce electrical signals which are interpreted as images composed of dots on a computer screen. The density of the target tissue determines the intensity of the echo, which in turn determines the brightness of its dot on the screen. The image is updated continuously by the continuous firing of multiple crystals within the transducers, and a real-time image is thus created. The frame rate is the rate at which the image is updated.

A variety of ultrasound transducers have been developed for use in obstetric ultrasound. The curvilinear transducer is most often used in obstetrics because it combines the most useful features of older sector and linear array transducers. The waves emitted by this transducer create a wedge-shaped area of imaging. Transducers for transvaginal imaging allow us to get closer to the target, an especially useful tool for the imaging of the small structures of early pregnancy and in patients with obesity.

The frequency of the sound waves generated is measured in cycles per second, or Hertz (Hz). Transabdominal transducers are generally 3.5 to

7 MHz, whereas transvaginal transducers can be up to 9 MHz. The higher the frequency, the better the resolution and image quality. However, penetration is better with lower-frequency transducers. The use of a coupling agent, such as water-soluble gel, is necessary because ultrasound waves travel poorly through air, and the gel creates an acoustic interface between the transducer and the patient.

Ultrasound has the ability to alter tissue by vibration or by inducing temperature changes; these are collectively known as bioeffects. To minimize the potential for bioeffects, it is important to keep the acoustic output at the minimal possible level, a process termed "as low as reasonably achievable (ALARA)." The Food and Drug Administration (FDA) has mandated that modern ultrasound equipment include two safety measures in its visual display to reflect the two main bioeffects:

1. Thermal index—a measure of the effect of ultrasound on increasing the temperature in target tissue
2. Mechanical index—a measure of the nonthermal effects ultrasound may have on target tissue, usually resulting from the interaction with microscopic gas bubbles, termed cavitation

By maintaining these indices at less than one, the chance of adverse effect on fetal tissue is minimized.

FIRST TRIMESTER

Ultrasound serves many roles in the first trimester. It is used to confirm viability in pregnancies in which this may be an issue. Patients with high rates of early spontaneous abortion, such as those with bleeding in the first trimester or those with pregnancies complicated by uncontrolled diabetes mellitus or severe renal disease are followed with ultrasound to confirm ongoing pregnancy. Ultrasound is used in the surveillance of pregnancies conceived by assisted reproductive technologies. Viability is confirmed by the demonstration of cardiac activity on ultrasound, either by 2D, M-mode or Doppler sonography, on either vaginal or abdominal ultrasound. Anembryonic gestation is diagnosed by the absence of a fetal pole or by the lack of cardiac activity within the fetal pole. Cardiac activity is usually visualized by the time the embryo measures 5 mm by transvaginal sonography.

The diagnosis of multifetal gestation is easily made on first-trimester ultrasound. Importantly, early ultrasound allows for greater ease in the evaluation of the chorionicity of the gestation. Precise knowledge regarding the chorionicity is very important in the counseling and surveillance of multifetal gestation.

The first sign of pregnancy on ultrasound is the gestational sac. In cases of ectopic pregnancy, however, a pseudosac, representing a collection of fluid within the uterus, may be visualized despite the extrauterine position of the gestation. The first definitive sign of intrauterine pregnancy is the yolk sac, first visualized transvaginally by about 5 weeks' gestation. When this is seen, ectopic pregnancy can be ruled out, except in the extremely rare case of heterotopic pregnancy. By 6 weeks, a fetal pole with cardiac activity can be seen on transvaginal ultrasound. By the time the serum beta human chorionic gonadotrophin (β-hCG) reaches 1200-2000 mIU/ml a fetal pole should be seen. If it is not, ectopic pregnancy or miscarriage should be suspected, depending on the clinical presentation.

One of the most important tasks in obstetrics is to establish the estimated date of delivery (EDD). Many subsequent decisions during pregnancy depend on this accurate estimation. Measurement of the fetal pole in the first trimester accurately dates the pregnancy within 5 to 7 days. This measurement is called the crown-rump length (CRL) and it is highly reproducible (Figure 3-1, *A* and *B* and Table 3-1). When the EDD by last menstrual period (LMP) differs from the EDD by CRL by more that 7 days, the CRL dating is favored. Ultrasonic estimation of gestational age has been demonstrated to be more accurate than menstrual dating, especially in the first trimester. Estimation of gestational age by measurement of the gestational sac alone is not accurate.

Evaluation of fetal anatomy in the first trimester has been reported and can be very accurate. This may be especially important in obese patients, in whom it is not expected that second-trimester transabdominal ultrasound will offer a high yield. However, knowledge of embryology is important, so as not to confuse normal development (e.g., physiologic herniation of the bowel) with pathology (e.g., omphalocele). An early sign of anomaly can be a CRL that is smaller than expected for that gestational age.

The newest application of first trimester ultrasound is in the screening for aneuploidy and structural malformations. Nuchal translucency (NT) is a term used to describe the sonolucent area in the back of the neck of the fetus (Figure 3-2). Two large trials have demonstrated that the measurement of the NT coupled with serum screening in the first trimester is able to predict

Figure 3-1

A, Crown-rump length of a 10-week embryo. The calipers are placed at the tip of the "rump" and the flat part of the "crown." **B,** Crown-rump length of a 12-week embryo. Note that anatomic elements such as the face, brain, spinal column, and limbs are more visible at this age.

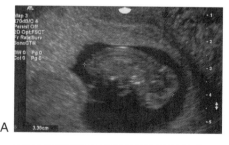

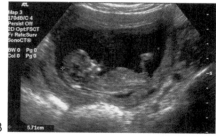

Table 3-1

Gestational Age by Crown-Rump Length (CRL)

CRL (cm)	Weeks	CRL	Weeks	CRL	Weeks
0.2	5.7	4.2	11.1	8.2	14.2
0.4	6.1	4.4	11.2	8.4	14.3
0.6	6.4	4.6	11.4	8.6	14.5
0.8	6.7	4.8	11.6	8.8	14.7
1.0	7.2	5.0	11.7	9.0	14.9
1.2	7.4	5.2	11.9	9.2	15.1
1.4	7.7	5.4	12.0	9.4	15.3
1.6	8.0	5.6	12.2	9.6	15.4
1.8	8.3	5.8	12.3	9.8	15.6
2.0	8.6	6.0	12.5	10.0	15.9
2.2	8.9	6.2	12.6	10.2	16.1
2.4	9.1	6.4	12.8	10.4	16.3
2.6	9.4	6.6	12.9	10.6	16.5
2.8	9.6	6.8	13.1	10.8	16.7
3.0	9.9	7.0	13.2	11.0	16.9
3.2	10.1	7.2	13.4	11.2	17.1
3.4	10.3	7.4	13.5	11.4	17.3
3.6	10.5	7.6	13.7	11.6	17.5
3.8	10.7	7.8	13.8	11.8	17.7
4.0	10.9	8.0	14.0	12.0	17.9

Adapted from Cunningham FG, Leveno KL, Bloom SL et al., editors: *Williams Obstetrics*, New York, 2005, McGraw Hill.

90% to 95% of fetuses with trisomy 21. Even in the absence of aneuploidy, an increased NT, especially in the form of a cystic hygroma, is still associated with anomalies, such as Noonan syndrome. These studies also demonstrated a significant association of increased NT with cardiac disease.

Ultrasound in the first trimester should always include evaluation of the maternal adnexa and careful assessment for the presence of pelvic masses and uterine anomalies. The corpus luteum of pregnancy, a normal finding, is easily visualized on first-trimester ultrasound and is characterized by a "ring" of Doppler-identified vascular flow in its periphery. Other masses, such as dermoid cysts and other ovarian tumors, can also be identified. Uterine leiomyomata

Figure 3-2

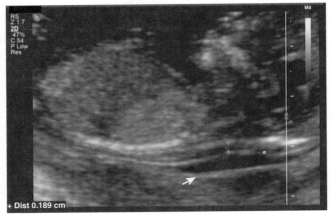

The nuchal translucency is measured in the mid-sagittal plane. The fetus occupies at least 75% of the image. The fetal neck is in a neutral position and the amnion is observed to be separate *(arrow)*. The measurement is taken at the widest place and the calipers are placed on the inner border.

Box 3-1   Indications for First-Trimester Ultrasound

To confirm the presence of an intrauterine pregnancy
To evaluate a suspected ectopic pregnancy
To define the cause of vaginal bleeding
To evaluate pelvic pain
To estimate gestational age
To diagnose or evaluate multiple gestations
To confirm cardiac activity
As an adjunct to chorionic villus sampling, embryo transfer, or localization and
    removal of an intrauterine device
To evaluate maternal pelvic masses or uterine abnormalities
To evaluate suspected hydatidiform mole

From ACOG Committee on Practice Bulletins: ACOG Practice Bulletin No. 58, Ultrasonography in pregnancy, *Obstet Gynecol* 104:1449-58, 2004 and American Institute of Ultrasound in Medicine: AIUM Practice guideline for the performance of an antepartum obstetric ultrasound examination, *J Ultrasound Med* 22(10):1116-25, 2003.

65

should be numbered and measured and their location clearly noted so that they may be followed during gestation as needed. The position of a gestational sac in a bicornuate or septate uterus should be assessed. Finally, the presence or absence of fluid in the cul-de-sac should be documented.

A summary of indications for first-trimester ultrasound is presented in Box 3-1.

SECOND AND THIRD TRIMESTERS

More than 80% of American women undergo at least one ultrasound during pregnancy, and the majority of these are performed in the second trimester. The value of routine ultrasound for all pregnant women has been debated extensively and is still controversial. Randomized and observational trials conducted in the 1980s and 1990s yielded conflicting results concerning the utility of routine ultrasound in pregnancy. Current American College of Obstetrics and Gynecologists (ACOG) recommendations do not mandate any specific number of ultrasound examinations for each pregnant woman but rather adhere to the guidelines put forth by the National Institutes of Health (NIH) in 1984. These indications are summarized in Box 3-2.

Estimation of Gestational Age

As mentioned previously, accurately assessing the gestational age during pregnancy is one of the obstetrician's key tasks. This becomes especially relevant in the second trimester, for example, with serum screening for aneuploidy. This screening is called the triple or quad screen and uses a combination of maternal serum alpha-fetoprotein, hCG, and unconjugated estriol, sometimes with the addition of inhibin. Screening for aneuploidy is totally dependent on its timing during pregnancy, and the most common cause of an abnormal quad screen is incorrect dating of pregnancy. Measurement of different anatomical landmarks, referred to as biometry, is used to estimate gestational age in the second trimester. This is then correlated to the EDD calculated by LMP. If biometry differs from LMP dating by more than 2 weeks in the mid-trimester, EDD based on biometry is favored. Measurements should always be correlated

---

Box 3-2 Indications for Ultrasonography in Pregnancy

Estimation of gestational age for patients with uncertain clinical dates, or verification of dates for patients who are to undergo scheduled elective repeat cesarean delivery, indicated induction of labor, or other elective termination of pregnancy

Evaluation of fetal growth

Vaginal bleeding of undetermined etiology in pregnancy

Evaluation of incompetent cervix

Abdominal and pelvic pain

Determination of fetal presentation

Suspected multiple gestation

Adjunct to amniocentesis

Significant uterine size and clinical dates discrepancy

Pelvic mass

Suspected hydatidiform mole

Adjunct to cervical cerclage placement

Suspected ectopic pregnancy

Suspected fetal death

Suspected uterine abnormality

Biophysical evaluation for fetal well-being

Suspected polyhydramnios or oligohydramnios

Suspected abruptio placentae

Adjunct to external version from breech to vertex presentation

Estimation of fetal weight or presentation in premature rupture of membranes or premature labor

Evaluation of abnormal serum screening value

Follow-up observation of identified fetal anomaly

Follow-up evaluation of placental location for identified "placenta previa"

History of previous congenital anomaly

Evaluation of fetal condition in late registrants for prenatal care

From ACOG Committee on Practice Bulletins: ACOG Practice Bulletin No. 58, Ultrasonography in pregnancy, *Obstet Gynecol* 104:1449-58, 2004 and American Institute of Ultrasound in Medicine: AIUM Practice guideline for the performance of an antepartum obstetric ultrasound examination, *J Ultrasound Med* 22(10):1116-25, 2003.

---

to previous ultrasound measurements if these are available—the earlier an ultrasound is performed, the more accurate it is in estimating gestational age. The measurements used for biometry include the following:

1. Biparietal diameter (BPD) and head circumference (HC). The level at which these measurements is obtained should include several landmarks, including the cavum septum pellucidum and the thalami, and is commonly referred to as the transthalamic view (Figure 3-3). The cerebellar hemispheres should not be visualized in this view. The BPD measurement is taken from the outer edge of the proximal bone to the inner edge of the bone on the opposite side. The HC is taken just outside the bony rim of the calvarium. The BPD is the most accurate method of estimation of gestational age in the second trimester, with a variation of only 7 to 10 days. However, the accuracy of the BPD is attenuated in cases in which the shape of the head varies. For example, the head may be flattened (dolichocephalic) in breech presentation or with oligohydramnios, falsely decreasing the BPD. The HC may be more accurate in this scenario.

Figure 3-3

The biparietal diameter (BPD) and head circumference (HC) at the transthalamic view. The *open arrow* is pointing to the thalami. The *closed arrow* indicates the cavum septum pellucidum.

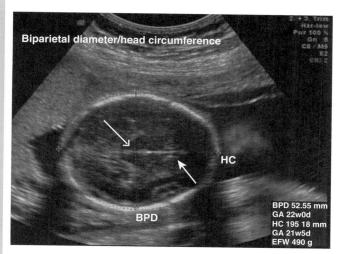

2. Femur length (FL). This measurement is used after 14 weeks' gestation. The femur should fill the screen and the distal femoral epiphyses should be visualized, although it is not included in the measurement (Figure 3-4). The calipers are placed on the outer surfaces of the femoral shaft. Variation in the measurement is 7 to 11 days.

3. Abdominal circumference (AC). A transverse, cross-sectional image of the abdomen is taken at the level of the stomach, portal vein, and the intrahepatic portion of the umbilical vein (Figure 3-5). This correlates with the largest transverse plane of the fetal abdomen. The circumference encircles the entire abdomen, including the skin, and may be taken either directly or indirectly by measuring two perpendicular planes and calculating the circumference. The AC has a wider variation than the above measurements, up to 2 weeks; however, it may be more sensitive in the diagnosis of fetal growth disturbances.

Figure 3-4

The femur length (FL).

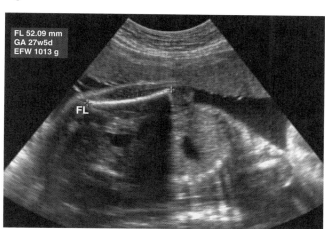

Figure 3-5

The abdominal circumference (AC). The *open arrow* indicates the portal vein and the *closed arrow* the stomach bubble.

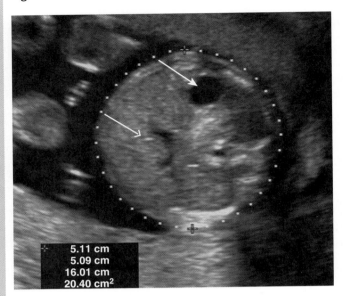

5.11 cm
5.09 cm
16.01 cm
20.40 cm²

Because of the variation and margin of error inherent in each of these independent measurements, a combination of measurements is more accurate than one alone. Formulas such as the Hadlock equation give an estimation of the gestational age based on the measurements supplied and how they predict the estimated fetal weight for that gestation. Moreover, serial measurements are more accurate than one single measurement.

Other anatomical measurements can also be used to assess gestational age. The transcerebellar diameter (TCD) in millimeters reflects the gestational age in weeks up to 24 weeks (Figure 3-6). After 24 weeks, the measurement correlates indirectly and, in cases in which gestational age is in question, it is helpful in giving an estimation. This is especially useful in cases in which the BPD cannot be used, such as with anencephaly and other disorders of the fetal calvarium. The interocular diameter is sometimes used and is obtained by moving caudally from the

Figure 3-6

Transcerebellar diameter (TCD) approximates gestational age when measured at less than 24 weeks' gestation. *CEREB*, cerebellum.

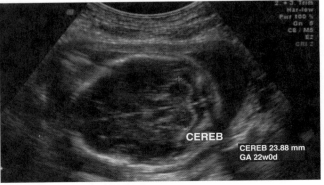

CEREB

CEREB 23.88 mm
GA 22w0d

BPD plane until the orbits are visualized. This plane is also useful for assessing symmetry of the eyes. The foot length can be used to estimate gestational age (Figure 3-7). This measurement is taken from the end of the first toe to the outer edge of the heel. Gestational age can also be estimated through measurement of the long bones of the fetal extremities, the most easily obtained being the humerus. Measurement of the distal bones can be more challenging because of fetal movement. Of these, the tibia is the favored measurement. The tibia and fibula are differentiated by the lateral position of the fibula. The ulna is seen to extend past the radius at the proximal joint, whereas they end together in the distal. Discrepancies between the growth of the long bones and growth of the head and/or abdomen may lead to the diagnosis of a skeletal dysplasia.

Estimation of Fetal Weight

Estimation of fetal weight is accomplished by applying formulas to the biometric measurements obtained during the ultrasound. The most common is the Hadlock formula, which incorporates HC, AC, and FL to give an estimated fetal weight within a 15% range of error. The estimated fetal weight (EFW) is then compared with established nomograms to give a percentile for growth by gestational age. Each ultrasound unit should use nomograms specific to its population, because there can be considerable variation by geographic and ethnic group.

Large for gestational age (LGA) refers to growth greater than the 90th percentile. Macrosomia is defined as weight greater than 4000 to 4500 g, regardless of gestational age, a point at which the risk of birth trauma increases greatly. Unfortunately, ultrasound estimates at these extremes of fetal weight have a greater range of variation than those in normally grown fetuses, up to 20%. In addition, clinical estimation of fetal weight (by abdominal examination and symphysiofundal measurement) is closely correlated to ultrasound estimation, and thus the utility of ultrasound in the management of macrosomia is still limited.

Small for gestational age (SGA) refers to growth at below the 10th percentile and may represent normal variations in growth potential. On the other hand, intrauterine growth restriction (IUGR), especially when seen in

Figure 3-7

Foot length measured from heel to toe.

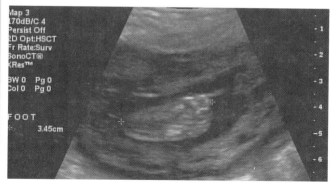

conjunction with oligohydramnios, implies pathology and is variably defined, with thresholds varying from the 3rd to the 10th percentile. Ultrasound has been used extensively in the management of fetuses with growth restriction. This topic is covered in Chapter 8.

Anatomical Survey

The components of the anatomical survey are outlined here. Transabdominal imaging is usually sufficient; however, transvaginal ultrasound may aid in the evaluation of an obese woman's fetus. If an anomaly is identified, a careful search for other abnormalities should be made. Common fetal anomalies are discussed in Chapter 7.

1. Head: The normal shape of the fetal head is an oval and is appreciated best at the level of the BPD (see Figure 3-3). A rim of bone should be seen around the entire head, thus excluding acrania or anencephaly. The structure of the brain is evaluated in the transverse, coronal, sagittal, and axial planes. The presence of midline structures and symmetry is ascertained. The transventricular views allows for assessment of the size and shape of the ventricles, as well as the appearance of each choroid plexus (Figure 3-8). Cysts are commonly seen within the choroid plexus in the midtrimester and may represent a normal variant. However, they are also seen more often in fetuses with trisomy 18, and a careful search should be undertaken for other findings associated with this disorder (see later). The midsagittal view allows for assessment of the corpus callosum, the major connection between the two hemispheres of the brain. In this view, it appears as a sonolucent band between two echogenic bands (Figure 3-9). Agenesis of the corpus callosum is often associated with other anomalies such as ventriculomegaly and some genetic syndromes, but its diagnosis antenatally can be very challenging. The transcerebellar view examines the posterior fossa contents: the dumbbell-shaped cerebellum, fourth ventricle, and cisterna magna (Figure 3-10, *A*).

   The ventricles are commonly measured at their atria. In the case of ventriculomegaly, defined as more than 2 to 4 SD from normal (usually >1 cm), the choroids may appear "dangling" or suspended from the walls of the ventricles. The most common causes of antenatally detected ven-

Figure 3-8

The posterior ventricle is measured at its atrium. The choroid plexus *(arrow)* appears homogenously echogenic. Note that the proximal ventricle is difficult to visualize because of shadowing from the cranium; this is the normal appearance.

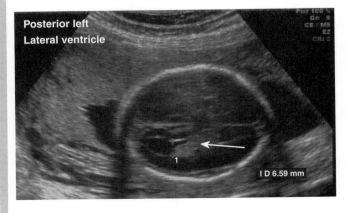

Figure 3-9

Midline sagittal image demonstrating the normal appearance of the corpus callosum *(arrow)*.

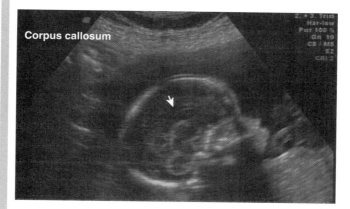

triculomegaly are neural tube defects, aqueductal stenosis, holoprosencephaly, and abnormalities of the fourth ventricle. Neural tube defects are associated with two abnormalities of the posterior fossa (Figure 3-10, *B*):

- The "lemon sign" refers to a triangular deformation of the head anteriorly, likely resulting from downward traction caused by the outward protrusion of the defect.
- The "banana sign" occurs when the cerebellar hemispheres are compressed and drawn down toward the upper spine resulting from this downward traction, also known as an Arnold-Chiari malformation.

Figure 3-10

A, The posterior fossa demonstrating the cerebellum, cisterna magna (CM), and nuchal fold (NF). **B,** The posterior fossa of a fetus with a neural tube defect. The "lemon sign" refers to the abnormal shape of the head. The "banana sign" *(arrow)* refers to the abnormal shape of the cerebellum. Compare with Figure 3-10A.

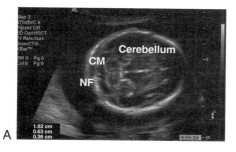

A

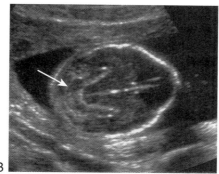

B

Holoprosencephaly refers to a spectrum of abnormalities resulting from abnormal or incomplete development of the prosencephalon, the embryonic forebrain. A single large ventricle with forebrain dysgenesis and abnormalities of the fetal face characterizes its most severe form, alobar holoprosencephaly (Figure 3-11). Aqueductal stenosis is usually a diagnosis of exclusion but may lead to progressive and severe dilation of the ventricles. The presence of cerebellar dysgenesis and dilation of the fourth ventricle, referred to as the Dandy-Walker malformation, may lead to compression of the third and fourth ventricle, with subsequent noncommunicating ventriculomegaly. This diagnosis is not made before the normal fusion of the cerebellar vermis, which occurs at approximately 18 weeks' gestation.

2. Neck: The nuchal thickness, the fold at the back of the neck, is measured from the calvarium behind the cisterna magna to the skin edge (see Figure 3-10, A). Its prominence (usually >5-6 mm) at a gestational age of less than 20 weeks is associated with aneuploidy (see later). Cystic hygroma refers to a particular kind of a thickened nuchal fold, which is made up of multiple cystic masses of differing size and shape (Figure 3-12). At least one third of fetuses with cystic hygroma will have other anomalies detectable by ultrasound. Another important cause of an increased nuchal fold may be as part of generalized skin and scalp edema, as seen in immune and nonimmune fetal hydrops.

3. Face: The fetal face, including the nose and lips, can be well visualized by imaging in multiple levels in the coronal and transverse planes (Figure 3-13). Facial clefts involving the palate, lips, or both are best seen in these views. The profile is seen in a sagittal plane and allows for the assessment of the nasal bone and the dimensions of the face (Figure 3-14). The absence of the nasal bone has been considered a marker of trisomy 21, although data in this regard are limited. The profile view is most important for the detection of micrognathia, which can be associated with a number of chromosomal and non-chromosomal anomalies. The discovery of facial anomalies leads to a

Figure 3-11

A case of alobar holoprosencephaly showing fusion of the thalami *(arrow)* and a single large ventricle. The cerebellum (measured) also appears abnormal.

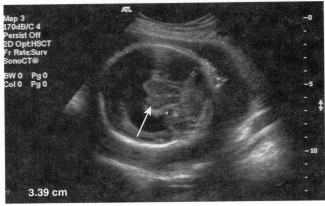

Figure 3-12

Cystic hygroma creating an increased nuchal fold. Compare with Figure 3-10, *B*. The *arrows* denote the cystic septations that characterize cystic hygromas.

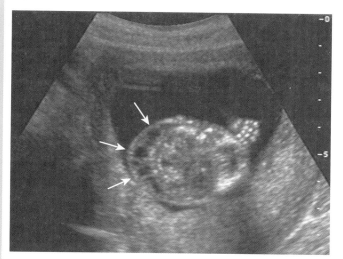

Figure 3-13

The fetal face—nose, lips, and chin.

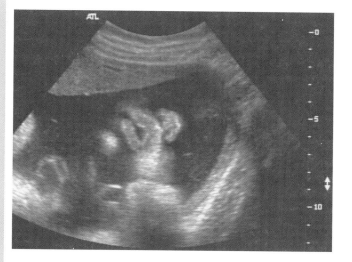

Figure 3-14

The fetal profile demonstrating a normal nasal bone *(arrow).*

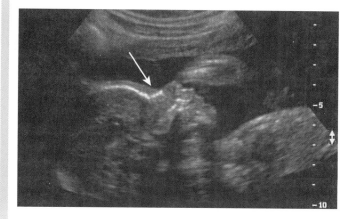

careful evaluation for other anomalies. In fact, the abnormalities of the face often reflect the abnormalities of the underlying intracranial structures—this is demonstrated best in the case of holoprosencephaly, characterized by disordered forebrain development and lack of midline structures. The fetal face in this case is also abnormal in the midline, as manifested by the presence of a single orbit (cyclopia) and abnormal noselike projection (proboscis), both in the midline.

4. Thorax: In the transverse view of the thorax, the ribs can be clearly visualized encircling the ovoid cavity (Figure 3-15). Abnormalities in the shape and size of the thorax are seen in most skeletal dysplasias. The fetal lungs are best seen after the first trimester. They are visualized as diffusely mildly echogenic areas on either side of the heart. However, in the presence of a congenital diaphragmatic hernia, the thoracic cavity may be filled with intraabdominal contents. To exclude this anomaly, a sagittal view can be obtained that demonstrates the heart and stomach on different sides of an intact diaphragm (Figure 3-16). Masses in the thoracic cavity are usually pulmonary in origin, most commonly cystic adenomatoid malformation (CAM) or bronchopulmonary sequestration. A feeding vessel from the systemic vasculature characterizes the latter.

The four-chamber view of the heart is taken in a transverse plane just superior to the diaphragm (see Figure 3-15). The heart should fill approximately one third of the thorax. The atrial and ventricular chambers should be assessed for size and shape—normally the two atria and the two ventricles are similar in size. The right ventricle is closer to the anterior chest wall, and the ventricular wall is slightly thicker, and the moderator band can be seen at the apex. The tricuspid valve is slightly closer to the apex of the heart than the mitral valve. The left atrium is closest to

Figure 3-15

The transverse view of the thorax with the four-chamber view of the heart. *Arrow* in the left ventricle.

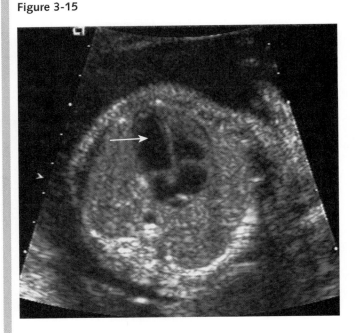

Figure 3-16

The diaphragm in the sagittal plane. The heart and stomach (Stom) are seen on either side.

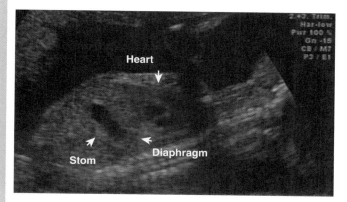

the fetal spine. An echogenic intracardiac focus (EIF) is a bright area, generally in the left ventricle but occasionally bilateral or right-sided, located just below the mitral or tricuspid valves (Figure 3-17). It maintains its echogenicity when the gain is brought down to a level that permits only the visualization of bone. An EIF has been associated with aneuploidy in some series (see later). The four-chamber view also allows for assessment of the cardiac axis, which should be 45 degrees to the left of the midline.

From the four-chamber view, the transducer is moved slightly toward the right fetal shoulder, bringing the left ventricular outflow tract (LVOT), or aortic outflow tract, into view (Figure 3-18). The interventricular septum should be seen continuing as the anterior wall of the aorta. Rotation from the LVOT back toward the other side brings the right ventricular outflow tract (RVOT) or pulmonary outflow tract into view (Figure 3-19). The LVOT and RVOT should be seen crossing each other. The aortic arch and the ductal arch can be identified in the sagittal and parasagittal planes (Figure 3-20, *A* and *B*). The aortic arch is commonly described as

Figure 3-17

Echogenic intracardiac focus (EIF, *arrow*) in the left ventricle. Its echogenicity is similar to that of the ribs.

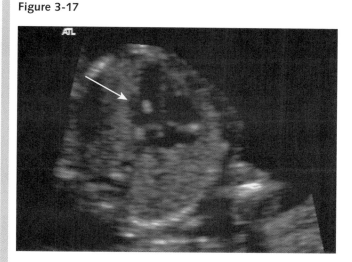

75

Figure 3-18

The left ventricular outflow tract (LVOT). The *arrow* is at the level of the aortic valve.

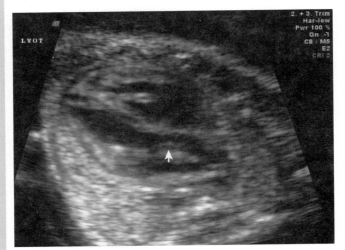

Figure 3-19

The right ventricular outflow tract (RVOT). The *arrow* is at the level of the pulmonary valve.

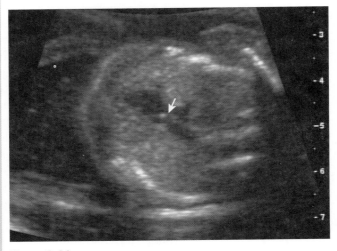

Figure 3-20

A, The aortic arch. The head vessels arising from the aorta are clearly demonstrated *(arrow).* **B,** The ductal arch.

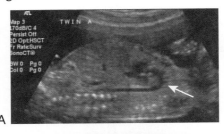

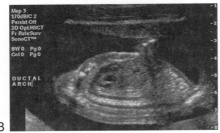

a candy cane, and the ductal arch resembles a hockey stick. Doppler imaging can be used to help identify these arches.

5. Abdomen: The gastrointestinal tract normally contains fluid and thus should be more easily visualized on ultrasound. The stomach should be seen on the left side of the body, and is visualized in virtually all fetuses after 14 weeks' gestation (see Figure 3-5). Inability to identify the stomach is because of a lack of fluid within it. This finding is associated with disorders such as tracheoesophageal fistulae and neurogenic disorders of fetal swallowing and should be investigated carefully. Conversely, duodenal atresia leads to obstruction and accumulation of fluid within the stomach and proximal duodenum (the "double bubble" sign). The appearance of the bowel should be assessed—hyperechoic bowel has been associated with anomalies such as cystic fibrosis, trisomy 21, and intrauterine hemorrhage.

Visualization of the insertion of the umbilical cord into the ventral wall rules out anomalies such as omphalocele and gastroschisis (Figure 3-21, A and B). The kidneys can be seen as paraspinous masses as early as 14 weeks (Figure 3-22). The renal pelves are measured in the anteroposterior diameter from a transverse view of the kidneys. The diagnosis of pyelectasis depends on the gestational age of the fetus, but is generally made when the anteroposterior (AP) diameter is greater than 4 mm. The bladder should be seen as a separate echolucent area in a sagittal plane that allows for concurrent visualization of the stomach. Obstruction in the urinary tract leads to fluid accumulation, readily seen on ultrasound as dilation. The level of the obstruction dictates the extent and location of the dilation.

Figure 3-21

A, Transverse view of the abdomen demonstrating the normal insertion of the umbilical cord *(open arrow)* into the ventral wall of the fetus. The *closed arrow* denotes the fetal spine. **B,** Sagittal view of the umbilical cord insertion *(open arrow).* The *closed arrow* denotes the fetal spine.

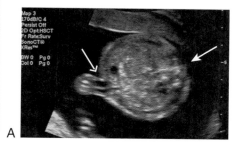

A

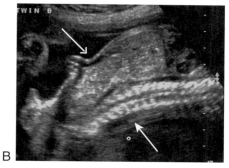

B

Figure 3-22

Transverse view of the abdomen at the level of the kidneys. The *arrows* show the renal pelves on either side of the fetal spine.

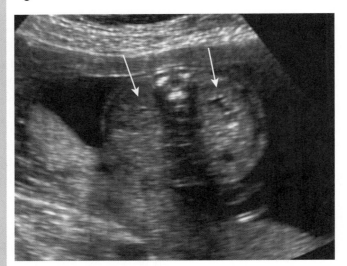

The adrenals can be appreciated just superior to kidneys. Color Doppler evaluation at the level of the bladder will show the two umbilical arteries on either side, diving posteriorly to join the iliac arteries (Figure 3-23).

6. Spine: The fetal spine should be examined throughout its cervical, thoracic, lumbar, and sacral regions (Figure 3-24). The sagittal plane allows for optimal evaluation of the skin overlying the spine. In a breech fetus, transvaginal ultrasound may be used to assess the sacral spine more completely. Ultrasound is very accurate in the identification of open neural tube defects, so much so that a search for a neural tube defect because of elevated maternal serum alpha-fetoprotein (MSAFP) usually ends with a negative ultrasound.

7. Extremities: All four limbs should be distinctly visualized on second-trimester ultrasound. The femurs are measured as described previously.

Figure 3-23

Color Doppler of the umbilical vessels dividing around the bladder *(arrow)*.

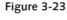

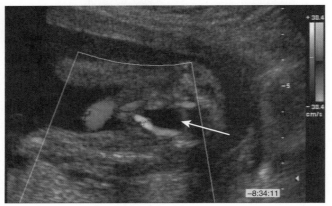

Figure 3-24

A sagittal image demonstrating the sacral, lumbar, and thoracic spine.

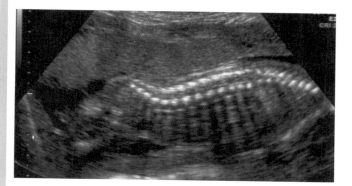

If a growth disorder is suspected, measurement of the distal long bones should be undertaken. Their growth is correlated with standard growth curves as well as with the expected growth for that particular fetus. The hands should be seen to open and close (Figure 3-25). Persistently clenched fists can be associated with aneuploidy (see later). The feet and lower legs are normally at right angles to each other. Loss of this relationship may indicate clubbing of the feet. Excessive edema of the feet, leading to abnormal curvature and a "rocker-bottom" appearance, is also associated with aneuploidy. The extremities should be seen moving freely with both extension and flexion positioning. Persistent positioning raises the suspicion of neurologic disorders such as arthrogryposis.

8. Gender: Depending on the fetal position, gender can often be identified in the second trimester. In multiple gestations, the identification of

Figure 3-25

Normal fetal hand. Each digit is visualized and the hand is open.

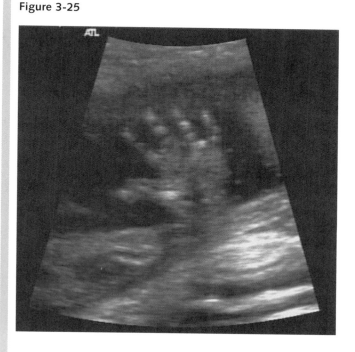

fetuses of differing gender confirms the diagnosis of dizygosity and dichorionicity.

Screening for Aneuploidy— The Genetic Sonogram

The finding of a major anomaly, such as a cardiac defect, overlapping fingers, micrognathia, omphalocele, and growth restriction (as seen in trisomy 13 or 18) greatly increases the risk of aneuploidy and is often an indication for more invasive testing, such as amniocentesis. However, over the years, a number of minor anomalies, referred to as "soft markers" have been associated to varying degrees with an increased risk of aneuploidy. A search for these ultrasound markers is undertaken at the time of second-trimester ultrasound, commonly referred to as the genetic sonogram. These markers are summarized in Table 3-2 and are more clearly defined previously. Because these soft markers alone are not sensitive for the detection of aneuploidy, they are used an adjunct to serum screening. Thus the combination of second-trimester serum screening and the genetic sonogram can identify 80% to 85% of fetuses with trisomy 21. Some, such as the increased nuchal thickness, are stronger predictors than others. Their presence modifies the patient's a priori risk of aneuploidy, that is, her risk before the ultrasound. The a priori risk may be based on age alone, although more often it is based on serum screening. The finding of a soft marker for aneuploidy may increase a patient's risk enough that she may seek more definitive testing, such as amniocentesis. Many authors believe that the utility of the genetic sonogram is the identification of fetuses at a lower risk of aneuploidy, in that the absence of any markers is associated with a decreased risk (0.22-0.6) for aneuploidy. Markers are only valid when identified before 20 weeks' gestation.

Assessment of Fetal Well-Being

Often the status of the fetus must be assessed in the third trimester. Different parameters are used to predict fetal well-being. The most basic is the amniotic fluid volume (AFV). This measurement varies by gestational age, and peaks in the thirty-fifth to thirty-sixth weeks of gestation. Three methods exist to estimate the AFV:

1. Maximum vertical pocket (MVP): The deepest pocket of amniotic fluid in the uterus is identified and measured vertically. A normal measurement is a pocket greater than 2 cm deep.
2. Amniotic fluid index (AFI): The uterus is divided into four quadrants. The deepest vertical pocket in each quadrant is measured in centimeters.

Table 3-2

Likelihood Ratio (LR) for Each Ultrasonographic Marker to Predict Trisomy 21 When Identified as an Isolated Abnormality

Marker	LR (95% CI)
Thickened nuchal fold	11 (5.5-22)
Echogenic bowel	6.7 (2.7-16.8)
Shortened humerus	5.1 (1.6-16.5)
Shortened femur	1.5 (0.8-2.8)
EIF	1.8 (1.0-3.2)
Renal pyelectasis	1.5 (0.6-3.6)

Adapted from Nyberg et al: Isolated sonographic markers for detection of fetal Down syndrome in the second trimester of pregnancy, *J Ultrasound Med* 20:1053, 2001. © American Institute of Ultrasound in Medicine.
CI, Confidence interval; *EIF*, echogenic intracardiac focus.

The sum of the measurements is equal to the AFI. Figure 3-26 shows the trend in AFI by gestational age.

3. Subjective assessment: A subjective assessment by an experienced sonologist or sonographer may be accurate in addition to the other methods of measurement of the fluid.

Both the MVP and the AFI are valid measures of AFV. The MVP is favored in multiple gestations in which division of each sac into four quadrants is more difficult. Figure 3-26 shows the change in AFI over gestation.

The AFV is one part of the biophysical profile (BPP), a five-part test of fetal well-being. The ultrasound parameters of the BPP are as follows:

1. Fetal movement
2. Fetal tone
3. Fetal breathing
4. AFV

The fifth parameter is the nonstress test (NST).

Evaluation of the Placental and Umbilical Cord

The position of the placenta is accurately assessed with ultrasound (Figure 3-27). Transvaginal ultrasound can exclude placenta previa definitively. Other disorders of the placenta, such as placental masses or abnormal cord insertions, can also be evaluated with ultrasound. Figure 3-28 shows a normal placental cord insertion. There is increasing interest in the use of ultrasound in the antenatal detection of placenta accreta. Sonography, however, is not useful in the assessment for placental abruption, a diagnosis that is made via clinical assessment.

The umbilical cord should be evaluated for number of vessels and for the presence of abnormal masses. The cord is made up of two arteries and one vein and these can be seen in cross section on ultrasound (Figure 3-29). Its insertion into the ventral wall of the fetus and into the placenta should be

81

Figure 3-26

Change in amniotic fluid index (AFI) over gestation. (From Cunningham FG, Leveno KL, Bloom SL et al., editors: *Williams Obstetrics*, ed. 22, New York, 2005, McGraw Hill. © The McGraw-Hill Companies, Inc.)

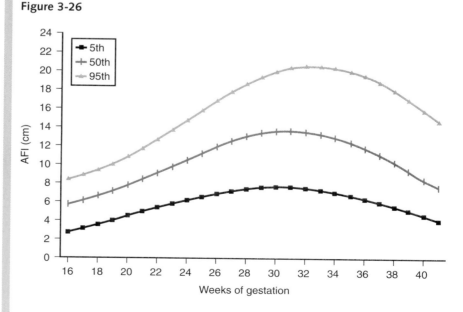

- 5th
- 50th
- 95th

AFI (cm)

Weeks of gestation

Figure 3-27

Abdominal ultra-sound of the placenta in the lower uterine segment. The cervix is clearly visualized and the placenta is not in its proximity.

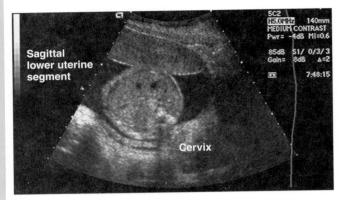

82

Normal umbilical cord insertion into the placenta.

Figure 3-28

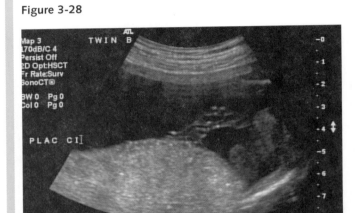
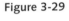

Figure 3-29

Cross section of the umbilical cord show-ing three vessels.

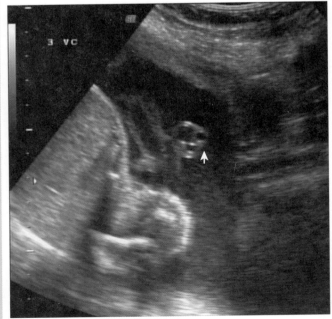

noted. A number of masses have been noted within the cord, including cysts, aneurysms, lymphangiomas, and varices. Doppler velocimetry of the cord is used in the evaluation of IUGR (see Chapter 8).

SUMMARY AND CONCLUSION

Box 3-3 summarizes the elements that should be evaluated and documented during ultrasound examinations performed in the second and third trimesters.

ACKNOWLEDGMENT

We gratefully acknowledge the contributions of Wendy Shaffer, RDMS, in collecting the images used in this chapter.

Box 3-3   **Elements of the Obstetric Ultrasound Examination**

83

Fetal life, number, and presentation
For multiple gestations, chorionicity
Placental location, appearance, and relationship to the internal os
Documentation of the number of vessels in the umbilical cord
Amniotic fluid volume, both subjective and objective measures
Gestational age and estimated fetal weight
Fetal anatomy, including, but not limited to, cerebral ventricles, spine, stomach, urinary bladder, umbilical cord insertion site, renal anatomy
Evaluation of the maternal uterus and adnexal structures

KEY POINTS

1. Ultrasound imaging is used throughout pregnancy and is the most commonly used diagnostic modality in pregnancy.

2. The basis of diagnostic ultrasound is that sound waves generated by a transducer composed of crystals of a piezoelectric material reflect off a target tissue and, on their return to that transducer, induce electrical signals that are interpreted as images composed of dots on a computer screen.

3. The frequency of the sound waves generated is measured in cycles per second, or Hertz (Hz): the higher the frequency, the better the resolution and image quality; lower frequency allows for better penetration.

4. No adverse effects of obstetric ultrasound on the developing fetus have been documented and ultrasound is considered to be safe in pregnancy. Ultrasound equipment includes two safety measures in its visual display: the thermal index and the mechanical index, which are both maintained at less than one.

5. In the first trimester, ultrasound is used for a number of indications, including confirmation of viability and location, surveillance of pregnancies conceived by assisted reproductive technologies, diagnosis of multifetal gestation and evaluation of the chorionicity of the gestation, establishing the estimated date of delivery (EDD), early evaluation of fetal anatomy, and screening for aneuploidy and structural malformations. The maternal adnexa should also be evaluated by ultrasound in the first trimester.

KEY POINTS—cont'd

6. Measurement of different anatomical landmarks, referred to as biometry, is used to estimate gestational age in the second trimester. The measurements used for biometry include the biparietal diameter (BPD), the head circumference (HC), the femur length (FL), and the abdominal circumference (AC).

7. Estimation of fetal weight is accomplished by applying formulas to the biometric measurements obtained during the ultrasound. The most common is the Hadlock formula, which incorporates HC, AC, and FL to give an estimated fetal weight within a 15% range of error.

8. The targeted antenatal ultrasound includes a complete anatomical survey including visualization, measurement, and characterization of the fetal head, neck, face, thoracic and abdominal cavities, spine, and extremities.

9. The genetic sonogram refers to the sonographic evaluation of the fetus in search for markers of aneuploidy, which may include major anomalies in addition to "soft markers," minor anomalies that have been associated to varying degrees with an increased risk of aneuploidy. Because these soft markers alone are not sensitive for the detection of aneuploidy, they are used an adjunct to serum screening.

10. Different parameters are used to predict fetal well-being via ultrasound in the third trimester. The most basic is the amniotic fluid volume (AFV), which is measured by maximum vertical pocket (MVP), amniotic fluid index (AFI), or subjective assessment.

11. The AFV is one part of the biophysical profile (BPP), a five-part test of fetal well-being. The ultrasound parameters of the BPP are fetal movement, tone, breathing, and AFV. The fifth parameter is the nonstress test (NST).

12. The position and appearance of the placenta and umbilical cord should be assessed during the ultrasound examination. Transvaginal ultrasound can exclude placenta previa definitively.

SUGGESTED READING

ACOG Committee on Practice Bulletins: ACOG Practice Bulletin #58: Ultrasonography in pregnancy, *Obstet Gynecol* 104:1449-58, 2004.

American Institute of Ultrasound in Medicine: AIUM practice guideline for the performance of an antepartum obstetric ultrasound examination, *J Ultrasound Med* 22(10):1116-25, 2003.

Benacerraf BR et al: Sonographic scoring index for prenatal detection of chromosomal abnormalities, *J Ultrasound Med* 11:449, 1992.

Bianchi DW, Crombleholme TM, D'Alton ME, editors: *Fetology: diagnosis and management of the fetal patient*, New York, 2000, McGraw-Hill.

Cunningham FG, Leveno KL, Bloom SL et al., editors: *Williams Obstetrics*, New York, 2005, McGraw Hill.

Hadlock FP et al: Estimation of fetal weight with the use of head, body and femur measurements—a prospective study, *Am J Obstet Gynecol* 151:333, 1985.

Malone FD et al: First-trimester or second-trimester screening, or both, for Down's syndrome, *N Engl J Med* 353:2068, 2005.

Nicolaides K: Screening for chromosomal defects, *Ultrasound Obstet Gynecol* 21:313, 2003.

Nyberg DA et al: Isolated sonographic markers for detection of fetal Down syndrome in the second trimester of pregnancy, *J Ultrasound Med* 20:1053, 2001.

Wapner R et al: First-trimester screening for trisomies 21 and 18, *N Engl J Med* 349:1405, 2003

ANOMALIES OF THE VENTRAL WALL

Ana Monteagudo and Ilan E. Timor-Tritsch

Defects of the ventral wall (abdominal wall defects) are relatively common malformations. The fetal anterior ventral (abdominal) wall can be consistently imaged from nine postmenstrual weeks. In cases of an isolated anomaly, good prognosis is usually the case. These anomalies are associated with increased maternal serum alpha-fetoprotein (MSAFP) and many come to light during the workup of an elevated study. In fetuses affected with these anomalies, a thick nuchal translucency is a common finding during the first trimester.

PHYSIOLOGIC MIDGUT HERNIATION

Up to the fourth to fifth week of development the embryo is relatively flat and subsequently begins to fold. Four folds occur: cephalic, caudal, and right and left lateral, which converge at the site of the umbilicus. The lateral folds will form the abdominal wall.

During this period there is also rapid growth of the intestines and the liver; this rapid growth results in the abdominal cavity temporarily becoming too small to accommodate all of its contents. During the sixth week of development (or 8 weeks from the last menstrual period), the bowel protrudes into the extraembryonic coelom of the umbilical cord. This temporary herniation is called the physiologic midgut herniation (PMH), which is sonographically evident between the ninth and eleventh postmenstrual weeks.

Reduction of the PMH occurs by the twelfth postmenstrual week. Beyond the twelfth week a midgut herniation is no longer physiologic; therefore, if present in a well-dated pregnancy, it should be considered pathologic (Figure 4-1). The diagnosis therefore should be a bowel-containing omphalocele.

In contrast to the fetal bowel, the liver does not follow a physiologic migration outside the abdominal cavity during development. Hence, the liver is never present in the PMH. If, however, the lateral folds fail to close, a large abdominal wall defect is created, through which the abdominal cavity contents, including the liver, can herniate. The result is a liver-containing omphalocele, which, because of the previously mentioned fact, can be diagnosed even before the twelfth postmenstrual week.

Figure 4-1

Physiologic midgut hernia. The hyper-echoic loops of bowel are seen within the root of the abdominal insertion of the cord at 10 postmenstrual weeks *(arrow)*.

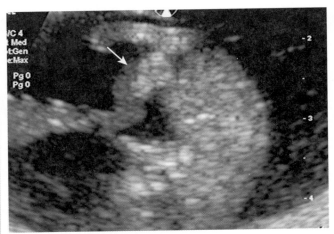

OMPHALOCELE

An omphalocele is a median abdominal wall defect in which the bowel has failed to return to the abdominal cavity and remains in the extraembryonic coelom of the umbilical cord. Of these, the simple bowel-containing ompha-locele is the most common. At times the liver may also be present within the omphalocele sac. The defect usually occurs at the level of the umbilical cord, with the cord inserting at the apex of the defect. The omphalocele is covered by peritoneum. Very rarely, the membrane covering the omphalocele may rupture during the pregnancy; if this happens it is difficult to separate it from a gastroschisis.

There are two types of omphalocele: *liver-containing* (or giant omphalocele) and *bowel* (nonliver)-*containing omphalocele*.

1. In the *bowel-containing omphalocele*, only bowel is present in the hernia. The sonographic diagnosis of this type of omphalocele can only be reli-ably made after 12 postmenstrual weeks, because before the twelfth week it is difficult to differentiate it from the PMH. In approximately 40% to 60% of the cases a chromosomal abnormality such as trisomy 18, 21, or 13 is present.

2. In the *liver-containing omphalocele*, both the bowel and the liver (or part of it) are present in the omphalocele sac. In cases of liver-containing omphalocele, the sonographic diagnosis can be made before the twelfth postmenstrual week. Sonographically, a liver containing omphalocele can be diagnosed during the first trimester, as early as 9 to 10 postmenstrual weeks, if a mass with the consistency of liver, measuring greater than 5 to 10 mm in diameter, is imaged within the area of the PMH (Figure 4-2). In contrast to the bowel-containing omphalocele, this type of an omphalocele is usually associated with a normal karyotype.

In addition to the chromosomal abnormalities, fetuses with omphalocele have other associated malformations. In as many as 50% of the cases a con-genital heart defect may be present, as well as a wide range of anomalies,

Figure 4-2

Two different fetuses with omphalocele. **A,** A liver-containing omphalocele diagnosed at 12 postmenstrual weeks and 4 days. **B,** In the sac of the hernia *(arrow)*, the bowel (B) and the liver (L) are seen side-by-side.

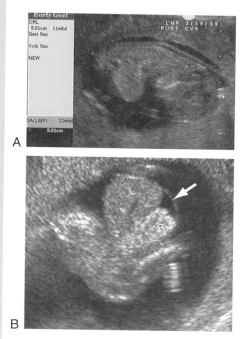

A

B

including gastrointestinal, genitourinary, neural tube defects, and intrauterine growth restriction. Also, in fetuses with increased nuchal translucency, even in the presence of normal chromosomes the prevalence of omphalocele is 10 times higher than in the general population.

Delivery by cesarean section is controversial; however, many pediatric surgeons recommend that all fetuses with omphalocele and an extracorporeal liver be delivered by cesarean section.

Approximately 4% of fetuses with omphalocele have Beckwith-Wiedemann syndrome (BWS). This syndrome encompasses a cluster of disorders that have in common the following features: omphalocele, macroglossia, visceromegaly, and neonatal hypoglycemia. This syndrome is caused by mutation in the chromosome 11p15.5 region (Figure 4-3). The mode of inheritance is complex. Possible patterns include autosomal dominant inheritance with variable expressivity, contiguous gene duplication at 11p15, and genomic imprinting resulting from a defective or absent copy of the maternally derived gene.

Figure 4-3

Beckwith-Wiedemann syndrome. **A,** The liver-containing omphalocele. Note the small amount of ascites surrounding the liver and clearly demonstrating the peritoneal covering. **B,** Macroglossia *(arrow)*.

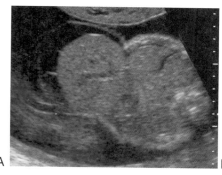

A

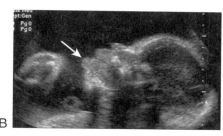

B

GASTROSCHISIS

Gastroschisis refers to a defect of the abdominal wall usually to the right of the umbilicus through which evisceration of the intestinal organs has occurred. It is theorized that gastroschisis is the result of a vascular compromise of either the umbilical vein or the omphalomesenteric artery. Gastroschisis has been diagnosed as early as the twelfth postmenstrual week (Figure 4-4). Gastroschisis, unlike omphalocele, is not associated with an increased incidence of chromosomal aneuploidy.

The fetus with gastroschisis, as well as the one with an omphalocele, should be followed with serial ultrasounds for (1) fetal growth; however, the abdominal circumference (AC) is of little value and other biometric parameters need to be used to assess growth; (2) amniotic fluid volume because oligohydramnios may occur; and (3) assessment of the bowel rigidity ("lead pipe" appearance), which may result from the exposure to the amniotic fluid, and assessment for bowel obstruction. Elective delivery by cesarean section is controversial.

The majority of infants with gastroschisis survive. The prognosis is usually good because it is not associated with chromosomal or other malformations. However, neonates with gastroschisis may have associated complications such as decreased bowel motility and obstruction. At times the exposed bowel has to be resected. Surgical replacement of the bowel into the abdominal cavity may take a multistaged approach.

Figure 4-4

Gastroschisis at 14 postmenstrual weeks. **A,** Note the hyperechoic bowel loops *(arrow)* not covered by membrane. **B,** On a horizontal (axial) section the hallmark features of the diagnosis of gastroschisis is evident. The bowel is extruded on the side of the normally inserting cord vessels *(arrow)*. **C,** A case of gastroschisis at 32 postmenstrual weeks. Note the free-floating cross sections of the bowel in the amniotic fluid.

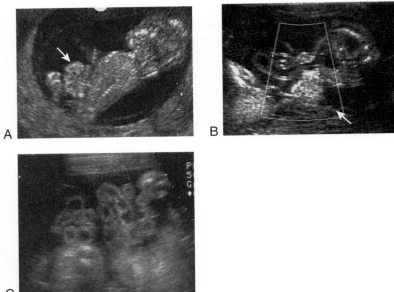

ECTOPIA CORDIS

Ectopia cordis is a rare and usually lethal defect. The heart is partly or completely exposed on the surface of the thorax. It results from failure of fusion of the lateral folds in the thoracic area during the sixth postmenstrual week. The diagnosis of ectopia cordis has been diagnosed and reported as early as the 12 to 14 postmenstrual weeks. It can be part of other, complex abnormalities.

PENTALOGY OF CANTRELL

Pentalogy of Cantrell is another rare and complex malformation in which ectopia cordis can occur as a result of a thoracoabdominal defect. The five anomalies encompassed in pentalogy of Cantrell are (1) median supraumbilical abdominal defect, (2) defect of the lower sternum, (3) deficiency of the diaphragmatic pericardium, (4) deficiency of the anterior diaphragm, and (5) intracardiac abnormality. This malformation has been diagnosed as early as the eleventh postmenstrual week. Pentalogy of Cantrell has been associated with trisomy 18, 13, and 21. In addition, cystic hygroma has also been reported with pentalogy of Cantrell. The prognosis for the fetus with pentalogy of Cantrell is poor.

89

SHORT UMBILICAL CORD SYNDROME (BODY STALK ANOMALY)

The short umbilical cord syndrome is a lethal and rare malformation, which occurs as a result of failure of fusion of the lateral folds that is believed to originate during the sixth postmenstrual week.

In this malformation the abdominal organs lie outside the cavity. The organs are contained within a sac, which is covered by amnioperitoneal membrane and is attached directly to the placenta. The umbilical cord in these cases may be totally absent or significantly shortened and severe kyphoscoliosis may be present. The limbs, face, and cranium are also affected (Figure 4-5). The anomaly can be diagnosed from the first to early second trimester of the pregnancy.

CLOACAL EXSTROPHY OR OEIS SYNDROME

Cloacal exstrophy is a rare anomaly. In some cases it may be fatal because of the severity of the anomalies. In milder forms corrective surgery is a possibility. The pathogenesis is the result of a lack of development of the urorectal septum and subsequent failure of the separation of the urogenital sinus from the rectum.

Multiple anomalies are usually present. Because of its association with the following anomalies, **O**mphalocele, **E**xstrophy of the bladder, **I**mperforate anus, and **S**pinal defects, the term OEIS syndrome at times is used to refer to this entity. The alpha-fetoprotein will be increased in both the maternal serum and the amniotic fluid, and the amniotic fluid acetyl cholinesterase level is increased as well. Prenatal diagnosis of this anomaly is possible from the early part of the second trimester of the pregnancy.

Figure 4-5

Body stalk (short cord) anomaly diagnosed at 12 weeks and 4 days. **A,** Oligohydramnios and large bladder is evident. **B,** The entire length of the two-vessel cord was 3.5 cm.

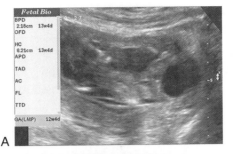

A

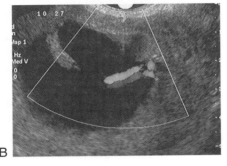

B

KEY POINTS

1. The physiologic midgut herniation can be imaged by ultrasound between the ninth and eleventh weeks of gestation.
2. Omphaloceles occur at the level of the umbilicus and usually are covered by peritoneum.
3. Gastroschisis is a right paraumbilical defect. The herniated bowel is not covered by peritoneum.
4. Maternal serum alpha-fetoprotein (MSAFP) is elevated in cases of abdominal wall defects.
5. Lethal defects of the abdominal wall include ectopia cordis and short umbilical cord syndrome.

SUGGESTED READING

Nyberg DA et al., editors: *Diagnostic imaging of fetal anomalies*, Philadelphia, 2003, Lippincott Williams & Wilkins, pp 507-602.

ANOMALIES OF THE FETAL FACE

Ana Monteagudo and Ilan E. Timor-Tritsch

Anomalies of the face can occur as an isolated finding but are often associated with chromosomal aneuploidy, such as trisomy 18 and 13, as well as nonchromosomal syndromes. In many instances when a brain anomaly is encountered, a facial anomaly is also seen. This is especially true when we are dealing with a brain anomaly such as holoprosencephaly (see Chapter 6). When a facial anomaly is imaged, a targeted scan of the fetus as well as genetic counseling and testing is indicated. In addition, no targeted fetal brain scan is complete without a careful evaluation of the fetal face.

For a full understanding of facial anomalies one should consult the classic textbooks of developmental embryology.

CLEFT LIP AND PALATE

Cleft lip not only is the most common facial anomaly but also is among the most common anomalies affecting the developing fetus, with a reported incidence of 1 per 1000 live births. In up to 80% of the cases, cleft lip is unilateral rather than bilateral, and most of the affected fetuses are male. Unilateral cleft lip is more commonly located on the left side. Developmentally, a continuous upper lip is formed by 8 weeks when the medial nasal and maxillary processes fuse. Failure of fusion of the medial nasal and maxillary processes will result in a cleft lip affecting one or both sides.

Cleft palate with or without cleft lip has a reported incidence of 1 in 2500 live births and more commonly affects female fetuses. The palate develops from the primary and the secondary palate. Its development starts at 7 postmenstrual weeks but is not complete until 14 postmenstrual weeks. Cleft palate results from failure of the mesenchymal masses in the lateral palatine process to fuse. Clefts may be unilateral or bilateral. Cleft lip and palate can be diagnosed during the early part of the second trimester.

In the literature, there are several sonographic markers that have been described to help in the detection of cleft lip:

1. The detection of an *echogenic median mass*, which actually is the premaxillary protrusion of the "curled-up" soft tissue (philtrum) present between the bilateral cleft (at times osseous and dental structures may be

Figure 5-1

A three-dimensional rendering of the face in a fetus with bilateral cleft lip.

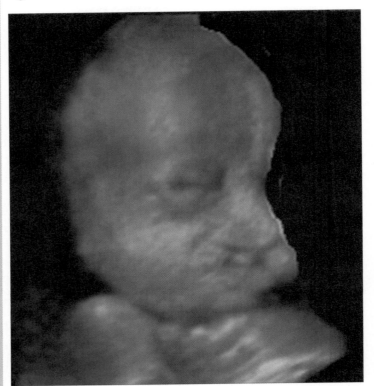

present within this mass as well). This mass can be imaged either in the median plane or in the coronal plane and can be especially useful in the second trimester to detect this anomaly.

2. A second sonographic marker is *pseudoprognathism*. This refers to a relative protrusion of the mandible as compared with the maxilla imaged on the sagittal or a paramedian section, which passes through the cleft lip and palate. This marker can be detected and used for the prenatal diagnosis of cleft lip from the early part of the second trimester.

At present, three-dimensional (3D) ultrasound is commonly used to image this defect (Figure 5-1). When this anomaly is imaged, genetic counseling and a search for other anomalies must be undertaken.

OCULAR ANOMALIES

Ocular anomalies affecting the developing fetus have been reported during the twelfth to eighteenth postmenstrual weeks using transvaginal sonography. Isolated anomalies affecting the developing fetal eye are rare, and in most cases anomalies are associated with other malformations, especially those of the developing brain (alobar holoprosencephaly) and with chromosomal aneuploidy (trisomy 13) and nonchromosomal syndromes.

Conditions such as hypertelorism and hypotelorism, anophthalmia, and microphthalmia have been diagnosed from 12 to 16 postmenstrual weeks by measuring the interocular distance, ocular diameter, and biocular distance. All of these measurements can be made in a single transverse section at the plane of the orbits.

Inner orbital diameter (IOD) is defined as the distance between the medial border of one orbit and the medial border of the opposite orbit.

Outer orbital diameter (OOD) is defined as the distance between the lateral border of one orbit and the lateral border of the opposite orbit.

Hypertelorism is defined as the orbits too far apart. In hypertelorism, the interorbital diameter (IOD) measurement falls above the 95th percentile, but the outer orbital diameter (OOD) is within the normal limits.

Hypotelorism is defined as the orbits too close together. In hypotelorism, both the IOD and the OOD fall two standard deviations below the mean.

Microphthalmia is defined as the orbital measurement below the 5th percentile for the gestational age.

Cyclopia is defined as fused orbits and is usually part of a complex anomaly such as holoprosencephaly.

THE FETAL LENS

The fetal lens can be imaged consistently from the twelfth postmenstrual week. The sonographic appearance of the normal lens is that of a hyperechogenic ring with a sonolucent core located within the fetal orbits. The lens is best viewed in an anterior coronal section of the face. The hyaloid artery can be seen posterior to the lens as a thin echogenic line between the lens and the posterior aspect of the lens. The hyaloid artery is best imaged in a paramedian section through the orbits. This artery regresses completely after 25-29 postmenstrual weeks. If persistently seen, brain anomalies or trisomy 21 should be ruled out.

Fetal cataracts or opacification of the lens has been diagnosed in utero. Congenital cataracts are commonly inherited in an autosomal dominant fashion, but are also the result of in utero infections, especially rubella, during the sixth to ninth postmenstrual weeks. The lens affected with cataracts no longer has its typical sonographic appearance of a hyperechogenic ring with a clear anechoic center, but it has a variety of appearances such as a thick, irregular, or crenated border; a dense homogenous echogenic center; or clusters of hyperechogenic material. Using these sonographic appearances, congenital cataracts have been diagnosed from the early part of the second trimester. In a fetus we scanned that was at risk for autosomal dominant cataracts (50% chance), we were able to diagnose the cataracts during the twelfth week of pregnancy.

KEY POINTS

1. The majority of cases of cleft lip are unilateral left-sided defects.
2. Cleft lip and palate can be diagnosed during the second trimester of the pregnancy using sonography.
3. Ocular anomalies are commonly associated with brain malformations as well as chromosomal and nonchromosomal syndromes.
4. Congenital fetal cataracts can be diagnosed in utero using sonography.
5. Three-dimensional ultrasound is useful in the evaluation and counseling of patients carrying fetuses with cleft lip and palate.

SUGGESTED READINGS

Benacerraf BR: *Ultrasound of fetal syndromes*, New York, 1998, Churchill Livingstone, pp 1-10, 360-1.

Nyberg DA et al. editors: *Diagnostic imaging of fetal anomalies*, Philadelphia, 2003, Lippincott Williams & Wilkins, pp 335-379.

Timor-Tritsch IE, Monteagudo A, Cohen HL, editors: *Ultrasonography of the prenatal and neonatal brain*, ed 2, New York, 2001, McGraw-Hill, pp 107-111, 277-313, 315-329.

6

ANOMALIES OF THE FETAL CENTRAL NERVOUS SYSTEM

Ana Monteagudo and Ilan E. Timor-Tritsch

Prenatal diagnosis of fetal anomalies was made possible thanks to ultrasound. Over the last 30 years sonographically aided prenatal diagnosis has moved slowly from the third to the early part of the second trimester and, in certain cases, into the first trimester of the pregnancy. This evolution (or revolution) is the result of the ever-changing and improving ultrasound technology available to examine the fetus. Currently, we are able to scan the fetal central nervous system (CNS) using transabdominal sonography (TAS), transvaginal sonography (TVS), three-dimensional sonography (3D), real-time three-dimensional sonography (4D), and Doppler techniques for the interrogation of vessels.

CNS ANOMALIES

Neural Tube Defects

Neural tube defects (NTDs) occur as a result of failure of the neural tube to close. The resulting defect can occur anywhere along the neural tube, and the spectrum of the defects ranges from anencephaly to sacral spina bifida. NTDs occur in approximately 1.4 to 2 per 1000 pregnancies. However, there are fluctuations in the incidence as a function of both genetic background and nutritional status. To prevent these defects, it is recommended that all women capable of becoming pregnant should consume 400 μg of folic acid daily. If a woman has had a prior child with an NTD or belongs to a high-risk group, the recommended dose of folic acid is 4 mg daily.

Maternal Serum Alpha-Fetoprotein (MSAFP)

In the United States, all pregnant women are routinely offered screening with MSAFP for NTDs at 16 to 18 postmenstrual weeks. Among low-risk women, MSAFP screening results in the detection of 80% to 90% of cases of fetal open NTDs. MSAFP levels are expressed as multiples of the normal median (MoM). An abnormal value is one that exceeds 2.5 MoM. Elevated MSAFP levels are associated with NTDs and a variety of other conditions. The higher the MSAFP, the more likely that the fetus will be affected with an anomaly. The AFP molecule enters the amniotic fluid via fetal urination, gastrointestinal tract secretions, or transudation from exposed blood vessels. It enters the maternal circulation by either diffusion across the placenta or diffusion across the amnion. In the normal pregnancy, the highest concentrations of AFP are found within the fetal serum (measured in milligrams), with the next highest value in the amniotic fluid (measured in micrograms), and the lowest concentration in the maternal serum (measured in nanograms). To adequately assess the MSAFP values, knowledge of an accurate fetal age is necessary. This is important to note because even in the event of an open NTD the concentration of AFP in the amniotic fluid will decrease with advancing gestational age; such a decrease may place the value in the range of a normal but much younger fetus.

Open neural tube defects are those in which the neural tissue is exposed and covered only by the thinnest of membranes; therefore the lesion is directly in contact with the amniotic fluid. In these cases, the AFP will be abnormally increased in the both the amniotic fluid and in the maternal serum (MSAFP).

Closed neural tube defects are those in which the defect is covered by skin or a thick membrane. Therefore the neural tissue is not in direct contact with the amniotic fluid. The AFP cannot freely diffuse across the lesion; therefore the MSAFP level will be within normal limits. In these cases the prenatal diagnosis is established when an abnormality is detected during the ultrasound examination.

Exencephaly-Anencephaly

Exencephaly-anencephaly is part of the spectrum of the open NTDs. The initial event in this sequence is *dysraphia*, or failure of the neural groove to close in the rostral region. This results in *exencephaly (acrania)*, in which the well-developed brain is exposed to amniotic fluid. As the result of this abnormal exposure, the unprotected brain sloughs off into the amniotic fluid, leading to *anencephaly* in the fetal period.

Exencephaly, or acrania, can be diagnosed by ultrasound during the first trimester (has been reported as early as the twelfth postmenstrual week). Using transvaginal sonography, the integrity of the fetal cranium and the amount of ossification can be determined early because ossification of the cranium begins and subsequently accelerates after the ninth postmenstrual week of development. The first trimester exencephalic fetus has an abnormally shaped head with anechoic spaces within the disintegrating brain. The outer shape of the head is often bilobed; this appearance has been compared with the shape of the head of Mickey Mouse (Figure 6-1, *A* and *B*).

Beyond the first trimester, the fetal facial bones, the lack of the cranium, and the exposed heterogeneous brain becomes more obvious and the "classical" appearance of anencephaly is seen.

Anencephaly is the most common of the NTDs, occurring in about 1 per 1000 births, and is always an open defect. The malformation is characterized by partial or total absence of the brain in conjunction with a missing cranial vault. Anencephaly, similarly to exencephaly, is a lethal malformation. In pregnancies that proceed beyond the first trimester, polyhydramnios

Figure 6-1

Exencephaly at 11 postmenstrual weeks. **A**, The head is abnormally shaped. Due to the absent cranium, the brain is exposed. **B**, This is a three-dimensional (3D) reconstruction of the same fetus.

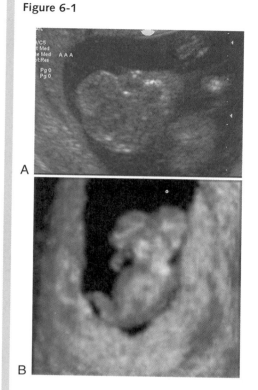

A

B

develops in about a half of the cases because of decreased fetal swallowing. Using sonography, especially TVS, the anencephalic fetus can be definitively identified by the end of the first trimester (twelfth postmenstrual week), although in some cases this diagnosis has been made earlier, at 9 to 10 postmenstrual weeks. When measuring the crown-rump length (CRL), these fetuses usually have size-date discrepancy or they measure below the fifth percentile for the gestational age.

Iniencephaly

Iniencephaly is a rare, lethal developmental anomaly. By many it is considered more as an anomaly of the upper cervical spine and the occipital bone than a CNS anomaly. Its three main features are a *defect in the occiput* involving the foramen magnum; retroflexion *of the entire spine*, which forces the fetus to look upward with its occiput directed toward the lumbar region; and *open spinal defects* of variable degrees. Associated malformations are common and include hydrocephaly, microcephaly, ventricular atresia, holoprosencephaly, polymicrogyria, agenesis of the cerebellar vermis, occipital encephalocele, diaphragmatic hernia, thoracic cage deformities, urinary tract anomalies, cleft lip and palate, omphalocele, and polyhydramnios. Sonographic findings are as follows: on the median plane the head appears large and held in retroflexion, the neck is not visualized, and the spine is usually lordotic. In some cases, a posterior cephalocele may be present in the occipital area; on transverse sections the U-shaped vertebrae typical of an open spinal defect is evident. On axial sections the head circumference may be several standard deviations below the mean and consistent with microcephaly. Biometry, in well-dated pregnancies, will show a size-date discrepancy. The sonographic diagnosis can be made from the late first to the early second trimester.

Cephalocele (Encephalocele)

Cephaloceles are usually midline cranial defects in which there is herniation of the brain and/or its meninges through a defect in the skull. When the cephalocele sac contains brain tissue, it is termed an encephalocele; if only cerebrospinal fluid (CSF) is present, it is referred to as a meningocele.

The cephalocele may involve the occipital, frontal, parietal, orbital, nasal, or nasopharyngeal region of the head. They are usually isolated lesions, but in a small percentage of cases they may be a part of a nonchromosomal or chromosomal syndrome. The typical sonographic appearance of a cephalocele is a defect of the bony skull with a protruding saclike structure. The sac may be anechoic and contain only contain CSF or may contain brain tissue or a combination of both (Figure 6-2). Similar to exencephaly-anencephaly, sonographic diagnosis can be made from the late first to the early second trimester.

Meckel or Meckel-Gruber syndrome (MGS) is an autosomal recessive condition mapped to chromosome 17 in which a cephalocele is often seen. Because of its 25% recurrence rate it is important to distinguish this syndrome from sporadic occipital cephaloceles, which may carry only a 1% to 3% recurrence rate. The classical triad of Meckel syndrome involves an *occipital cephalocele, bilateral polycystic kidneys,* and *postaxial polydactyly.* To make the diagnosis of MGS, at least two of the three major signs must be present. Of the three, the cystic dysplastic kidneys are the most consistent anomaly. The kidneys are enlarged up to 10 to 20 times larger than normal, are hyperechogenic, and contain multiple small cysts measuring between 2 and 5 mm. The dysplastic kidneys have impaired renal function; therefore oligohydramnios is present. The oligohydramnios resulting from the bilateral dysplastic kidneys in turn results in pulmonary hypoplasia; therefore, MGS is a lethal anomaly. Prenatal diagnosis of MGS can be made during the first and early second trimesters of the pregnancy.

Figure 6-2

Posterior cephalocele. Brain tissue is extruding through the bony skull through an opening in the parieto-occipital fissure.

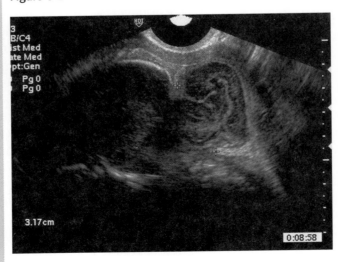

Walker-Warburg syndrome (WWS) is another autosomal recessive syndrome in which a cephalocele may be present. The sonographic features of WWS are lissencephaly (smooth brain), cerebellar hypoplasia, and Dandy-Walker cyst and ocular abnormalities. The Dandy-Walker malformation (DWM) and the ventriculomegaly are common findings. Both usually become evident at around 15 to 17 postmenstrual weeks. In contrast, lissencephaly can be suspected before but can only be diagnosed reliably after the twenty-eighth week of gestation because the normal fetal brain is relatively smooth (no gyri and sulci, only some of the fissures) until 28 to 32 weeks, when rapid brain growth occurs. Other sonographic findings include polyhydramnios and intrauterine growth restriction (IUGR) (Figure 6-3, A through D).

Figure 6-3

Walker-Warburg syndrome—the features of the syndrome. **A,** The posterior fossa shows the Dandy-Walker malformation. **B,** Posterior encephalocele. **C,** Ventriculomegaly. **D,** Lissencephaly.

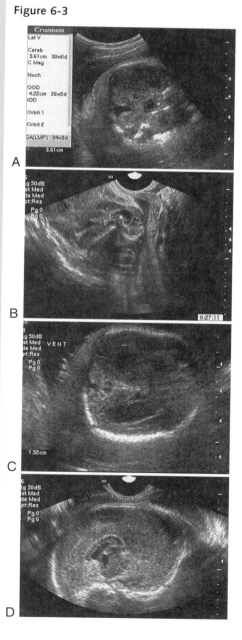

The prognosis for the neonate/infant with WWS is poor because these infants are profoundly mentally retarded. They usually die within the first year of life.

Spinal Dysraphism

Spinal dysraphism or spina bifida is characterized by an open NTD with protrusion of the spinal contents through a bony defect. The incidence of myelomeningocele in the United States is 0.2 to 0.4 per 1000 live births. *Myelocele* refers to a midline plaque of neural tissue (neural placode) that is flush with the surface and is not covered by skin. In contrast, *myelomeningocele* is a bulging defect in which the elevated neural plate and meninges are contiguous laterally with the subcutaneous tissue. Ten percent to 15% of spinal dysraphic defects are closed, and normal skin covers the bony defect. Therefore these defects will not result in an elevated MSAFP. Most lesions (80%) occur in the lumbar area of the spine, with the cervical and sacral areas accounting for the rest (about 20%).

Ultrasound has a high sensitivity (greater than 80%-90%) to diagnose spinal defects even without knowledge of the MSAFP results. The clues to the sonographic diagnosis are (1) on the sagittal view, irregularities of the bony spine may be seen, with a bulging within the posterior contour of the fetal back or obvious disruption of the fetal skin contours (Figure 6-4, *A* and *B*); (2) on transverse sections, the open vertebrae has a U-shape; and (3) in the coronal section, the affected bony segment shows a divergent configuration replacing the normal parallel lines of the normal vertebral arches. The sonographic diagnosis can be made from the early second trimester.

Figure 6-4

Spina bifida. **A,** The sagittal section of the sacral spine shows the meningocele sac covered with skin; therefore the maternal serum alpha-fetoprotein (MSAFP) was within the normal range. **B,** Three-dimensional surface rendering of the lesion. This picture may be important during the counseling session with the parents. In addition, it may aid the pediatric neurosurgeon to understand the extent of the lesion.

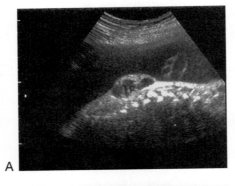

A

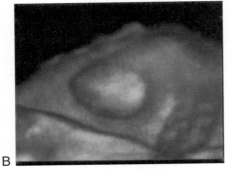

B

Determining the site and the extent of the spinal lesion is important because it correlates with the neurologic outcome of the fetus. The higher and larger the lesion, the more severe the neurologic dysfunction the neonate will have. A volume can be obtained with 3D ultrasound, and the transparency or x-ray display can be used to easily image the skeleton. The ribs can be counted, and, using the twelfth rib as a reference, the location and extent of the defect can be determined.

Additional clues to spinal defects can be found in the fetal head, namely, *"the lemon sign"* (depression of the frontal bones on an axial section of the head), *"the banana sign"* (the curved appearance of the impacted cerebellum with obliteration of the cisterna magna), and hydrocephaly (Figure 6-5, *A* through *B*). The lemon sign is present in virtually all cases between 16 to 24 postmenstrual weeks, but after 24 weeks of gestation the lemon sign is a less reliable marker of spinal defect. The banana sign is present in almost all cases of spinal dysraphism; however, after 24 postmenstrual weeks cerebellar absence is more commonly seen.

Arnold-Chiari type II malformation refers to the combination lemon sign plus the banana sign plus hydrocephaly in conjunction with a spinal defect. It is present in almost every case of thoracolumbar, lumbar, and lumbosacral myelomeningocele. The hydrocephaly probably results from either the hindbrain malformation that blocks the flow of CSF through the fourth ventricle or posterior fossa or from aqueductal stenosis that is often seen in these cases.

Other brain or spinal abnormalities that may be seen with myelomeningocele include relative microcephaly, agenesis of the corpus callosum (AGCC), diastematomyelia, congenital scoliosis or kyphosis, and hip deformities.

Figure 6-5

The cranial signs of spina bifida. **A,** The "lemon" shaped skull with the typical indent at the temporal bone *(arrows).* **B,** The impacted cerebellum assumes the shape of a banana, hence the term "banana sign."

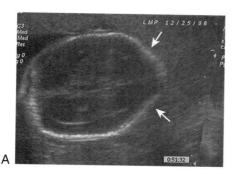

A

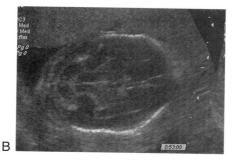

B

Congenital Hydrocephaly

Ventriculomegaly is defined as dilatation of the ventricular system in the presence of normal fetal intraventricular pressures not secondary to atrophy of the brain. It is accepted that the transverse diameter of a fetal lateral ventricle, when measured in the axial plane at the level of the glomus of the choroid plexus using transabdominal sonography, is normal up to 10 mm. Between 10 and 13 mm it is considered to be borderline in size. Some allow the upper limit to be 15 mm and still consider borderline ventriculomegaly. Beyond 15 mm is clearly an abnormal measurement.

Hydrocephaly is defined as dilatation of the ventricular system resulting from an increased amount of CSF with increased intraventricular pressures with or without enlargement of the cranium not secondary to atrophy of the brain. Usually the ventricle size is greater than 15 mm. In addition to the increased size of the lateral ventricle, the choroid plexus becomes thin and floats within the dilated ventricle ("dangling choroid plexus sign") (Figure 6-6, A and B).

Hydrocephaly can be grouped into two general types; namely, the noncommunicating and the communicating types.

Noncommunicating hydrocephaly refers to the fact that there is an obstruction of the CSF flow leading to the ventricular dilatation above the obstruction. Aqueductal stenosis is the most common form of the noncommunicating hydrocephaly. This can be the result of genetic diseases, infections, space-occupying lesions, or exposures to teratogens and accounts for about half of the cases of hydrocephaly. DWM accounts for 13% of the noncommunicating cases of hydrocephaly.

Communicating hydrocephaly, the hydrocephaly resulting from extraventricular causes, is the second most common cause of hydrocephaly,

Figure 6-6

Ventriculomegaly. **A,** An axial section reveals the extreme dilation of the lateral ventricles, both measuring more than 18 mm. The dangling choroid is also seen *(arrow)*. **B,** A parasagittal section reveals the dilatation of all three horns of the lateral ventricle.

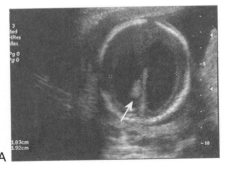

A

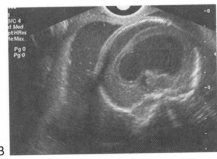

B

accounting for about a third of all cases. In this general group, Arnold-Chiari malformation, encephalocele, and congenital absence of the arachnoid granulations are among the causes of hydrocephaly. Also in this group are other less common causes of hydrocephaly such as AGCC, arachnoid cysts, and aneurysm of the vein of Galen. Polyhydramnios is present in 30% of the cases of hydrocephaly.

The prognosis for fetuses with ventriculomegaly or hydrocephaly depends on the presence or absence of associated anomalies or chromosomal aneuploidy. Associated anomalies are common and can be intracranial as well as extracranial. Of the extracranial anomalies, cardiac anomalies have been reported in approximately 20% of fetuses. In the presence of other cranial or extracranial anomalies, the prognosis for the fetus/neonate may be poor depending on the severity of the associated anomaly, and developmental delay may range from mild to severe, again related to the presence or absence of other anomalies.

The prognosis for isolated borderline hydrocephaly or mild ventriculomegaly (lateral ventricles measuring between 10-15 mm) is good in most cases, with minimal or mild developmental delays seen in the minority of the cases.

The recommended workup for ventriculomegaly or hydrocephaly should include genetic counseling with an amniocentesis to rule out chromosomal abnormalities, a detailed anatomical survey, viral titers to rule out infection (cytomegalovirus [CMV] and toxoplasmosis), and serial scans to reassess the intracranial anatomy and determine if the finding is persistent or progressive.

Midline Anomalies

Holoprosencephaly

Holoprosencephaly is a malformation sequence that results from failure of the prosencephalon to differentiate into the cerebral hemispheres and lateral ventricles between the fourth to eighth postmenstrual weeks. In holoprosencephaly a spectrum of the anomalies exists, which ranges from a complete failure of cleavage of the prosencephalon to partial failure, namely *alobar, semilobar,* and *lobar holoprosencephalies.* In addition to the brain malformation, variable degrees of facial dysmorphism may be present. Microcephaly may be present in all three types of holoprosencephaly.

Alobar holoprosencephaly is the most severe type. The malformation consists of a lack of the normal midline structures. The ultrasound reveals a single brain ventricle with absence of the falx cerebri. A single undivided thalami is apparent. There is AGCC and cavum septi pellucidi. The brain itself is small. The face may reveal severe facial dysmorphism that includes hypertelorism, midline facial defect(s), cyclopia, ethmocephaly, and cebocephaly. This type of holoprosencephaly can be reliably diagnosed during the first trimester (Figure 6-7, *A* through *C*).

Semilobar holoprosencephaly is characterized by some degree of brain cleavage. The ultrasound findings are not as striking as those of the alobar type and include posterior, partially separated lateral ventricles and cerebral hemispheres. There are partially fused thalami. On the coronal plane the choroid plexus covers the thalami in a contiguous fashion, looking like a "mustache." Anteriorly a single ventricular cavity is evident. The face

Figure 6-7

Alobar holoprosencephaly. **A,** Note the fused thalami *(arrow)*. **B,** The proboscis is one of the signs of the malformation *(arrow)*. **C,** Three-dimensional rendering of the face. The only orbit *(arrow)* is seen below the proboscis *(double arrow)*.

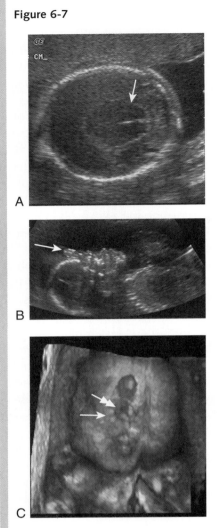

may reveal some degree of facial dysmorphism such as hypertelorism and midline facial defects. Semilobar holoprosencephaly can be diagnosed during the later part of the first trimester and definitively during the early part of the second trimester.

Lobar holoprosencephaly sonographically is the most difficult type of holoprosencephaly to diagnose because of its subtle findings. Sonographically on the mid coronal plane the interhemispheric fissure and the falx cerebri are present; the corpus callosum may be absent, hypoplastic, or normal; the septum pellucidum is absent; and there may be midline fusion of the cingulate gyrus. The frontal horns are fused and have a flat roof that freely communicates with the third ventricle. Lobar holoprosencephaly cannot be diagnosed during in the first trimester; its diagnosis has to wait until about the twentieth week because its most consistent feature, the absence of the cavum septum pellucidi, cannot reliably be imaged before that time of the pregnancy. Its most important differential diagnostic entity is septo-optic dysplasia.

Agenesis of the Corpus Callosum and Cavum Septi Pellucidi

Agenesis of the corpus callosum (AGCC) can be *complete or partial*, depending on the stage of development at which growth was arrested. The corpus callosum begins to develop anterior to the interventricular foramina (Monroe) during the later part of the first trimester (about 12 weeks of gestation). Then it grows upward and backward, in a C shape, as the primitive cerebral hemispheres grow laterally and then posteriorly. By 19 to 20 weeks' gestation the entire corpus callosum can be sonographically imaged. The total or partial lack of this structure can occur as an isolated anomaly; however, 80% of the cases have other associated malformations. Most cases of AGCC are sporadic, but several genetic disorders and chromosomal disorders have been associated with it. Partial AGCC usually involves its posterior portion because of its embryologic development and may also be associated with other malformations.

Sonographic diagnosis of AGCC is made when complete absence of the corpus callosum is imaged on a median section of the brain (Figure 6-8, *A* and *B*). On the median section the gyri and sulci have an abnormal structural pattern in which they appear to be radiating in a perpendicular fashion from the dilated third ventricle in a "sunburst" pattern. When color Doppler is applied looking at the median plane, the pericallosal artery, which usually hugs the superior aspect of the corpus callosum, is absent as well (Figure 6-8, *C* and *D*). On an oblique section the frontal horns appear narrow and laterally displaced, and the atria and occipital horns appear slightly dilated (colpocephaly). The coronal section demonstrates a wide interhemispheric fissure that communicates with the third ventricle, the lateral ventricles are widely separated and have a distinctive configuration similar to the horns on a "viking helmet," and the thalami are widely separated because of the dilated third ventricle. The cavum septi pellucidi in cases of complete AGCC is absent (see Figure 6-8, *B*).

Agenesis of the cavum septi pellucidi may occur as an isolated abnormality or associated with other brain malformations such as septo-optic dysplasia (de Morsier syndrome), holoprosencephaly, Chiari type II malformation, and abnormalities of the corpus callosum. The sonographic finding of the absent cavum septi pellucidi on the coronal section appears as a box-shaped hypoechoic area just below the corpus callosum, similar to the sonographic picture of lobar holoprosencephaly.

Dandy-Walker Malformation

DWM results from a cystic dilatation of the fourth ventricle with dysgenesis or complete agenesis of the cerebellar vermis and, often associated hydrocephaly. Evidence suggests that DWM represents a complex developmental anomaly of the fourth ventricle occurring around the sixth to seventh postmenstrual week, which accounts for the concurrent anomalies present in this syndrome. The incidence of DWM has been estimated to be 1 in 30,000 births. DWM may occur as part of a mendelian disorder (i.e., Meckel syndrome), can be associated with chromosomal aneuploidy (i.e., 45 X, triploidy), can result from environmental exposures (i.e., rubella, alcohol), can be multifactorial (i.e., congenital heart defect, NTDs), and can occur as a sporadic defect (i.e., holoprosencephaly).

Figure 6-8

Agenesis of the corpus callosum. **A,** On the median section, no corpus callosum or cavum septi pellucidi is seen. **B,** On a posterior coronal section, the distended posterior horns are seen (colpocephaly). The echogenic dangling choroid is also obvious *(arrows)*. **C,** Color Doppler reveals a bizarre blood supply to the brain in this median section of the brain. The pericallosal artery is not seen. **D,** A normal brain (median section) is shown for comparison. The pericallosal artery (PCA) *(arrow)* is seen above the corpus callosum.

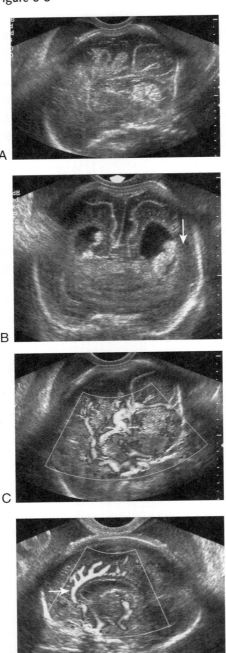

A recent classification of DWM has been introduced based on postnatal neuroimaging studies. In this classification, DWM is separated into the *classic malformation, the Dandy-Walker variant* (small defect in the cerebellar vermis without dilatation of the cisterna magna), and *the mega-cisterna magna* (large cisterna magna without cerebellar abnormalities).

Sonographic findings in the classic malformation are as follows: on the coronal and the median planes, there is a large cyst of the posterior fossa, which is contiguous with the fourth ventricle; an elevated tentorium; and dilatation of the third and the lateral ventricles (Figure 6-9, *A* through *C*). Differentiation between a DWM and an arachnoid cyst of the posterior fossa relies on the demonstration of a hypoplastic vermis and the connection of the cyst with the fourth ventricle.

It is important to realize that there are developmental changes in the area of the cerebellum and most importantly in the cerebellar vermis. The vermis does not reach its "final" shape until the sixteenth to twentieth postmenstrual weeks. Therefore before this time in the pregnancy the fourth ventricle communicates through a wide opening with the cerebello-medullary cistern (also know as cisterna magna), resembling the typical appearance of the DWM. It is therefore important not to call this relatively wide opening by mistake (or ignorance!) vermian dysgenesis or a variant of Dandy-Walker syndrome. One should wait and follow up on this finding and reevaluate the brain at 20 to 22 postmenstrual weeks. In most cases during the repeat scan a normal vermis will be detected.

Figure 6-9

Dandy-Walker malformation. **A,** The vermis is replaced by a fluid-filled larger cisterna magna. The splayed cerebellar hemispheres are also seen *(arrows)*. **B,** A slightly lower section depicts the large fluid-filled "cystlike" space. **C,** The median section reveals the upward displaced tentorium *(arrow)* and the dilated, fluid-filled posterior fossa.

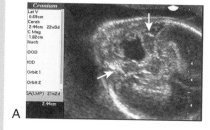

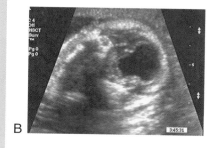

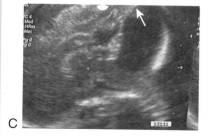

Choroid Plexus Cysts

Choroid plexus cysts (CPCs) are common findings during the second trimester of pregnancy. Their reported incidence during the second trimester is 0.18% to 3.6% of all fetuses scanned. They may be visualized during the late first trimester; however, their prevalence during the first trimester has not yet been determined (Figure 6-10). CPCs are usually asymptomatic and benign. They usually resolve by the mid-trimester and have been associated with both a normal and an abnormal fetal karyotype. CPCs are thought to result from filling of the neuroepithelial folds with CSF.

The typical sonographic appearance of a CPC is that of a small (usually less than 1 cm), sonolucent structure with well-delineated borders located within the choroid plexus (see Figure 6-10). CPCs have a wide range of appearances, from unilateral single cysts to bilateral septate and multiple cysts.

Once a CPC is imaged, a targeted scan should follow. Attention should be given to the appearance of the fetal hands and to the cardiac anatomy. In addition, knowledge of the first or second trimester maternal serum screen can help triage which patients may need further consultations (genetic) and testing (amniocentesis). In the literature, there is a wide range of opinions regarding the need for a fetal karyotype in the presence of a CPC. Some authors recommend that all cases should be offered genetic testing, whereas others believe that only in the presence of an associated congenital anomaly is genetic testing justified.

Arachnoid Cysts

Similar to CPCs, arachnoid cysts are localized collections of CSF in the arachnoid membrane–containing regions of the brain. However, unlike CPCs, they have not been associated with chromosomal aneuploidy. In the arachnoid cyst, the CSF is located within the layers of the arachnoid membrane, which may or may not communicate with the subarachnoid space.

The sonographic appearance of an arachnoid cyst is that of an anechoic cystic mass with thin, smooth walls lying adjacent to the cerebral hemispheres, cerebellum, or brainstem (Figure 6-11). The cysts are usually located

Figure 6-10

Choroid plexus cysts (bilateral).

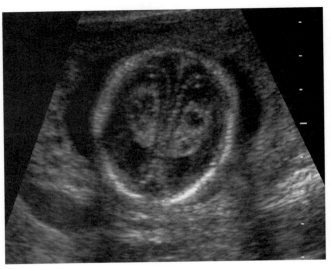

Figure 6-11

A small arachnoid cyst in the quadrigeminal cistern (arrow).

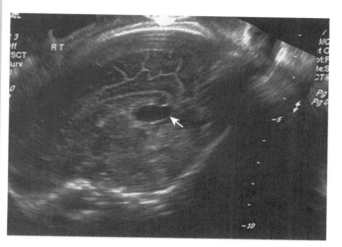

on the convex surface of the brain, most commonly close to the cerebral fissures within the anterior, middle, and posterior fossa. However, they can be seen in other places such as the quadrigeminal cistern and in the cisterna ambiens, above the cerebellum. Once an arachnoid cyst is diagnosed, a careful evaluation of the neuroanatomy is indicated. Although arachnoid cysts can be isolated lesions, they may be associated with other brain malformations such as AGCC, deficient cerebellar lobulation, and Arnold-Chiari type I malformation. Many of these associated findings do not become sonographically apparent until the late second trimester of pregnancy. A large cyst can cause hydrocephaly because of its mass, causing obstruction to the flow of the CSF. Arachnoid cysts do not communicate with the lateral ventricles.

Sonographic diagnosis of arachnoid cysts can be made from the early part of the second trimester. Once a fetus has been diagnosed with this finding, serial ultrasounds scan are recommended to assess growth of the cyst, if any, and to detect hydrocephaly, especially in cases in which the size of the cyst is progressive.

Aneurysms of the Vein of Galen

The vein of Galen is a median structure that drains the blood from the inferior sagittal sinus and continues into the straight sinus. Aneurysms of the vein of Galen are rare arteriovenous malformations of the brain. They may cause obstruction of the ventricular system at the level of the aqueduct of Silvius, resulting in hydrocephaly.

The sonographic appearance (gray-scale) of the aneurysm in the midsagittal plane is that of a large, well-defined, supratentorial, anechoic nonpulsatile structure running from the splenium of the corpus callosum above the cerebellum all the way posterior to the bony cranium. In the coronal plane, the aneurysm appears as an anechoic round, cystic centrally located structure. When color Doppler is applied, the structure fills with bright color(s) because of the turbulent flow within the dilated cavity. Other sonographic findings include hydrops fetalis secondary to high-output congestive heart failure and polyhydramnios.

The prognosis for the fetus/neonate depends on the severity and the time of presentation of the cardiovascular symptomatology. Development of high-output failure in utero or before 3 months of life is usually lethal despite medical and surgical treatments.

Microcephaly

Microcephaly is usually diagnosed when the fetal head size falls below three standard deviations from the mean. Microcephaly can occur as a result of an autosomal recessive trait, as part of a chromosomal syndrome (e.g., trisomies 13 and 18), or as a result of environmental factors such as infections (CMV), intrauterine alcohol exposure, intrauterine anoxia, maternal metabolic diseases, or abnormality of the skull (e.g., craniosynostosis).

The sonographic diagnosis of microcephaly is based on biometric measurements of the fetal head. In well-dated pregnancies in which the head circumference falls below three standard deviations from the mean, microcephaly must be entertained. Once this diagnosis is made, a detailed fetal neuroscan is indicated because microcephaly is associated with other brain anomalies such as AGCC, ventriculomegaly secondary to brain atrophy, lissencephaly, porencephaly, and holoprosencephaly.

The prognosis of a microcephalic fetus relates to the severity of associated anomalies and to the size of the head. Unfortunately, isolated microcephaly cannot be diagnosed until the late second or third trimester, when the growth of the fetal head slows down significantly.

Schizencephaly

Schizencephaly represents a spectrum of destructive lesions affecting the brain. Schizencephaly, lately considered as a type of porencephaly, is a rare developmental disorder in which brain clefts are usually present. The clefts may be bilateral or unilateral. Their pathogenesis is not clear, but they are believed to arise from an in utero ischemic event.

Sonographic findings include the presence of bilateral or unilateral brain clefts and ventriculomegaly. Two types of schizencephaly have been described. In Type I there are small symmetrical clefts in which the lips of the clefts are fused within a pia-ependymal seam that is continuous with the ependyma of the lateral ventricle. Type 2 has more extensive clefts, which extend from the ventricle to the surface of the brain. The clefts are wedge shaped and extend outward to reach the bones of the skull.

The prognosis for the fetus/neonate with schizencephaly depends on whether or not the clefts are bilateral or unilateral. In cases of bilateral clefts, the neonates/infants are commonly developmentally and speech delayed and have corticospinal dysfunction. Those with unilateral clefts (Figure 6-12, *A* and *B*) are often paralyzed on one side of the body and may have normal intelligence. In general, individual with schizencephaly may also have microcephaly, mental retardation, hemiparesis or quadriparesis, hypotonicity, and seizures, and some may have hydrocephaly.

Hydran-encephaly

Hydranencephaly is believed to be the result of either an in utero cerebral brain infarction resulting from bilateral carotid artery occlusion or primary agenesis of the neural wall. The cerebellum, midbrain, thalami, and basal ganglia are usually preserved.

Figure 6-12

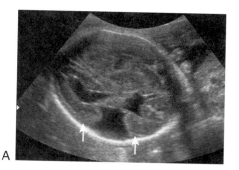

A

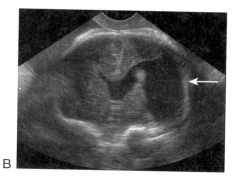

B

Unilateral open lip schizencephaly. **A,** The subarachnoid space is contiguous with the lateral ventricle. The edges of the cortex are rounded *(arrows).* This is an axial section. **B,** On this mid-coronal section, the gaping connection between the brain surface and the left lateral ventricle *(arrow)* is visible. (Courtesy of Dr. Courtney Stephenson.)

Sonographic findings include macrocephaly, a large fluid-filled intracranial cavity with variable amount of echogenicity. No cerebral cortex is present, but there is partial preservation of portions of the occipital lobe. The falx cerebri is usually intact. The midbrain and basal ganglia are variably preserved. The differential diagnosis includes severe hydrocephaly, alobar holoprosencephaly, and porencephaly. Polyhydramnios is usually present. Prognosis for the neonate is poor and most die within the first year of life.

Lissencephaly, Pachygyria, Microgyria, and Heterotopias

Lissencephaly, pachygyria, microgyria, and heterotopies result from disturbances in migration of the neuroblast to the forming cerebral cortex. Depending on when the disturbance or insult occurred, the resulting cortex will completely lack gyri and sulci (lissencephaly) (see Figure 6-3, *D*), may have a few coarse gyri (pachygyria), may have multiple small gyri (microgyria), or have fragments of gray matter present in an abnormal location of the brain (heterotopias). All children with this type of migrational disorder are neurologically impaired.

Lissencephaly or agyria (smooth brain) is a rare developmental anomaly of the brain characterized by incomplete or failure of neuronal migration to occur during 12 to 24 postmenstrual weeks, resulting in a lack of gyri and sulci development.

Transvaginal sonography allows imaging of the surface of the cerebral hemispheres and can facilitate the in utero diagnosis of lissencephaly. Usually these fetuses will have microcephaly and ventriculomegaly. A detailed neuroscan may reveal a relatively straight midline echo corresponding to the interhemispheric fissure, the subarachnoid space and the lateral sulcus

(Sylvian fissures) will appear wide (similar to the appearance of the fetal brain before 20 weeks gestation), and there may be complete or partial AGCC. A scan of the face will reveal dysmorphism. In addition, a search for other non-CNS anomalies is important because anomalies such as duodenal atresia, urinary tract abnormalities, congenital heart defects, polydactyly, and ear anomalies may be found.

Lissencephaly has been divided into two types. Type I is associated with facial dysmorphism, and in some patients there is a deletion of chromosome 17p13 (Miller-Dieker syndrome). In type II lissencephaly, there is associated hydrocephaly and dysgenesis of the cerebellum, and it is usually part of a syndrome. Prenatal diagnosis of lissencephaly probably cannot be reliably made until 26 to 28 postmenstrual weeks, when the normal gyri and sulci become well defined, because up to this time the normal fetal brain has a relatively smooth appearance.

Prognosis for the neonate is poor, with death usually occurring within the first 2 years of life. All children with lissencephaly suffer from severe mental retardation, and almost all have seizures.

Infections Affecting the CNS: CMV and Toxoplasmosis

CMV infection is the most common infection affecting the developing human fetus. It is estimated that approximately 3000 to 4000 infants are born yearly with symptomatic disease and an additional 30,000 to 40,000 with asymptomatic disease. Fetal infection can result from a primary maternal infection, from reinfection, or from a reactivation of a latent infection. Primary maternal infection during the pregnancy may be asymptomatic, but it results in a 30% to 40% risk of intrauterine transmission. The prognosis for the fetus is worse if infection occurs in the first trimester. Diagnosis of a primary disease during pregnancy can be made by documented seroconversion or the presence of CMV-specific immunoglobulin M (IgM) antibodies.

The classical CNS sonographic finding of fetuses with CMV is bilateral periventricular hyperechogenicities (calcifications). However, there are also branching linear echogenic areas in the thalami, as well as microcephaly, hydrocephaly, cerebellar hypoplasia, large cisterna magna, lissencephaly, paraventricular cysts, and ischemic destructive lesions such as porencephaly, hydranencephaly, and polymicrogyria. Non-CNS sonographic findings include growth restriction (IUGR), hydrops, oligohydramnios, hepatomegaly, and splenomegaly.

The prognosis for the neonate/infant with in utero CMV relates to the severity of the intracranial abnormalities. Approximately 95% of the infants with microcephaly and intracranial "calcifications" will either die or exhibit major neurologic sequelae such as developmental delay, seizures, deafness, and motor deficits. Of course, children with "milder" neurologic signs will have a better prognosis.

Prenatal diagnosis of fetal CMV infection relies on a combination of diagnostic tests, which includes sonography, and amniotic fluid studies (viral culture or a polymerase chain reaction [PCR]). Unfortunately, at present no drug therapy is available to treat fetal CMV infection.

Toxoplasmosis is the result of a transplacental infection with the parasite *Toxoplasma gondii*. The most common source of infection in the human is from the domesticated cat or by the ingestion or handling of contaminated meat. The incidence of congenital toxoplasmosis ranges from 0.5 to 2.0 per 1000 live births.

The risk and the severity of fetal infection are dependent on when during the pregnancy the primary maternal infection was contracted. Infection during the first and second trimester results in approximately 20% to 25% of the fetuses becoming infected, whereas infection during the third trimester results in infection in up to 65%. However, the severity of the disease decreases from approximately 75% severe infection in the first trimester to 0% in the third trimester. The diagnosis of maternal primary disease is made based on documentation of seroconversion, a marked increased in antibody titers, or the presence of toxoplasmosis-specific IgM.

The intracranial sonographic findings of fetal toxoplasmosis include hyperechogenic foci or calcifications, hydrocephaly, microcephaly, brain atrophy, and hydranencephaly. The intracranial calcifications in fetal toxoplasmosis are multifocal and are present in many areas of the brain such as the basal ganglia, periventricular area, white matter, and cerebral cortex. Prenatal diagnosis of fetal toxoplasmosis relies on sonography, amniotic fluid studies (culture and PCR), and fetal blood sampling for the determination of toxoplasmosis-specific IgM.

Fetal therapy includes the treatment of the mother with spiramycin in cases of primary infection during the pregnancy. But once fetal infection has been documented, a combination of pyrimethamine, sulfadiazine, and folinic acid is recommended.

The prognosis for the fetus and subsequent neonate affected with toxoplasmosis relates to the severity of the neuropathology. Only about 10% of neonates with severe neurologic features are normal on follow-up. The remainder suffers from mental retardation, seizures, spastic motor deficits, and severe visual impairment.

KEY POINTS

1. Closed neural tube defects are covered by skin or a thick membrane. They are not associated with increased maternal serum alpha-fetoprotein.
2. Anencephaly can be diagnosed during the first trimester of the pregnancy.
3. Some cephaloceles are associated with autosomal recessive conditions.
4. Eighty percent of cases of spinal dysraphism occur in the lumbar region of the spine.
5. The Dandy-Walker malformation is difficult to diagnose in utero. In cases in which a vermian defect is suspected, a repeat scan at 20 to 22 weeks of gestation is suggested to reassess the diagnosis.

SUGGESTED READINGS

Cheschies N: ACOG Practice Bulletin #44: *Int J Gynaecol Obstet* 83:123-33, 2003.

Nyberg DA et al. editors: *Diagnostic Imaging of Fetal Anomalies.* Philadelphia, 2003, Lippincott Williams & Wilkins, pp 221-319, 907-911.

Timor-Tritsch IE, Monteagudo A, Cohen HL, editors: *Ultrasonography of the Prenatal and Neonatal Brain,* ed 2. New York, 2001, McGraw-Hill, pp 13-276.

7

COMMON FETAL ANOMALIES: THE FETAL HEART

Svena Julien and Joshua Copel

FETAL CIRCULATION

The goal of fetal echocardiography is to diagnose congenital heart disease (CHD). CHD includes a wide array of structural abnormalities that vary significantly in severity and prognosis. In this chapter we review basic fetal circulation and the goals of prenatal cardiac assessment. We then detail the most commonly encountered cardiac anomalies.

In utero the placenta acts as the organ of oxygenation. Blood leaving the placenta has a hemoglobin oxygen saturation of 80% to 85%. From the placenta, blood enters the umbilical vein and travels toward the liver. The liver receives 50% of this flow. The other 50% bypasses the liver via the ductus venosus. Blood from the lower extremities, liver, and ductus venosus enters the heart via the inferior vena cava (IVC). Streaming of the highly oxygenated ductal flow occurs in the IVC and right atrium. This blood is preferentially shunted to the left atrium via the foramen ovale. Blood in the left atrium then enters the left ventricle and leaves the heart via the ascending aorta. The coronary, innominate, left carotid, and left subclavian arteries receive about two thirds of left ventricular (LV) output, which has an oxygen saturation of about 65%.

The IVC, superior vena cava (SVC), and coronary sinus empty into the right atrium. Blood that is not shunted to the left atrium enters the right ventricle. This blood leaves the heart via the main pulmonary artery (PA). Eight percent of the combined ventricular output travels to the right and left pulmonary arteries while the remainder is shunted across the ductus arteriosus to the descending aorta. The oxygen saturation of blood in the descending aorta is 55%.

ULTRASOUND EVALUATION

The goal of the cardiac examination is to identify CHD in the fetus. This can be accomplished using a systematic evaluation of the heart that includes the following:

1. Identify the position of the heart in the body
2. Identify the cardiac chambers

3. Identify the atrioventricular (AV) connections
4. Identify the ventriculo-arterial connections

First, the fetal head and spine should be located to establish the left and the right sides of the fetal body. Next, the abdominal visceral situs is determined. The stomach should occupy the left side of the upper abdomen with the spleen behind it, the gallbladder should be on the right, and the umbilical vein should be seen hooking toward the right as it enters the fetal liver. This is termed situs solitus. When the viscera are reversed (stomach on the right, liver on the left), the term used is situs inversus. Situs inversus totalis is reversal of the contents of both the abdomen and thorax, whereas situs ambiguous refers to abnormal location of stomach or heart (e.g., in the midline).

One should locate the fetal abdominal landmarks including the stomach, portal sinus, aorta, spine, and IVC in an axial plane. Scanning further cephalad will reveal the four-chamber view of the heart. In this view, the heart should occupy nearly one third of the cross-sectional area of the chest. Normally the fetal heart is on the left side of the thorax with the apex to the left anterior at about a 45-degree angle from the midline. The right atrium and ventricle are anterior to the left atrium and ventricle. The ventricular apices should lie at the same level, and the ventricles should be of equal size. In dextrocardia, the heart will be on the right side of the chest with the apex facing the right chest wall. Mesocardia is used to describe the heart that occupies the central position in the heart. The apex points to the anterior chest wall in this case. It is important to note that external compression and rightward displacement of the heart by a diaphragmatic hernia or lung mass is termed dextroposition rather than dextrocardia.

The four-chamber view of the heart is best obtained in a transverse, or axial, view of the fetal chest (Figure 7-1). In this view, the chamber sizes and AV connections may be visualized. The atria should be of near equal size. The interatrial septum and foramen ovale are noted (Figure 7-2). Often the valve of the foramen ovale can be seen in the left atrium. The AV junction should be evaluated. The insertion of the tricuspid valve is located closer to the cardiac apex on the interventricular septum than the insertion of the mitral valve. The AV valves should move freely and independently.

Although the ventricular sizes should be nearly equal, the morphology is different. The left ventricle is smooth-walled and takes the shape of a "V." The right ventricle is more "U" shaped and has a coarse appearance because of its trabeculated walls. The moderator band is a coalescence of the muscles with the interventricular septum near the apex of the right ventricle that may give the chamber a slightly foreshortened appearance.

Next, apical and long axis views of the heart should be obtained. This allows visualization of the interventricular and interatrial septa. It is important to obtain a lateral and an apical view because the apical four-chamber view may not show the intact septum because it relies on lateral resolution of the ultrasound beam, which is never as detailed as views using axial resolution. The long-axis view will demonstrate the great vessels, and the AV and ventriculo-arterial connections (Figure 7-3). In the normal heart, the anterior wall of the ascending aorta is continuous with the interventricular septum and the posterior wall is continuous with the mitral valve, forming the left ventricular

Figure 7-1

Transverse view of the normal four-chamber heart. The moderator band is seen at the apex of the right ventricle (left side of image).

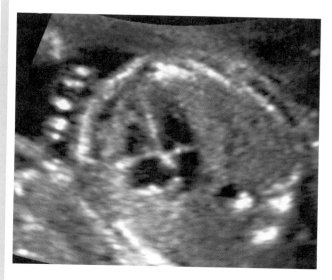

outflow tract (LVOT). The ascending aorta courses superiorly and the three branches to the head and neck may be seen. From slight rotation of the transducer in the direction of the fetal left side, the pulmonary trunk and descending aorta should be visualized. In the normal heart, the right ventricular outflow tract (RVOT) should arise from the right ventricle to form the main pulmonary trunk. Rotation of the transducer to image the left and right outflow tracts will also demonstrate the great vessels in a cross pattern as seen in Figure 7-4.

A short-axis view of the heart should complement the long-axis view. This view is perpendicular to the long axis and is parallel to the fetal

Figure 7-2

Four-chamber cardiac view. The valve of the foramen oval is seen within the left atrium. The interventricular septum is intact and the moderator band is seen in the right ventricle (right side of image).

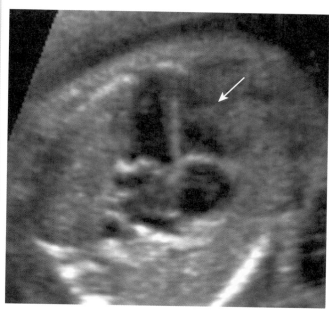

Figure 7-3

Long-axis view of the normal heart. The aorta is visualized as it leaves the left ventricle.

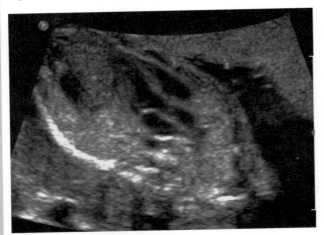

spine. The short-axis view will demonstrate the most proximal area of the great vessels, the aortic arch, and is most useful in defining the relationship between the main PA, ductus arteriosus, and descending aorta (Figure 7-5).

Finally, color Doppler and M-mode may be used to evaluate flow patterns, chamber size, and function. These modalities are not part of the routine fetal screening cardiac examination but may be used during an echocardiography examination. They are also useful in the assessment of arrhythmias and in the determination of ventricular wall thickness.

Figure 7-4

Normal image of the great vessel crossing. The aorta and pulmonary artery cross as they exit the respective ventricles.

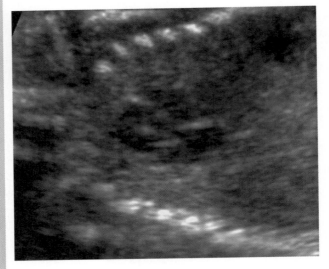

Figure 7-5

Short-axis view of the normal heart. The pulmonary artery leaves the right ventricle and bifurcates in the left and right pulmonary arteries.

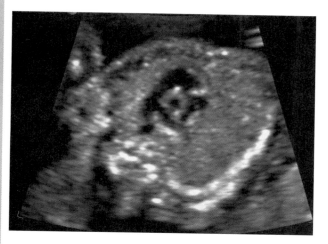

EPIDEMIOLOGY

The most common congenital lesions include ventricular septal defects (VSDs), tetralogy of Fallot, and transposition of the great vessels. The incidence of CHD in the general population is 8 per 1000 live births. However, many authors believe that this is an underestimation of the fetal incidence because of failure to identify all losses of anomalous fetuses.

The inheritance of CHD is thought to be multifactorial. Single-gene disorders account for 1% to 2% of CHD. The same is true for environmental factors such as maternal use of antiseizure medications or consumption of excess amounts of alcohol. However, the incidence of aneuploidy in fetuses with CHD is as high as 35% (Box 7-1).

The risk of recurrent CHD for a couple that has already had an affected child is 2% to 5%. This risk increases to 10% to 15% after a second sibling is affected. If the mother has CHD, the risk of CHD in the offspring is 5% to 12%, whereas it is 1.3% to 5% if the father is affected. Although no specific data are available in the literature, the risk of CHD when the affected family member is *not* a first-degree relative is likely to be the same as that of the general population.

COMMON CARDIAC LESIONS

Ventricular Septal Defect

VSDs are the most common congenital heart lesion found in the first year of life. They account for 30% of all CHD. Early in development, there is a foramen in the muscular interventricular septum. This foramen is closed when the muscular ventricular septum fuses with the endocardial cushions and forms the area termed the membranous portion of the septum. This area then fuses with the aortico-pulmonary septum by the seventh

Box 7-1   Indications for Echocardiography

- Parent with CHD
- Sibling with CHD

Maternal Conditions
- Pre-gestational diabetes mellitus
- Drug exposure
  - Antiseizure medications including
    1. Phenytoin
    2. Valproic acid
    3. Carbamazepine
  - Lithium
  - Retinoic acid

- Alcohol consumption
- PKU
- Anti-ro (SSA) or anti-la (SSB) antibodies

Fetal Conditions
- Chromosomal anomalies
  - Trisomy 21
  - Trisomy 13
  - Trisomy 18
- Polyhydramnios
- Nonimmune hydrops fetalis
- Arrhythmias
- Major fetal anomalies:
  - Diaphragmatic hernia
  - Omphalocele
  - Increased nuchal translucency ($\geq$3.0 mm)
- Abnormal four-chamber view

week of development. Failure of complete fusion results in one type of VSD. The most common location for a VSD is in the membranous portion of the septum. On ultrasound, a deficiency of tissue is visualized within the interventricular septum on the long- and short-axis views of the ventricles (Figure 7-6).

Defects in the muscular portion of the ventricular septum are less common and are often multiple. These defects may be located anywhere along the interventricular septum from the insertion of the tricuspid valve to the apex of the heart. Even moderate-sized defects may be difficult to identify on sonogram.

In utero, the VSD does not have an adverse impact on the fetal cardiovascular system because there are normal shunts from the right to left and the pressure in the ventricles is equal. However, an increase in the systemic arterial pressure and a drop in the pulmonary arterial pressure accompany the transition from fetal to neonatal circulation. Over time, this will lead to a left to right shunt and consequently pulmonary vascular congestion. If this shunt is uncorrected, a right to left shunt will eventually develop, with pulmonary hypertension and development of Eisenmenger syndrome.

When a small VSD is present, the neonate is usually observed without intervening, because 60% of muscular defects and 25% of membranous

Figure 7-6

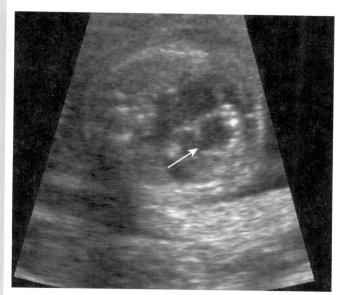

Large VSD *(arrow)*. The right vetricle appears dilated. The interventricular septum is truncated and does not reach the interarterial septum.

defects will close spontaneously by age 6 years. If the VSD has not closed by this age, surgical correction may be considered.

When a VSD is suspected during a routine sonogram, a detailed sonogram and formal fetal echocardiogram should be performed. Counseling must include a discussion of amniocentesis because of the increased risk of extracardiac and chromosomal anomalies. The pediatric cardiology team should assist in the diagnosis, counseling, and antenatal management.

Atrioventricular Septal Defect

By 6 weeks of embryonic life, the interatrial and interventricular septa grow toward the endocardial cushions to divide the heart into four chambers. Failure of these structures to coalesce at the level of the superior ventricular septum and inferior atrial septum (central fibrous body) leads to an atrioventricular septal defect (AVSD). The insertion of both the tricuspid and mitral valves on the interventricular septum are at the same level (if the septum reaches that level), and the single AV valve has five leaflets. The partial form of AVSD arises from a defect in the ostium primum with bridging tissue across the valve structure. There is usually no VSD, but there is a persistent connection between the atria, and the AV valves are separate. Often the mitral valve has three leaflets but is functional.

On ultrasound (Figures 7-7 and 7-8), the interatrial septum is either very underdeveloped or completely absent. The AV valves meet at the same level, whereas normally the tricuspid valve inserts onto the ventricular septum closer to the cardiac apex than does the mitral valve. A complete anatomical survey and echocardiogram should be performed to exclude other anomalies. Trisomy 21 is found in 57% to 72% of fetuses with an AVSD, so an amniocentesis should be offered.

In utero, the fetus may tolerate the lesion. However, there is a risk of valvular insufficiency leading to congestive failure, as evidenced by fetal hydrops. The

Figure 7-7

Complete atrioventricular septal defect (AVSD). Note the large common atrium. The atrioventricular (AV) valve appears to be a single band between the atrium and two ventricles. There is also a small ventricular septal defect (VSD) present in this fetus.

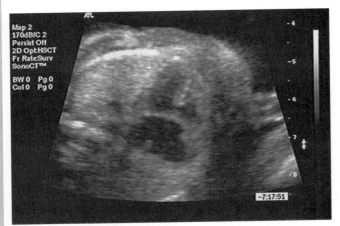

transition to neonatal circulation is accompanied by an increase in left atrial and ventricular pressure. Although neonates may initially do well, increasing pulmonary congestion from the higher pressure left ventricle sending flow to the low-resistance pulmonary circulation will eventually lead to the decision for surgical repair. Left to right shunting may lead to pulmonary hypertension after many years. In addition, the location of the defect predisposes the fetus to AV block and other conduction system abnormalities.

The prognosis for a fetus with AVSD depends on the extent of the defect and the presence of congestive heart failure (CHF). Massive valve insufficiency and congestive failure in utero confer a poor prognosis. The mortality rate is near 80% for a neonate who develops CHF. Fetuses born with an AVSD will need surgical correction of the lesion. Timing of the correction is

Figure 7-8

Transposition of the great vessels. The pulmonary artery and aorta are aligned in a parallel fashion. AO, Aorta; LV, left ventricle; PA, pulmonary artery; RV, right ventricle.

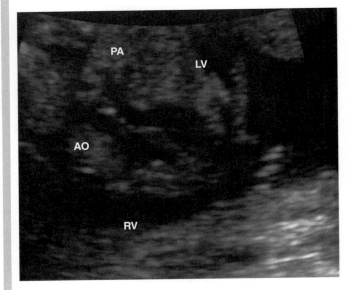

determined by the severity of the lesion and the development of pulmonary congestion related to increased pulmonary flow. Well-tolerated lesions may be corrected in infancy usually before 24 months of age. More severe lesions need to be corrected before the development of irreversible pulmonary vascular damage, and surgical correction of the lesion is curative. This cardiac defect does not warrant changes in the intrapartum obstetric management, but pediatric cardiology should be alerted to evaluate the neonatal transitional circulation and establish long-term follow-up after delivery.

Tetralogy of Fallot

Tetralogy of Fallot is a complex defect in the rotation, development, and partitioning of the truncus conus. The aorta is shifted anteriorly over a VSD, and that shift in the position of the aorta narrows the pulmonary outflow portion of the right ventricle. Right ventricular (RV) hypertrophy is usually not seen in utero but is the result of the obstruction to RV output after birth. Formation of an intact ventricular septum is dependent on the rotation of the truncus (which forms the aorta and main PA) and fusion with the muscular and membranous portions of the interventricular septum. The great vessels are formed from the division of the truncus conus. Failure of the conus to rotate and fuse with the interventricular septum results in a VSD while unequal portioning of the conus results in a stenotic PA trunk and enlarged aortic root.

123

Tetralogy is suspected when an enlarged aorta is noted to be overriding the ventricular septum with a VSD and a small pulmonary trunk. A careful complete cardiac and anatomical survey should be performed when this defect is suspected. There may be varying degrees of pulmonic stenosis depending on when in gestation the lesion is identified. Over the course of gestation, the stenosis may worsen.

The prevalence of the microdeletion of the long arm of chromosome 22 (22q) is 5% to 10% in fetuses with tetralogy of Fallot. This heart defect is also seen more commonly in trisomy 18, trisomy 21, and other autosomal trisomies; therefore an amniocentesis should be offered when tetralogy is suspected on sonogram.

In utero, the defects are well tolerated. At birth, the systemic pressure increases while the pressure in the pulmonary vascular bed falls. The degree of pulmonary stenosis determines the degree of shunting from right to left through the VSD. The prognosis for these patients depends on the extent of the RV outflow obstruction and the presence of persistent cyanosis. Neonatal surgical correction is necessary for survival if the degree of pulmonic stenosis warrants it, but if there is adequate pulmonic flow repair may be delayed into infancy with survival greater than 95%. The pediatric cardiology service should be involved in the antenatal period and delivery should occur at an institution that can provide surgical care if needed.

Transposition of the Great Arteries

Transposition of the great vessels may be either complete (dextro) transposition or "congenitally corrected" with AV and ventriculoarterial discordance. In complete transposition, there are normal AV connections, but the LV outflow is directed to the PA while the RV outflow is directed into the aorta. During embryonic development, the truncus arteriosus must rotate before its division in order for the great vessels to be properly aligned. Failure of this rotation results in complete transposition. The aorta is located anterior and to the right of the PA and the vessels lie in parallel. Systemic oxygenation is maintained by communication between the two systems, including a patent ductus arteriosus and interatrial (i.e., foramen ovale) or interventricular connections (i.e., VSD, if one is present).

Congenitally corrected transposition occurs when the embryonic cardiac tube fails to loop properly so that the morphologic left ventricle is located anteriorly and to the right while the morphologic right ventricle is oriented posteriorly and to the left. The truncus arteriosus divides properly and the great vessels are aligned with the aortic trunk arising from the posterior (morphologic right) ventricle and the pulmonary trunk arising from the anterior (morphologic left) ventricle. The great vessels are oriented in series as in the normal heart. Because they are aligned in series, there is systemic flow of oxygenated blood.

The diagnosis of transposition of the great vessels is suspected when the long- and short-axis views of the great vessels fail to demonstrate the normal crossing pattern. Instead, the vessels are parallel to one another (Figure 7-8). Often other cardiac anomalies are present, necessitating a detailed sonogram. Although aneuploidy is rare in the setting of transposition with an intact septum, amniocentesis should be considered if other anomalies are found. Serial scans should be performed given the risk of the development of CHF.

The fetus tolerates TGA well in utero because the normal fetal circulation is a parallel system. However, in cases of complete transposition, survival in the neonatal period is not possible unless there are adequate connections between the two circulatory patterns. An atrial septal defect (ASD), VSD, patent ductus, or patent foramen ovale must persist. The treatment is medical therapy to maintain a patent ductus arteriosus and often balloon atrial septostomy (Rashkind procedure) followed by surgery in the early neonatal period. For cases of congenitally corrected transposition, no surgical intervention is warranted because the systemic circulation is maintained. As with other complex congenital cardiac lesions, the pediatric cardiology team should be involved early in the antenatal course and delivery should occur at a tertiary care center.

Hypoplastic Left Heart Syndrome

Hypoplastic left heart syndrome (HLHS) is characterized by the presence of a small left ventricle with varying degrees of function in the presence of mitral and/or aortic valve stenosis or atresia. The result is minimal flow within the left ventricle, which renders it hypoplastic. The right ventricle is responsible for the total cardiac output. The PA supplies systemic circulation as blood is shunted across the ductus arteriosus to the descending aorta normally, and retrograde flow through the aortic isthmus supplies the head and neck vessels and the coronaries.

HLHS is suspected when the left ventricle is much smaller than the right and has poor contractility. In early acute aortic obstruction, the left ventricle may transiently dilate, with echogenic walls and little visible contractility. On echocardiography the aorta may appear to be small. The right ventricle may appear to be hypertrophic. A complete survey of the heart and other anatomy should take place as is the case with other cardiac anomalies, and an amniocentesis should be considered. The fetus should have serial sonograms given the risk of hydrops from overload of the right ventricle. Recently, some have suggested that early disease may be amenable to intrauterine intervention by aortic valve balloon dilation. However, valvuloplasty is still in the experimental stages and is only offered at specialized centers.

This lesion is well tolerated prenatally, because the right heart is able to provide adequate cardiac output and the physiologic shunts remain open. The transition to neonatal life is accompanied by the closure of the foramen ovale and ductus arteriosus. The ductus serves as the bridge between the right ventricle and the systemic circulation. Therefore closure results in circulatory collapse and death unless surgical intervention occurs. The treatment is surgical correction in the early neonatal period, usually by the multistage Norwood repair or by cardiac transplantation. Delivery should occur at a tertiary care center, which has been shown to improve mortality and morbidity in affected infants, and the pediatric cardiology team should be involved early in the antenatal course.

Pulmonary Stenosis

Pulmonary stenosis is an obstruction of the outflow from the right ventricle. Stenosis is usually the result of fusion of the commissures of the valve. The stenosis is characterized by the location of the obstruction and may be at, below, or above the valve. Stenosis may lead to increased work by the right ventricle, causing RV hypertrophy.

It is difficult to definitively diagnose pulmonary stenosis in utero. Comparison of flow patterns across the PA and aorta may suggest pulmonary stenosis. In addition, PA stenosis is suspected when the diameter of the PA is markedly smaller than that of the aorta (Figure 7-9).

Figure 7-9

Pulmonary stenosis. Note the discrepancy in the diameter of the aorta versus the pulmonary artery. The pulmonary artery is very small and is outlined by the calipers. The aorta is superior to the pulmonary artery in this view.

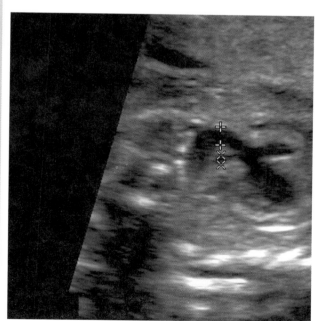

In utero, the fetus may tolerate the lesion well, but an echocardiogram should be performed in the early neonatal period. If critical obstruction is present, valvuloplasty will be needed in the early postnatal period. Some progression of the lesion occurs in utero, and some fetuses will develop frank hypoplastic right heart syndrome. Serial sonograms are important to define progression and change leading up to delivery. As with other lesions, the pediatric cardiology service should be an integral part of the antenatal and immediate neonatal care.

KEY POINTS

1. The incidence of congenital heart disease (CHD) is 8 per 1000.
2. There is an increased risk of CHD with an affected first-degree relative.
3. The indications for fetal echocardiography include an affected sibling or parent and fetal and maternal conditions.
4. The most common CHD found in the first year of life is a ventricular septal defect.
5. Prenatal diagnosis should be followed with neonatal echocardiogram in the first days of life.
6. Most defects are well tolerated in utero.
7. Transition from fetal to neonatal circulation may exacerbate the shunt caused by the defect and may lead to damage to the pulmonary vascular bed.
8. The pediatric cardiology team should be involved in the prenatal period.
9. Delivery of the neonate with a complex cardiac defect should occur at a tertiary care center with adequate neonatal support services.

SUGGESTED READING

Abuhamad A: *A Practical Guide to Fetal Echocardiography.* Philadelphia, 1997, Lippincott-Rawen.

Callen PW: *Ultrasonography in Obstetrics and Gynecology,* ed 4. Philadelphia, 2000, Saunders.

Friedman AH, Fahey JT: The transition from fetal to neonatal circulation: normal responses and implications for infants with heart disease. *Semin Perinatol* 17:106, 1992.

Hess DB, Hess LW: *Fetal Echocardiography.* Stamford, CT, 1999, Appleton and Lange.

Moore KL, Persaud TV: *The Developing Human: Clinically Oriented Embryology,* ed 7. Philadelphia, 2003, Saunders.

Romero R et al: *Prenatal Diagnosis of Congenital Anomalies.* Norwalk, CT, Appleton and Lange.

8

ABNORMAL FETAL GROWTH: INTRAUTERINE GROWTH RESTRICTION

Michael Y. Divon and Yoni Barnhard

Numerous advances in perinatal medicine have contributed to a dramatic drop in perinatal mortality rates. This medical progress now challenges the perinatal community to focus on the prevention of severe morbidity in the newborn. This residual neonatal morbidity often appears in the form of intrauterine growth restriction (IUGR). Despite extensive research efforts resulting in a deeper appreciation of the pathophysiology of IUGR and the development of sensitive diagnostic tools, the greatest risk of adverse perinatal outcome still occurs among growth-restricted fetuses with birth weights below the third percentile for gestational age. Fetal interventions to maximize neonatal outcome have not demonstrated efficacy in small clinical trials. This emphasizes the fact that IUGR is not a single disease entity but a physical condition that results from a broad variety of pathogenic mechanisms. Hopefully, novel therapeutic modalities will lead to a decrease in the morbidity and mortality that result from impaired fetal growth.

DEFINITION

Birth weight is the most accessible and reliable measure of the newborn and it is the most commonly used indicator of fetal growth. The adequacy of intrauterine growth is determined by comparing the birth weight of the newborn with an expected norm for gestational age. Fetal size and fetal growth, however, are often confused in clinical practice. IUGR denotes a pathologic process stemming from growth restriction. In contrast, small for gestational age (SGA) identifies the infant whose birth weight is below an arbitrary percentile for gestational age. The tenth percentile is most widely used for this purpose; however, some authors have suggested that the 3rd percentile be used for this definition. Using birth weight criteria as the gold standard for intrauterine growth, however, presents a few problems. SGA fetuses thus fall into three categories (Box 8-1). Most small fetuses are otherwise normal. These fetuses

Box 8-1	Classification of Small for Gestational Age Fetuses
Type	**Description**
1	Constitutionally small fetuses (not at risk for IUGR)
2	Growth restricted (intrinsic to the fetus)
3	Growth restricted (extrinsic to the fetus)

IUGR, Intrauterine growth restriction.

are not at risk for the sequelae of IUGR. The second group includes fetuses that are growth restricted owing to factors intrinsic to the fetus; this group often is classified as symmetrically growth restricted (Box 8-2). These fetuses have suffered an insult that is fixed at the time of detection and in most cases is irreversible. This group includes those with chromosomal abnormalities, structural defects, or an early intrauterine insult from infection or exposure to certain illicit drugs or other toxins. These intrinsic factors affect the fetus in a manner that may limit any benefit from early delivery. The third group includes those fetuses affected by extrinsic abnormalities such as maternal hypertension, maternal collagen vascular disease, or placental insufficiency; they often are classified as asymmetrically growth restricted. These fetuses, in theory, may benefit from detection and therapy, including early delivery, by providing a more conducive environment to growth outside the uterus.

Early-phase growth disturbance often culminates in symmetric growth restriction. Because growth in this phase is primarily because of cell hyperplasia, restriction of growth results in a lower cell count with a resulting symmetrically small newborn. This pattern is often seen in growth disturbances associated with chromosomal anomalies, congenital malformations, and early transplacental infections. In the asymmetric type, the growth rate of the fetal trunk is smaller than that of other organs. This is caused by relative depletion of the actively growing liver, combined with decreased subcutaneous fat deposition. Third-trimester growth abnormalities, particularly those associated with extrinsic factors, restrict growth during the hypertrophic growth phase and are usually characterized by preferential perfusion of fetal organs, resulting in asymmetrical growth restriction. These intrinsic and extrinsic factors often present in the antenatal period as symmetric and asymmetric growth restriction, respectively. These patterns of diminished growth may

Box 8-2	Causes of Intrauterine Growth Restriction

Intrinsic Factors
- Chromosomal abnormalities
- Congenital structural defects
- Infection
- Drugs and medications

Extrinsic Factors
- Maternal disease
- Placental abnormalities
- Uterine abnormalities

overlap and can be difficult to distinguish. A maternal vascular disease beginning early in pregnancy may cause symmetric growth restriction. In addition, some genetic diseases may be associated with severe asymmetric growth. Likewise, an asymmetrically growth-restricted fetus may become symmetric once brain sparing or linear growth is no longer maintained.

CLASSIFICATION

Numerous approaches to differentiate the fetus with growth restriction from the small but otherwise healthy fetus have been proposed. Some criteria pertain to fetal evaluation; others can only be used in the neonate (Box 8-3). This is critical for preventing unnecessary obstetrical interventions. As many as 70% of fetuses who weigh below the 10th percentile for gestational age are small simply because of constitutional factors such as body mass index, genetic makeup, female gender, or maternal ethnicity; they are not at high risk of perinatal mortality and morbidity. By comparison, a malnourished fetus whose birth weight is slightly greater than the 10th percentile may be misclassified as appropriately grown and at low risk of adverse perinatal outcome, even though its weight may be far below its genetic potential.

Quantitatively, normal singleton fetal growth increases from approximately 5 g/day at 14 to 15 weeks of gestation to 10 g/day at 20 weeks and 30 to 35 g/day at 32 to 34 weeks, after which the growth rate decreases.

INCIDENCE AND OUTCOME

The incidence of IUGR varies according to the population under examination, the geographic location, and the standard growth curves used as a reference. In general, approximately one third of all infants weighing less than 2500 g at birth have sustained IUGR, and approximately 4% to 8% of all infants born in developed countries are classified as growth restricted.

Despite advances in perinatal medicine, perinatal mortality and morbidity increase markedly as birth weight falls from the 10th to the 1st percentile. Overall, infants born between 38 and 42 weeks' gestation whose weights are between 1500 and 2500 g have perinatal mortality and morbidity 5 to 30 times that of infants whose weights are between

---

Box 8-3 Approaches in Differentiating Suspected Growth-Restricted Fetuses

- Customized optimal growth curve based on serial ultrasound measurements
- Use of multiple parameters, such as sonographically estimated fetal weight, amniotic fluid volume, and maternal blood pressure status
- Umbilical artery Doppler
- Neonatal morphometric parameters such as the ponderal index to identify the neonate with soft tissue wasting and diminished organ size
- Nucleated red blood cell counts on cordocentesis or from postnatal umbilical cords
- Postnatal growth patterns

the 10th and 90th percentile and substantially higher if the birth weight is less than 1500 g.

ETIOLOGY

The etiologies of IUGR can be divided into fetal, placental, and maternal factors. Fetal factors include genetic conditions and congenital anomalies. Placental factors tend to involve abnormally implanted or formed placentas with resulting reduced perfusion. Maternal factors include infection, nutrition, drug use, and underlying maternal medical conditions such as hypertension that affect uterine blood flow.

Fetal Factors

- Karyotypic abnormalities, such as trisomies, autosomal deletions, ring chromosomes, uniparental disomy, Turner syndrome, and confined placental mosaicism are the underlying etiology in 5% to 10% of IUGR.
- Genetic syndromes, such as Bloom, Cornelia de Lange, Dubowitz, and Russell-Silver, are associated with prenatal onset of IUGR.
- Skeletal dysplasias with associated long bone shortening.
- Major congenital anomalies, such as congenital heart defects, are often associated with restricted fetal growth.
- Mutations in the gene for insulin-like growth factor may affect both prenatal and postnatal growth.
- The growth curve for multiple gestations begins to deviate from the singleton curve early in the third trimester with the differences increasing from the thirty-fifth week until delivery. In addition, monozygotic twins have a lower birth weight and higher rates of congenital anomalies than dizygotic twins, which suggests that the etiology of these problems may be related to the monozygotic twinning process.

Placental Factors

- Structural placental factors, such as single umbilical artery, velamentous umbilical cord insertion, bilobate placenta, and placental hemangioma.
- Any mismatch between fetal nutritional or respiratory demands and placental supply can result in impaired fetal growth. This can occur with several placental abnormalities, including chronic inflammatory lesions, thrombophilia-related uteroplacental pathology, or abnormal placental implantation.
- An abnormal fetal-placental interaction may result in IUGR.

An indirect measurement of such inadequate fetal growth can be obtained from umbilical artery velocity waveforms. A relative decrease in end-diastolic velocity resulting in an increased S/D ratio identifies a specific placental microvascular lesion characterized by obliteration of small muscular arteries in the tertiary stem villi.

Maternal Factors

- Maternal vascular disease, with its associated decrease in uteroplacental perfusion, is believed to account for 25% to 30% of all IUGR infants. This includes hypertension, preeclampsia, chronic renal disease, and collagen vascular diseases.

- Congenital thrombophilic disorders, such as a prothrombin gene mutation and the acquired coagulopathy, antiphospholipid syndrome, have been implicated in IUGR.
- Severe and prolonged maternal starvation and modest degrees of malnutrition affect fetal growth. In addition, women who are underweight at the start of pregnancy or have poor weight gain during pregnancy are at higher risk of IUGR.
- Maternal hypoxemia resulting from chronic pulmonary disease, cyanotic heart disease, and severe chronic anemia (as with sickle cell anemia) are associated with fetal growth restriction.
- Fetal infection, especially with cytomegalovirus, may cause IUGR, particularly before 20 weeks' gestation. Other viruses and parasites (rubella, toxoplasmosis, varicella, and malaria) have been reported to increase the risk of IUGR.
- Maternal smoking may decrease fetal weight by up to 300 g, and drugs such as cocaine, heroin, and alcohol may influence fetal growth and development.
- Toxic exposures, including various medications such as Coumadin, anticonvulsants, and antineoplastic agents can produce IUGR with associated dysmorphic features.

In addition, several variables, including maternal birth weight, altitude, race, pregnancy at the extremes of reproductive life, and previous delivery of an IUGR infant have been demonstrated to be associated with fetal growth restriction.

DIAGNOSIS

Routine prenatal screening for IUGR involves recognizing etiologic risk factors and performing serial assessments. Reliability of the diagnosis requires accurate knowledge of the gestational age that is best assessed by performing a sonographic crown-rump length measurement in the first trimester. Fundal height measurements, ideally done serially by the same examiner, have been reported to be a useful screening method in the detection of IUGR fetuses. Although the clinical diagnosis of IUGR by physical examination alone is not sufficient to make or exclude the diagnosis, it may create an index of suspicion serving to initiate additional assessment.

At the current time, ultrasound evaluation of the fetus is considered the standard for the diagnosis of IUGR. A variety of sonographic parameters have been used to screen for and diagnose IUGR including:

- Fetal abdominal circumference (AC)
- Head circumference (HC)
- Biparietal diameter (BPD)
- Femur length (FL)

These parameters are converted to fetal weight estimates using several available formulae. This estimated fetal weight (EFW) is plotted against gestational age on a standard growth curve, allowing detection of the fetus whose weight is below the 10th percentile and mapping of serial fetal growth at 2- to 4-week intervals.

Most studies report a reduced AC is the most sensitive single morphometric indicator of IUGR. When fetal growth is compromised, the fetal AC is smaller than expected because of depletion of abdominal adipose tissue, combined with a profound decrease in glycogen storage in the liver. Equations that incorporate the AC, BPD, and FL seem to provide the most accurate estimates of fetal weight and are within 10% of the actual birth weight in 75% of patients with suspected IUGR.

The comparison of growth in some body organs relative to others has led to the development of a number of different morphometric ratios; however, neither the FL/AC nor the HC/AC has demonstrated a high enough sensitivity or positive predictive value to be used for screening purposes in the general population. Therefore these measurements are best used to confirm suspected asymmetric IUGR.

In addition to determining fetal morphometric measurements, sonography allows a qualitative assessment of amniotic fluid volume. The low sensitivity and high specificity of amniotic fluid volume as an indicator of IUGR have been demonstrated by several investigators. Therefore although oligohydramnios is a poor screening modality for IUGR, if oligohydramnios is noted in the absence of ruptured membranes or congenital anomalies, fetal weight should be ascertained; however, the accuracy of the sonographically estimated weight will be decreased and the true fetal weight likely underestimated.

Although fetal growth restriction results in a decrease in both adipose tissue and muscle mass, there are presently inadequate data to define the best site for these measurements or the sensitivity and specificity of these parameters in the prediction of IUGR. It is possible that in the future, three-dimensional volumetric fetal measurements will improve our ability to identify the IUGR fetus.

Continuous and adequate perfusion of the maternal and fetal sides of the placenta is necessary for normal fetal growth. IUGR is associated with diminished flow and abnormal Doppler velocity waveforms. Overall, Doppler studies are not useful for screening and diagnosis of the small fetus. However, these studies are helpful in identifying the small fetus that is at risk for an adverse perinatal outcome (nonreassuring intrapartum fetal status, cesarean section, neonatal intensive care unit [NICU] admission, and asphyxia). Thus they serve to distinguish the constitutionally small fetus from the IUGR fetus at risk for perinatal compromise. Abnormal umbilical artery diastolic flow thus helps identify early fetal compromise, thereby allowing for possible management options (intensive monitoring, corticosteroids, early delivery) that may reduce perinatal mortality. Other fetal vessels that have been studied for the prediction of IUGR include the fetal descending aorta and cerebral arteries. Measurement of the pulsatility index (PI) of the fetal descending aorta is not effective for screening and diagnosis of IUGR but may have a role in predicting the fetus beginning to decompensate from chronic hypoxia. Several studies have demonstrated that measurement of cerebral velocimetry did not improve the detection of IUGR, but may be a useful tool in assessing the IUGR fetus at increased risk of adverse perinatal outcome.

MANAGEMENT

There is little consensus in the literature as to what constitutes the most effective management strategy of IUGR. The ideal strategy will depend on gestational age at diagnosis, the severity of IUGR, the underlying etiology, and the probability of intact extrauterine survival in the institution's NICU.

There is a paucity of evidence from randomized trials that any specific antenatal treatment for the IUGR fetus is beneficial. Given multiple etiologies of IUGR, it is clear that any treatment modalities proposed must be tailored specifically to the underlying cause. Unfortunately, no intervention has been shown to be consistently efficacious in reducing perinatal mortality. These treatments include nutritional supplementation, pharmacologic manipulations aimed at improving blood flow such as heparin and low-dose aspirin, plasma volume expansion, and bed rest. Maternal hyperoxygenation may be useful, but its long-term use requires further study. The preterm, IUGR fetus should be treated with antenatal steroids to decrease the risk of neonatal pulmonary and central nervous system (CNS) morbidity if preterm delivery is anticipated.

Birth weight and gestational age remain the most important determinants of perinatal outcome and it is for this reason that management strategies of the IUGR fetus are so challenging. Serial ultrasound evaluation of fetal growth, fetal behavior as reflected by the biophysical profile, amniotic fluid volume, and impedance to blood flow in fetal vessels form the basis of evaluation of the fetal condition and decision making. The biophysical profile (BPP), of which amniotic fluid volume measurement and the nonstress tests are components, remains a useful tool in the serial evaluation of fetal well-being. In fact, semiweekly BPP testing is associated with a very low perinatal mortality rate of approximately 1 in 1000 live births. The evaluation of flow impedance through the umbilical cord by Doppler artery velocimetry can significantly reduce perinatal death and unnecessary induction of labor in the preterm IUGR fetus. In general, when the Doppler systolic/diastolic ratio remains within normal limits, the pregnancy can be followed with weekly Doppler evaluations. The BPP, or an NST and AFI, can be used either as an interval test between Doppler examinations or twice weekly.

When fetal testing is nonreassuring, the commonly accepted guidelines apply to IUGR as well. Growth-restricted fetuses with oligohydramnios warrant intensive fetal surveillance or possible delivery depending on the suspected etiology and gestational age. Evidence of fetal lung maturity may provide sufficient reassurance to proceed with delivery in many instances.

There is a risk involved in the serial evaluation of IUGR. The fallibility of assessment methods leaves open the possibility that the diagnosis will be incorrect or that the risk level will be inaccurately estimated. Performing serial antenatal testing twice weekly with interval growth assessment every 2 weeks allows abnormal tests to be corroborated and, ideally, fetal maturity to be achieved before intervention. Despite close fetal surveillance, the decision to intervene and deliver a premature IUGR fetus is difficult and must be determined for each case individually. Indications for delivery include (1) a pregnancy at 39 weeks' gestation or greater, (2) cessation of fetal growth as evidenced by ultrasound during a 2- to 3-week period, (3) fetal compromise with a risk of intrauterine death as determined by fetal testing, and (4) deterioration of an underlying maternal complication of pregnancy (Box 8-4).

There is a tendency toward increased recurrence of IUGR in subsequent pregnancies; however, antenatal management is routine unless a potentially treatable cause of IUGR is identified.

Timing of Delivery

The fetus should be delivered if the risk of fetal death exceeds that of neonatal death and such decision-making requires individualized assessment. Early delivery may result in an infant at risk for serious sequelae of prematurity, whereas delaying delivery may yield a hypoxic, acidotic infant. Both scenarios are associated with an increased risk for long-term neurologic sequelae.

The diagnosis of IUGR alone is not an indication for preterm delivery because the neonatal consequences of IUGR are more severe when compounded by prematurity. Indeed, IUGR has been shown to increase both mortality and morbidity among premature neonates. A 2004 study reviewed 29,916 prematurely born neonates and found that within each gestational age group from 25 to 32 weeks, IUGR was associated with increased mortality, necrotizing enterocolitis, need for respiratory support at 28 days of age, and retinopathy of the premature infant. These associations were significant even when corrected for by exposure to antenatal steroids, and mode of delivery. As the Growth Restriction Intervention Trial (GRIT) study demonstrated, the effect of delivering these patients early to prevent in utero hypoxemia versus delaying for as long as possible to increase maturity is a difficult clinical decision. The decision to delay delivery results in an increased number of stillbirths; however, earlier delivery results in an almost exactly equal number of additional perinatal deaths. Pregnancies complicated by IUGR should not extend beyond 40 weeks of gestation.

Intrapartum Management

Cesarean delivery of the IUGR fetus is reserved for the usual obstetric indications, with the most common indication being nonreassuring fetal status. A recommendation for an immediate cesarean section may include late decelera-

---

Box 8-4   Diagnosis of Intrauterine Growth Restriction

- Recognize risk factors
- Perform serial measurements of fundal height
- Perform serial sonographic assessment
- Estimated fetal weight (EFW)
- AFV
- Umbilical artery Doppler

tions, absent variability, and progressive moderate to severe variable decelerations, especially if accompanied by an acidotic fetal blood pH value. The judicious use of oxytocin for induction or augmentation of labor is safe when there is no contraindication for a vaginal delivery. If the well-being of the fetus is not compromised and if labor is progressing, the usual guidelines for diagnosing labor abnormalities should be followed. Continuous fetal heart rate monitoring is advisable and pediatricians should be present for the delivery. Cord blood pH and blood gas values should always be obtained to provide information regarding fetal status before delivery. It must be remembered that hypoxia and acidosis at delivery are not necessarily secondary to intrapartum events. Narcotic analgesics such as Demerol and morphine should be used cautiously because of their depressant effect on newborn respiration. Lumbar epidural anesthesia is the method of choice in most IUGR deliveries to reduce the effects of narcotics on newborn respiratory function.

NEONATAL OUTCOME

Neonatal outcomes are variable and relate to the etiology of IUGR, gestational age and birth weight, and antepartum and intrapartum factors. Overall, these newborns have a higher risk of neonatal mortality and cognitive and neurologic morbidity, particularly among those born very preterm. Regardless of gestational age, there may be an adverse impact in the IUGR newborn on cognitive function and neurobehavioral impairment. Epidemiologic studies suggest an increased incidence of learning deficits in these children and an increased association with spastic cerebral palsy. Several studies have demonstrated that an elevated nucleated red blood cell (NRBC) count may distinguish the fetus with growth restriction from the small but healthy fetus. In addition, an elevated NRBC count may independently predict adverse short-term neonatal outcome in IUGR fetuses. IUGR may also be a risk factor for the subsequent development of chronic hypertension, ischemic heart disease, and diabetes.

KEY POINTS

- Despite extensive research efforts, resulting in a deeper appreciation of the pathophysiology of IUGR and the development of sensitive diagnostic tools, the greatest risk of adverse perinatal outcome still occurs among growth-restricted fetuses with birth weights below the 3rd percentile for gestational age.
- IUGR denotes a pathologic process stemming from growth restriction. In contrast, SGA identifies the infant whose birth weight is below an arbitrary percentile for gestational age.
- As many as 70% of fetuses who weigh below the 10th percentile for gestational age are small simply because of constitutional factors such as body mass index, genetic makeup, female gender, or maternal ethnicity; they are not at high risk of perinatal mortality and morbidity.

KEY POINTS—cont'd

- Infants born between 38 and 42 weeks' gestation whose weights are between 1500 and 2500 g have perinatal mortality and morbidity 5 to 30 times that of infants whose weights are between the 10th and 90th percentile.
- The etiologies of IUGR can be divided into fetal, placental, and maternal factors.
- At the current time, ultrasound evaluation of the fetus is considered the standard for the diagnosis of IUGR.
- Birth weight and gestational age remain the most important determinants of perinatal outcome and it is for this reason that management strategies of the IUGR fetus are so challenging.
- The diagnosis of IUGR alone is not an indication for preterm delivery because the neonatal consequences of IUGR are more severe when compounded by prematurity.
- Cesarean delivery of the IUGR fetus is reserved for the usual obstetric indications, with the most common indication being nonreassuring fetal status.
- Neonatal outcomes are variable and relate to the etiology of IUGR, gestational age and birth weight, and antepartum and intrapartum factors.

SUGGESTED READINGS

American College of Obstetricians and Gynecologists (ACOG): *Intrauterine Growth Restriction*. Washington, DC, 2000, ACOG.

Creasy R, Resnik R: Intrauterine growth restriction. In Creasy R, Resnik R, editors: *Maternal-Fetal Medicine*. New York, 1999, WB Saunders, pp 569-585.

Divon MY, editor: *Clinical Obstetrics and Gynecology: Intrauterine Growth Restriction*. Vol 40, No 4, 1997.

Divon MY, editor: *Abnormal Fetal Growth*. New York, 1991, Elsevier.

Resnik R: Intrauterine growth restriction. *Obstet Gynecol* 99:490, 2002.

9

MANAGEMENT OF OLIGOHYDRAMNIOS AND POLYHYDRAMNIOS

Robert Gagnon and Michael G. Ross

DEFINITION

Amniotic fluid volume may be defined using quantitative or semiquantitative techniques. In human pregnancy, normal amniotic fluid changes have been described by Brace and Wolf, referencing prior studies that used indicator dilution techniques. These results suggest that there is a progressive increase in amniotic fluid volume from a mean of 30 ml at 10 weeks to 190 ml at 16 weeks, peaking at 780 ml at 32 to 35 weeks' gestation; thereafter, amniotic fluid volume progressively decreases to approximately 550 ml at 42 weeks. The wide biologic variability in the amniotic fluid volume with advancing gestational age makes an absolute volume criterion for oligohydramnios or polyhydramnios inappropriate. Accordingly, amniotic fluid volume abnormalities are best defined as a volume below the 5th percentile or above the 95th percentile for gestational age. In clinical practice, ultrasonographic assessment of amniotic fluid volume is used as an estimate of amniotic fluid volume and it is an integral part of the biophysical profile, the most commonly used ultrasound-based antenatal test of fetal well-being.

Amniotic fluid volume may be estimated by quantifying the largest single vertical measurement (known as the maximum vertical pocket or single deepest pocket [SDP]) of amniotic fluid without a loop of umbilical cord. With these criteria, oligohydramnios has been defined as a SDP that does not exceed 1 or 2 cm in two perpendicular planes. Conversely, polyhydramnios has been defined as a minimum of one pocket of amniotic fluid that measures 8 cm in two perpendicular planes (Box 9-1).

The most common assessment of amniotic fluid volume is the amniotic fluid index (AFI), which is applicable only in singleton pregnancies. The pregnant uterus is divided in four equal quadrants and the SDP of fluid within each quadrant is summed. When using the AFI, oligohydramnios is defined as an index less than 5 cm and polyhydramnios is commonly defined as an index of either more than 18 or more than 24 cm.

Box 9-1

Oligohydramnios is usually defined as an amniotic fluid index of less than 5 cm or a maximum pocket of amniotic fluid that measures less than 1 cm or less than 2 cm in two perpendicular planes. Conversely, polyhydramnios is defined as an amniotic fluid index of more than 18 cm or more than 24 cm or a single pocket of amniotic fluid that measures more than 8 cm in two perpendicular planes.

ETIOLOGY

It is important to have a basic understanding of the pathways for amniotic fluid movement. In early gestation, before the establishment of fetal urine production and fetal swallowing, the most likely mechanism for amniotic fluid maintenance is an active transport of solute by the amnion into the amniotic space, with water moving passively down the solute gradient and osmolality gradient. After 17 to 18 weeks, the excretion of fetal urine and later respiratory secretion of fluid become the major sources, and fetal swallowing the major clearance mechanism of amniotic fluid. As a result, even with congenital absence of fetal kidneys, amniotic fluid volume may appear normal before 17 weeks' gestation. After 18 weeks, bilateral renal agenesis or lethal forms of bilateral multicystic kidney disease usually result in oligohydramnios. Fetal micturition at term has been estimated to be between 500 and 1200 ml/day depending on the methodology used. It has long been recognized that fetal pulmonary hypoplasia is associated with oligohydramnios due to renal agenesis, resulting in Potter's syndrome, a lethal anomaly. Recent experiments in fetal sheep have indicated that fetal hypoxia does not reduce urine production. Thus oligohydramnios associated with placental insufficiency may be because of increased intramembranous absorption of water into the fetal and maternal vascular compartments rather than reduced fetal urine production (Box 9-2).

Premature rupture of membranes is defined as rupture of the chorioamnionic membranes before the onset of labor. This complication of pregnancy, occurring preterm, is responsible for approximately 30% of all premature deliveries. Oligohydramnios seen on ultrasonography is usually confirmatory. Indomethacin treatment also has been associated with the development of oligohydramnios secondary to decreased fetal urine production, particularly if used for several days. The onset of oligohydramnios during long-term administration of indomethacin is unpredictable.

Box 9-2

Recent experiments of severe placental insufficiency in fetal sheep have shown that oligohydramnios associated with placental insufficiency is not due to a reduction in fetal urine production but more likely to increased intramembranous absorption of water into the fetal and maternal vascular compartments.

Box 9-3

Esophageal atresia, duodenal atresia (30% risk of trisomy 21), jejunal atresia, or large bowel obstruction are associated with polyhydramnios that usually develop after 25 weeks' gestation.

Polyhydramnios has been associated with maternal diabetes, particularly poor maternal glycemic control. It is usually believed that polyhydramnios occurs because of excessive fetal urine production; however, only 32% of diabetic pregnant women demonstrated an increase in fetal urine production, perhaps a result of relative fetal glycosuria. Inability of the fetus to swallow due to a major central nervous system anomaly, that is, anencephaly, esophageal atresia, duodenal atresia (30% risk of trisomy 21), jejunal atresia, or large bowel obstruction, is associated with polyhydramnios that usually develops after 25 weeks' gestation (Box 9-3). As a rule, with fetal gastrointestinal tract obstruction, the more proximal the obstruction, the more severe the polyhydramnios because amniotic fluid swallowed is reabsorbed within the small and large bowel. With severe acute polyhydramnios, premature rupture of membranes with ensuing premature delivery may ensue. Nonimmune hydrops, diaphragmatic hernia, and myotonic dystrophy are less common fetal conditions associated with polyhydramnios. Approximately 50% of cases of polyhydramnios are idiopathic, without any obvious cause identified. The incidence of chromosomal anomalies associated with polyhydramnios has been reported as high as 8% to 10%. In multiple gestations with monochorionic placentation, approximately 15% of these pregnancies are complicated with twin-to-twin transfusion syndrome characterized by oligohydramnios in the donor twin and polyhydramnios in the recipient twin. There is growing evidence that optimal management of twin-to-twin transfusion syndrome may involve fetoscopic laser ablation of communicating arteriovenous anastomosis with better neurologic outcome in survivors than those treated with amnioreduction. Table 9-1 summarizes the most common causes of disorders of amniotic fluid volume.

Table 9-1

Etiologies of Amniotic Fluid Volume Abnormalities

Oligohydramnios	Fetal renal agenesis
	Severe placental insufficiency
	Bilateral multicystic kidney disease
	Posterior urethral valve
	Premature rupture of membranes
	Donor twin in twin-to-twin transfusion syndrome
Polyhydramnios	Maternal diabetes
	Fetal macrosomia
	Central nervous system anomaly
	Gastrointestinal tract obstruction
	Nonimmune hydrops
	Myotonic dystrophy
	Recipient twin in twin-to-twin transfusion syndrome
	Circulatory system anomaly

PATHOGENESIS

The regulation of amniotic fluid volume is still not completely understood. In the later half of pregnancy, potential amniotic fluid volume regulatory pathways include the following: the two major inflows into the amniotic sac include fetal urine production and fetal lung fluid secretion, and the two major outflows include fetal swallowing and the intramembranous pathway. In the absence of fetal anomalies, if there is a regulatory mechanism for amniotic fluid volume homeostasis, it is likely through modulation of intramembranous flow. This pathway involves exchange of water and solutes between amniotic fluid and fetal blood; under normal conditions, intramembranous flow approximates 200 ml/day.

Late in gestation when amniotic fluid volume averages 700 to 800 ml, 1000 ml of fluid flows into the amniotic compartment, and 1000 ml leaves the amniotic compartment daily. Therefore only minor to moderate aberrations in fluid flows during a period of days could readily lead to oligohydramnios or polyhydramnios. Recent observations from Brace et al. in sheep suggest that the primary mechanism that mediates intramembranous solute fluxes is bulk flow rather than passive osmosis. During fetal hypoxia without placental damage, there is a progressive fetal polyuria with relatively small changes in amniotic fluid volume, suggesting an increase in intramembranous absorption. Further, as noted previously, we have shown in sheep that severe placental insufficiency induced by fetal placental embolization causes oligohydramnios without any change in fetal urine production. These results provide evidence that the intramembranous pathway is responsible for oligohydramnios during such pathologic conditions.

In humans, there is no good correlation between maternal blood volume or composition and AFI. Thus, individual patient AFI variation is a result of factors other than maternal blood volume or composition. During twin-to-twin transfusion syndrome, the discordance in amniotic fluid volume primarily is due to a difference in fetal urine production rate between the donor, who has low urine output and oligohydramnios, and the recipient twin, who demonstrates high urine output and subsequent polyhydramnios.

CLINICAL PRESENTATION

History Making the correct diagnosis of oligohydramnios is essential for optimal outcome. Premature rupture of membranes may be indicated by a patient's history of a large gush of clear fluid from the vagina followed by persistent leakage. However, other potential explanations for discharge of fluid from the vagina include urinary leakage, excessive vaginal discharge, or silent dilatation of the cervix without premature rupture of membranes. Early signs of premature labor such as pelvic cramps and clinical signs of chorioamnionitis, including maternal fever, chills, malodorous vaginal discharge, and uterine tenderness, are important to document. Lethal hereditary renal anomalies (e.g., bilateral multicystic kidney disease) also may contribute to oligohydramnios. Thus, a detailed family history and family tree of previous stillbirth or early neonatal death may be performed if appropriate.

The clinical diagnosis of intrauterine growth restriction (IUGR) should be considered in patients presenting with oligohydramnios. Several factors might increase the clinician's index of suspicion about suboptimal fetal growth. Known risk factors for placental insufficiency, such as maternal smoking, maternal hypertensive disorder (Box 9-4), uncorrected cyanotic heart disease, diabetes type I with vascular disease, previous pregnancy with IUGR, previous history of thrombophilias, and lupus erythematosus, need detailed documentation. Early pregnancy viral infection (e.g., primary herpes, cytomegalovirus, toxoplasmosis) may also be responsible. Chromosomal anomalies may be present in 5% to 8% of all pregnancies complicated with IUGR, particularly if associated with normal amniotic fluid volume or polyhydramnios.

The development of polyhydramnios may first become evident as a pregnant woman presents complaining of increasing abdominal discomfort, onset of premature labor, or preterm premature rupture of membranes because of overdistention of the uterus. Alternatively, a rapidly enlarging abdomen may signify twin gestation, both a result of increased fetal mass and potential twin-to-twin transfusion syndrome. When following multiple gestations with monochorionic placentation, ultrasound to assess fetal growth and amniotic fluid volume may be performed at frequent intervals (e.g., every 2-4 weeks), beginning with fetal viability. Evidence for diagnosis of twin-to-twin transfusion syndrome includes (1) single monochorionic placenta, (2) polyhydramnios/oligohydramnios sequence, and (3) same-sex fetuses (Box 9-5).

Symptoms

As previously noted, there may or may not be any specific symptom associated with oligohydramnios or polyhydramnios until complications arise (e.g., oligohydramnios-associated intrauterine fetal death, polyhydramnios-associated premature rupture of membranes, or premature labor).

Laboratory Findings

Severe placental insufficiency and oligohydramnios may be associated with acquired thrombophilias, including the presence of antiphospholipid or anticardiolipin antibodies, lupus anticoagulant, or acquired activated protein C resistance. Under conditions of unexplained fetal growth restriction, inherited thrombophilias may be assessed for mutation of factor V Leiden resulting in activated protein C resistance, prothrombin gene mutation, hyperhomocysteinemia, antithrombin deficiency, and protein S deficiency. Maternal serology for both immunoglobulin (Ig) G and IgM for toxoplasmosis, cytomegalovirus, and herpes simplex may be determined to rule out recent infection that may be associated with IUGR.

Box 9-4

Several factors might increase the clinician's index of suspicion about suboptimal fetal growth. Known risks factors for placental insufficiency include maternal smoking and maternal hypertensive disorders.

Box 9-5

Evidence for diagnosis of twin-to-twin transfusion syndrome includes (1) single monochorionic placenta, (2) polyhydramnios/oligohydramnios sequence, and (3) same sex fetuses.

Standard investigations for premature rupture of membranes include a vaginorectal culture for group B streptococcus, complete blood count, and fetal health surveillance using fetal heart rate monitoring and/or biophysical profile as indicated. In cases of polyhydramnios, an oral glucose tolerance test is recommended to rule out gestational diabetes. Similarly, in women with diabetes type I and type II, tighter glycemic control may improve polyhydramnios. Once the diagnosis of oligohydramnios or polyhydramnios is established, management is dependent on the radiologic (ultrasound) findings and gestational age.

Radiologic Findings

Using the single largest pocket SDP of amniotic fluid, oligohydramnios has been variously defined. The AFI of less than 5 cm, and SDP less than 2 cm has resulted in oligohydramnios prevalence rates of 8% and 1%, respectively. Oligohydramnios can usually be attributed to five major causes, including anomalies and/or chromosome abnormalities, IUGR, postterm pregnancy, ruptured membranes, and iatrogenic.

The prevalence of congenital anomalies (4.5%-37%) and aneuploidy (up to 4%) is based on the size and selection criteria of the population studied. The majority of fetal anomalies resulting in oligohydramnios involve the urinary tract. Sonography can accurately depict the majority of significant renal anomalies resulting in oligohydramnios, including bilateral renal agenesis, bladder outlet obstruction, multicystic dysplastic kidneys, and infantile polycystic kidney disease. Renal agenesis is a difficult malformation to confirm as hypertrophied adrenal glands may be confused with normal kidneys. Failure to detect the renal arteries at the appropriate distance confirms the diagnosis of bilateral renal agenesis, whereas spontaneous filling and emptying of the fetal urinary bladder virtually excludes the diagnosis of bilateral renal agenesis. Demonstration of early symmetric IUGR suggests the possibility of an underlying chromosomal anomaly such as trisomy 18 or triploidy and requires a complete detailed fetal anatomy survey assessment. Genetic amniocentesis may be offered depending on ultrasound results. IUGR is suspected when the estimated fetal weight falls below the 10th percentile for the expected gestational age. The incidence of IUGR is 20% and 39% when the single largest pocket of amniotic fluid measures less than 2 cm and less than 1 cm, respectively. Umbilical artery Doppler may be considered with IUGR to assess placental function. When oligohydramnios is associated with postterm pregnancy, induction and delivery is generally indicated.

In the presence of preterm premature rupture of membranes, persistent oligohydramnios in the second trimester carries a poor prognosis. Severe oligohydramnios for more than 14 days at less than 25 weeks is associated with a 90% neonatal mortality. On the other hand, leakage of fluid following genetic amniocentesis has a more favorable prognosis. Finally, medications such as nonsteroidal antiinflammatory drugs and angiotensin-converting enzyme inhibitors may results in oligohydramnios and thus are not indicated in pregnancy unless benefits outweigh potential gains.

The prevalence of polyhydramnios is between 0.4% and 3% depending on the population studied. Semiquantitative assessment based on the largest pocket of amniotic fluid can be used to classify polyhydramnios into mild, moderate, and severe (>8cm, >12 cm, and >16 cm, respectively). Most often, polyhydramnios is mild and chronic, although the acute development of polyhydramnios may be associated with twin-to-twin-transfusion syndrome. As the severity of polyhydramnios increases, there is a greater likelihood of ultrasound detection of congenital anomalies. The most common anomalies include malformations of the gastrointestinal tract (40%), central nervous system (25%), cardiocirculatory system (22%), and urinary tract (13%).

143

DIFFERENTIAL DIAGNOSIS

Table 9-1 summarizes the most common causes for oligohydramnios and polyhydramnios; these causes are discussed in detail throughout the chapter.

TREATMENT AND EXPECTED OUTCOME

Oligohy-dramnios

The most common complications resulting from oligohydramnios include intrauterine fetal death, pulmonary hypoplasia, and various skeletal and facial deformities (oligohydramnios deformation syndrome). The ultimate prognosis depends on the underlying etiology, the severity of oligohydramnios, gestational age at diagnosis, and duration. Patients diagnosed with oligohydramnios during the second trimester have a higher incidence of major anomalies (50%) and a lower survival rate (10%) than when it is diagnosed during the third trimester (22% with anomalies and 85% survival) (Box 9-6). Neonates with skeletal deformities (talipes equinovarus, craniofacial deformities) have a higher mortality rate if there is associated severe pulmonary hypoplasia than those without the skeletal deformities.

Isolated oligohydramnios during the third trimester is not necessarily associated with poor outcome in the absence of fetal anomalies, although the fetal mortality rate is increased. In the absence of anomalies, the perinatal mortality rate reported by Chamberlain et al. was 10.9% when the largest

---

Box 9-6

Patients diagnosed with oligohydramnios during the second trimester have a higher incidence of major anomalies (50%) and a lower survival rate (10%) than when it is diagnosed during the third trimester.

pocket of fluid was less than 1 cm, and 3.8% when the largest pocket was less than 2 cm, as compared with 1.9% with normal amniotic fluid. If severe placental insufficiency is documented with IUGR and oligohydramnios, delivery is indicated with appropriate consideration of cesarean delivery.

Forced maternal hydration has been suggested to improve amniotic fluid volume, although there is very limited evidence to support such a strategy. Notably, maternal hydration would not be expected to alter amniotic fluid volume in pregnancies with fetal anomalies, whereas the response in the presence of preterm premature rupture of membranes is unknown. At the present time, bed rest and limited activity is the only established treatment, although the efficacy of these simple actions is similarly unknown. With preterm premature rupture of membranes, careful monitoring for early detection of signs and symptoms of chorioamnionitis is recommended. If chorioamnionitis develops, delivery should be expedited (Box 9-7) regardless of gestational age. If the cervix is open in the presence of preterm premature of membranes, cord prolapse is a potential but rare catastrophic event, particularly in nonvertex or unstable presentations. Long-term survival for infants delivered at more than 32 weeks is very good. In the absence of infection, elective induction at 32 to 36 weeks is recommended.

For patients with suspected IUGR, enhanced fetal health surveillance with one or more modalities (fetal heart rate monitoring, biophysical profile, umbilical artery Doppler) is recommended. When reversed end-diastolic velocity develops, if viability has been achieved, glucocorticoid administration followed by delivery may be considered because deteriorating placental function is associated with excessively high perinatal death rate.

Polyhydramnios

Treatment of polyhydramnios depends on the etiology and prognosis for effective treatment. Therapeutic amniocentesis is an option for the treatment of twin-to-twin transfusion syndrome. However, recent studies have indicated that fetoscopic laser ablation of the communicating blood vessels is of greater efficacy in severe cases. Medical treatment of polyhydramnios has been attempted using prostaglandin antagonists (i.e., indomethacin). However, recent information suggests an increased risk of intraventricular hemorrhage and pulmonary hypertension in neonates exposed to indomethacin for several days. Thus indomethacin should be used selectively (e.g., extreme prematurity) for treatment of polyhydramnios.

Box 9-7

With preterm premature rupture of membranes, careful monitoring for early detection of signs and symptoms of chorioamnionitis is recommended. If clinical chorioamnionitis develops, delivery should be expedited.

KEY POINTS

- The clinician must have a high index of clinical suspicion for IUGR in women with known risk factors.
- There is no proven effective treatment for oligohydramnios or polyhydramnios in singleton pregnancies.
- Twin-to-twin transfusion syndrome may be treated with therapeutic amniocentesis or fetoscopic laser ablation of the communicating vessels.
- Because of the incidence of congenital and chromosomal anomalies in singleton pregnancies with oligohydramnios or polyhydramnios, these patients may require a detailed fetal anatomy survey. Genetic amniocentesis may also be offered.
- More research is required to better understand amniotic fluid volume regulation.

SUGGESTED READINGS

Brace RA: Amniotic fluid dynamics. In Creasy RK, Resnik R, editors: *Maternal Fetal Medicine: Principles and Practice*. Philadelphia, 2004, Elsevier, pp 45-54.

Chamberlain PL, Manning FA, Morrison L, et al: Ultrasound evaluation of amniotic fluid volume. *Am J Obstet Gynecol* 150:245-249, 1984.

Hill LM, Sohaey R, Nyberg DA: Abnormalities of amniotic fluid. In Nyberg DA et al, editors: *Diagnostic Imaging of Fetal Anomalies*. Philadelphia, 2003, Lippincott Williams and Wilkins, pp 59-84.

10

RECURRENT PREGNANCY LOSS

Anna K. Sfakianaki and Charles J. Lockwood

Human reproduction is an inefficient process. Only 15% to 30% of fertilized oocytes result in viable pregnancy. The loss of a pregnancy before viability is referred to as miscarriage, or spontaneous abortion (SAb), and is the most common complication of pregnancy. Forty percent to fifty percent of conceptuses are lost before expected menses and 30% to 35% are lost at or following missed menses.

Approximately 2% of women have two consecutive pregnancy losses. Traditionally, recurrent pregnancy loss (RPL), which affects approximately 1% of couples, refers to the loss of three or more consecutive pregnancies. However, the risk of a third loss after two miscarriages is approximately 30%, whereas the risk after three losses is about 33%. Because this difference is very small, many clinicians will begin the evaluation of RPL after two losses. This approach may be especially useful in older women. Primary RPL refers to patients who have never achieved pregnancy, whereas secondary RPL refers to those in whom the miscarriages follow at least one normal pregnancy. The risk of miscarriage is lower in women who carry at least one pregnancy to term, whereas a history of miscarriage increases the chance of miscarriage in subsequent pregnancies. Maternal age is also a strong predictor of recurrent losses.

The workup of RPL is negative in more than 50% of patients. However, successful pregnancy occurs in up to 35% to 80% of couples who have been evaluated for RPL, regardless of the etiology and treatment. Couples with unexplained RPL have even higher chances of successful pregnancy. Counseling regarding the risk of recurrence depends on the etiology demonstrated.

This chapter outlines the causes of RPL (Box 10-1) and their potential therapies, where applicable.

CHROMOSOMAL ABNORMALITIES

Chromosomal abnormalities occur in 64% to 88% of isolated SAbs. Of these, 62% to 70% are autosomal trisomies, 8% to 20% are triploid or tetraploid, and 6% are related to chromosomal structural abnormalities. The prevalence of chromosomal abnormalities in RPL is at least 50% and is usually related to maternal age. In patients undergoing in vitro fertilization (IVF), preimplantation failure is associated with chromosomal abnormalities in 67% to

> **Box 10-1   Etiology of Recurrent Pregnancy Loss**
>
> - Chromosomal
> - Anatomic/uterine
> - Endocrine
> - Immunologic
> - Thrombophilic

85% of cases. Preimplantation karyotyping of embryos from recurrent abortion patients demonstrates a sixfold increased rate of monosomies. Recurrent aneuploidy can be demonstrated in more than two thirds of subsequent pregnancies after diagnosis in a first pregnancy.

The etiology of chromosomal abnormalities is not completely understood. Abnormalities that arise during the first meiotic division account for the majority of aneuploidy. The exact mechanism through which this occurs is under investigation. Genetic factors that are age-independent, such as fragile sites on chromosomes, inversions, and translocations, account for 3.5% to 4.4% of RPL from aneuploidy. Of these, translocations are most often found in RPL. There are two major types of translocations: reciprocal, in which two segments from different chromosomes are exchanged, and Robertsonian, in which there is fusion at the centromere of two acrocentric chromosomes. Balanced translocations may result in normal carriers but can lead to unbalanced rearrangements in offspring and thus miscarriage. Pregnancy loss is more common with maternal translocations.

Nutritional factors such as abnormal folate metabolism, elevated homocysteine levels (>18 micromol/L), lower erythrocyte folate levels (<160 mg/ml), and low vitamin B_6 levels (<49 nmol/L) are all linked to RPL. Age-related decreased telomerase activity that leads to shorter telomeres may cause meiotic failure and nondisjunction.

When possible, genetic evaluation of aborted material should be undertaken in women who experience consecutive miscarriages. This is possible at dilation and curettage for anembryonic gestations or embryonic demise; however, if the patient completes the miscarriage on her own this is not always possible. In couples with more than three consecutive losses, karyotype of both partners should be performed, looking for translocations that may affect pregnancy.

Patients in whom a genetic factor is suspected may benefit from folate and/or vitamin B_6 therapy. Couples with proven translocations may undergo IVF and preimplantation genetic diagnosis (PGD) with transfer of only genetically normal embryos. The use of IVF with PGD in older mothers with RPL because of recurrent aneuploidy has been recommended by some experts, but at least one study has suggested that it is not effective. Finally, these patients can undergo IVF using donated gametes (egg or sperm).

INFECTIOUS DISEASES

Although infection is a frequent cause of poor pregnancy outcome later in pregnancy, no consistent association between infection and RPL has been demonstrated. Neither *Chlamydia* nor *Mycoplasma* species, common causes of preterm birth and other complications after the first trimester, has been conclusively identified as a cause of RPL. These may, however, be associated with nonrecurrent or sporadic pregnancy loss.

UTERINE FACTOR

Müllerian Tract Anomalies

Congenital anomalies of the müllerian tract manifest as a spectrum of findings, from partial septa to complete duplication of the upper reproductive tract (Figure 10-1). Often these anomalies are noted as incidental findings at routine obstetric ultrasound or at delivery; however, they are found in 10% to 15% of patients with RPL. The one anomaly that has been repeatedly associated with RPL is uterine septum, which occurs when there is a failure of resorption in the midline. It has been postulated that septa lead to miscarriage through a mechanism of "poor" implantation, but this explanation lacks biologic plausibility. Although resection of the septum has been recommended in patients with RPL, it has not been studied in a rigorous fashion. The American College of Obstetrics and Gynecologists (ACOG) does not recommend any surgical corrections on women with müllerian anomalies unless attempt at pregnancy has been made and has failed.

Uterine Fibroids

Fibroids are classically described by their location with respect to the uterine wall. Subserosal fibroids are located on the exterior aspect of the uterus and do not involve the endometrial cavity. Intramural fibroids are entirely within the myometrial thickness and similarly do not impinge on the interior of the uterus. Submucosal fibroids, however, extend into the cavity and may distort its contours. In this location they act in a similar fashion to uterine septa, leading to abnormal implantation and/or vascular supply and recurrent miscarriage. Hysteroscopic resection of submucosal fibroids is straightforward; however, no prospective study has evaluated its efficacy in the treatment of RPL.

The diagnosis of uterine abnormalities can be achieved through sonohysterography, hysterosalpingogram (HSG), or hysteroscopy. Each technique is associated with particular benefits. Sonohysterography is an ultrasound-based procedure in which the instillation of sterile saline allows better visualization of the shape of the uterine cavity. Importantly, the exterior of the uterus may also be evaluated, allowing the distinction between septate and bicornuate uterine anomalies. Three-dimensional ultrasound is a promising new modality for this latter indication. HSG also allows evaluation of intra-uterine pathology; however, it involves the use of radiocontrast dye and is limited in its ability to assess the contour of the fundus. Hysteroscopy, like HSG, allows assessment only of the inside of the uterus. However, operative hysteroscopy may also be used in the treatment of submucous fibroids, septa, and synechiae.

Magnetic resonance imaging is emerging as tool for the evaluation of uterine anomalies. It is particularly useful in the workup of myometrial pathology, including fibroids and adenomyosis.

Figure 10-1

The classification of müllerian anomalies. Congenital anomalies of the müllerian tract manifest as a spectrum of findings, from partial septa to complete duplication of the upper reproductive tract. *DES*, Diethylstilbestrol. (From Speroff L, Fritz MA: *Clinical Gynecologic Endocrinology and Infertility,* ed 7. Philadelphia, 2005, Lippincott Williams and Wilkins.)

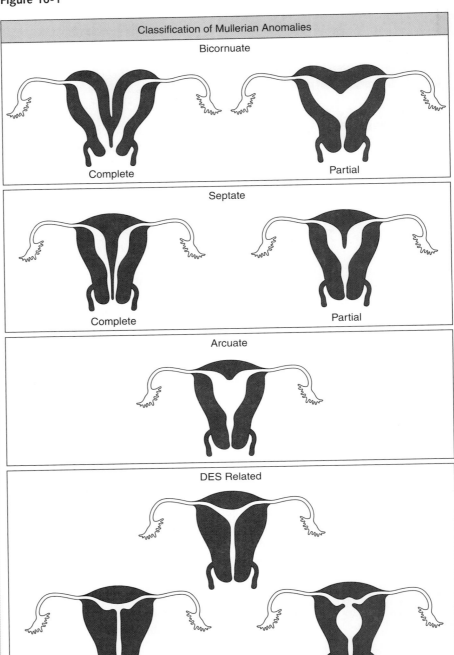

ENDOCRINE CAUSES

Thyroid Disease

RPL is not associated with subclinical hypothyroidism or adequately treated thyroid disease. Untreated thyroid disorders are associated both with infertility and recurrent miscarriage. There is controversy regarding the utility of screening asymptomatic women with RPL for thyroid disease.

Diabetes

Poorly controlled diabetes mellitus has been consistently associated with early pregnancy loss. The correlation seems to be dose-dependent: higher hemoglobin A1C values are associated with higher rates of miscarriage. There is no association between RPL and well-controlled diabetes. Screening for diabetes is not warranted in the absence of symptoms of hyperglycemia.

Insulin Resistance

Insulin resistance is also associated with RPL, and polycystic ovarian syndrome (PCOS) has been associated with SAb. This may be mediated via an impaired fibrinolytic response as evidenced by the fact that women with PCOS and RPL have elevated levels of plasminogen activator inhibitor (PAI-1). Elevated levels of PAI-1 may impede trophoblast implantation and invasion mediated by urokinase-type plasminogen activator. Other potentially embryotoxic factors found in excess in PCOS patient's follicular fluid include glucose, insulin-like growth factor-1 (IGF-1), and androgen levels. Polycystic ovaries alone do not predict the risk of miscarriage. However, obesity is independently associated with pregnancy loss. Retrospective and small case-control studies have shown that therapy with metformin reduces the risk of RPL in women with PCOS from 42% to 62% to 26% to 29%. Larger prospective studies are necessary to confirm this association.

Luteal Phase Defects

In the first trimester, the corpus luteum produces progesterone, which provides the hormonal support necessary for the maintenance of early pregnancy. Abnormalities in this mechanism may lead to pregnancy loss. The prevalence of luteal phase defect, in which there is a relative deficiency in progesterone, is 25% in RPL patients. Unfortunately there are no definitive diagnostic criteria, and there are conflicting reports regarding the benefit of progesterone therapy in these patients. A meta-analysis of trials of progesterone therapy for RPL did not demonstrate a benefit. In addition, luteal phase defect is also seen in women who subsequently carry pregnancies to term. One therapy that is currently under investigation is human chorionic gonadotropin (hCG). A Cochrane review suggested that this therapy may reduce the risk of pregnancy loss; however, more research is needed.

Hyperprolactinemia

Elevated prolactin levels have been associated with RPL, and treatment with bromocriptine has been shown, in at least one study, to increase the likelihood of normal pregnancy.

IMMUNOLOGIC FACTORS

Alloimmune Losses

The acceptance of the fetal and placental allograft by the maternal immune system results from trophoblast expression of nonimmunogenic HLA-G; Fas ligand; immunosuppressive agents such as hCG, PAPP-A, and progesterone; and increased maternal cortisol levels. In theory, maternal rejection of the fetus should result in RPL. However, the failure of multiple trials of immunomodulatory therapy suggests that this simple scenario is unlikely. Randomized controlled trials of maternal immunization with paternal antigens have yielded conflicting results. Subsequent meta-analyses came to opposite conclusions, with one showing increased rates of live births in treatment groups and the other showing no difference. These studies have been limited by methodologic inconsistencies. Tests have been developed for maternal anti-paternal leukocyte "blocking" antibodies; however, these are neither sensitive nor specific, as patients without maternal anti-paternal leukocyte antibodies have normal pregnancies and patients with the antibodies may miscarry. Meta-analysis of trials of intravenous immunoglobulin therapy also shows no difference in outcomes; however, analysis was not done to distinguish effects in patients with primary versus secondary RPL. In summary, this information suggests that well-designed prospective trials of immunomodulatory therapy for RPL are needed.

Natural Killer Cells

Another potential theory of placental immunopathology focuses on natural killer (NK cells), lymphocytes that are part of the innate immune system. The presence of elevated levels of NK cells in the uterine mucosa is putatively associated with RPL, although their presence in peripheral blood is not. Indeed, we have shown that uterine NK cells express a very different repertoire of genes than those in the circulation. Moreover, the Moffett laboratory at the University of Cambridge has reported that decreased decidual NK cell activity may be associated with impaired endovascular trophoblast invasion, fetal growth restriction, and preeclampsia. Thus the precise role of uterine NK cells in mediating adverse pregnancy outcomes remains uncertain.

Antiphospholipid Antibody Syndrome (APLS)

The autoimmune disorder APLS can be a catastrophic disease and is associated with arterial and venous thrombosis or RPL and with laboratory abnormalities (Box 10-2). APLS may occur as a primary condition or as a secondary syndrome in women with underlying autoimmune disorders. Ten percent to fifteen percent of patients with RPL have APLS, which is also associated with later pregnancy complications including preeclampsia, growth restriction, and fetal death. Some studies suggest that APLS is more often associated with loss after 10 weeks' gestation. In APLS, antibodies to proteins binding to negatively charged phospholipids on the membranes of endothelial cells impair the normal anticoagulant properties and enhance coagulation, leading to progressive thrombosis. When these thromboses occur in the placenta, thrombus formation, infarction, and vasculopathy

---

Box 10-2   Preliminary Classification Criteria for Antiphospholipid Syndrome

Clinical criteria

1. Vascular thrombosis

   One or more clinical episodes of arterial, venous, or small vessel thrombosis in any tissue or organ. Thrombosis must be confirmed by imaging or doppler studies or histopathology, with the exception of superficial venous thrombosis. For histopathologic confirmation, thrombosis should be present without significant evidence of inflammation in the vessel wall.

2. Pregnancy morbidity

   (a) One or more unexplained deaths of a morphologically normal fetus at or beyond the tenth week of gestation, with normal fetal morphology documented by ultrasound or by direct examination of the fetus, or

   (b) One or more premature births of a morphologically normal neonate at or before the thirty-fourth week of gestation because of severe preeclampsia or eclampsia or severe placental insufficiency (18,19), or

   (c) Three or more unexplained consecutive spontaneous abortions before the tenth week of gestation, with maternal anatomic or hormonal abnormalities and paternal and maternal chromosomal causes excluded.

In studies of populations of patients who have more than one type of pregnancy morbidity, investigators are strongly encouraged to stratify groups of subjects according to a, b, or c above.

Laboratory criteria

1. Anticardiolipin antibody of IgG and/or IgM isotype in blood, present in medium or high titer on two or more occasions at least 6 weeks apart, measured by a standardized enzyme-linked immunosorbent assay for β_2-glycoprotein I–dependent anticardiolipin antibodies (7,20).

2. Lupus anticoagulant present in plasma on two or more occasions at least 6 weeks apart, detected according to the guidelines of the International Society on Thrombosis and Hemostasis (Scientific Subcommittee on Lupus Anticoagulants/Phospholipid-Dependent Antibodies) (21), in the following steps:

   (a) Prolonged phospholipid-dependent coagulation demonstrated on a screening test, e.g., activated partial thromboplastin time, kaolin clotting time, dilute Russell's viper venom time, dilute prothrombin time, Textarin time.

   (b) Failure to correct the prolonged coagulation time on the screening test by mixing with normal platelet-poor plasma.

   (c) Shortening or correction of the prolonged coagulation time on the screening test by the addition of excess phospholipid.

   (d) Exclusion of other coagulopathies, e.g., factor VIII inhibitor or heparin, as appropriate.

Definite antiphospholipid antibody syndrome is considered to be present if at least one of the clinical criteria and one of the laboratory criteria are met.

From Wilson WA et al: International consensus statement on preliminary classification criteria for definite antiphospholipid syndrome: report of an international workshop. *Arthritis Rheum* 42:1309-11, 1999.

lead to complications during pregnancy. These antibodies also activate complement in the decidua, promoting inflammation and impaired trophoblast invasion.

The basic tests in the evaluation for APLS are lupus anticoagulant, immunoglobulin (Ig) G or IgM antibodies to ß2-glycoprotein I, and anticardiolipin IgG or IgM antibodies. The antibodies must be present in moderate to high levels. For the diagnosis to be made, the tests must be positive on two occasions at least 6 weeks apart. Some clinicians evaluate for APLS only in patients with both RPL and later pregnancy complications.

A recent meta-analysis examined the therapy for RPL resulting from APLS. Aspirin in combination with prophylactic dose heparin, either unfractionated or low molecular weight, was shown to increase the live birth rate in women with APLS. In women with a history of thrombosis, full anticoagulation with heparin is recommended. Therapy should continue to 6 weeks postpartum. Aspirin is not effective in the treatment of unexplained recurrent miscarriage.

Antinuclear Antibodies (ANAs)

In the absence of other clinical or laboratory findings, women with an isolated positive ANA do not demonstrate higher rates of recurrent miscarriages. Treatment of these women with aspirin is not effective; therefore, testing for ANA is not recommended in the evaluation of RPL.

THROMBOPHILIAS

Although in theory disorders that cause thrombosis within the placenta can cause RPL, the epidemiologic data are conflicting. Interpretation of studies is difficult because of varying definitions of pregnancy loss by gestational age. Inherited thrombophilias, such as the factor V Leiden mutation and the prothrombin G20210A mutation, have not been consistently linked to recurrent early pregnancy loss at less than 10 weeks' gestation. However, after 10 to 14 weeks' gestation, the inherited thrombophilias do appear to be modestly associated with pregnancy loss.

SUMMARY: EVALUATION OF RPL

It is important to remember that couples who are being evaluated for RPL have high levels of depression and stress. Some studies have indicated that psychological support may decrease the rates of unexplained miscarriage. Finally, patients should be reassured that even without treatment, successful pregnancy occurs in the majority of cases.

KEY POINTS

1. Spontaneous abortion is the most common complication of pregnancy. Forty percent to fifty percent of conceptuses are lost before expected menses, and 30% to 35% are lost at or following missed menses.
2. Traditionally, RPL refers to the loss of three or more consecutive pregnancies; however, many clinicians will begin the evaluation of RPL after two losses, because the risk of a third loss after two miscarriages is approximately 30%, whereas the risk after three losses is about 33%. This approach may be especially useful in older women.

KEY POINTS—cont'd

3. The risk of miscarriage is lower in women who carry at least one pregnancy to term, whereas a history of miscarriage increases the chance of miscarriage in subsequent pregnancies. Maternal age is also a strong predictor of recurrent losses.

4. The major causes of RPL are chromosomal, anatomic/uterine, endocrine, immunologic, and thrombophilic.

5. The evaluation of couple with RPL should include the following:

   - Parental karyotypes
   - Uterine evaluation with sonohysterography, HSG, and/or hysteroscopy
   - Evaluation for APLS: lupus anticoagulant, anticardiolipin antibodies, antibodies to ß2-glycoprotein I
   - A workup for inherited thrombophilias if the losses have occurred after 10 weeks
   - Serum prolactin level

6. The workup of RPL is negative in more than 50% of patients. However, successful pregnancy occurs in up to 35% to 80% of couples who have been evaluated for RPL, regardless of the etiology and treatment.

SUGGESTED READINGS

ACOG Practice Bulletin #68: Antiphospholipid syndrome. *Obstet Gynecol* 106:1113, 2005.

ACOG Practice Bulletin: Management of recurrent pregnancy loss. Number 24, February 2001. (Replaces Technical Bulletin Number 212, September 1995). American College of Obstetricians and Gynecologists. *Int J Gynaecol Obstet* 78:179, 2002.

Baart EB, Martini E, van den Berg I, et al: Preimplantation genetic screening reveals a high incidence of aneuploidy and mosaicism in embryos from young women undergoing IVF. *Hum Reprod* 21:223, 2006.

Daya S, Gunby J: The effectiveness of allogeneic leukocyte immunization in unexplained primary recurrent spontaneous abortion. Recurrent Miscarriage Immunotherapy Trialists Group. *Am J Reprod Immunol* 32:294, 1994.

Empson M, Lassere M, Craig JC, Scott JR: Recurrent pregnancy loss with antiphospholipid antibody: a systematic review of therapeutic trials. *Obstet Gynecol* 99:135, 2002.

Lockwood CJ: Inherited thrombophilias in pregnant patients: detection and treatment paradigm. *Obstet Gynecol* 99:333, 2002.

Oates-Whitehead RM, Haas DM, Carrier JA: Progestogen for preventing miscarriage. *Cochrane Database Syst Rev* CD003511, 2003.

Porter TF, LaCoursiere Y, Scott JR: Immunotherapy for recurrent miscarriage. *Cochrane Database Syst Rev* CD000112, 2006.

Rai R, Regan L: Recurrent miscarriage. *Lancet* 368:601, 2006.

Roque H et al: Maternal thrombophilias are not associated with early pregnancy loss. *Thromb Haemost* 91:290, 2004.

11

PRETERM PREMATURE RUPTURE OF THE FETAL MEMBRANES

Thomas F. McElrath

DEFINITION

Preterm premature rupture of the fetal membranes (PPROM) is one of the most common preterm complications of pregnancy on any busy tertiary antenatal service. It is defined as the spontaneous rupture of fetal membranes in the interval when neonatal viability is possible—typically between 23 and 37 weeks' gestation with modern neonatal intensive care unit (NICU) care. Because the neonate could potentially survive once delivered, management of the patient presenting with PPROM fundamentally involves an assessment of the risks versus the benefits of continued intrauterine development balanced against potential neonatal morbidities after delivery. This balance requires that the practitioner be familiar with both the gestational age–specific morbidities associated with preterm delivery and the potential interventions that can be offered after clinical presentation to minimize these complications.

This discussion also refers to a second form of membrane rupture called "midtrimester PPROM." In this presentation, amniorrhexis occurs between 16 and 23 weeks' gestation or before immediate fetal viability. This form of membrane rupture receives less attention in this discussion and, unless otherwise noted, the abbreviation PPROM refers to the former of the two conditions. Neither of these presentations should be confused with premature rupture of fetal membranes, which is defined as the occurrence of amniorrhexis after 37 weeks but before the onset of uterine contractions. This third presentation of membrane rupture is a normal variant of term labor and is not considered in this discussion.

EPIDEMIOLOGY

Preterm premature membrane rupture is associated with one third of all preterm deliveries. Perinatal epidemiologists have exerted a great deal of effort during the past four decades attempting to define specific patient characteristics associated with an increased risk of PPROM. One of the most widely cited risk factors for PPROM is the occurrence of PPROM in a prior pregnancy. Depending on the population studied and the exclusion criteria used, the risk of reoccurrence is between 13% and 32%. This observation is not, however, useful in clarifying the etiology of PPROM because it simply implies a tautology and does not help clarify an underlying causal pathway. Noting that a condition is likely to reoccur does not explain why it occurred in the first place.

The epidemiology of PPROM is complex and characterized by multiple risk factors. Among these, one of the most highly correlated is the occurrence of genital tract infection. Several authors have noted that women with PPROM are more likely to have pathologic microorganisms cultured from their amniotic fluid than those with other forms of preterm delivery. The identification of amniotic fluid inflammatory markers at the time of second trimester amniocentesis is associated with an increased risk of PPROM. This observation suggests that chronic, subclinical intrauterine inflammation may contribute to the pathology of preterm amniorrhexis long before clinical presentation. Others have observed that ascending infection from the lower genital tract is also associated with the risk of PPROM. Women with vaginitis or cervicitis concurrent with pregnancy have long been known to be at increased risk of PPROM. The presence of bacterial vaginalis, gonococcus, *Chlamydia*, *Gardnerella*, and *Trichomonas* in the first or second trimester is associated with a dramatically increased risk of PPROM. This risk is increased further if multiple infections are present at the same time. Postpartum endometritis is more common among women delivering after PPROM, suggesting a higher incidence of antepartum intrauterine infection. Genital tract infection is highly associated with the occurrence of PPROM and may, in fact, be causative in the pathology of amniorrhexis rather than simply associative. Microbial contamination of the fetal membranes could elicit both proteases and local inflammatory responses that in turn degrade membrane stability. However, a wide variety of other risk factors has also been identified and should be considered in the epidemiology of preterm amniorrhexis. Box 11-1 presents a set of acknowledged risk factors for PPROM.

It should be noted, however, that despite four decades of investigation of PPROM epidemiology, no investigators have yet managed to assemble a risk-scoring system that allows the prediction of PPROM at close to a clinically useful level. At best, most risk-scoring systems have a positive predictive value of 10% to 30%.

Midtrimester PPROM shares most of the epidemiologic risk factors with PPROM. However, iatrogenic amniorrhexis after amniocentesis represents a risk factor more commonly associated with midtrimester PPROM than with PPROM itself. The outcomes after iatrogenic amniorrhexis are favorable, with 90% of cases spontaneously resealing and allowing the subsequent reaccumulation of amniotic fluid.

Box 11-1   Risk Factors for Preterm Premature Rupture of the Fetal Membranes

Social and Demographic
Low economic status
Limited access to or use of health care
History of mental illness
African-American racial identification
Poor social supports/single motherhood
Extremes of maternal age (<18 or >40 yr)
Low maternal educational attainment

Behavioral
Tobacco use
Substance abuse

Health Related
Poor nutritional status/low body mass index
Corticosteroid use
Bacterial vaginitis
Sexually transmitted disease (gonorrhea, syphilis)
Urinary tract infection
Collagen vascular disorder

Cervical
In utero DES exposure
Premature cervical dilatation/effacement
Prior cone biopsy

Uterine
Premature uterine activity
Uterine anomaly
Excessive uterine distention
Chronic vaginal bleeding

DES, Diethylstilbestrol.

ETIOLOGY

The fetal membranes are made up of multiple layers, with the innermost layer being the cuboidal amniotic cells and the outermost layer being the chorion laeve. Intermediate layers of acellular connective tissue composed predominantly of interlinked collagen type I and III give the membranes their tensile strength. From a functionally simplistic point of view, both PPROM and midtrimester PPROM could result either from the intrinsic weakness of the collagen matrix or an acquired degradation to the structural integrity and strength of this matrix. For example, patients with inherited collagen deficiencies are at a marked increased risk of PPROM. Similarly, patients requiring chronic administration of corticosteroids for rheumatologic disorders during pregnancy are also at increased risk of PPROM potentially resulting from the effects of corticosteroids on collagen deposition.

Evidence also implicates transcervical bacterial contamination of the fetal membranes in the pathology of PPROM. The production of bacterially secreted metalloproteinases in close proximity to the acellular layer of the fetal membranes might degrade the collagen cross-links and thereby reduce the structural integrity of the membranes. Unfortunately, routine screening for vaginitis or vaginosis appears to be of little or no benefit in preventing PPROM in low-risk patients, and treatment may paradoxically increase the risk of preterm delivery.

CLINICAL PRESENTATION

The effective management of preterm amniorrhexis begins with the correct diagnosis. Figure 11-1 presents a schematic diagnostic algorithm to be considered in the management of PPROM. The majority of patients will note a gush of clear or yellow-tinged fluid. Less often, a patient may present complaining of a persistent slow leak unrelated to her voiding pattern. The correct diagnosis can be made in more than 90% of cases purely on patient history alone. Most cases of preterm amniorrhexis will be unheralded, although a history of first or second trimester vaginal bleeding can occasionally be elicited. Abdominal trauma can also cause membrane rupture, although the history of extremely forceful abdominal trauma, such as a motor vehicle accident, would be evident from other concurrent clinical circumstances.

Figure 11-1

Algorithm for physical examination evaluation of preterm premature rupture of the fetal membranes (PPROM). *FFN,* Fetal fibronectin.

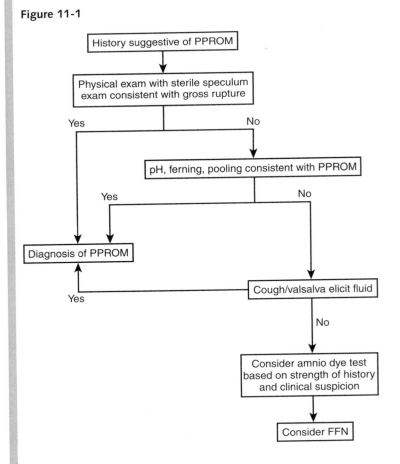

Clinical suspicion for PPROM must be confirmed by the presence of amniotic fluid in the vagina. This is most often accomplished with a sterile speculum examination of the cervix. Occasionally, the volume of fluid will overwhelm visualization of the cervix and thus confirm the diagnosis. This dramatic presentation is, however, relatively uncommon in the setting of either PPROM or midtrimester PPROM. Most often, the diagnosis will be confirmed by the simultaneous observation of the following:

1. The presence of a pool of fluid in the posterior fornix (pooling)
2. An increase in the physiologic pH of the vagina (nitrazine positive)
3. Ferning on thin film microscopy

If the presence of pooling is not immediately obvious, it can sometime be elicited by instructing the patient to cough several times while the cervix is kept under direct visual examination. Chemical detection of an increase in this pH, traditionally performed with nitrazine paper, would also strongly suggest the presence of amniotic fluid. The nitrazine test has a 99% positive and a 96% negative predictive value with respect to membrane rupture. The examiner should be aware, however, that a misleading positive change in the coloring of nitrazine paper can be elicited in the presence of blood, semen, or alkaline urine—all of which exist at a physiologic pH above 6.0. A sample of the pooled fluid should be air-dried on a glass slide, then examined for the fractal-like presence of fern fronds. These fronds are created by the crystallization of the proteins in the amniotic fluid as it dries. The ferning test has a 98% positive and a 92% negative predictive value. Care must be taken, however, to distinguish the long and lacelike appearance of amniotic fluid ferns from the shorter, stubbier ferns of cervical mucus. This distinction is not always obvious and can lead to an incorrect suspicion of amniorrhexis.

Additionally, at the time of sterile speculum examination, the cervix should be observed for the presence and extent of dilatation and effacement. The presence of a fetal part or portion of the umbilical cord must also be excluded. The patient should be assessed for the presence of uterine activity, the presentation of the fetus, the fetal heart rate, and any abdominal or uterine tenderness. A baseline complete blood count should also be obtained at this time. Cervical culture for *Chlamydia* and gonococci and vaginal culture for Group B streptococcus should also be obtained immediately after the confirmation of amniorrhexis. If the patient is beyond 32 weeks' gestation, a sample of the vaginal pool may be aspirated and submitted for fetal lung maturity testing. If the gestation is beyond 18 weeks, a negative fetal fibronectin excludes amniorrhexis. A variety of modifications of the nitrazine test and other point-of-care detections of intraamniotic biomarkers are either presently on the market or in premarket testing.

Digital examination of the cervix should be limited to an absolute minimum. The risk of intrauterine infection increases proportionally with each digital examination performed after amniorrhexis. On presentation with suspected PPROM, a digital examination should be deferred if at all possible until amniorrhexis has been ruled out. If PPROM is confirmed, usually the cervix can be adequately evaluated during the sterile speculum examination.

Routine examination of the cervix outside of active labor should be vigorously discouraged unless fetal heart rate instability suggests possible fetal or cord prolapse.

If the presence of PPROM cannot be adequately excluded on physical examination or if the strength of a suggestive history does not match an equivocal examination, then a dye test can be performed. This test is performed under ultrasound guidance and assumes that a sufficient pocket of intraamniotic fluid can be identified. The patient is asked to insert a standard tampon. An amniocentesis is performed and 10 ml of normal saline mixed with 1 ml indigo carmine is injected. After 30 minutes the tampon is removed and inspected for blue staining. The presence of blue staining would indicate membrane rupture, whereas its absence effectively excludes amniorrhexis. Greenish staining on the tampon can give equivocal results if the tampon was either left in place too long or the cervix is sufficiently dilated that transudate can weep across the exposed membranes. The patient should also be warned that her urine will have a greenish tint for several hours after the test. If the patient is beyond 32 weeks' gestation, the examiner should consider obtaining fluid for fetal lung maturity before injecting the dye.

Ultrasound typically plays an adjunctive role in the diagnosis of PPROM largely by confirming the presence of oligohydramnios in the setting of a patient with a suspicious history and supportive physical examination. The serendipitous observation of oligohydramnios on ultrasonic examination should be evaluated with an examination encompassing the features described previously. If the diagnosis of PPROM has already been confirmed, then an ultrasound examination should be performed:

1. To confirm viability
2. To evaluate fetal presentation
3. To estimate fetal weight
4. To estimate the volume of residual fluid
5. To confirm placentation

The risk of intrauterine infection is inversely related to the volume of residual fluid. This is due to the antimicrobial properties of the fluid itself and the physical cleansing effect of an ongoing efflux of fluid through the cervix that limits retrograde bacterial contamination. Ultrasound can also be crucial in distinguishing PPROM from other fetal anatomic sources of oligohydramnios.

TREATMENT AND EXPECTED OUTCOMES

The first principle of treating PPROM is to understand the range of expected outcomes not only to counsel the patient but also to maintain an appropriate level of clinical vigilance. Many of the risks, such as infection and sepsis, are shared by both mother and fetus. Many others, however, such as the risk of cerebral palsy, are borne by the fetus alone. This discussion begins by detailing the maternal risks, then moves to discuss the fetal risks and additional consideration of the unique circumstances of midtrimester PPROM.

Any mother with PPROM is at risk of a common set of complications, including preterm delivery, intrauterine infection, postpartum endometritis, an increased risk of placental abruption, and abdominal delivery. The risk of preterm delivery, whether spontaneous or iatrogenic, is greatly increased in the setting of PPROM. The latency interval between membrane rupture and delivery is inversely related to the gestational age at amniorrhexis. Less than 26 weeks, the median latency interval is 7 days. Between 28 and 34 weeks, the median latency decreases to 24 hours with 90% of deliveries occurring within 7 days. For comparison, at term the median interval is 12 to 18 hours with 90% of deliveries occurring within 24 hours. The shortening of the latency interval with increasing gestational age suggests that the pathophysiologic mechanisms either causing amniorrhexis or linking amniorrhexis with uterine activity are likely to change with advancing gestational age.

The risk of clinical chorioamnionitis also increases as a function of gestational age but not as a function of latency interval. The contemporary obstetrical literature contains multiple definitions of clinical chorioamnionitis. One of the most commonly cited is the occurrence of a combination of the following: fetal tachycardia, maternal tachycardia, maternal pyrexia ($\geq 38°$ C), or maternal fundal tenderness. Many clinicians will also interpret regular painful uterine contractions or a purulent cervical discharge as signs of clinical chorioamnionitis as well. Approximately 25% of all cases of PPROM will ultimately exhibit signs of clinical chorioamnionitis. For gestational ages less than 24 weeks, the incidence of clinical chorioamnionitis increases to approximately 40%. Unlike at term, when the incidence of clinical chorioamnionitis increases in proportion to the latency interval, the incidence of clinical chorioamnionitis does not appear to be a clear function of latency among patients with PPROM. This may, in part, be a function of the increased number of cervical exams endured by patients at term.

Among women who experience clinical chorioamnionitis in the setting of PPROM, approximately 40% will go on to experience postpartum endometritis. Postpartum endometritis is commonly characterized by pyrexia, particularly in the setting of fundal tenderness. Oddly enough, in light of the lack of a relation between latency interval and the risk of clinical chorioamnionitis, there appears to be inverse relation between the risk of postpartum endometritis and the latency interval. The shorter the latency interval, the greater the risk of postpartum endometritis. This inverse relation suggests a difference in the etiology of intrauterine infection in the setting of PPROM with the cases of shorter latency being associated with an established and fulminant intrauterine infection at the time of delivery.

The increased risk of intrauterine infection associated with PPROM is familiar to most contemporary clinicians. However, many clinicians fail to appreciate the increased risk of placental abruption and associated hemorrhage that also accompanies PPROM. Overall, placental abruption will occur in approximately 10% of cases of PPROM versus only about 1% of cases within the general obstetrical population. The risk of PPROM-associated abruption is inversely related to the gestational age of amniorrhexis, with an incidence of 40% to 50% before 20 weeks' gestation, 30% between 24 and 28 weeks, and a gradual decline thereafter. The underlying cause of PPROM-associated abruption is unclear. It may be as simple as the mechanical shearing of the placenta associated with uterine decompression. Recent evidence suggests, however, that abruption may also be an inflammatory phenomena associated with intrauterine infection. This second hypothesis is intriguing in that it suggests that rupture—whether through the membranes (as in PPROM) or through the placenta itself (as in abruption)—may be a generalized inflammatory phenomenon.

There are a common set of risks to the fetus and neonate after PPROM. The character of these risks changes depending on whether the amniorrhexis occurs in the midtrimester or after viability. In general, neonatal survival after midtrimester PPROM ranges between 10% and 40% with a direct relation to the gestational age at amniorrhexis. Table 11-1 displays several recent studies documenting the rates of neonatal survival after midtrimester PPROM. The direct relationship between gestational age and neonatal survival after midtrimester PPROM is likely to be a result of the longer latency intervals at the earlier gestational ages. With a median latency after midtrimester PPROM of greater than a week, those pregnancies that persist into the viable period will have a much greater chance of survival than those that deliver before viability. The potential for survival also increases in proportion to the amount of residual amniotic fluid. For PPROM between 15 and 28 weeks, severe, moderate, and mild oligohydramnios are associated with survival rates of 43%, 69%, and 74%, respectively. The positive association between residual amniotic fluid and neonatal survival is likely to be the result of the decreased risk of cord accident and intraamniotic infection associated with increased amniotic fluid volumes.

In cases of midtrimester PPROM after amniocentesis, the risks of neonatal mortality and adverse morbid outcome return to baseline if the membranes spontaneously reseal and the amniotic fluid volume reaccumulates. There does not appear to be a residual risk associated with resolved iatrogenic amniorrhexis.

With the loss of amniotic fluid, the fetus is deprived of its unrestricted environment in which pressure is evenly distributed across all body surfaces. After amniorrhexis, chest excursion and limb mobility are reduced and the risks of pulmonary hypoplasia and limb deformation are increased. Not surprisingly, the risk of both conditions increases inversely in relation to the amount of residual amniotic fluid. Pulmonary hypoplasia results from the deformation of the fetal thorax during the critical canicular stage of lung

Table 11-1

Survival by Gestational Age at Midtrimester Preterm Premature Rupture of the Fetal Membranes

Author	Weeks	Survival (%)
Farooqi et al., 1998[1]	14-19	40
	20-25	92
Falk et al., 2004[2]	20-21	13
	22-23	55
Yang et al., 2004[3]	<23	12
	23	60

development when the acinus ramifies from the terminal bronchioles. This process is necessary for the lung to attain sufficient surface area to support respiration and can be inhibited by the application of exogenous pressure. The overall incidence of pulmonary hypoplasia with midtrimester PPROM is 9%. The neonatal mortality rate associated with pulmonary hypoplasia ranges between 70% and 90%. The incidence of pulmonary hypoplasia falls rapidly with advancing gestational age. At 16 weeks, the incidence is approximately 80%, whereas by 26 weeks the incidence has fallen to less than 1%. There is an approximate 50% reduction in the odds of pulmonary hypoplasia with each additional week of gestation.

The incidence of limb deformation also increases after PPROM in the midtrimester but is not as closely linked to gestational age as is the risk of pulmonary hypoplasia. The incidence of limb deformation is approximately 7% after midtrimester PPROM with an increased incidence after 14 days of latency. The risk is inversely associated with the residual volume of amniotic fluid. For severe oligohydramnios the risk of limb deformation is approximately 50%. Fortunately, however, limb deformation is not associated with an increased risk of neonatal death and often does not require more than physical therapy for successful treatment.

The fetal consequences of PPROM change after 23 weeks' gestation as the pregnancy progresses beyond the midtrimester and the fetus becomes potentially viable. Fetal morbidity in this gestational age range is predominantly a function of both gestational age and intrauterine infection. The incidence of the major neonatal morbidities decreases with increasing gestational age at delivery. Although the gestational age at the time of amniorrhexis will be important in the occurrence of some forms of neonatal morbidity, particularly the risk of infection, the type and incidence of most postbirth complications will be primarily a function of the gestational age when the delivery actually occurs. Specifically, the risk of neonatal respiratory distress (nRDS) is a function of the age at delivery. The incidence of nRDS is almost universal if delivery occurs between 23 and 28 weeks with severity being much greater in the earlier gestational ages, when it is often the limiting factor for overall neonatal survival. After 28 weeks, the incidence of nRDS falls in a linear fashion to about 2% to 3% in the 36-week age range. After 36 weeks, the incidence remains low but never completely drops to zero. There are occasional cases of nRDS even in babies born at term.

Necrotizing enterocolitis (NEC), a pathology specific to the preterm neonate with an unclear etiology that might be partly infectious in nature, is also most common in the earlier gestational age ranges. NEC occurs in approximately 2% to 8% of all premature neonates but is dramatically less common after 32 weeks' gestation. At the extreme, therapy for NEC includes surgical resection of the bowel and can lead to life-long "short-gut" related gastrointestinal and nutritional complications. NEC can, however, be managed medically with a deferral of enteral feeding—a management that may affect neonatal growth but does reduce the need for surgical intervention.

The incidence of damage to the neonatal brain either through intraventricular or intraparenchymal hemorrhage or through the nonhemorrhagic

165

loss of white matter mass is also a major source of extreme-prematurity–related neonatal morbidity. The spectrum of neurologic damage includes an increased risk of mental retardation and cerebral palsy. The incidence of neurologic anomaly on neonatal head ultrasound ranges between 6% and 12% of all extremely premature neonates and the incidence falls dramatically with delivery after the twenty-eighth week of gestation. Although the etiology of this form of neonatal neurologic damage is unclear, the role of intrauterine or intrapartum hypoxia appears to be more limited than has classically been assumed. Instead, the risk of neurologic damage in the extremely premature neonate appears to be more closely correlated with the occurrence of intrauterine inflammation, and a pathologic role of intrauterine inflammatory cytokinemia has been hypothesized.

Other morbidities are also common to these early gestational ages. These include retinopathy of prematurity, hypoglycemia, and hyperbilirubinemia. Retinopathy of prematurity is a disorder involving the proliferation of the microvasculature within the retina and can be associated with loss of visual acuity or blindness. Both hypoglycemia and hyperbilirubinemia can be associated with neurologic damage and mental retardation if not managed appropriately.

After PPROM, there is a loss of the membranous barrier to ascending transcervical infection and loss of the continuity of the intrauterine environment. In addition to possible neurologic damage, as noted previously, the neonatal consequences of intrauterine infection include sepsis, pneumonia, and localized conjunctivitis. These risks are greater if the neonate is delivered before 30 to 32 weeks' gestation when immune competence is typically attained. The risk of neonatal sepsis is approximately 5% in pregnancies complicated by PPROM. This risk increases to 20% if there is clinical evidence of chorioamnionitis before delivery.

Given that many of the risks for both intrauterine and neonatal morbidity decrease with advancing gestation, the gestational age at presentation becomes a key consideration in the management of the patient presenting with PPROM. The clinician will be more likely to tolerate risks of infection and intrauterine morbidity at 23 to 24 weeks because of the overwhelmingly poor prognosis for survival at these extremely low gestational ages. However, all else being equal, a patient presenting after 34 weeks would be managed less conservatively because the risks of infection and intrauterine morbidity are outweighed by the good prognosis for morbidity-free survival after delivery. Management therefore must strike a gestational age specific balance between intrauterine risk and extrauterine morbidity.

MANAGEMENT

Hospitalization should be considered standard management for patients diagnosed with PPROM. The majority of respondents to a recent survey conducted within the Society of Maternal Fetal Medicine indicate that they routinely hospitalize their patients diagnosed with PPROM for the duration of the pregnancy. American College of Obstetricians and Gynecologists guidelines do allow for home management of stable, compliant patients with sufficient support at home to allow both rest and the rapid presentation to medical evaluation should their status deteriorate. However, given the rapidity and subtlety with which clinical chorioamnionitis can present, it is the practice at most tertiary teaching institutions to hospitalize patients presenting with PPROM after 23 weeks. The justification for this policy is that expectant management would no longer be indicated in the setting of clinical chorioamnionitis and that the risk of neonatal sepsis and morbidity will be reduced if delivery is effected expediently. Having the patient under the supervision of experienced antenatal staff presumably allows this to occur more quickly. Patients with midtrimester PPROM may be managed as outpatients because fetal viability and subsequent morbidity are not clinical expectations.

The point at which the expectant management of PPROM patients should end and they should be electively delivered is not clear. A recent survey of maternal-fetal medicine practitioners indicates that the majority of providers are electively delivering their expectantly managed patients in the thirty-fourth week of gestation. This relatively advanced gestational age avoids many of the major morbidities of prematurity associated with the earlier gestational ages while minimizing the ongoing background risk of clinically evident intrauterine infection and potential cord accident. Elective delivery after 32 weeks' gestation in the setting of a positive screen for fetal lung maturity has been demonstrated as a means of avoiding the ongoing risk of intrauterine infection associated with expectant management. Amniotic fluid can be obtained via amniocentesis if an adequate fluid pocket can be visualized. Alternatively, it can be obtained as a vaginal pool specimen during a sterile speculum examination. Both sources yield equivalent positive and negative predictive values. The evaluation of creatinine levels in the vaginal pool specimen should be considered to exclude contamination with urine and the associated risk of a false-negative screen.

The administration of antenatal corticosteroids for the enhancement of lung maturity should be offered to all patients presenting with PPROM after the attainment of fetal viability. The National Institutes of Health consensus committee suggests that there is insufficient evidence for the benefits of antenatal corticosteroids after 32 weeks' gestation to warrant their routine administration, although administration may be considered if amniotic fluid screening suggests immature fetal lung development. It is common practice within most tertiary teaching hospitals to routinely offer a single course of antenatal steroids to patients between 23 and 32 weeks' gestation unless screening suggests the presence of fetal lung maturity. Decisions regarding the administration of steroids to patients with immature fetal lung screens between 32 and 34 weeks' gestation are typically left to the discretion of the individual provider. There is presently no evidence for the administration of multiple courses of antenatal steroids and this practice should best be pursued in the context of an approved research protocol.

The administration of prophylactic broad-spectrum antibiotics to patients presenting with PPROM has become the hallmark of contemporary PPROM management. A recent survey of maternal-fetal medicine practitioners notes that 99% of respondents use a prophylactic antibiotic protocol in their management of PPROM. A variety of antibiotic protocols have been published in the obstetrical literature (Table 11-2). These protocols tend to be broad-spectrum because the intrauterine infection associated with PPROM tends to be polymicrobial with an overrepresentation of atypical species. On average, the administration of prophylactic antibiotics to patients presenting with PPROM increases the latency interval 5 to 7 days with an associated reduction in the incidence of nRDS, neonatal sepsis, and other complications of prematurity. The use of prophylactic antibiotics has also been associated with a reduction in clinical chorioamnionitis and postpartum endometritis. Criticisms have been raised that many of the early prophylactic antibiotic trials were performed before the routine use of antenatal corticosteroids. Critics have suggested that antibiotics might not have as dramatic a benefit if steroids were used routinely. Recent work, however, has included both antenatal steroids and prophylactic antibiotics and demonstrates a benefit to antibiotic prophylaxis in addition to that of the steroids administration. Several recent trials have also compared the more conventional 7-day course of antibiotic prophylaxis to a shorter 3-day course. These studies did not observe a difference in the latency interval or incidence of neonatal morbidity with the shorter course.

The risks of antibiotic prophylaxis are minimal. Several authors have noted an increase in complaints of nausea, vomiting, and abdominal pain among patients receiving prophylaxis, particularly if erythromycin is one of the agents. An increase in the incidence of candidiasis in both the

Antibiotic Prophylaxis
in Premature Rupture
of Membranes

Table 11-2

Author	No.	Antibiotic
Amon et al., 1988	82	Ampicillin IV/PO
Morales et al., 1989	165	Ampicillin IV
Johnston et al., 1990		Mezlocillin Ampicillin IV/PO
McGregor et al., 1991	54	Erythromycin
Christmas et al., 1992	56	Ampicillin Gentamicin Clindamycin
Mercer and Arheart, 1995	220	Erythromycin base
Lockwood et al., 1992	75	Piperacillin
Blanco et al., 1993	306	Cefizox
Owen et al., 1993	117	Ampicillin, erythromycin base
Lovett et al., 1997	112	Unasyn
Mercer et al., 1997	614	Ampicillin/erythromycin

Modified from Creasy R, Resnik R, Iams R: *Maternal fetal medicine*, 5 ed, Philadelphia, Saunders, 2004.

mother and neonate has also been reported. There is also some evidence that the use of Augmentin may be associated with an increased incidence of NEC in the neonate and for this reason many practitioners have steered away from this agent. The use of prophylactic antibiotics has been associated with an altered microbial resistance pattern in several tertiary neonatal intensive care units.

Compared with the use of antibiotics, both the use of tocolytics and the antenatal monitoring after amniorrhexis are areas of management that remain much less studied and formalized. Seventy-three percent of surveyed maternal-fetal medicine practitioners respond that they routinely use tocolysis after PPROM. However, the vast majority of these providers indicate that they would only administer tocolysis for the first 48 hours of hospitalization until the patient has received a full course of antenatal steroids. Tocolytics in the setting of PPROM should be used with caution. Any attempts at tocolysis should only be pursued after the practitioner has thoroughly excluded the possibility of clinical chorioamnionitis. Consideration should also be given to the types of tocolytics administered. Agents that have antipyretic properties, such as indomethacin, or that might elevate the maternal heart rate could unnecessarily confuse the presentation of clinical chorioamnionitis and complicate management.

How a patient should be monitored during her latency interval after PPROM is not generally agreed on and seems to vary regionally within the United States. Most practitioners would agree that the patient should be examined regularly for fundal tenderness, fever, or maternal tachycardia. Complaints of frank vaginal bleeding, a purulent component to the vaginal discharge, or new malaise should prompt additional evaluation. The fetal heart rate should also be regularly assessed for evidence of fetal tachycardia. However, there is no consensus regarding the type or frequency of fetal monitoring after PPROM. Some institutions use daily nonstress testing, whereas others rely on kick-count assessment. There is no consensus in the contemporary literature as to the optimal mode or frequency of antenatal testing.

The management of amniorrhexis in the patient with a cervical cerclage in place is similar to that of a patient without a cerclage. The cerclage should be immediately removed if there is evidence of clinical chorioamnionitis or progress into active labor. Early reports in relatively small samples suggested that there might be an increased risk of intrauterine infection and the consequences of neonatal sepsis among patients who were managed with the cerclage in place after PPROM. Several later and larger reports suggest that this risk was overstated and that there does not appear to be a difference in neonatal outcome if the cerclage is retained or removed. The management can therefore be individualized with reference to the original indication for the cerclage placement.

KEY POINTS

1. Amniorrhexis should be confirmed by physical examination, with the possible use of an intraamniotic dye test if the diagnosis is equivocal.
2. Patients should be managed with hospitalization, a minimum of digital cervical examinations, routine assessment for the signs and symptoms of clinical chorioamnionitis, and an immediate progress toward delivery if chorioamnionitis is suspected.
3. Antenatal antibiotics prolong latency in patients presenting with PPROM while lowering both maternal and neonatal morbidity.
4. A single course of antenatal corticosteroids should be administered to patients presenting with PPROM between 23 and 32 weeks' gestation to reduce the neonatal consequences of prematurity.
5. Tocolysis should be considered only once clinical chorioamnionitis has been excluded.
6. The ideal mode of fetal assessment after PPROM remains unclear.
7. Patients with a mature fetal lung screen after 32 weeks should be considered for delivery. In most cases, patients should be delivered by 34-35 weeks, without regard to fetal lung maturity, given the risk of infection.

REFERENCES

1. Farooqi A, Holmgrem PA, Engberg S, Serenius F: Survival and 2-year outcome with expectant management of second-trimester rupture of membranes. *Obstet Gynecol* 92(6):895-901, 1998.
2. Falk SJ, Campbell LJ, Lee-Parritz A, Cohen AP, Ecker J, Wilkins-Haug L, Lieberman E: Expectant management in spontaneous preterm premature rupture of membranes between 14 and 24 weeks' gestation. *J Perinatol* 24(10):611-6, 2004.
3. Yang LC, Taylor DR, Kaufman HH, Hume R, Calhoun B: Maternal and fetal outcomes of spontaneous preterm premature rupture of membranes. *J Am Osteopath Assoc* 104(12):537-42.

SUGGESTED READINGS

ACOG Practice Bulletin. *Premature Rupture of Membranes.* 1998, American College of Obstetricians and Gynecologists, Washington, DC.
Mercer BM et al: Antibiotic therapy for reduction of infant morbidity after preterm premature rupture of the membranes: a randomized controlled trial. *JAMA* 278:989, 1997.
National Institutes of Health. National Institutes of Health Consensus Development Conference Statement: Effect of corticosteroids for fetal maturation on perinatal outcomes. February 28-March 2, 1994. *Am J Obstet Gynecol* 173:246, 1995.
Ramsey PS et al: Contemporary management of preterm premature rupture of membranes (PPROM): a survey of maternal-fetal medicine providers. *Am J Obstet Gynecol* 191:1497, 2004.

12

PRETERM LABOR AND BIRTH

Mert Ozan Bahtiyar and Charles J. Lockwood

OVERVIEW

Preterm birth (PTB) is defined as delivery before 37 0/7 weeks of gestation. In the United States, PTB is the second most common cause for neonatal mortality and morbidity, surpassed only by congenital malformations. Despite advances in diagnosis, the incidence of PTB is higher than ever before, at approximately 12.5%.

Approximately half of all PTB occur secondary to preterm labor (PTL), one third are because of preterm premature rupture of the membranes (PPROM), and one fifth are iatrogenic because of obstetrical or medical complications.

ETIOLOGY

The etiology of PTB is not clearly understood; however, four primary processes are thought to be responsible for PTL and delivery (Box 12-1).

Activation of the Maternal or Fetal Hypothalamic-Pituitary-Adrenal Axis

Premature activation of the hypothalamic-pituitary-adrenal (HPA) axis can initiate PTL (Figure 12-1, *A* and *B*).

Corticotropin-releasing hormone (CRH) is released by the hypothalamus, but, during pregnancy, it is also expressed by placental and chorionic trophoblasts, amnion, and decidual cells. It stimulates the secretion of adrenocorticotropic hormone (ACTH) from the pituitary, which then promotes the release of cortisol from the adrenal. In the maternal HPA axis, cortisol inhibits hypothalamic CRH and pituitary ACTH release, creating a negative feedback loop. In contrast, cortisol stimulates CRH release in the decidua, trophoblast, and membranes. CRH, in turn, further drives maternal and fetal HPA activation, establishing a potent positive feedback loop. In addition CRH also enhances prostaglandin production by amnion, chorion, and decidua. Prostaglandins stimulate CRH release from the decidua, trophoblast, and membranes, thus creating a second positive feedback loop for CRH secretion. The rise in prostaglandins is ultimately thought to result in parturition. There is also some evidence that CRH can directly affect the myometrium (see Figure 12-1, *A*).

Box 12-1   Etiology of Preterm Labor

- Activation of HPA axis
- Infection
- Decidual hemorrhage
- Pathologic uterine distention

HPA, Hypothalamic-pituitary-adrenal.

Fetal pituitary ACTH secretion stimulates adrenal synthesis of dehydro-epiandrosterone sulfate (DHEA), which is converted to 16-hydroxy-DHEA-S in the fetal liver. Placental CRH also can augment fetal adrenal DHEA production directly. The placenta converts these androgen precursors to estrone (E1), estradiol (E2), and estriol (E3), which in turn activate the myometrium by increasing gap junction formation, oxytocin receptors, prostaglandin

Figure 12-1

A, During pregnancy corticotropin-releasing hormone (CRH) is released by the hypothalamus and placental chorionic trophoblast, amnion, and decidual cells. It stimulates the secretion of adrenocorticotropic hormone (ACTH) from the pituitary, which then promotes the release of cortisol from the adrenal. In the maternal hypothalamic-pituitary-adrenal (HPA) axis, cortisol inhibits hypothalamic CRH and pituitary ACTH release, creating a negative feedback loop. In contrast, cortisol stimulates CRH release in the decidua-trophoblast-membranes compartment. CRH, in turn, further drives maternal and fetal HPA activation, establishing a potent positive feedback loop. In addition CRH also enhances

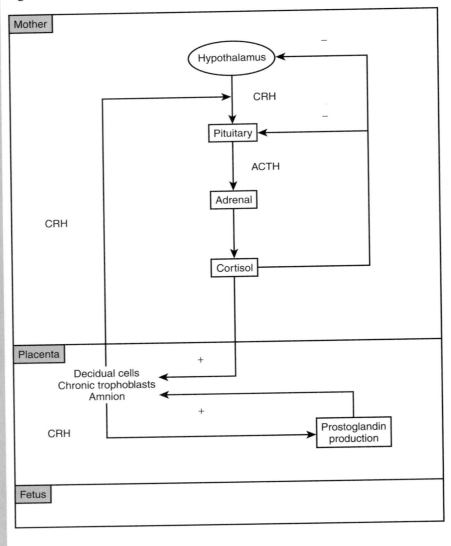

prostaglandin production by amnion, chorion, and decidua. Prostaglandins stimulate CRH release from the decidua-trophoblast-membranes compartment, creating a second positive feedback loop for CRH secretion. The rise in prostaglandins ultimately results in parturition. Furthermore, CRH can directly affect the myometrium. **B,** Fetal pituitary ACTH secretion stimulates adrenal synthesis of dehydro-epiandrosterone sulfate (DHEA), which is converted to 16-hydroxy-DHEA-S in the fetal liver. Placental corticotropin-releasing hormone (CRH) also can augment fetal adrenal DHEA production directly. The placenta converts these androgen precursors to estrone (E1), estradiol (E2), and estriol (E3), which, in turn, activate the myometrium by increasing gap junction formation, oxytocin receptors, prostaglandin activity, and enzymes responsible for muscle contraction (myosin light chain kinase, calmodulin).

Figure 12-1, cont'd

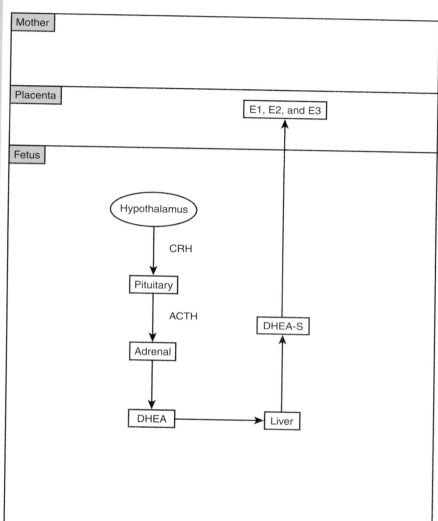

activity, and enzymes responsible for muscle contraction (myosin light chain kinase, calmodulin) (see Figure 12-1, *B*).

Infection

Evidence shows a link between spontaneous PTL and both systemic and ascending genital tract infections. Both clinical and subclinical chorioamnionitis are much more common in preterm than term deliveries, and may account for 50% of PTBs before 30 weeks of gestation.

The maternal and/or fetal inflammatory response to amniochorionic-decidual infection is likely the final common pathway for triggering preterm labor/delivery. This response is mediated by activated macrophages and granulocytes that induce proinflammatory substances, such as cytokines (e.g., interleukins 1, 6, 8; tumor necrosis factor; granulocyte colony-stimulating factor) and matrix metalloproteinases.

Eventually, cytokines directly stimulate prostaglandin E2 and F2 production and inhibit their metabolism in the amniochorionic-decidual compartment. Prostaglandins ripen the cervix and cause uterine contractions at all gestational ages. On the other hand, metalloproteinases (e.g., collagenase, gelatinase, elastase, and stromelysin) weaken membranes and ripen the cervix by disrupting the normally rigid collagen matrix.

In addition to inducing an inflammatory response, some organisms (e.g., *Pseudomonas, Staphylococcus, Streptococcus, Bacteroides,* and *Enterobacter*) are capable of producing proteases, collagenases, and elastases that can degrade the fetal membranes. Bacteria also produce phospholipase A2 (which leads to prostaglandin synthesis) and endotoxin, substances that stimulate uterine contractions and can cause PTL.

Despite these findings, it has not been established that antibiotic therapy can prevent PTL in these cases.

Decidual Hemorrhage

Vaginal bleeding from decidual hemorrhage is associated with a high risk of both PTL and premature rupture of the membranes (PROM). Vaginal bleeding in more than one trimester increases the risk of PPROM sevenfold. Through a series of reactions, tissue factor, which is the primary cellular mediator of hemostasis, interacts with factor Va, factor X, and cofactor Va. This complex interaction eventually generates thrombin. Thrombin, by binding to decidual membrane receptors, regulates expression of proteases and metalloproteinases, which play a role in PPROM and PTL. It appears that progestin inhibits this process.

Pathologic Uterine Distention

Multiple gestation, polyhydramnios, and other causes of excessive uterine distention are well-described risk factors for PTL. Enhanced stretching of the myometrium induces the formation of gap junctions, upregulation of oxytocin receptors, and production of prostaglandin E2 and F2 and myosin light chain kinase, which are critical events preceding uterine contractions and cervical dilation.

RISK FACTORS

Numerous risk factors for PTL and PTB have been reported. A causal association between these risk factors and PTB has been difficult to establish because many PTBs occur among women with no risk factors at all (Box 12-2).

History of Prior PTB

Prior PTB is the strongest risk factor for future PTB, although most women who have had a PTB will have subsequent pregnancies of a normal duration. The risk of PTB is highest when the previous PTB was in the penultimate pregnancy or there is a history of multiple PTBs.

Box 12-2   Risk Factors for Preterm Labor and Birth

- History of preterm birth
- Multifetal gestation
- Vaginal bleeding
- Infection
- Asymptomatic bacteriuria
- Periodontal disease
- Genetic
- Induced abortion
- Interpregnancy interval
- Delayed ovulation

Women who have history of prior spontaneous PTB are more than twice as likely to have a PTB in the next gestation than are women with no history of prior spontaneous PTB (22% vs. 9%). In addition, women whose prior spontaneous PTB was at 23 to 27 weeks of gestation have an even higher rate of recurrent PTB (27%). If both the first and second births were preterm, the risk of recurrent PTB is as high as 28%. Term births decrease the risk of PTB in subsequent pregnancies.

Approximately one half of the recurrent PTBs occur within 1 week of the gestational age of the prior delivery and 70% occur within 2 weeks.

Multifetal Gestation

Multiple pregnancy accounts for 17% of all births less than 37 weeks of gestation, 23% of all early births less than 32 weeks, 24% of all infants of birth weight less than 2500 g, and 26% of all very low birth weight infants (less than 1500 g). The incidence of multiple gestations has increased as assisted reproductive technology (ART) using superovulation and in vitro fertilization has become widely available and successful in achieving pregnancy.

In the United States, twin births increased from 18.9 per 1000 live births in 1980 to 32.2 per 1000 live births in 2004. The rate of triplet and higher-order multiple births increased more than fourfold from 37 per 100,000 live births in 1980 to 177 per 100,000 live births in 2004.

The mechanism for PTL in multiple gestations, and particularly higher-order multiple gestations, may be related to uterine distension, increased intrauterine volume, or related complications such as cervical incompetence. However, there may also be specific causes related to the endocrine environment produced by superovulation or the multiple pregnancy. For example, multiple gestations produce a proportionately increased amount of estrogen, progesterone, and sex steroids compared with singleton pregnancies. Increased steroid production in multiple pregnancies may play a role in initiation of PTL.

Vaginal Bleeding

Recurrent decidual hemorrhage presenting as vaginal bleeding anytime in pregnancy is associated with a threefold increase in the adjusted relative risk for PTB because of PTL. In addition, vaginal bleeding in more than one trimester carries a sevenfold increase in the risk of PPROM. The risk of PTB is even higher (100-fold) in women experiencing vaginal bleeding in more than one trimester who also have a previous pregnancy complicated by PPROM.

Infection

Multiple studies have shown an association between infection/inflammation and PTB. Histologic evidence indicates chorioamnionitis in the placentas of 20% to 75% of PTBs and positive membrane cultures in 30% to 60% of such patients. The rate increases with decreasing gestational age: 15% at 28 to 32 weeks, 8% at 33 to 36 weeks, and 5% after 36 weeks of gestation.

Microorganisms associated with PTL are capable of either directly producing prostaglandins or producing phospholipase A2, resulting in increased production of prostaglandins. Prostaglandins are uterotonic and contribute to cervical softening.

Asymptomatic bacteriuria has long been associated with PTB. Treatment of asymptomatic bacteriuria decreases the incidence of preterm and low birthweight births.

Periodontal disease and periodontal pathogens in amniotic fluid have been associated with a variety of adverse pregnancy events, including low birth weight, PTB, fetal growth restriction, preeclampsia, and fetal death.

Treatment of periodontal disease is associated with a significant reduction in PTB. On the other hand, at least one study has refuted the finding that clinical periodontal disease is a potential risk factor for PTB.

PTL/PTB has been associated with many infections in addition to asymptomatic bacteriuria, including Group B streptococci, *Chlamydia trachomatis,* bacterial vaginosis, *Neisseria gonorrhoeae, Ureaplasma urealyticum,* and *Trichomonas vaginalis.* However, placebo-controlled trials have shown either a modest or no effect of antibiotic treatment on prolonging gestation and, in the case of asymptomatic *T. vaginalis,* appeared to cause harm.

Although treatment of these infections to prevent PTB is not recommended (except for asymptomatic bacteriuria and in some women with bacterial vaginosis), treatment is indicated in symptomatic women and for prevention of complications from and spread of sexually transmitted infections (i.e., *C. trachomatis, N. gonorrhoeae*).

Cervical and Uterine Factors

There is an inverse relationship between cervical length and gestational age at delivery. Ablative and excisional procedures have been associated with increased risks of late miscarriage and PTB. When a large amount of collagen is removed during cervical conizations, decreased tensile strength of the cervix and susceptibility to PTL and delivery may result.

Congenital and acquired uterine malformations are associated with PTB and the risk depends on the specific abnormality. A PTB rate of 17% has been reported for unicornuate uterus. Women with uterine duplication abnormalities are also at higher risk of PTB than women with normal uteri (29% vs. 3%).

The relationship between PTB and uterine leiomyoma is more complicated and is largely based on observational studies. The presence of a large fibroid (i.e. $\geq$ 5 to 6 cm) appears to be the factor that best correlates with an increased risk of PTB. The mechanism for PTL and delivery is thought to be decreased uterine luminal volume and/or cervical incompetence.

PTB resulting from a uterine septum, bicornuate uterus, intrauterine adhesions, and fibroids may be amenable to treatment by surgical correction of the abnormality.

Prenatal Care and Lifestyle Issues

The absence of prenatal care has been consistently identified as a risk factor for PTL and delivery, but it is less clear whether this association is causal or a marker for other factors that contribute to PTB. Intensive prenatal care has not been shown to decrease the risk of PTB.

Maternal substance abuse increases the risk of PTB. Cocaine is the most common substance identified. Alcohol and toluene are additional substances associated with an increased risk of PTL. The risk of PTB is 25% in women who use multiple drugs. In addition, cigarette smoking has a dose-dependent relationship with the risk of PTB.

PREDICTION OF PTL AND DELIVERY

Traditional methods for predicting women destined to deliver preterm relied on obstetrical history, demographic factors, or premonitory symptoms that were neither sensitive nor specific. Various laboratory and technologic tools were developed, but these have also been unable to reliably distinguish between women who will and will not deliver preterm.

Women with a prior spontaneous PTB are at high risk for recurrence. Although obstetrical history is useful for predicting the duration of a subsequent gestation, it cannot be used in primigravidas, who comprise approximately 40% of deliveries in the United States.

Biochemical Markers

The most clinically useful biochemical approach to differentiating women who are at high risk for impending PTB from those who are not at high risk is measurement of fetal fibronectin (fFN) in the cervicovaginal secretions.

Fetal Fibronectin

Fibronectins are large molecular weight (450 kD) glycoproteins found in the plasma and extracellular matrix. A unique fibronectin identified in amniotic fluid, extracts of placental tissue, and malignant cell lines is called fFN. fFN is thought to be a "trophoblast glue" that promotes cellular adhesion at uterine-placental and decidual-fetal membrane interfaces. It is released into cervicovaginal secretions when the extracellular matrix of the chorionic/decidual interface is disrupted.

The fFN assay has been used in two ways. The first is to predict the risk of PTB in symptomatic patients. The second use is to identify asymptomatic women, usually in a high-risk group (e.g., previous preterm delivery, multiple gestation), who are most likely to deliver preterm.

Candidates for testing should have intact fetal membranes, cervical dilatation less than 3 cm, and gestational age between 24 0/7 and 34 6/7 weeks. Samples are collected from secretions in the posterior fornix or external cervical os using a swab. Manipulation of the cervix (digital or ultrasound examination, coitus within 24 hours) and intravaginal preparations (e.g., lubricants, medications) should be avoided before obtaining the sample because they can cause a false-positive result. An fFN concentration greater than 50 ng/ml is considered positive.

Systematic reviews indicated that highest sensitivity (77%) was achieved in symptomatic women who delivered within 7 days; specificity was 87% for absence of delivery within 7 or 14 days. In asymptomatic women, fFN was less predictive of PTB. The positive predictive value for PTB within 7 to 10 days is only 13% to 30% but with a negative predictive value of at least 99%.

Salivary Estriol

Circulating maternal estrogens are primarily derived from placental conversion of fetal adrenal-derived dehydroepiandrosterone, whose concentration reflects fetal HPA axis activation. Estrogens prepare the uterus for labor by binding to myometrial receptors to enhance synthesis of gap junctions (connexin 43) formation, oxytocin receptor mRNA levels, prostaglandin F2-alpha activity, and myosin light chain kinase and calmodulin expression. Priming of the myometrium is initiated by a surge in maternal estradiol secretion, which has been observed 9 days before the onset of both preterm and term labor. Both plasma and amniotic fluid of patients with premature contractions who deliver prematurely show elevated estradiol concentrations compared with those with false labor delivering at term.

Human studies have not shown consistent changes in the plasma or urinary levels of progesterone and estrogen immediately before the initiation of labor. Measurement of unbound estrogen, which can be detected as salivary estriol, suggests a large rise in estriol production before delivery, with a lesser increase or plateau in progesterone production.

A salivary E3 test was developed for clinical use in the prediction of risk for spontaneous PTL. A single salivary E3 concentration ≥ 2.1 ng/ml had sensitivity, specificity, and positive and negative predictive values of 57%, 78%, 9%, and 98%, respectively, for the prediction of PTB (<37 weeks). The positive predictive value (PPV) was enhanced if the woman had a second positive test (PPV 19%) or belonged to a group at high risk (Creasy score >10) for PTB (PPV 14% after one and 26% after two positive tests).

A significant rise of mean salivary E3 level is only observed in patients with PTL between 30 and 37 weeks, not those laboring before 30 weeks. Therefore this test has reduced effectiveness for identifying patients at risk for PTD before 30 weeks of gestation, precisely the group at highest risk for perinatal morbidity and mortality.

The test is not predictive of PTD in women who have been treated with glucocorticoid therapy and has not been evaluated in pregnancies with multiple gestations, placental abruption, PROM, incompetent cervix, or fetal growth restriction.

Test results are not available for 72 hours, so the high negative predictive value cannot be used to assist in decisions concerning the immediate care of the patient.

The American College of Obstetricians and Gynecologists Committee on Obstetric Practice does not currently recommend this test for screening women with PTL.

Cervical Length

Shortened cervical length determined by transvaginal ultrasonography is predictive of PTD. Although a shortened cervix can represent normal biologic variability, it may also result from effacement related to pathologic processes such as inflammation, hemorrhage, premature contractions, or uterine overdistension.

Routine use of cervical ultrasonography for prediction of PTB in asymptomatic women is not currently recommended because of controversy regarding the length that should provoke an intervention and the lack of effective interventions.

By comparison, measurement of cervical length may be useful in management of symptomatic women when the diagnosis of PTL is uncertain. As a general guideline, PTB is unlikely if the cervix is longer than 30 mm but should be considered in women with contractions if the cervix is less than 30 mm and particularly in those with cervices less than 15 to 20 mm. A long cervical length, especially greater than 35 mm, is suggestive of a low likelihood of spontaneous PTD, even in the presence of other risk factors for PTB.

Cervical Length Combined with fFN

Whether the patient is symptomatic or not changes the predictive ability of fFN in combination with cervical length assessment by transvaginal ultrasound.

Asymptomatic Women

The sensitivity and positive predictive values for each test (cervical length and fFN) or both tests combined for PTB before 35 weeks of gestation is low in asymptomatic low-risk women.

Nulliparous women with positive fFN screening results (>50 ng/ml) and a short cervix (<25 mm) are at higher risk of PTD before 35 weeks because of PPROM than gravida without these risk factors (11.1% vs. 0.9%). Multiparous women with these risk factors and a previous PTD caused by PPROM have a 25% risk of recurrent PTD from PPROM.

Women with both a positive fFN result and a short cervix are at substantially increased risk of spontaneous PTD (33.3%) before 28 to 30 weeks of gestation, whereas those with either marker alone have an intermediate risk of PTD (6.2%). Women without either marker are at low risk (1.3%).

Among patients with a previous PTD, the recurrence risk in women with a positive fFN and cervical length less than 25 mm or less than 35 mm at 24 weeks was 65% and 25%, respectively. If the fFN was negative, the recurrence rate at these cervical lengths was 25% and 7%, respectively. The risk of recurrence increased as cervical length shortened in both fetal fFN-positive and fFN-negative women.

Symptomatic Women

In women with preterm contractions, sonographic cervical length assessment, followed by fFN if the cervix is short, improves the ability to distinguish between women who will and will not deliver within 7 or 14 days. Women with cervical length ≥30 mm are unlikely to deliver preterm and measuring fFN does not enhance the predictive value of ultrasound examination in these women. By comparison, if the cervix is less than 30 mm in length, the risk of delivery within 7 days with negative and positive fFN results is 11% and 45%, respectively; the risk of delivery within 14 days is 13% and 56%, respectively. Delivery within 7 days occurs in 75% of women with cervical length less than 15 mm and positive fFN.

Women with cervical length greater than 30 mm are unlikely to deliver within 7 days and the addition of fFN testing does not significantly improve the predictive value of cervical length measurement alone. A two-step testing can be done: initially an fFN sample is collected and set aside for testing pending ultrasound result. Then sonographic assessment of the cervix is performed with functional canal length less than 20 mm as a positive result and greater than 31 mm as a negative one. fFN testing is then performed only in patients with a length of 21 to 31 mm. Two-step testing has overall sensitivity, specificity, and positive and negative predictive values of 86%, 90%, 63%, and 97%, respectively, for predicting delivery within 28 days. The combined use of the cervical sonography and fFN testing predicts preterm delivery with higher sensitivity and negative predictive value than any of the methods alone.

Home Uterine Activity Monitoring

Home uterine activity monitoring (HUAM) was devised as a means for early detection of PTL. The rationale was that early detection of increased contraction frequency would allow early intervention with tocolytic drugs and thereby lead to improved rates of labor inhibition and prolongation of pregnancy. Unfortunately there is only a weak relationship between the maximum frequency of contractions and preterm delivery.

Although the United States Food and Drug Administration has approved this device for use in women with a prior PTB, both the U.S. Preventive Services Task Force and the American College of Obstetricians and Gynecologists have concluded that there are insufficient data supporting a benefit from HUAM. HUAM is not recommended because it is not an effective technique for prevention of preterm delivery.

DIAGNOSIS

Signs and symptoms of early PTL include menstrual-like cramping, constant low backache, mild uterine contractions at infrequent and/or irregular intervals, and bloody show. These signs and symptoms are nonspecific and often noted in women whose pregnancies go to term.

The diagnosis of PTL is generally based on clinical criteria of regular painful uterine contractions accompanied by cervical dilation and/or effacement. Suggested specific criteria include persistent uterine contractions (four every 20 minutes or eight every 60 minutes) with documented cervical change or cervical effacement of at least 80% or cervical dilatation greater than 2 cm.

Digital cervical examination has limited reproducibility between examiners, especially when changes are not pronounced; therefore, some centers evaluate cervical length via transvaginal ultrasound to confirm the diagnosis. A short cervix has been variously defined as less than 2.0 cm, 2.5 cm, or 3.0 cm.

PTL is one of the most common reasons for hospitalization of pregnant women, but identifying women with preterm contractions who will deliver preterm is an inexact process. In one systematic review, approximately 30% of PTLs spontaneously resolved. Others have reported 50% of patients hospitalized for PTL deliver at term.

TREATMENT

Candidates for Treatment

Treatment of an acute episode of idiopathic PTL does not abolish the underlying etiology of PTL. Therefore the goals when treating this condition are as follows:

1. Delay delivery so that corticosteroids can be administered.
2. Allow safe transport of the mother, if indicated, to a facility that can provide an appropriate level of neonatal care if the patient delivers preterm.
3. Prolong pregnancy when there are underlying, self-limited causes of labor, such as pyelonephritis or abdominal surgery, that are unlikely to cause recurrent PTL.

There are no evidence-based guidelines for when to initiate treatment for PTL or universally agreed on criteria for making this diagnosis. The general prerequisites for beginning labor-inhibiting therapy are as follows:

1. Presence of PTL—This diagnosis is generally based on clinical criteria of regular painful uterine contractions accompanied by cervical dilation and/or effacement. Suggested specific criteria include persistent uterine contractions (four every 20 minutes or eight every 60 minutes) with documented cervical change or cervical effacement of at least 80% or cervical dilatation greater than 2 cm.
2. Gestational age less than 34 weeks—The lowest gestational age for which inhibition of PTL should be considered is controversial; there are no data from randomized trials. Fifteen weeks gestational age has been arbitrarily selected by many investigators because it defines a point at which early pregnancy loss is less attributable to karyotypic abnormality. Others use 20 weeks for the same reason and because delivery before this age is considered a spontaneous abortion rather than a PTB.

There is some consensus for the upper gestational age limit of 34 weeks because perinatal morbidity and mortality are too low to justify the potential maternal and fetal complications and costs associated with the inhibition of labor.

Contraindications to labor inhibition are as follows:

1. Intrauterine fetal demise
2. Lethal fetal anomaly
3. Nonreassuring fetal assessment
4. Severe intrauterine growth restriction with reversed Doppler flow at the ductus venosus and umbilical artery

181

5. Chorioamnionitis
6. Maternal hemorrhage with hemodynamic instability
7. Severe preeclampsia or eclampsia

Known or suspected fetal pulmonary maturity is not necessarily a contraindication to tocolysis because there are nonpulmonary morbidities associated with PTB. As an example, a 30-week fetus with a mature amniotic fluid test is still at risk for intraventricular hemorrhage, sepsis, hyperbilirubinemia, and other morbidities unrelated to hyaline membrane disease. These fetuses could potentially benefit from prolongation of pregnancy and the nonpulmonary benefits of glucocorticoid therapy.

Inhibition of PTL is less effective when cervical dilatation is advanced (greater than 3 to 4 cm). Tocolysis can still be considered in these cases, especially when the goal is to administer antenatal corticosteroids or safely transport the mother to a tertiary care center.

Inhibition of PTL is not effective in the presence of intraamniotic infection. Although there is universal agreement that tocolysis is contraindicated in the presence of overt infection and may be harmful, there is no consensus on whether women in PTL should be evaluated for subclinical infection. Moreover, the appropriate tests for diagnosis of subclinical infection have not been determined.

Treatment Strategies

Bed Rest, Hydration, and Sedation

There are no well-designed randomized studies evaluating the efficacy of bed rest for prevention or treatment of PTL in singleton pregnancy. A Cochrane review concluded there was no evidence either supporting or refuting the use of bed rest at home or in hospital to prevent PTB. Routine bed rest does not prolong gestation in twins, but this observation does not address the use of bed rest for inhibition of PTL. Randomized studies have shown that neither intravenous hydration nor sedation reduces the rate of PTB in women with PTL.

Corticosteroids

A course of antenatal corticosteroids is administered to decrease the risks associated with PTB. The benefits of antenatal glucocorticoid administration include reduction in the risks of neonatal respiratory distress syndrome, intraventricular hemorrhage, necrotizing enterocolitis, and mortality. A benefit of this therapy is initially observed approximately 18 hours after giving the first dose, with maximal benefit occurring 48 hours after the first dose; thus the primary benefit of treating an acute episode of PTL, even for a brief period, is to allow time for the administration and action of corticosteroids (betamethasone, two doses of 12 mg given intramuscularly 24 hours apart).

Tocolytics

Tocolytics are classes of medications that are used mainly to relax the myometrium. Each category has its disadvantages that have to be taken into account before administration.

Beta-Adrenergic Receptor Agonists

Ritodrine and terbutaline are the two examples of beta-adrenergic receptor agonists. They cause myometrial relaxation by binding with beta-2 adrenergic receptors and increasing intracellular adenyl cyclase. An increase in intracellular cyclic AMP activates protein kinase and results in the phosphorylation of intracellular proteins. The resultant drop in intracellular free calcium interferes with the activity of myosin light chain kinase. Interference with myosin light chain kinase inhibits the interaction between actin and myosin, and thus myometrial contractility is diminished.

Many of the maternal side effects of the beta-adrenergic receptor agonists are related to their cross-reactivity with beta-1 adrenergic receptors. Stimulation of beta-1 adrenergic receptors increases maternal heart rate and stroke volume. Stimulation of beta-2 adrenergic receptors causes peripheral vasodilatation and diastolic hypotension (as well as bronchial relaxation). The combination of these two cardiovascular effects leads to tachycardia, palpitations, and a lowered blood pressure.

Common side effects include chest discomfort, shortness of breath, palpitations, tremor, and anxiety. Rarely myocardial ischemia and pulmonary edema complicates beta-adrenergic therapy. Pulmonary edema likely occurs as a result of fluid overload or increased vascular permeability resulting from infection, inflammation, or preeclampsia. Therefore clinicians should pay meticulous attention to cumulative fluid intake and urine output during beta-adrenergic agonist administration and perform serial pulmonary examinations.

Beta-adrenergic receptor agonists have important metabolic effects as well, including hypokalemia, hyperglycemia, and lipolysis. Glucose and potassium concentrations should be monitored during drug administration.

Beta-adrenergic receptor agonists cross the placenta. Fetal effects, such as fetal tachycardia and neonatal hypoglycemia have been reported.

Labor inhibition with a beta-adrenergic receptor agonist is contraindicated among women with cardiac disease because of potent chronotropic effects. Women with poorly controlled hyperthyroidism or diabetes mellitus should likewise not receive this class of labor-inhibiting agents. Well-controlled diabetes mellitus is not a contraindication to beta-adrenergic receptor agonist therapy, as long as glucose and potassium concentrations are followed carefully and regulated. The final decision in these situations requires balancing the perceived benefit of delaying the delivery with potential side effects of treatment.

In the United States, terbutaline sulfate is the most commonly used beta-adrenergic receptor agonist for labor inhibition therapy.

For the management of acute PTL, terbutaline can be administered subcutaneously by intermittent injection. The dose for intermittent injections is variable: 0.25 mg can be administered every 20 to 30 minutes for up to four doses or until tocolysis is achieved.

Magnesium Sulfate

The precise mechanism of magnesium's effects on uterine contractions has not been completely elucidated. Magnesium likely competes with calcium at the level of the plasma membrane voltage-gated channels.

There is no evidence of a clinically important tocolytic effect for magnesium sulfate; the drug does not significantly reduce the proportion of women delivering within 48 hours.

Rapid infusion of magnesium sulfate causes diaphoresis, flushing, and warmth. Nausea, vomiting, headache, visual disturbances, and palpitations can also occur. Dyspnea or chest pain may be symptoms of pulmonary edema, a rare side effect of magnesium sulfate administration. Magnesium toxicity is related to serum concentration: loss of deep tendon reflexes occurs at 8 to 10 mEq/L, respiratory paralysis at 10 to 15 mEq/L, and cardiac arrest at 20 to 25 mEq/L. Magnesium infusion also causes hypocalcemia, which rarely may become symptomatic (tetany, delirium, electrocardiographic [ECG] abnormalities).

Magnesium freely crosses the placenta. Maternal therapy causes a slight decrease in baseline fetal heart rate and fetal heart rate variability, which is not clinically significant.

Magnesium sulfate tocolysis is contraindicated in women with myasthenia gravis. It also should not be used in women with known myocardial compromise or cardiac conduction defects because of its antiinotropic effects. It can be used with caution in patients who are already on calcium channel blockers.

Magnesium is eliminated by the kidneys; therefore women with impaired renal function may develop magnesium toxicity at the usual doses of administration. Urine output and deep tendon reflexes should be closely monitored. Evaluation of serum magnesium concentration should be performed as needed. Calcium gluconate (1 g intravenously) may be administered to counteract magnesium toxicity.

Magnesium sulfate is usually administered as a 4 to 6 g intravenous load over 20 minutes, followed by a continuous infusion of 2 to 4 g/hour. The infusion rate is titrated based on assessment of contraction frequency and maternal toxicity. Serial serum magnesium concentrations may be helpful in titrating the dose.

Calcium Channel Blockers

Calcium channel blockers directly block the influx of calcium ions through the cell membrane. They also inhibit release of intracellular calcium from the sarcoplasmic reticulum and increase calcium efflux from the cell.

Nifedipine is a peripheral vasodilator, and thus may cause symptoms such as nausea, flushing, headache, dizziness, and palpitations. Nifedipine also decreases mean arterial pressure because of arteriolar smooth muscle relaxation. This is often accompanied by a reflex increase in heart rate.

Calcium channel blockers are contraindicated in women with known hypersensitivity to the drug and should be used with caution in women with left ventricular dysfunction or congestive heart failure. The concomitant use of a calcium channel blocker and magnesium could act synergistically to suppress muscular contractility, which could result in respiratory paralysis.

An optimal nifedipine dosing regimen for treatment of PTL has not been defined. A common approach is to administer an initial loading dose of 30 mg orally, followed by an additional 20 mg orally in 90 minutes. An alternative regimen is to administer 10 mg orally every 20 minutes for up to 4 doses, followed by 20 mg orally every 4 to 8 hours.

Cyclooxygenase Inhibitors

Cyclooxygenase (COX or prostaglandin synthase) is the enzyme responsible for conversion of arachidonic acid to prostaglandins, which are critical in parturition. Prostaglandins enhance the formation of myometrial gap junctions and increase available intracellular calcium by raising transmembrane influx and sarcolemmal release of calcium. Cyclooxygenase exists in two isoforms, COX 1 and COX 2. COX 1 is constitutively expressed in gestational tissues, whereas COX 2 is the inducible form. COX 2 is the isoform that dramatically increases in the decidua and myometrium during term and preterm labor.

Cyclooxygenase inhibitors decrease prostaglandin production by either general inhibition of cyclooxygenase or specific inhibition of COX 2, depending on the agent. Indomethacin, a nonspecific COX inhibitor, is the most commonly used tocolytic in this class. Maternal side effects, including nausea, esophageal reflux, gastritis, and emesis, are seen in approximately 4% of patients treated with indomethacin for PTL. Platelet dysfunction may occur with the use of nonsteroidal antiinflammatory drugs. Other alterations of maternal cardiovascular physiology are minimal. The primary fetal concerns with use of indomethacin are constriction of the ductus arteriosus and oligohydramnios. Premature narrowing or closure of the ductus arteriosus can lead to pulmonary hypertension, tricuspid regurgitation, and persistent fetal circulation. Several cases of premature ductal closure have been reported in pregnancies in which the duration of indomethacin exposure exceeded 48 hours; however, this complication has not occurred in fetuses exposed to short-term indomethacin treatment. This is more likely to occur if indomethacin is used after 32 weeks of gestation.

Maternal administration of indomethacin also causes a reduction in amniotic fluid volume. Fetal urine output is reduced because of indomethacin's ability to enhance the action of vasopressin and reduce renal blood flow. For this reason, indomethacin has been used as a medical therapy for symptomatic polyhydramnios. In women with normal amniotic fluid volumes, indomethacin treatment of PTL can result in oligohydramnios.

Neonatal complications implicated to be associated with in utero indomethacin exposure include bronchopulmonary dysplasia, necrotizing enterocolitis, patent ductus arteriosus, and intraventricular hemorrhage. However, these associations are controversial.

Maternal contraindications to cyclooxygenase inhibitors include platelet dysfunction or bleeding disorder, hepatic dysfunction, gastrointestinal ulcerative disease, renal dysfunction, and asthma (in women with hypersensitivity to aspirin).

The dose of indomethacin for labor inhibition is given as a 50 to 100 mg loading dose, followed by 25 mg orally every 4 to 6 hours. Fetal blood concentrations are 50% of maternal values, but the half-life in the neonate is substantially longer than that in the mother (15 and 2.2 hours, respectively).

If indomethacin is continued for longer than 48 hours, sonographic evaluation for oligohydramnios and narrowing of the fetal ductus arteriosus is warranted at least weekly. Evidence of oligohydramnios or ductal constriction should prompt discontinuation of this therapy.

Oxytocin Receptor Antagonists

Atosiban is a selective oxytocin-vasopressin receptor antagonist, which is not available in the United States. It competes with oxytocin for binding to oxytocin receptors in the myometrium and decidua, thus preventing the increase in intracellular free calcium that occurs when oxytocin binds to its receptor.

A Cochrane review of randomized trials of oxytocin receptor antagonists found that atosiban did not reduce the incidence of PTB more than placebo; however, atosiban use resulted in fewer and less severe side effects.

The U.S. Food and Drug Administration has not approved the use of atosiban for tocolysis because of concerns about the drug's safety when used in fetuses of less than 28 weeks of gestation. It is available for clinical use in Europe.

PREVENTION

There are few potentially beneficial interventions to prevent a recurrent PTL and PTB. One of the most promising interventions is the supplementation of progesterone to mothers with history of prior PTB. There is increasing evidence that progesterone supplementation can reduce the rate of PTB in high-risk women. When women at high-risk for preterm delivery (prior history of preterm delivery) are given weekly intramuscular injections of 17 alpha-hydroxyprogesterone caproate (250 mg) beginning at 16 to 20 weeks of gestation and continuing until 36 weeks, the risk of delivery at less than 37 weeks significantly reduces by approximately 33%. Progesterone-exposed infants had less perinatal morbidity, with significantly reduced rates of necrotizing enterocolitis, intraventricular hemorrhage, and need for supplemental oxygen. There was no evidence of virilization of female offspring, which was a theoretic concern of this therapy.

Although supplemental progesterone appears to be effective in preventing PTB in some high-risk women, it should not be seen as a panacea. An analysis of 2002 national birth certificate data demonstrated that even if all eligible women received progesterone prophylaxis, it would only reduce the overall PTB rate in the United States by approximately 2% (from 12.1% to 11.8%). This is because only 22.5% of PTBs in 2002 were recurrent and prophylaxis only reduces the incidence of recurrent PTB by 33%. In addition, it has been shown that supplemental progesterone is beneficial in twin pregnancies to prevent PTL. However, it is not known if supplemental progesterone is effective in patients with acute PTL without history of PTB.

KEY POINTS

1. PTB is the second most common cause for neonatal mortality and morbidity, following congenital malformations, and accounts for 12.4% of all deliveries.

2. The etiology of PTB is not clearly understood; however, four primary processes, (1) activation of maternal or fetal HPA axis, (2) infection, (3) decidual hemorrhage, and (4) pathologic uterine distention, are thought to be responsible from the pathologic process.

3. Prior PTB is the strongest risk factor for recurrent PTB.

4. There is an inverse relationship between cervical length and gestational age at delivery.

5. Prediction of PTB is an imperfect science. History of prior PTB and cervical fFN testing combined with cervical length assessment are the best predictors.

SUGGESTED READINGS

Goldenberg RL et al: The National Institute of Child Health and Human Development Maternal-Fetal Medicine Units Network. Preterm prediction study: sequential cervical length and fetal fibronectin testing for the prediction of spontaneous preterm birth. *Am J Obstet Gynecol* 182:636, 2000.

Iams JD et al: The National Institute of Child Health and Human Development Maternal Fetal Medicine Unit Network. The length of the cervix and the risk of spontaneous premature delivery. *N Engl J Med* 334:567, 1996.

Iams JD et al., the National Institute of Child Health and Human Development Network of Maternal–Fetal Medicine Units: frequency of uterine contractions and the risk of spontaneous preterm delivery. *N Engl J Med* 346:250, 2002.

Klebanoff MA et al: The National Institute of Child Health Human Development Network of Maternal–Fetal Medicine Units. Failure of metronidazole to prevent preterm delivery among pregnant women with asymptomatic *Trichomonas vaginalis* infection. *N Engl J Med* 2001; 345:487-493, Aug 16, 2001.

Lockwood CJ et al: Fetal fibronectin in cervical and vaginal secretions as a predictor of preterm delivery. *N Engl J Med* 325:669, 1991.

Meis PJ et al., the National Institute of Child Health and Human Development Maternal–Fetal Medicine Units Network: Prevention of recurrent preterm delivery by 17 alpha-hydroxyprogesterone caproate. *N Engl J Med* 348:2379, 2003.

Sibai B et al: Maternal Fetal Medicine Units Network of the National Institute of Child Health and Human Development. Plasma CRH measurement at 16 to 20 weeks' gestation does not predict preterm delivery in women at high-risk for preterm delivery. *Am J Obstet Gynecol* 193(3 Pt 2):1181, 2005.

13

CERVICAL CERCLAGE: INDICATIONS, CONTRAINDICATIONS, AND TECHNIQUES

Nastaran Foyouzi and Errol R. Norwitz

Cervical insufficiency (or cervical incompetence) is defined as the inability to support a pregnancy until term because of a functional defect of the cervix. It is characterized clinically by acute, painless dilatation of the cervix usually in the mid-trimester culminating in prolapse and/or premature rupture of the membranes (PROM) with resultant preterm and often previable delivery. It is estimated that cervical incompetence complicates from 0.1% to 2% of all pregnancies[1] and is thought to be responsible for approximately 15% of habitual immature deliveries between 16 and 28 weeks of gestation.[2]

ETIOLOGY OF CERVICAL INSUFFICIENCY

In most cases, the etiology of cervical incompetence is unknown. Some known causes include müllerian abnormalities that can be either congenital (e.g., congenital cervical hypoplasia) or drug-induced (in utero diethylstilbestrol [DES] exposure), traumatic (prior surgical or obstetric trauma), and connective tissue abnormalities (including Ehlers-Danlos syndrome). Interestingly, a prior history of first-trimester abortion does not appear to be a risk factor for cervical incompetence.[3-6]

Although the causes underlying many of the congenital anomalies of the female reproductive tract are unclear, it has been well documented that prenatal exposure to maternally ingested DES at a particular stage in embryonic life results in abnormal uterine, cervical, and vaginal development. The most common resultant congenital anomalies include cervical hypoplasia, cervical insufficiency leading to preterm birth, and vaginal adenosis with an increased risk of clear-cell adenocarcinoma of the vagina.[7] Recent studies suggest that DES may exert this teratogenic effect by inducing alterations in *HOXA9* or *10* gene expression during in utero reproductive tract development.[8]

CERVICAL ANATOMY AND PHYSIOLOGY

Embryologically, the body and cervix of the uterus are derived from fusion and recanalization of the paramesonephric (müllerian) ducts, a process that is complete by the fifth month of pregnancy. The cervix (which means "neck" in Latin) is the narrow, most caudal portion of the uterus. It measures approximately 3 to 4 cm in length in the adult nulligravida and is contiguous with the inferior aspect of the uterine corpus (body). The point of juncture is known as the isthmus.

Histologically, the cervix consists of fibrous connective tissue, muscle, and blood vessels. Muscular connective tissue constitutes approximately 15% of the cervical stroma but is not uniformly distributed throughout the cervix. Muscular connective tissue constitutes approximately 30%, 18%, and 7% of the upper, mid, and lower thirds of the cervix, respectively.[9] Conversely, the fibrous connective tissue content of the cervical stroma increases as one moves from the external os to the uterine corpus, and it is this component that is believed to confer tensile strength to the cervix. Defects in tensile strength at the cervico-isthmic junction are thought to lead to cervical insufficiency.

DIAGNOSIS OF CERVICAL INSUFFICIENCY

The diagnosis of cervical insufficiency is a clinical one, with evidence of fetal membranes bulging through a partially dilated cervix in an asymptomatic (nonlaboring) patient in the second trimester of pregnancy. More typically, a retrospective and presumptive diagnosis is made on the basis of a characteristic history of silent dilatation of the cervix followed by PROM and a relatively painless, rapid labor with delivery of a living but extremely immature and often previable infant. On inspection in the nonpregnant state, the cervix may appear shortened with a patulous os or may be deformed with lacerations that sometimes extend to the vaginal fornix. Several studies have suggested that, in the nonpregnant state, such findings as the passage of a no. 16 Foley catheter or no. 8 Hegar dilator through the cervix, an abnormally wide uterocervical canal on hysterosalpingogram (≥8 mm at the level of the internal os), and/or evidence of cervical trauma with marked anatomic distortion are suggestive of cervical insufficiency.[10] However, the weight of evidence in the literature suggests that the diagnosis of cervical insufficiency cannot be made before pregnancy. Because their predictive value is not clear, such prepregnancy tests should not routinely be recommended. It is also unclear whether such women will benefit from prophylactic cerclage.

Real-time sonographic evaluation of the cervix has demonstrated a strong inverse correlation between cervical length and preterm birth.[11,12] In light of these data, an alternative strategy that has developed for the identification of asymptomatic pregnancies at increased risk of preterm birth because of premature cervical effacement and/or dilatation is serial vaginal assessment and/or transvaginal sonographic cervical length measurements.[13,14] Whether there are interventions that can abrogate the risk of preterm birth in women with an abnormally shortened residual cervical length at 22 to 24 weeks' gestation is not known.

Although several treatments have been recommended over the years with variable success rates (e.g., vaginal pessary placement), the generally accepted treatment for cervical insufficiency is to attempt to strengthen the intrinsically weakened cervix through the surgical placement of a cervical cerclage (stitch).[13]

CERVICAL CERCLAGE

Cervical cerclage has become the mainstay for the management of cervical insufficiency but remains one the more controversial surgical interventions in obstetrics. This is primarily not only because it is rare to find a patient that has a classical history for cervical insufficiency but also because the majority of patients with a history suggestive of cervical insufficiency will deliver subsequent pregnancies at term even in the absence of obstetric intervention. Only 15% to 30% of women with a prior pregnancy loss resulting from cervical insufficiency will have a recurrence of this complication in a subsequent pregnancy.[1,2]

Indications for Cervical Cerclage

Since the introduction of cervical cerclage in 1955,[15] it has undergone many changes with regard to techniques, indications, and postoperative care. Cervical cerclage may be placed either prophylactically or emergently.

Prophylactic (Elective) Cervical Cerclage

Placement of a prophylactic cervical cerclage is indicated in women with a history of prior recurrent mid-trimester pregnancy loss and/or preterm delivery resulting from cervical insufficiency. Several randomized trial studies have shown no benefit of prophylactic cerclage in improving perinatal outcome.[16,17] Aside from a small reduction in preterm birth rates at less than 33 weeks' gestation in the largest trial,[18] a recent meta-analysis that evaluated pregnancy outcome of elective cerclage in six randomized clinical trials revealed no overall reduction in pregnancy loss or preterm delivery rates.[16,17,19] In light of these data, a recently published American College of Obstetricians and Gynecologists (ACOG) guideline suggests that elective cerclage be performed only in patients with three or more unexplained second-trimester pregnancy losses or preterm deliveries remote from term.[20] In patients with a history of fewer than three second-trimester pregnancy losses, cervical cerclage is not supported by evidence-based studies and the use of serial transvaginal ultrasound surveillance may be a more judicious approach.[20]

The role of prophylactic cerclage in multiple pregnancies is still controversial. There is no question that women with multiple pregnancies are at increased risk of preterm delivery; however, there is no consistent evidence that prophylactic cerclage is of any benefit in uncomplicated twin pregnancies.[19,21,22] The questions as to whether or not all DES-exposed women should be offered a prophylactic cerclage also remains controversial. Most clinicians believe that a history of in utero DES exposure alone (without a history of prior pregnancy loss) is not an indication for prophylactic cerclage placement, but further studies are required to clarify this issue.[20]

A prophylactic cervical cerclage is placed most commonly between 13 and 16 weeks of gestation.[20] Late first-trimester cerclage placement has become more popular because there is a less than 1% chance of spontaneous pregnancy loss if fetal heart tones are present and if no gross fetal structural anomalies are noted on early ultrasound.[2,23]

Emergent (Salvage) Cervical Cerclage

The primary indication for an emergent cervical cerclage is premature effacement and/or dilatation of the cervix (with or without prolapsing of the fetal membranes) in the absence of labor before 28 weeks' gestation. Asymptomatic women with sonographic evidence of cervical shortening and/or funneling may also benefit from emergent cervical cerclage placement, although the data in this regard are controversial.

Contraindications to Cervical Cerclage

Contraindications to cervical cerclage placement are listed in Box 13-1. These can be divided into two categories: absolute and relative contraindications. Intraamniotic infection is an absolute contraindication to cerclage placement. The presence of bacteria on Gram stain or a positive culture from preoperative amniocentesis is associated with a failure rate of more than 90%.[24,25] However, preoperative amniocentesis cannot be recommended in all such patients.

In the absence of any contraindications to expectant management (e.g., intraamniotic infection) and with extensive patient counseling, it may not be unreasonable to place a cerclage. According to ACOG,[20] if transvaginal sonography before 16 to 20 weeks of gestation identifies an abnormally shortened cervix (typically defined as <2.0 cm), the examination should be

---

Box 13-1   Contraindications to Cervical Cerclage Placement

Absolute Contraindications
- Chorioamnionitis
- Labor
- PROM
- Active vaginal bleeding
- Fetal demise
- Fetal anomaly incompatible with life
- Life-threatening maternal condition that precludes anesthesia
- Gestational age ≥28 weeks

Relative Contraindications
- Placenta previa
- IUGR
- Mucopurulent cervical discharge with membrane opacification
- Fetal membranes prolapsing through the cervical os
- Gestational age 24≥ weeks

IUGR, Intrauterine growth retardation; *PROM*, premature rupture of the membranes.

repeated in 1 to 2 weeks. However, if a short cervix is identified at or after 20 weeks of gestation, prompt assessment is necessary to exclude preterm labor and chorioamnionitis. ACOG supports cervical cerclage placement up to 28 weeks' gestation.[20] However, many practitioners would not recommend emergent cervical cerclage placement beyond the limit of fetal viability (defined as 24 weeks), because the potential for harm probably outweighs the potential benefit.[1,26]

Technical Considerations

Preoperative Considerations

Once the decision has been made to proceed with cervical cerclage placement, there are several technical considerations that need to be addressed. An ultrasound examination should be performed before cerclage placement to exclude gross structural anomalies (e.g., anencephaly) and/or fetal demise. Any urinary or genital tract infection should be identified and treated. Cultures for gonorrhea and *Chlamydia* should be taken if the patient is at high risk and/or if these tests have not been done recently. Testing for perineal Group B streptococcal carrier status is not indicated. Antibiotic treatment should be initiated immediately if vaginal cultures are positive, and treatment should be completed before elective cerclage placement. Every effort should be made to exclude intraamniotic infection (chorioamnionitis) before emergent cerclage placement. The vast majority of these infections result from bacteria ascending from the vagina. The diagnosis of intraamniotic infection is based on the presence of at least two of four characteristic clinical manifestations (oral temperature >100.4° F, maternal tachycardia, fetal tachycardia, uterine contractions, and tenderness). A foul discharge (pus) emanating from the cervix on speculum examination is pathognomonic of intrauterine infection. Amniocentesis is not recommended for all women presenting with an advanced cervical examination in the mid- to late-second trimester but may be indicated if the clinical setting is concerning (e.g., an unexplained elevation in maternal white blood cell count or sustained fetal tachycardia) or if infection with *Listeria monocytogenes* is suspected.

Prophylactic broad-spectrum antibiotics (ampicillin 2 g or cefazolin 1 g intravenous [IV] given 30 minutes before surgery) are recommended for emergent cerclage placement because of the risk of intraamniotic infection. However, there are insufficient data to recommend prophylactic antibiotics for prophylactic cerclage placement, and empirical evidence suggests that they are not required. Prophylactic tocolysis may be used to inhibit transient uterine contractions associated with cerclage placement, but there is no objective evidence that tocolysis improves outcome. Tocolysis is generally unnecessary for elective cervical cerclage placement at less than 16 weeks' gestation. The lack of clear benefit for antibiotic and tocolytic therapy after cerclage suggests that these drugs should be used with caution.[20] Indomethacin (100 mg rectally 30 minutes before surgery) is commonly administered before emergent (but not prophylactic) cerclage because this drug diminishes procedure-induced elevations in prostaglandin levels that, in theory, may lead to preterm contractions and labor. Indomethacin (25 mg orally every 6 hours) is generally continued for 24 to 48 hours postoperatively.

Risks and benefits of the procedure should be discussed in detail, and written consent obtained. Regional anesthesia is preferred, because of the decreased maternal morbidity as compared with general endotracheal anesthesia. Moreover, women recovering from general anesthesia are more likely to retch and put undue strain on the stitch. Confirmation of fetal viability is required both immediately before and after the procedure, either by auscultation or by ultrasound.

If the fetal membranes are found to be prolapsing through the external os, the risk of iatrogenic rupture of the fetal membranes may be as high as 40% to 50%. Trendelenburg position,[27] backfilling the bladder,[28,29] placement of a 30-ml Foley catheter[30] or moistened sponge forceps into the cervical os,[31] and/or therapeutic amniocentesis[32,33] have all been used to reduce the fetal membranes before cerclage placement with varying results.

Operative Considerations

The choice of cervical cerclage is best left to the discretion of the obstetric care provider. A transvaginal cervical cerclage is placed around the cervix via a vaginal approach; a transabdominal cerclage is performed through an abdominal incision. The object of both procedures is to reinforce and increase the tensile strength on an intrinsically weakened cervix. Although a transabdominal cerclage can often be placed at a more favorable position close to the cervico-isthmic junction whereas a transvaginal cerclage often ends up distal to the internal os, there is no evidence that one approach is superior to the other. The most common transvaginal procedures are the McDonald and Shirodkar cerclage. Careful patient selection and the experience of the surgeon are far more important determinants of success than the choice of suture technique. However, under certain circumstances, one or other technique may be preferable. For example, if the cervix is very short or lacerated, a Shirodkar cerclage may be technically easier to place. Considerably more skill is required to place a Shirodkar cerclage, and this may be why it is the less popular of the two commonly used techniques.

- **McDonald cerclage** refers to a transvaginal purse-string suture placed around the cervix as high as possible without dissection of the bladder or rectum (Figure 13-1). When placing such a cerclage, the cervix is pulled toward the surgeon and manipulated with one or two ring forceps placed on the anterior and posterior lips. A needle loaded with heavy nonabsorbable suture material (no. 1 or 2 polypropylene or braided nylon) is inserted at the 12 o'clock position, as high as possible at the junction of the rugated vaginal mucosa and the smooth-walled cervix. Four to six bites are taken circumferentially around the cervix in a purse-string fashion. Each bite should be deep enough to extend midway into the cervical stroma but not into the endocervical canal. The two ends of the suture are then tied securely and cut, leaving the ends long enough to grasp when it is time to remove the cerclage. A second McDonald cerclage may be necessary if the first stitch did not result in optimal closure of the cervix. This often occurs when placing an emergent cerclage in a woman with cervical effacement and prolapsed membranes. In such a setting, it is usual to leave both stitches in place until removal later in pregnancy.

Figure 13-1

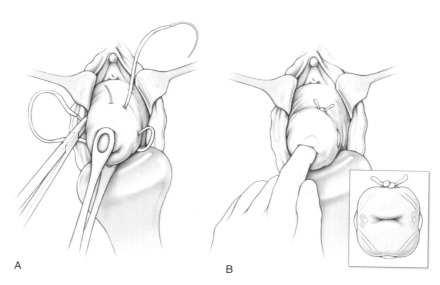

A   B

McDonald cerclage. **A,** When placing a McDonald cerclage, the cervix is pulled toward the surgeon and a purse-string suture placed circumferentially around the cervix as high as possible without dissection of the bladder or rectum. **B,** The two ends of the suture are then secured (in this case, anteriorly) and the integrity of the endocervical canal is checked.

195

- **Shirodkar cerclage** is performed transvaginally using a 5-mm Mersilene tape (or heavy suture) placed around the cervix at the level of the internal os after surgically reflecting the bladder anteriorly and the rectum posteriorly. The bladder should be emptied with a catheter to facilitate visualization of the cervix. The cervix is pulled toward the surgeon with one or two ring forceps while an assistant retracts the vaginal sidewalls. A 1- to 2-cm vertical or transverse incision is made on the posterior cervix at the junction of the rugated vaginal mucosa and the smooth-walled cervix using either a scalpel or electrosurgery. The incision may be facilitated by better defining the surgical planes through a prior injection of 1 to 2 ml of sterile saline. The rectum is then dissected off the posterior cervix using blunt dissection with a finger, sponge on a stick, or peanut on a long clamp. The same procedure is repeated anteriorly to dissect the bladder off the anterior cervix. The dissection should be carried back far enough to allow the insertion of the uterosacral and cardinal ligaments onto the cervix to be palpated at the level of the internal os. Electrosurgery may be used to control small bleeders. Long curved Allis or Teale clamps are then used to grasp and approximate the lateral edges of the anterior and posterior incisions and paracervical tissue. Two atraumatic (blunted) needles premounted with a single 5-mm Mersilene band are used for the cerclage. The tip of one needle is introduced anteriorly at the lateral edge of the incision at the level of or as close as possible to the internal os and threaded submucosally adjacent to the cervical stroma and medial to the cervical branches of the uterine vessels to emerge at the lateral edge of the posterior incision. The same procedure is performed on the opposite side with the other needle, and the two ends are tied firmly using four to six square knots (Figure 13-2). The tails of the suture should be left long. The decision of whether to tie the stitch anteriorly or posteriorly should be left to the discretion of the

Figure 13-2

Shirodkar cerclage.
A, When placing a
Shirodkar cerclage,
the cervix is pulled
toward the surgeon
and a 5-mm Mersi-
lene tape (or heavy
suture) is placed
around the cervix at
the level of the inter-
nal os after surgically
reflecting the bladder
anteriorly and the
rectum posteriorly.
B, The two ends of
the suture are then
secured (in this case,
anteriorly) and the
integrity of the
endocervical canal
is checked.

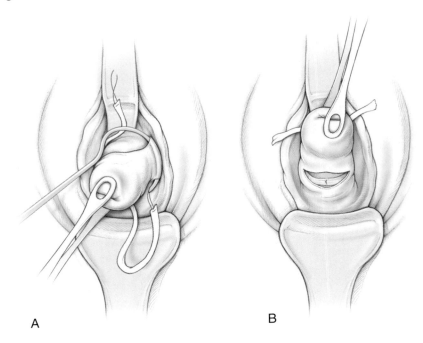

A   B

operator. In general, it is easier to place and remove the cerclage if the
knot is placed anteriorly, although there are rare instances of such a
knot causing bladder discomfort and even eroding into the bladder. Following Shirodkar cerclage placement, the vaginal mucosa may be reap-
proximated with a fine chromic catgut suture, although this is not necessary if hemostasis is good. Moreover, it is not recommended to bury
the ends of the knot below the mucosa or to anchor the tape to the cervix because this will make removal of the stitch before delivery more difficult. Alternatively, if cesarean delivery is planned, the Shirodkar cerclage can be left in place postpartum for use in a future pregnancy. In
such cases, it is recommended that the knot be buried completely under
the vaginal mucosa to minimize vaginal discharge. In pregnancies complicated by cervical insufficiency and in which a transvaginal cerclage
has previously failed or is not technically feasible, transabdominal cervical cerclage offers the possibility of a successful outcome.

- **Transabdominal cervical cerclage** is usually performed under general or regional anesthesia with the patient in the supine or modified li-
thotomy position. The abdominal cavity is entered through a transverse
or vertical incision and the peritoneal reflection of the bladder is opened
to expose the cervico-isthmic junction. The uterine vessels can be palpated between the thumb and forefinger, and should be drawn laterally
away from the uterus to expose the avascular space immediately adjacent to the cervico-isthmic junction. This maneuver can be facilitated by
having an assistant gently elevate the uterus out of the pelvis to provide

optimum exposure of the vessels and isthmus. Gentle uterine manipulation is particularly important when the uterus is gravid. A 15-cm long 5-mm Mersilene band is passed through the avascular space between the lateral wall of the uterus and the ascending and descending branches of the uterine arteries at the level of the cervico-isthmic junction (Figure 13-3). This can be achieved by loading the suture onto a needle or by creating a tunnel through the posterior leaf of the broad ligament using a long right-angled forceps or Moynihan clamp. Care should be taken not to injure nearby veins. The identical procedure is repeated on the opposite side. The Mersilene band should be wrapped around the uterine isthmus at the level of the uterosacral ligament insertions, made to lie flat against the uterus, tied to slightly compress the intervening tissue, and secured anteriorly with a triple square knot. The ends can be sutured to the band with fine nonabsorbable sutures. Intraoperative ultrasound is occasionally used to monitor the fetal heart rate to ascertain that blood flow through the uterine artery has not been compromised by the procedure and to ensure that the membranes are above the level of the cerclage.

197

Figure 13-3

Transabdominal cervical cerclage. When placing a transabdominal cerclage, the abdominal cavity is entered and the peritoneal reflection of the bladder opened to expose the cervico-isthmic junction. A 15-cm long 5-mm Mersilene band is passed through the avascular space between the lateral wall of the uterus and the ascending and descending branches of the uterine arteries at the level of the cervico-isthmic junction on both sides. The Mersilene band is wrapped around the uterine isthmus and secured to slightly compress the intervening tissues.

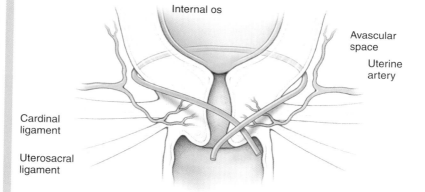

Internal os

Avascular space

Uterine artery

Cardinal ligament

Uterosacral ligament

Postoperative Recommendations

In the immediate postoperative period, patients should be warned that they may experience symptoms of spotting, cramping, and/or dysuria (because of minor muscle injury from the vaginal wall retractors), all of which should abate within a few days. Once a cerclage is in place, weekly or bi-weekly follow-up visits for cervical examinations are probably sufficient in the absence of clinical symptoms. Cervical assessment may be by simple bi-manual examination or by ultrasound. Bed rest and "pelvic rest" (no coitus, tampons, or douching) are usually recommended until a favorable gestational age is reached but without proven benefit. Any vaginal fluid leakage should be evaluated immediately for possible preterm PROM. In the absence of obstetric complications, the cerclage is usually removed electively in the office at around 37 weeks' gestation (late enough to avoid preterm delivery but early enough to avoid laboring with a cerclage in place). Earlier removal may be necessary in the event of premature uterine contractions to avoid cervical lacerations and/or uterine rupture. Removal of cerclage can often be achieved in the office without analgesia, although on occasion it may be necessary to return to the operating room for removal. This is more common with a Shirodkar cerclage and may be because of the knot being buried under the vaginal mucosa or to infiltration of the Mersilene band by cervical granulation tissue. In general, patients can be sent home after cerclage removal to await the onset of labor.

Complications of Cervical Cerclage

The complications of cervical cerclage are presented in Box 13-2. They can be categorized as early (<48 hours after the procedure) or late (≥48 hours). The most common complications are suture displacement, rupture of membranes, and chorioamnionitis, and their incidence varies widely in relation to the timing and indications for the cerclage. Emergency cerclage is associated

---

Box 13-2   Complications of Cervical Cerclage

Early Complications (<48 hr)
- PROM
- Excessive blood loss (requiring blood transfusion)
- Pregnancy loss (abortion)
- Complications from anesthesia.

Late Complications (≥48 hr)
- Cervical laceration
- Chorioamnionitis
- Cervical stenosis
- IUGR
- Fetal demise
- Placental abruption
- Thrombophlebitis
- Bladder pain
- Migration of suture
- Increased obstetric intervention including higher rates of admission to hospital, administration of oral tocolytics, induction of labor, and cesarean delivery
- Puerperal infection

IUGR, Intrauterine growth retardation; *PROM,* premature rupture of the membranes.

with higher incidence of morbidity as a result of cervical shortening and exposure of the fetal membranes to the vaginal ecosystem.[20] In addition to the known risks of laparotomy, transabdominal cervical cerclage can be complicated by rupture of membranes, chorioamnionitis, or intraoperative hemorrhage from the uterine veins when the cerclage is tunneled between the bifurcation of the uterine artery. Life-threatening complications such as uterine rupture and maternal septicemia are extremely rare but have been reported with all type of cerclage.[20]

Cervical cerclage is also associated with increased obstetric intervention, including higher rates of admission to hospital, administration of oral tocolytics, induction of labor, and cesarean delivery. Puerperal infection occurs in approximately 6% of patients with cerclage, which is twice as common as the incidence in gestational age-matched controls without cerclage.[21] For this reason, it is important that cervical cerclage be performed only in women with a clear indication.

199

CURRENT CONTROVERSIES

Transabdominal Cerclage

Transabdominal cerclage appears to be a safe and effective procedure for reducing the incidence of mid-trimester pregnancy loss in select patients with cervical insufficiency. It has not been shown to be more effective than transvaginal cerclage, and it is a far more morbid procedure that requires a laparotomy and subsequent cesarean delivery. The specific criteria to evaluate the indications for a transabdominal cerclage are congenitally short or extensively amputated cervix, marked scarring of the cervix, deeply notched multiple cervical defects, penetrating lacerations of the fornix, subacute cervicitis, wide or extensive cervical conization, cervico-vaginal fistulas, and one or more previous transvaginal cerclage failures. The main advantage of the transabdominal cervico-isthmic procedure is the placement of the non-absorbable suture at the level of the internal os, which avoids the placement of a foreign body within the vagina with the subsequent risk of ascending lower genital tract infection.[34] The major objection to this procedure is the need for multiple laparotomies (cerclage and subsequent caesarean section at 37 to 39 weeks of gestation after confirmation of fetal lung maturity) despite the ability to leave the band in place between pregnancies. The technical skill and experience of the operator are crucial to the success of the procedure.[35] The laparoscopic approach has the advantage of obviating the need for a laparotomy, reducing abdominal wall trauma, and minimizing recovery time. Such procedures (especially gasless laparoscopy) appear to be safe for both mother and fetus. However, the inability to cannulate the cervical os and the increased size of uterus leading to reduced exposure make the laparoscopic procedure more difficult during pregnancy.[35-37]

Transabdominal cerclage placement is usually recommended either before conception or during early pregnancy (11-14 weeks). Placement of the cerclage later in pregnancy may be difficult because of the size of the uterus. The stitch can be removed at the time of cesarean delivery or left in place if future pregnancies are planned. In the event of a fetal loss in the first trimester, cervical dilation and evacuation of the uterus can be safely and effectively performed without removal of the cerclage. It is not clear whether these procedures can be successfully accomplished for a second trimester pregnancy loss. It may also be technically feasible to remove the cerclage through a transvaginal colpotomy, thereby permitting vaginal delivery. In practice, however, this technique is far more difficult than reported and is not generally recommended.

Removal of a Transvaginal Cerclage Following Rupture of Membranes

The presence of a cerclage does not appear to increase the incidence of preterm PROM remote from placement. On occasion, however, preterm PROM will occur with a cerclage in place. The decision of whether or not to remove the cerclage in such patients remains controversial. Retention of the cerclage may prolong latency, thereby allowing for a more favorable gestational age at delivery. Alternatively, a retained cerclage may provide a nidus for infection. Therefore some authors recommend immediate cerclage removal regardless of gestational age in cases of PROM.[38] In contrast, a more recent retrospective analysis of pregnancy outcome in patients with preterm PROM and preexisting cerclage between 24 and 35 weeks' gestation suggested that the decision to remove or retain the cerclage did not affect latency or perinatal outcome. Moreover, comparison of the cerclage patients with control subjects with preterm PROM but no cerclage suggested that gestational age at presentation was the most important determinant of pregnancy outcome.[39] It is reasonable therefore to individualize the decision of whether or not to remove the cerclage in the setting of preterm PROM.

Cervical Cerclage for a Shortened Cervix

Sonographic evaluation of the cervix has demonstrated a strong inverse correlation between cervical length and preterm delivery.[12,40] If the cervical length is less than 10th percentile for gestational age, the pregnancy is at a sixfold increased risk of delivery before 35 weeks.[11] A cervical length of 15 mm or less at 23 weeks occurs in less than 2% of low-risk women but is predictive of delivery before 28 weeks and 32 weeks in 60% and 90% of cases, respectively.[11] The ability of transvaginal ultrasound to identify women at risk of cervical incompetence and thereby preterm birth may be increased by measuring the response of the cervix to transfundal pressure.[40] Whether parturient identified by such tests as being at high-risk of preterm birth will benefit from cervical cerclage remains unclear. There are several retrospective studies suggesting that cervical cerclage placement in asymptomatic women with short cervical length on endovaginal ultrasound may improve perinatal outcome.[12,41-43] However, more recent studies suggest that cerclage does not prevent preterm delivery in women at high risk for this outcome on the basis of cervical shortening.[44-46] Indeed, in a recent clinical trial from the United Kingdom of 253 women with shortened cervical length (≤15 mm) at 22 to 24 weeks who were randomized to either cervical cerclage (n = 127) or expectant management (n = 126) showed that insertion of a Shirodkar cerclage did not substantially reduce the risk of early preterm delivery.[46]

CONCLUSIONS

Cervical insufficiency is a diagnostic dilemma. Unfortunately, it is not possible to predict with any certainty which women with a history of cervical insufficiency will have a successful subsequent pregnancy without needing a cerclage or which will have a complication from cerclage placement. Moreover, there have been very few large, prospective, randomized, controlled studies to determine the efficacy of the various surgical methods. Until such data are available, cervical cerclage placement should be used judiciously and only after extensive and comprehensive patient counseling.

KEY POINTS

1. Cervical insufficiency (cervical incompetence) refers to the inability to support a pregnancy until term because of a functional defect of the cervix.
2. It is a clinical diagnosis with evidence of membranes bulging through a partially dilated cervix in an asymptomatic (nonlaboring) patient in the second trimester of pregnancy; the diagnosis cannot be made before pregnancy.
3. Risk factors include congenital müllerian abnormalities, in utero DES exposure, traumatic abnormalities (prior surgical or obstetric trauma), and connective tissue abnormalities; most cases have no known cause.
4. Placement of a cervical cerclage (stitch) has become the mainstay for the management of cervical insufficiency, but a prior history of two or more prior unexplained midtrimester pregnancy losses is the only absolute indication for elective (prophylactic) cerclage placement.
5. Placement of an emergent (salvage) cervical cerclage is of no proven benefit over bed rest alone.
6. Cervical shortening on transvaginal ultrasound is associated with an increased risk of preterm birth, but placement of a cervical cerclage in this setting does not appear to prevent preterm birth or improve perinatal outcome.

REFERENCES

1. Norwitz ER GM, Repke JT: Cervical cerclage—elective and emergent. *ACOG Update* 24:1, 1999.
2. Shortle B, Jewelewicz R: Cervical incompetence. *Fertil Steril* 52:181, 1989.
3. Harlap S et al: A prospective study of spontaneous fetal losses after induced abortions. *N Engl J Med* 301:677, 1979.
4. Cousins L: Cervical incompetence, 1980. a time for reappraisal. *Clin Obstet Gynecol* 23:467, 1980.
5. Harlap S et al: A prospective study of spontaneous fetal loss after induced abortion. *N Engl J Med* 301:677, 1979.
6. Cousins L: Cervical incompetence, 1980. A time for reappraisal. *Clin Obstet Gynecol* 23:467, 1980.
7. *Novak's Gynecology*, ed 13. Philadelphia, 2002, Lippincott Williams & Wilkins.
8. Block K et al: In utero diethylstilbestrol (DES) exposure alters Hox gene expression in the developing müllerian system. *FASEB J* 14:1101, 2000.

9. DN D: The fibrous nature of the human cervix, and its relation to the isthmic segment in gravid and nongravid uteri. *Am J Obstet Gynecol* 53:541, 1947.

10. ACOG criteria set: Cervical cerclage. Number 17, October 1996. Committee on Quality Assessment of the American College of Obstetricians and Gynecologists. *Int J Gynaecol Obstet* 56:211, 1997.

11. Iams JD et al: The length of the cervix and the risk of spontaneous premature delivery. National Institute of Child Health and Human Development Maternal Fetal Medicine Unit Network. *N Engl J Med* 334:567, 1996.

12. Heath VC et al: Cervical length at 23 weeks of gestation: prediction of spontaneous preterm delivery. *Ultrasound Obstet Gynecol* 12:312, 1998.

13. *Danforth's Obstetrics and Gynecology* [electronic resource]. Philadelphia, 1999, Lippincott Williams & Wilkins.

14. Al-Azemi M et al: Changing trends in the obstetric indications for cervical cerclage. *J Obstet Gynaecol* 23:507, 2003.

15. Shirodkar VN: A new method of operative treatment for habitual abortions in the second trimester of pregnancy. *Antiseptic* 52:299, 1955.

16. Lazar P et al: Multicentred controlled trial of cervical cerclage in women at moderate risk of preterm delivery. *Br J Obstet Gynaecol* 91:731, 1984.

17. Rush RW et al: A randomized controlled trial of cervical cerclage in women at high risk of spontaneous preterm delivery. *Br J Obstet Gynaecol* 91:724, 1984.

18. Drakeley AJ, Roberts D, Alfirevic Z: Cervical cerclage for prevention of preterm delivery: meta-analysis of randomized trials. *Obstet Gynecol* 102:621, 2003.

19. Dor J et al: Elective cervical suture of twin pregnancies diagnosed ultrasonically in the first trimester following induced ovulation. *Gynecol Obstet Invest* 13:55, 1982.

20. Ressel GW et al: ACOG releases bulletin on managing cervical insufficiency [Comparison of cerclage and cerclage pessary in the treatment of pregnant women with incompetent cervix and threatened preterm delivery] Relationship between tumor necrosis factor-alpha genotype and success of emergent cerclage. *Am Fam Physician* 69(2): 436, 439, 2004.

21. Final report of the Medical Research Council/Royal College of Obstetricians and Gynaecologists multicentre randomised trial of cervical cerclage. MRC/RCOG Working Party on Cervical Cerclage. *Br J Obstet Gynaecol* 100:516, 1993.

22. Parilla BV, Haney EI, MacGregor SN: The prevalence and timing of cervical cerclage placement in multiple gestations. *Int J Gynaecol Obstet* 80:123, 2003.

23. Kurup M, Goldkrand JW: Cervical incompetence: elective, emergent, or urgent cerclage. *Am J Obstet Gynecol* 181:240, 1999.

24. Mays JK et al Amniocentesis for selection before rescue cerclage. *Obstet Gynecol* 95:652, 2000.

25. Romero R et al: Infection and labor. VIII. Microbial invasion of the amniotic cavity in patients with suspected cervical incompetence: prevalence and clinical significance. *Am J Obstet Gynecol* 167(4 Pt 1):1086, 1992.

26. MacDougall J, Siddle N: Emergency cervical cerclage. *Br J Obstet Gynaecol* 98:1234, 1991.

27. Olatunbosun OA, Dyck F: Cervical cerclage operation for a dilated cervix. *Obstet Gynecol* 57:166, 1981.

28. Scheerer LJ et al: A new technique for reduction of prolapsed fetal membranes for emergency cervical cerclage. *Obstet Gynecol* 74(3 Pt 1):408, 1989.

29. Oleszczuk J et al: [Amniocentesis and mother's bladder overfilling in operative treatment of advanced cervical incompetence] Amnioreduction in emergency cerclage with prolapsed membranes: comparison of two methods for reducing the membranes [Variations of the Holman method for reducing prolapsed fetal membranes]. *Ginekol Pol* 72:1116, 2001.

30. Sher G: Congenital incompetence of the cervical os: reduction of bulging membranes with a modified Foley catheter. *J Reprod Med* 22:165, 1979.

31. McDonald IA: Suture of the cervix for inevitable miscarriage. *J Obstet Gynaecol Br Emp* 64:346, 1957.

32. Goodlin RC: Cervical incompetence, hourglass membranes, and amniocentesis. *Obstet Gynecol* 54:748, 1979.

33. Locatelli A et al: Amnioreduction in emergency cerclage with prolapsed membranes: comparison of two methods for reducing the membranes [Variations of the Holman method for reducing prolapsed fetal membranes]. *Am J Perinatol* 16: 73, 1999.

34. McGregor JA et al: Preterm birth and infection: pathogenic possibilities. *Am J Reprod Immunol Microbiol* 16:123, 1988.

35. Gallot D et al: Experience with three cases of laparoscopic transabdominal cervico-isthmic cerclage and two subsequent pregnancies. *BJOG* 110:696, 2003.

36. Scarantino SE et al: Laparoscopic removal of a transabdominal cervical cerclage. *Am J Obstet Gynecol* 182:1086, 2000.

37. Lesser KB, Childers JM, Surwit EA: Transabdominal cerclage: a laparoscopic approach. *Obstet Gynecol* 91(5 Pt 2): 855, 1998.

38. Ludmir J, Bader T, Chen L, Lindenbaum C, Wong G: Poor perinatal outcome associated with retained cerclage in patients with premature rupture of membranes. *Obstet Gynecol* 84:823, 1994.

39. McElrath TF et al: Perinatal outcome after preterm premature rupture of membranes with in situ cervical cerclage. *Am J Obstet Gynecol* 187:1147, 2002.

40. Guzman ER et al: A new method using vaginal ultrasound and transfundal pressure to evaluate the asymptomatic incompetent cervix. *Obstet Gynecol* 83:248, 1994.

41. Guzman ER et al: Longitudinal assessment of endocervical canal length between 15 and 24 weeks' gestation in women at risk for pregnancy loss or preterm birth. *Obstet Gynecol* 92:31, 1998.

42. Hibbard JU, Snow J, Moawad AH: Short cervical length by ultrasound and cerclage. *J Perinatol* 20:161, 2000.

43. Althuisius SM et al: Cervical incompetence prevention randomized cerclage trial (CIPRACT): study design and preliminary results. *Am J Obstet Gynecol* 183:823, 2000.

44. Berghella V et al: Prediction of preterm delivery with transvaginal ultrasonography of the cervix in patients with high-risk pregnancies: does cerclage prevent prematurity? *Am J Obstet Gynecol* 181:809, 1999.

45. Hassan SS et al: Does cervical cerclage prevent preterm delivery in patients with a short cervix? *Am J Obstet Gynecol* 184:1325; discussion 1329, 2001.

46. To MS et al: Cervical cerclage for prevention of preterm delivery in women with short cervix: randomised controlled trial. *Lancet* 363:1849, 2004.

14

POSTTERM PREGNANCY

Nastaran Foyouzi and Errol R. Norwitz

The timely onset of labor and delivery is an important determinant of perinatal outcome. Both preterm and postterm births are associated with higher rates of perinatal morbidity and mortality than pregnancies delivering at term. Postterm (prolonged) pregnancy refers to a pregnancy that has extended to or beyond a gestational age of 42.0 weeks (294 days; estimated date of delivery [EDD] plus 14 days) from the first day of the last normal menstrual period (LMP). The term *post-dates* is poorly defined and, as such, is best avoided.

INCIDENCE

The incidence of postterm pregnancy is dependent on the population mix (including the percentage of primigravid women, women with pregnancy complications, and the incidence of preterm birth) and on the local practice patterns (e.g., the rate of elective cesarean delivery and of routine induction of labor).[1] Overall in the United States, approximately 10% (range, 3%-14%) of all singleton pregnancies continue beyond 42 weeks of gestation, and around 4% (2%-7%) will continue beyond 43 completed weeks in the absence of obstetric intervention.[2-4] The lowest incidence of postterm pregnancy is reported in studies using routine ultrasonography for confirmation of gestational age. Errors in gestational age dating based on standard clinical criteria (e.g., last normal menstrual period and uterine size) contribute to inaccurate diagnosis.

ETIOLOGY

The majority of postterm pregnancies have no known cause. Primiparity and prior postterm pregnancy are the most common identifiable risk factors for prolongation of pregnancy.[1-3] Rarely, postterm pregnancy may be associated with placental sulfatase deficiency or fetal anencephaly (in the absence of polyhydramnios).[3] Male gender also predisposes to prolongation of pregnancy.[5]

RISK FACTORS

Postterm pregnancy is associated with both fetal and maternal risks,[6-10] which are summarized in Table 14-1 and Table 14-2.

Fetal Risks

Perinatal mortality (stillbirths plus early neonatal deaths) at 42 weeks of gestation is twice that at term (4-7 vs. 2-3 per 1000 deliveries) and increases fourfold at 43 weeks and five- to sevenfold at 44 weeks.[9-11] Uteroplacental insufficiency, asphyxia (with and without meconium aspiration), intrauterine infection, and anencephaly all contribute to the excess perinatal deaths, although postterm anencephaly is essentially nonexistent with modern obstetrical care.[12] Postterm pregnancy is an independent risk factor for low 5-minute Apgar scores and fetal acidosis.[13]

Postterm infants have higher birth weights than term infants, with a higher incidence of fetal macrosomia (defined as an estimated fetal weight ≥4500 g): 2.5% to 10% versus 0.8% to 1%.[14,15] Complications associated with fetal macrosomia include prolonged labor, cephalopelvic disproportion, and shoulder dystocia with resultant risks of orthopedic or neurologic injury.

Approximately 20% of postterm fetuses have "fetal dysmaturity (postmaturity) syndrome," which describes infants with characteristics of chronic intrauterine growth restriction from uteroplacental insufficiency.[16-18] These pregnancies are at increased risk of umbilical cord compression from oligohydramnios, nonreassuring fetal antepartum or intrapartum assessment, meconium aspiration, short-term neonatal complications (hypoglycemia, seizures, respiratory insufficiency), and probably long-term neurologic sequelae. Postterm fetuses are at increased risk of death within the first year of life,[19-21] although the reason for this is not clear.

Maternal Risks

Maternal risks of prolonged pregnancy include an increase in labor dystocia (9%-12% vs. 2%-7% at term), an increase in severe perineal injury that appears to be related to fetal macrosomia (3.3% vs. 2.6% at term), and a doubling

Table 14-1

Fetal Risks of Postterm Pregnancy

Morbidity	Incidence*	
	Postterm (%)	Term (%)
Stillbirth and early neonatal death	0.4-0.7	0.2-0.3
Uteroplacental insufficiency	20-40	??
Asphyxia and fetal distress	8	5
Macrosomia	2.5-10	0.8-1
Fetal postmaturity syndrome	20	33
Meconium aspiration	37.7	12.5

*Data from Alexander JM, McIntire DD, Leveno KJ: Forty weeks and beyond: pregnancy outcomes by week of gestation. *Obstet Gynecol* 96:291, 2000; Treger M et al: Post-term pregnancy: should induction of labor be considered before 42 weeks? *J Matern Fetal Neonatal Med* 11:50, 2002; Olesen AW, Westergaard JG, Olsen J: Perinatal and maternal complications related to postterm delivery: a national register-based study, 1978-1993. *Am J Obstet Gynecol* 189:222, 2003.

Maternal Risks of
Postterm Pregnancy

Table 14-2

Morbidity	Incidence*	
	Postterm (%)	Term (%)
Labor dystocia	9.5-11	2-7
Severe perineal injury	3.3	2.6
Increased rate of cesarean delivery	25	15
Postpartum hemorrhage	10	8
Labor dysfunction	11.9	9.4

*Data from Alexander JM, McIntire DD, Leveno KJ: Forty weeks and beyond: pregnancy outcomes by week of gestation. *Obstet Gynecol* 96:291, 2000; Treger M et al: Post-term pregnancy: should induction of labor be considered before 42 weeks? *J Matern Fetal Neonatal Med* 11:50, 2002; Olesen AW, Westergaard JG, Olsen J: Perinatal and maternal complications related to postterm delivery: a national register-based study, 1978-1993. *Am J Obstet Gynecol* 189:222, 2003.

in the rate of cesarean delivery.[22-24] Cesarean delivery is associated with higher risks of complications such as endometritis, hemorrhage, and thromboembolic disease.

MANAGEMENT

Management of postterm pregnancy includes such issues as the following:

* Accurate gestational age assessment in early pregnancy
* Antenatal fetal surveillance

Accurate Gestational Age Assessment

The diagnosis of prolonged pregnancy requires accurate determination of the gestational age. The EDD is best determined early in a pregnancy. Although the patient's recollection of the first day of her LMP is the best clinical determinant of the EDD, only 70% of women can recall the date of their LMP. The introduction of ultrasound has helped enormously in the confirmation of gestational age because, even in patients who do recall their LMP, the EDD may still be inaccurate by several days.[25] Several studies suggest that routine early ultrasound examination would lower the number of pregnancies judged to be postterm by around 50% to 70% and therefore minimize unnecessary intervention.[26-29] However, this practice has not been recommended as a standard of prenatal care in the United States.

The American College of Obstetricians and Gynecologists (ACOG)[28] no longer describes any specific upper limit of gestational age for expectantly managed pregnancies.[3] Many physicians now induce labor routinely between weeks 41 and 42 weeks and do not allow pregnancy to extend beyond 43 weeks of gestation.

Antenatal Fetal Surveillance

Fetal surveillance may be used while awaiting the onset of labor or spontaneous ripening of the cervix before elective induction. The pitfalls of the use of antenatal testing in this setting are twofold. On the one hand, false-positive tests commonly lead to interventions that are unnecessary and potentially hazardous to the gravida. On the other hand, no program of fetal testing has been shown to date to eliminate the risk of stillbirth. The optimal gestational age for the initiation of fetal testing has not been established. ACOG recommends that antepartum fetal surveillance be initiated by 47 weeks of gestation, without a specific recommendation regarding the type of test or frequency.[3] Options for evaluating fetal well-being include maternal assessment of fetal movement ("kick-counts"), nonstress testing with or without amniotic fluid volume assessment, the biophysical profile (BPP) or modified BPP, the oxytocin challenge test, or a combination of these modalities.[3,30] Most authorities would advise twice-weekly testing with some evaluation of amniotic fluid volume at least weekly.[31,32] Recently, Magann et al.,[33] in a prospective randomized trial of postterm pregnancies, showed that assessment of amniotic fluid by measuring the single deepest pocket is a better test for clinical evaluation of amniotic fluid volume than the amniotic fluid index (AFI). AFI identified twice as many pregnancies as being "at risk" as compared with the single deepest pocket technique, and yet the percentage of pregnancies developing fetal intolerance in labor was the same in both groups.

TIMING OF ELECTIVE DELIVERY

Delivery is typically recommended when the risks to the fetus by continuing the pregnancy are greater than those faced by the neonate after birth. High-risk patients (summarized in Box 14-1) should not be allowed to progress into the postterm period because, in these pregnancies, the balance appears to shift in favor of delivery at around 38 to 39 weeks of gestation. Management of low-risk pregnancies is more controversial. Because delivery cannot always be brought about readily, maternal risks and considerations are more apt to confound this decision. Factors that need to be considered include results of antepartum fetal assessment, favorability of the cervix (Bishop score), gestational age, and maternal preference. Any decision should only be made after a detailed discussion of the risks, benefits, and options of expectant management with antepartum monitoring versus labor induction.

Delivery should be effected immediately if there is evidence of oligohydramnios or fetal compromise on antepartum fetal testing.[34,35] Oligohydramnios may result from uteroplacental insufficiency or decreased fetal urinary output[36] and may predispose to umbilical cord compression, thereby leading to intermittent fetal hypoxemia, meconium passage, or meconium aspiration. Adverse pregnancy outcome (nonreassuring fetal heart rate tracing, neonatal intensive care unit [NICU] admission, low Apgar) is more common when oligohydramnios is present.[36-39] Frequent assessment appears important because amniotic fluid can become drastically reduced within 24 to 48 hours.[40]

Favorable Cervix

Labor is generally induced in postterm pregnancies in which the cervix is favorable regardless of parity. In 1964, E.H. Bishop described a standardized method of identifying patients whose cervix were considered favorable for induction.[41] Interestingly, the original intent of his scoring system was to

---

Box 14-1 High-Risk Pregnancies

Maternal Factors
- Antiphospholipid syndrome
- Hemoglobinopathies (e.g., sickle cell disease, thalassemia)
- Cyanotic heart disease
- Chronic renal disease
- Chronic pulmonary disease
- Thromboembolic disease
- Diabetes (including both pregestational and gestational diabetes)
- Hypertension

Uteroplacental Factors
- Premature rupture of membranes
- Oligohydramnios and polyhydramnios
- Placenta abruption
- Placenta previa and vasa previa
- Prior "classical" hystrotomy

Fetal Factors
- Previous unexplained fetal demise
- Moderate to severe isoimmunization
- Intrauterine growth restriction
- Decreased fetal movements
- Multiple gestation (especially monozygous twins or dizygous twins with growth discordance)
- Nonreassuring fetal testing
- Intraamniotic infections
- Fetal structural anomaly

characterize the cervical condition of multiparous patients before induction of labor to prevent iatrogenic prematurity. The Bishop score was modified by Friedman et al.[42] in 1966, and five characteristics of the cervix were described that correlated with the success of labor induction. These five characteristics are cervical dilatation, effacement, consistency, position, and station (Table 14-3). Subsequent studies have shown that an increase in Bishop score is associated with a shortening in all phases of labor, and a reduction in the risk of failed induction and subsequent cesarean delivery. In general, the single most important factor in predicting the success of induction is cervical dilatation. In a nulliparous patient, a "closed" cervix is the worst prognostic sign, irrespective of all other factors.[43]

Table 14-3

Bishop Score

Parameters	Score			
	0	1	2	3
Dilatation (cm)	Closed	1-2	3-4	≥5
Effacement (%)	0-30	40-50	60-70	≥80
Station	−3	−2	−1 or 0	+1 or +2
Consistency	Firm	Medium	Soft	
Cervical position	Posterior	Mid-position	Anterior	

Unfavorable Cervix

Both expectant management and labor induction are associated with low complication rates in low-risk postterm gravida. However, there appears to be a small advantage to labor induction at 41 weeks of gestation, regardless of parity or method of induction. The introduction of preinduction cervical maturation has resulted in fewer failed and serial inductions, lower fetal and maternal morbidity, a shorter hospital stay, lower medical cost, and possibly a lower rate of cesarean delivery in the general obstetric population.[3,44-46] These agents are summarized in Box 14-2. In addition, findings of several meta-analyses suggest that routine induction at 41 weeks' gestation has fetal benefit without incurring additional maternal risks resulting from a higher rate of cesarean delivery.[21,47-49] However, this conclusion has not been universally accepted.[23,47]

Intrapartum Management

Most authors recommend continuous electronic fetal monitoring in labor for these pregnancies because of a higher risk of intrapartum fetal heart rate abnormalities and passage of meconium.[6]

Risks of Induction of Labor

Two potential complications of labor induction are iatrogenic prematurity and failed induction leading to cesarean delivery. Of these, iatrogenic prematurity can be minimized by using strict criteria for gestational age and estimation of fetal lung maturity, if indicated. Failed induction can also be minimized by using more effective cervical ripening agents. It is believed that preinduction cervical maturation results in fewer failed inductions, fewer serial inductions, lower fetal and maternal morbidity rates, shorter hospital stays, lower medical costs, and possibly lower rates of cesarean deliveries.[21]

PROGNOSIS

At 1 and 2 years of age, the general intelligence quotient, physical milestones, and frequency of intercurrent illnesses is the same for normal term infants and those from prolonged pregnancies.[17]

Box 14-2   Methods of Cervical Ripening—Pharmacologic Methods

- Hormonal techniques
  1. Prostaglandin E_2 (PGE_2)
  2. Prostaglandin E_1 (PGE_1)
  3. Oxytocin
  4. Estrogen
- Steroid receptor antagonists
  1. RU-486 (Mifepristone)
  2. ZK-98299 (Onapristone)
- Hygroscopic dilators
  1. Laminaria
  2. Lamicel
  3. Dilapan
- Balloon catheter
- Amniotomy
- Membrane stripping
- Mechanical dilators

CONCLUSION

The risks of routine induction in the era of cervical ripening agents are lower than previously reported. The risk of fetal death is also low, but not zero, in expectantly managed, carefully monitored pregnancies. For these reasons, most clinicians favor a policy of routine induction at 41 weeks of gestation.

KEY POINTS

- Postterm (prolonged) pregnancy refers to a pregnancy that has extended to or beyond 42 weeks (294 days) of gestation.
- Accurate gestational age dating is critical to the diagnosis of postterm pregnancy.
- Risk factors include primiparity, a prior postterm pregnancy, placental sulfatase deficiency, and fetal anencephaly (in the absence of polyhydramnios); most cases have no known cause.
- Postterm pregnancy is associated with significant risks to the fetus, including stillbirth, meconium aspiration syndrome, intrapartum asphyxia (low 5-minute Apgar score and fetal acidosis), fetal macrosomia (leading to shoulder dystocia with resultant risks of orthopedic or neurologic injury), and neonatal encephalopathy.
- Postterm pregnancy is also associated with significant risks to the mother, including increased risks of labor dystocia and cesarean delivery, severe perineal injury, and postpartum hemorrhage.
- Routine induction of labor at 41 weeks' gestation is a safe, effective, and cost-effective way of preventing the fetal and maternal complications associated with postterm pregnancy.

211

REFERENCES

1. Alfirevic Z et al: Management of post-term pregnancy: to induce or not? Management of preterm labour. Safety of hormone treatment unproved. *Br J Hosp Med* 52:218, 1994.
2. Gynecologists ACoOa: Diagnosis and management of postterm pregnancy. 1989, American College of Obstetricians and Gynecologists; Technical bulletin No.130.
3. ACOG practice patterns. Management of postterm pregnancy. Number 6, October 1997. American College of Obstetricians and Gynecologists. *Int J Gynaecol Obstet* 60:86, 1998.
4. Bergsjo P: Post-term pregnancy. In *Progress in Obstetrics and Gynecology*, Vol 5. Edinburgh, 1985, Churchill Livingstone.
5. Divon MY et al: Male gender predisposes to prolongation of pregnancy. *Am J Obstet Gynecol* 187:1081, 2002.
6. Knox GE, Huddleston JF, Flowers CE Jr: Management of prolonged pregnancy: results of a prospective randomized trial. *Am J Obstet Gynecol* 134:376, 1979.
7. Yeh SY, Read JA: Management of post-term pregnancy in a large obstetric population. *Obstet Gynecol* 60:282, 1982.
8. Lagrew DC, Freeman RK: Management of postdate pregnancy. *Am J Obstet Gynecol* 154:8, 1986.
9. Feldman GB: Prospective risk of stillbirth. *Obstet Gynecol* 79:547, 1992.
10. Olesen AW, Westergaard JG, Olsen J: Perinatal and maternal complications related to postterm delivery: a national register-based study, 1978-1993. *Am J Obstet Gynecol* 189:222, 2003.
11. Bakketeig L, Bergsjo P: Effective care in pregnancy and childbirth. In Enkin M, Keirse M, Chalmers I, editors: *Post-term Pregnancy: Magnitude of the Problem.* Oxford, 1989, Oxford University Press.

12. Hannah M: Postterm pregnancy: should all women have labour induced? A review of the literature. *Fetal Matern Med Rev* 5(3), 1993.

13. Kitlinski ML et al: Gestational age-dependent reference values for pH in umbilical cord arterial blood at term. *Obstet Gynecol* 102:338, 2003.

14. Spellacy WN et al: Macrosomia—maternal characteristics and infant complications. *Obstet Gynecol* 66:158, 1985.

15. Rosen MG, Dickinson JC: Management of postterm pregnancy. *N Engl J Med* 326:1628, 1992.

16. Vorherr H: Placental insufficiency in relation to postterm pregnancy and fetal postmaturity. Evaluation of fetoplacental function; management of the postterm gravida. *Am J Obstet Gynecol* 123:67, 1975.

17. Shime J et al: The influence of prolonged pregnancy on infant development at one and two years of age: a prospective controlled study. *Am J Obstet Gynecol* 154:341, 1986.

18. Mannino F: Neonatal complications of postterm gestation. *J Reprod Med* 33:271, 1988.

19. Hilder L, Costeloe K, Thilaganathan B: Prolonged pregnancy: evaluating gestation-specific risks of fetal and infant mortality. *Br J Obstet Gynaecol* 105:169, 1998.

20. Cotzias CS, Paterson-Brown S, Fisk NM: Prospective risk of unexplained stillbirth in singleton pregnancies at term: population-based analysis. *BMJ* 319:287, 1999.

21. Rand L et al: Post-term induction of labor revisited. *Obstet Gynecol* 96(5 Pt 1):779, 2000.

22. Treger M et al: Post-term pregnancy: should induction of labor be considered before 42 weeks? *J Matern Fetal Neonatal Med* 11:50, 2002.

23. Alexander JM, McIntire DD, Leveno KJ: Forty weeks and beyond: pregnancy outcomes by week of gestation. *Obstet Gynecol* 96:291, 2000.

24. Alexander JM, DD MC, Leveno KJ: Prolonged pregnancy: induction of labor and cesarean births. *Obstet Gynecol* 97:911, 2001.

25. Duff C, Sinclair M: Exploring the risks associated with induction of labour: a retrospective study using the NIMATS database. Northern Ireland Maternity System. *J Adv Nurs* 31:410, 2000.

26. Neilson JP: Ultrasound for fetal assessment in early pregnancy. *Cochrane Database Syst Rev* (2): CD000182, 2000.

27. Ultrasonography in pregnancy. ACOG Technical Bulletin Number 187. December 1993. *Int J Gynaecol Obstet* 44:173, 1994.

28. ACOG: ACOG Practice Bulletin. Assessment of risk factors for preterm birth. Clinical management guidelines for obstetrician-gynecologists. Number 31, October 2001. (Replaces Technical Bulletin number 206, June 1995. Committee Opinion number 172, May 1996. Committee Opinion number 187, September 1997. Committee Opinion number 198, February 1998. and Committee Opinion number 251, January 2001). *Obstet Gynecol* 98:709, 2001.

29. Blondel B et al: Algorithms for combining menstrual and ultrasound estimates of gestational age: consequences for rates of preterm and postterm birth. *BJOG* 109:718, 2002.

30. Crowley P: Interventions for preventing or improving the outcome of delivery at or beyond term. *Cochrane Database Syst Rev* (2):CD000170, 2000.

31. ACOG practice bulletin. Antepartum fetal surveillance. Number 9, October 1999 (replaces Technical Bulletin Number 188, January 1994). Clinical management guidelines for obstetrician-gynecologists. *Int J Gynaecol Obstet* 68:175, 2000.

32. Norwitz ER RJ: *Management of Postterm Pregnancy.* ACOG practice bulletin 2004. 55.

33. Magann EF et al: Biophysical profile with amniotic fluid volume assessments. *Obstet Gynecol* 104:5, 2004.

34. Phelan JP et al: The role of ultrasound assessment of amniotic fluid volume in the management of the postdate pregnancy. *Am J Obstet Gynecol* 151:304, 1985.

35. Crowley P, O'Herlihy C, Boylan P: The value of ultrasound measurement of amniotic fluid volume in the management of prolonged pregnancies. *Br J Obstet Gynaecol* 91:444, 1984.

36. Oz AU et al: Renal artery Doppler investigation of the etiology of oligohydramnios in postterm pregnancy. *Obstet Gynecol* 100:715, 2002.

37. Tongsong T, Srisomboon J: Amniotic fluid volume as a predictor of fetal distress in postterm pregnancy. *Int J Gynaecol Obstet* 40:213, 1993.

38. Bochner CJ et al: Antepartum predictors of fetal distress in postterm pregnancy. *Am J Obstet Gynecol* 157:353, 1987.

39. Morris JM et al: The usefulness of ultrasound assessment of amniotic fluid in predicting adverse outcome in prolonged pregnancy: a prospective blinded observational study. *BJOG* 110:989, 2003.

40. Clement D, Schifrin BS, Kates RB: Acute oligohydramnios in postdate pregnancy. *Am J Obstet Gynecol* 157(4 Pt 1):884, 1987.

41. Bishop EH: Pelvic scoring for elective induction. *Obstet Gynecol* 24:266, 1964.

42. Friedman EA et al: Relation of prelabor evaluation to inducibility and the course of labor. *Obstet Gynecol* 28:495, 1966.

43. Wing DA: Elective induction of labor in the USA. *Curr Opin Obstet Gynecol* 12:457, 2000.

44. Keirse M, Chalmers. I: Methods for inducing labour. In Chalmers I EM, Keirse MJNC, editors: *Effective Care in Pregnancy and Childbirth.* Oxford, 1989, Oxford University Press.

45. Poma PA: Cervical ripening. A review and recommendations for clinical practice. *J Reprod Med* 44:657, 1999.

46. Xenakis EM et al: Induction of labor in the nineties: conquering the unfavorable cervix. *Obstet Gynecol* 90:235, 1997.

47. Menticoglou SM, Hall PF: Routine induction of labour at 41 weeks gestation: nonsensus consensus. *BJOG* 109:485, 2002.

48. Crowley P: Interventions for preventing or improving the outcome of delivery at or beyond term. In 1 I, editor: *The Cochrane Review,* Vol 1999. Oxford, 1999, The Cochrane Library.

49. Sanchez-Ramos L et al: Labor induction versus expectant management for postterm pregnancies: a systematic review with meta-analysis. *Obstet Gynecol* 101:1312, 2003.

15

MANAGEMENT OF MULTIPLE PREGNANCIES

Despina Mavridou, Errol R. Norwitz, Julian N. Robinson, and Hee Joong Lee

Approximately 1% to 3% of all pregnancies in the United States are multiple gestations. The vast majority (97%-98%) are twin pregnancies. Multiple pregnancies constitute significant risk to both mother and fetuses. Antepartum complications—including preterm labor, preterm premature rupture of the membranes (PPROM), intrauterine growth restriction (IUGR), intrauterine fetal demise (IUFD), gestational diabetes, and preeclampsia—develop in more than 80% of multiple pregnancies as compared with approximately 25% of singleton gestations. Multiple pregnancies also account for 9% to 12% of all perinatal deaths. This chapter reviews in detail the diagnosis, complications, and management of multiple pregnancies.

EPIDEMIOLOGY

Spontaneous twin pregnancies occur at a rate of approximately 1 in 80 gestations and spontaneous triplets at a rate of around 1 in 8000 gestations. However, multiple pregnancies are seen far more often and are becoming increasingly common in developed countries primarily because of the expanded use of fertility treatments and older maternal age at childbirth. In 2002, twin births accounted for 3.1% of all live births in the United States. The increased incidence in multifetal gestations is true also of higher-order multiple pregnancies (triplets and up), which now constitute 0.1% to 0.3% of all births. In the United States, multiple pregnancy rates have increased disproportionately among ethnic groups that commonly use artificial reproductive technologies (Caucasians) as compared with ethnic groups that use such interventions less commonly (African-American and Native American populations). Recent data suggest that 30% to 50% of twins and 75% of triplets occur after infertility treatment.

PHYSIOLOGY

Maternal Physiologic Adaptations to Multiple Pregnancy

Physiologic adaptations occur in the mother in response to the demands of pregnancy. These demands include support of the fetus (volume support, nutritional and oxygen supply, and clearance of fetal waste), protection of the fetus (from starvation, drugs, toxins), preparation of the uterus for labor, and protection of the mother from potential cardiovascular injury at delivery. All maternal systems are required to adapt; however, the quality, degree, and timing of the adaptation varies from one individual to another and from one organ system to another. Multiple gestations significantly affect the ability of the mother to adapt to the demands of pregnancy. These include the following:

- **Cardiovascular system:** Twin pregnancy is characterized by a more hyperdynamic circulation than singleton pregnancy. Compared with singleton pregnancy, twin pregnancies are associated with a 30% increase in blood volume (+1570 ml vs. +1960 ml, respectively) and a 20% increase in maternal cardiac output because of a greater increase in stroke volume (+15%) and heart rate (+3.5%).
- **Renal physiology:** Glomerular filtration rate increases by 50% by the end of the first trimester, resulting in a decrease in circulating blood urea nitrogen and creatinine levels. These functional changes are not significantly different between singleton and twin pregnancies, and levels return to normal after delivery. Rarely, the excessive enlarged uterus can lead to an obstructive uropathy.
- **Respiratory system:** Ventilatory drive (but not respiratory rate) is increased during pregnancy because of a direct stimulatory effect of progesterone. This leads to a state of hyperventilation as evidenced by an increase in minute ventilation, alveolar ventilation, and tidal volume. The net result is a reduction in maternal $PaCO_2$ from a nonpregnant level of 35 to 45 mmHg to 27 to 34 mmHg in pregnancy and an increase in bicarbonate excretion by the kidneys. Pregnancy therefore represents a state of compensated respiratory alkalosis. In twin pregnancies, exaggerated abdominal distention and loss of abdominal muscle tone leads to greater use of the accessory muscles during respiration, which may contribute to the increased complaints of dyspnea in such women but does not translate into any significant difference in respiratory physiology between singleton and multiple pregnancies.
- **Hematologic system:** The additional increase in circulating blood volume in multiple pregnancies results in an exaggerated dilutional (physiologic) anemia and thrombocytopenia.

Fetal Physiology

Birth outcomes for multiple pregnancies are determined by both zygosity and chorionicity. *Zygosity* refers to the genetic composition of the pregnancy. Twins are either dizygotic (derived from two separate embryos and therefore nonidentical in both genotype and phenotype [DZ]) or monozygotic (derived from a single embryo and thus identical [MZ]). Of all twins,

70% to 80% are DZ. MZ twinning is a random event occurring in approximately 1 in every 300 pregnancies. As a result, the incidence of MZ twins worldwide is approximately 4 to 5 per 1000 live births and is independent of race, maternal age, parity, and family history. The only factor that increases the incidence of MZ twinning is in vitro fertilization (IVF), likely because of the use of artificial embryo culture media and the use of assisted hatching techniques. The incidence of DZ twins, on the other hand, ranges widely around the world from 1.3 to 49 per 1000 live births. The factors influencing the incidence of DZ twinning are summarized in Table 15-1. The distinction between MZ and DZ twins can typically be made on examination of the placentae and fetal membranes after delivery; in some cases, however, it may be necessary to use blood type or even DNA testing to make the diagnosis.

Chorionicity refers to the number and arrangements of the fetal membranes (amnion and chorion) and is determined by zygosity and, in the case of MZ twins, by the timing of embryo division. In DZ twins, each fetus has its own placenta and fetal membranes. Placentation is therefore always dichorionic/diamniotic (Figure 15-1). MZ twins result from a single conceptus that divides into two, and placentation depends on the timing of that division. Division before day 3 postconception results in dichorionic/diamniotic placentation (30% of MZ twins), division between days 4 and 8 postconception results in monochorionic/diamniotic placentation (67%), division between days 9 and 12 postconception results in monochorionic/monoamniotic placentation (<3% with an overall incidence of 1 in 10,000 pregnancies), and division at

Risk Factors for Dizygous Multiple Pregnancies

Table 15-1

Risk Factor	Association
Assisted reproductive technologies	Ovulation induction with or without in vitro fertilization (IVF) increases the risk of DZ pregnancies
Ethnicity	Increased in African-American populations (1 in 70 pregnancies); lower in Caucasian (1 in 100 pregnancies) and Asian populations (1 in 155 pregnancies)
Maternal age and parity	Incidence of multiple pregnancies increases with increasing maternal age and parity
Family history of multiple pregnancy	Increased incidence of multiple pregnancies in women with a family history of DZ twins
Endogenous levels of gonadotropins	Serum levels of FSH/LH are higher in women with twins
Maternal weight and height	Increased incidence of multiple pregnancies with increasing BMI and maternal height
Seasonal variation	Increased delivery of twins in late summer (November to December) in Northern Hemisphere; translates into increased twin conception in late winter
Coital frequency	Possible increased incidence of twins with increased coital frequency

BMI, Body mass index; *DZ*, dizygous; *FSH*, follicle-stimulating hormone; *LH*, luteinizing hormone.

Figure 15-1

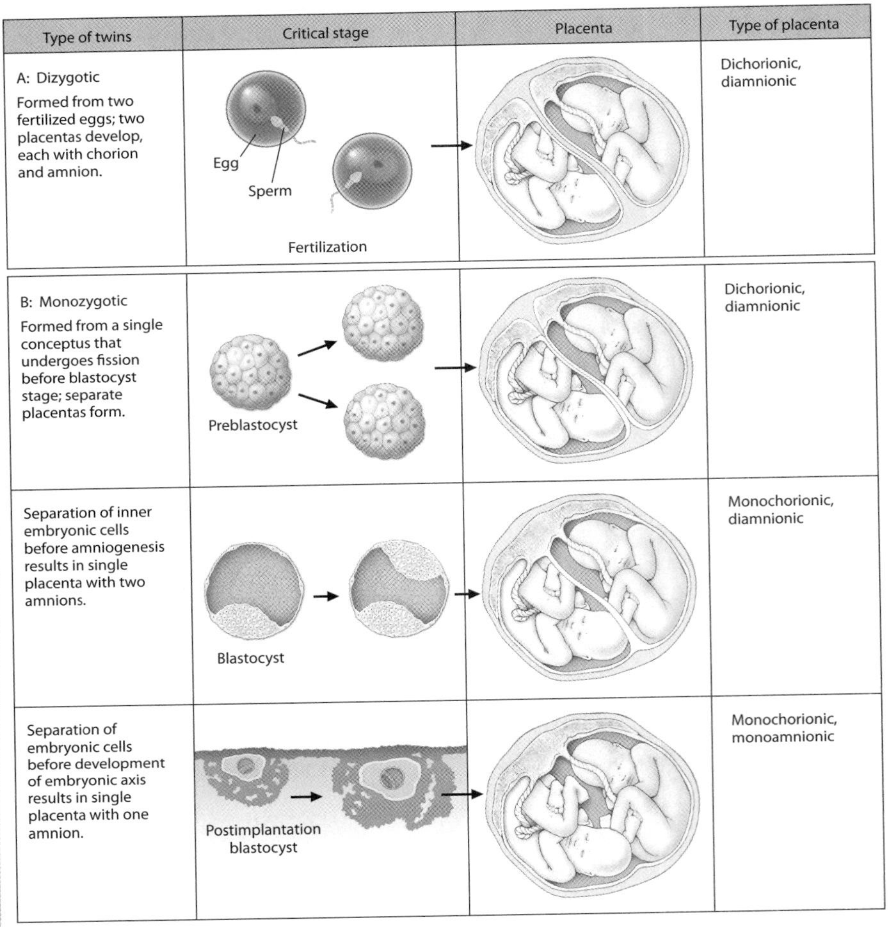

Chorionicity and zygosity in multiple pregnancies. **A,** Dizygotic twins form from separately fertilized eggs (pink and blue) resulting in two separate placentae, a chorion and an amnion. **B,** Monozygotic twins form from a single conceptus (pink) that divides into two. Division before the blastocyst stage (<3 days postconception) results in two separate placentae (dichorionic/diamniotic placentation). Division of the blastocyst before amniogenesis (days 4-8 postconception) results in a single placenta and two amnions (monochorionic/diamniotic placentation). Division after formation of the amnion but before development of the primitive streak (days 9-12 postconception) results in a single placenta with one amnion (monochorionic/monoamniotic placentation). (From Redline RW: Non-identical twins with a single placenta—disproving dogma in perinatal pathology. *N Engl J Med* 349:111-4, 2003. Copyright © 2003 Massachusetts Medical Society. All rights reserved.)

Type of twins	Critical stage	Placenta	Type of placenta
A: Dizygotic — Formed from two fertilized eggs; two placentas develop, each with chorion and amnion.	Egg / Sperm — Fertilization		Dichorionic, diamnionic
B: Monozygotic — Formed from a single conceptus that undergoes fission before blastocyst stage; separate placentas form.	Preblastocyst		Dichorionic, diamnionic
Separation of inner embryonic cells before amniogenesis results in single placenta with two amnions.	Blastocyst		Monochorionic, diamnionic
Separation of embryonic cells before development of embryonic axis results in single placenta with one amnion.	Postimplantation blastocyst		Monochorionic, monoamnionic

or after 13 days postconception results in conjoined twins (rare, with an overall incidence of 1 in 50,000 births). In general, monochorionic twins have a worse prognosis than their dichorionic counterparts. For this reason, it is important to determine the chorionicity of each multiple pregnancy as early as possible. This can be determined by ultrasound using several techniques depending on the gestational age (Figure 15-2).

COMPLICATIONS

Multiple gestations are associated with higher rates of almost every pregnancy-related complication, with the exceptions of postterm pregnancy and fetal macrosomia (Tables 15-2 and 15-3). Antepartum complications develop in more than 80% of multiple pregnancies as compared with approximately 25%

Ultrasound determination of chorionicity. Chorionicity is best determined by ultrasound examination before delivery. The presence on ultrasound of a male and female fetus, two separate placentae, and/or a thick dividing membrane (>2 mm) is suggestive of dichorionic/diamnionic placentation. In the first trimester, the presence of a sonographic "twin-peak" sign (a triangular projection of placental tissue into the intertwin membrane) is suggestive of dichorionic/diamniotic placentation. Monochorionic/diamniotic pregnancies, on the other hand, are more likely to have a single placenta and a thin dividing membrane on ultrasound, whereas monochorionic/monoamniotic pregnancies have no dividing membrane and may have evidence of cord entanglement.

Complications of Multiple Pregnancies

Figure 15-2

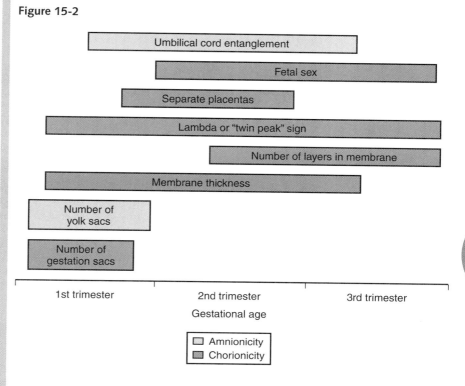

Table 15-2

Maternal Complications	Uteroplacental Complications	Fetal Complications
Spontaneous abortion	Placenta previa	Fetal growth discordance
Anemia	Placental abruption	Intrauterine growth restriction
Hyperemesis gravidarum	Preterm premature rupture of membranes	
Gestational diabetes		Intrauterine fetal demise of one or both twins
Preterm labor and birth	Cord entanglement	
Pregnancy-induced hypertension/preeclampsia	Postpartum hemorrhage	Congenital anomalies
		Malpresentation
Acute fatty liver of pregnancy		Twin-to-twin transfusion syndrome
Cesarean delivery		Twin reversed arterial perfusion (TRAP) syndrome

Mortality and
Morbidity in
Multiple Pregnancy

Table 15-3

Characteristics	Singletons	Twins	Triplets	Quadruplets
Gestational age (weeks)	39.5	35.5	32.2	29.9
Birth weight (grams)	3500 g	2347 g	1687 g	1309 g
IUGR (%)	<10%	14-25%	50%-60%	50%-60%
NICU admission (%)	<2%	25%	75%	100%
Major handicap (%)	0%	0%	20%	50%
Risk of cerebral palsy	—	Fourfold higher than singletons	Seventeenfold higher than singletons	—
Risk of infant mortality (death by 1 year of age)	—	Sevenfold higher than singletons	Twentyfold higher than singletons	—

Mean results are shown. Data from Russell RB et al: The changing epidemiology of multiple births in the United States. *Obstet Gynecol* 101:129, 2003; ACOG Practice Bulletin No. 56. Multiple gestation: Complicated twin, triplet, and higher-order multifetal pregnancy. *Obstet Gynecol* 104:869, 2004.
IUGR, Intrauterine growth restriction; *NICU*, neonatal intensive care unit.

of singleton gestations. Specific complications are discussed in detail in the following.

Maternal Complications

Spontaneous Pregnancy Loss

With early ultrasound, it has become apparent that the incidence of multifetal pregnancies is higher than previously appreciated. Approximately 14% (range, 8%-36%) of twins will reduce spontaneously to a singleton by the end of the first trimester. Many of these events go unrecognized. The phenomenon of the "vanishing twin" can occur before 14 weeks' gestation in a dichorionic/diamniotic twin pregnancy without any consequence for the remaining fetus and without any evidence of multiple gestation on subsequent antenatal evaluation. Fetal death even as late as the end of the first trimester can be followed by complete fetal resorption with no evidence of multiple conception at delivery or on pathologic examination of the placenta and fetal membranes. Death of one MZ twin is more likely to result in loss of the entire pregnancy.

Gestational Diabetes

Gestational diabetes is more common in twin pregnancies, but diagnosis and management are similar to that in singleton pregnancies.

Hypertensive Disorders of Pregnancy

Hypertensive disorders of pregnancy are a common cause of maternal death and are also associated with high perinatal mortality and morbidity rates, primarily because of iatrogenic prematurity. Both preeclampsia (gestational proteinuric hypertension) and pregnancy-induced hypertension are more common in twin compared with singleton pregnancies (approximately 12% vs. 5%-6% for both). The reason for this is not clear but may be related to an increase in placental mass. In addition, early severe preeclampsia and hemolytic anemia, elevated liver enzymes, and low platelet count (HELLP) syndrome are seen more often with multiple gestations. The diagnosis, management, and course of these conditions are not usually affected by fetal number. However, there have been isolated case reports of resolution of early severe preeclampsia upon the death of one twin.

Preterm Premature Rupture of Membranes (PPROM)

PPROM refers to rupture of the fetal membranes before the onset of contractions before 37 weeks' gestation. It is associated with 30% to 40% of preterm births and 10% of all perinatal mortality. PPROM complicates 2% to 4% of singleton and 7% to 10% of twin pregnancies. In multiple pregnancies, PPROM typically occurs in the presenting sac but can occur in the nonpresenting twin, especially after invasive procedures such as amniocentesis.

Latency (period from premature rupture of the fetal membranes [PROM] to delivery) is dependent on several factors: (1) gestational age (at term, 50% of women with PROM go into spontaneous labor within 12 hours and 95% within 72 hours; latency is generally longer if PROM occurs preterm, with 50% of women going into labor within 24-48 hours and 70%-90% within 7 days), (2) severity of oligohydramnios (severe oligohydramnios is associated with shortened latency period), and (3) number of fetuses (twins have a shorter latency period than singletons).

The management of PPROM should be similar in singleton and twin pregnancies. It should include documentation of fetal well-being, exclusion of intrauterine infection, broad-spectrum antibiotic therapy to prolong latency, and antenatal corticosteroids, if indicated. The National Institutes of Health (NIH) consensus statement on the benefit of antenatal corticosteroids for improving perinatal outcome in women at high-risk of preterm birth stated that, although randomized studies of antenatal corticosteroid therapy included only small numbers of multiple pregnancies, it is reasonable to treat women with multiple gestations as one would treat women with threatened premature delivery carrying a singleton. Rarely, the situation may arise when one fetus delivers vaginally, the cervix closes, and the pregnancy continues. Although such delayed interval deliveries are described, they should be regarded as high risk because of the risk of intrauterine infection, placental abruption, and preterm birth.

Neonatal complications are related primarily to prematurity, including respiratory distress syndrome (RDS), intraventricular hemorrhage (IVH), necrotizing enterocolitis (NEC), and sepsis. Overall, PPROM is associated with a fourfold increase in perinatal mortality and a threefold increase in neonatal morbidity. Maternal complications include increased cesarean delivery, intraamniotic infection, and postpartum endometritis. Studies comparing perinatal and neonatal outcomes after PPROM have shown no significant differences in twin versus singleton gestations, although infection is generally lower in the nonpresenting twin.

Preterm Labor and Birth

Preterm labor and birth occurs in 7% to 12% of all deliveries but accounts for more than 85% of all perinatal morbidity and mortality. Preterm labor represents a syndrome rather than a diagnosis because the etiologies are varied. Approximately 20% of preterm births are iatrogenic, meaning that they are indicated preterm births for either maternal or fetal complications. Spontaneous preterm labor and birth is the most common maternal complication of multiple pregnancies. The average length of gestation for singleton, twin, triplet, and quadruplet pregnancies is 40, 37, 33, and 29 weeks, respectively. Despite initial suggestions that pulmonary maturity may be accelerated in multiple pregnancies, subsequent studies have shown that neonatal outcome is similar for singletons, twins, and triplets who are matched for gestational age.

Several tests have been introduced in an attempt to identify women at high risk for preterm birth. Currently, the most reliable screening tests include sonographic measurement of cervical length and/or measurement of fetal fibronectin (fFN) in cervicovaginal secretions. *Cervical shortening on transvaginal ultrasound* can identify multiple pregnancies at risk for preterm birth, but the positive predictive value is low. There is currently no consistent evidence from prospective studies that routine serial sonographic cervical length measurements will reduce the incidence of preterm birth. fFN measured in the cervicovaginal discharge of women at 22-0/7 to 34-6/7 weeks' gestation is a useful marker for preterm birth in both singleton and twin pregnancies. There is no consistent evidence that routine use of fFN testing in asymptomatic multiple pregnancies can improve perinatal outcome.

Obstetric care providers are getting better at identifying women at risk of preterm birth; however, our ability to prevent these adverse outcomes is limited. A number of interventions have been recommended in an attempt to prevent preterm birth.

- **Bed rest**—Although bed rest (reduced activity) and hydration are often recommended to prevent preterm birth, randomized trials of hospitalization or bed rest in twin pregnancies have failed to show a prolongation of gestational age at delivery.
- **Antibiotics**—Although effective in the setting of PPROM, there is no role for broad-spectrum antibiotic therapy to prolong latency in preterm labor with intact membranes.
- **Cervical cerclage**—Prospective studies have shown no benefit to the use of cerclage in twin pregnancies whether they were placed empirically or in women with cervical shortening. There are too little data to comment on the use of cerclage in high-order multiple pregnancies.
- **Tocolytic drugs**—Although tocolytic therapy is often used in women with preterm labor, clinical trials have consistently shown that such agents are effective in prolonging delivery by only 24 to 48 hours. Women with multiple pregnancies are at particularly high risk of developing complications such as pulmonary edema because of their higher blood volume and lower colloid osmotic pressure. As such, tocolytic drugs should be used with caution in women with multiple gestations.

- **Progesterone supplementation**—Progesterone supplementation may prevent preterm birth in some women at high risk by virtue of a prior preterm delivery. Further investigations are needed to evaluate further the efficacy of progesterone supplementation for the prevention of preterm delivery in multiple pregnancies because earlier studies did not demonstrate a clear benefit in this cohort.

Fetal Complications

Intrauterine Fetal Demise

IUFD (stillbirth) is defined in the United States as fetal demise after 20 weeks' gestation but before delivery. The inability to identify fetal heart tones or the absence of uterine growth may suggest the diagnosis. Ultrasound is the gold standard to confirm IUFD by documenting the absence of fetal cardiac activity. Other sonographic findings in later pregnancy may include scalp edema, overlapping sutures, and fetal maceration. The rates of late fetal and infant death in multiple pregnancies are shown in Table 15-4. The twin infant death rate is fivefold higher than that of singletons (37 versus 7 per 1000 live births).

Death of Both Twins

Every effort should be made to avoid cesarean delivery in the setting of IUFD of both twins. As such, expectant management is often recommended. Latency (the period from fetal demise to delivery) varies depending on the underlying cause and gestational age. In general, the earlier the gestational age, the longer the latency period. However, many women find the prospect of carrying one or more dead fetuses distressing and want the pregnancy terminated as soon as possible. Management options include surgical dilatation and evacuation or induction of labor with cervical ripening, if indicated. Around 20% to 25% of women who retain a dead singleton for longer than 3 weeks will develop disseminated intravascular coagulopathy (DIC) because of excessive consumption of clotting factors. Delivery should therefore be effected within this time period. Whether this is true also of pregnancies complicated by the death of both twins is not known.

Death of a Co-Twin

The death of one twin after the first trimester occurs in 2.5% to 6.8% of twin pregnancies and confers an increased risk of major morbidity to the surviving twin, including IUFD, neurologic injury, multiorgan system failure, thrombosis, distal limb necrosis, placental abruption, and premature labor and birth. The prognosis for the surviving twin depends on the cause of death, gestational age, chorionicity, and time interval between death of the

Table 15-4

*Fetal and Infant Death Rates in Twin Gestations**

Outcome	Percent
Two surviving infants	93.7
One infant death, one surviving infant	2.3
Two infant deaths	1.5
One fetal death, one surviving infant	1.1
Two fetal deaths	1.1
One fetal death, one infant death	0.4

Data from Johnson CD, Zhang J: Survival of other fetuses after a fetal death in twin or triplet pregnancies. *Obstet Gynecol* 99:698, 2002.
*Both fetuses alive at 20 weeks of gestation; n = 150,386.

first twin and delivery of the second. DZ twin pregnancies do not share circulation, and the death of one twin may have little impact on the surviving twin. The dead twin may be resorbed completely or become compressed and incorporated into the membranes *(fetus papyraceus)*. DIC in the surviving fetus and/or mother is rare. It is therefore not necessary to monitor for maternal coagulopathy in the setting of a surviving fetus, although a platelet count and fibrinogen level are desirable before delivery. On the other hand, some degree of shared circulation can be demonstrated in almost all MZ twin pregnancies, and death of one fetus in this setting carries an increased risk of death of its co-twin. If it survives, the co-twin has a 20% to 40% risk of developing neurologic injury (multicystic encephalomalacia). Unfortunately, immediate cesarean delivery does not appear to protect the surviving twin from neurologic injury, and ultrasound and fetal testing may not be able to identify fetuses with multicystic encephalopathy. Therefore management of a surviving co-twin depends on chorionicity and gestational age. Fetal surveillance (kick counts, nonstress testing, biophysical profile) should be instituted on a regular basis and delivery considered in the setting of non-reassuring fetal testing or at a favorable gestational age. Vaginal delivery is a reasonable option in this setting, and cesarean delivery can be reserved for usual obstetric indications.

Intrauterine Growth Restriction

Birth weight is a function of both gestational age and rate of fetal growth. IUGR likely represents the clinical end-point of many different fetal, uteroplacental, and maternal conditions. The clinical diagnosis of IUGR is difficult enough in singleton pregnancies, in which physical examination will fail to identify more than 50% of growth-restricted fetuses, but it is essentially impossible in multiple pregnancies. IUGR in multiple pregnancies is therefore an ultrasound diagnosis that requires either an estimated fetal weight (EFW) less than the 3rd percentile (two standard deviations from the mean) for gestational age or an EFW less than the 10th percentile for gestational age, along with evidence of fetal compromise (usually oligohydramnios or abnormal umbilical artery Doppler velocimetry). Fetuses that are less than the 10th percentile without evidence of compromise should be referred to as small for gestational age (SGA) and not IUGR. Accurate gestational age dating is clearly critical for the diagnosis of IUGR.

The growth rate of twins is not significantly different from that of singletons in the first and second trimesters. Although controversial, most studies have described slower fetal growth after 30 to 32 weeks of gestation, which has been attributed to placental crowding and anomalous umbilical cord insertion. Although twins typically weigh less than singletons of the same gestational age, their weights usually remain within the range considered to be normal.

IUGR is a major risk factor for increased perinatal morbidity and mortality in twin pregnancies. Outcomes are generally worse if IUGR is seen in a MZ twin pregnancy or if both twins are IUGR. Neonatal morbidity (meconium aspiration syndrome, hypoglycemia, polycythemia, pulmonary hemorrhage) may be present in up to 50% of IUGR twin neonates. Long-term studies show a twofold increased incidence of cerebral dysfunction (ranging from minor learning disability to cerebral palsy [CP]) in IUGR infants delivered at term and an even higher incidence if the infant was born preterm. Bed rest and low-dose aspirin have not been shown to prevent IUGR. Principles of management include identification of women at risk, serial ultrasound examination of all twin pregnancies (every 2 weeks in MZ twins and every 3-4 weeks in DZ twins), early diagnosis, aggressive attempts to identify the etiology (especially preeclampsia), regular (usually twice-weekly) fetal surveillance once the diagnosis is made, and appropriate timing of delivery. Cesarean delivery can be reserved for the usual obstetric indications; however, up to 50% to 80% of IUGR fetuses will show evidence of nonreassuring fetal testing ("fetal distress") in labor, requiring cesarean delivery.

Fetal Growth Discordance

Like IUGR, fetal growth discordance (typically defined as a $\geq 20\%$ difference in EFW between fetuses of the same pregnancy) is a marker of growth abnormality and is associated with an increased risk of fetal death and neonatal mortality or morbidity. Significant risk factors for discordant growth include monochorionic placentation, preeclampsia, and antepartum bleeding. Fetal growth discordance is evident in 5% to 15% of twins and 30% of triplets and is associated with a sixfold increase in perinatal morbidity and mortality. For these reasons, all multiple pregnancies should be followed with serial ultrasound examinations throughout gestation. Growth discordance is also a strong marker for the presence of a SGA/IUGR neonate. In almost two thirds of discordant twin pairs, the smaller twin has a birth weight less than the 10th percentile. Twin pregnancies with growth discordance require regular fetal surveillance and delivery once a favorable gestational age is reached.

Congenital Anomalies

Because of the increased number of fetuses, congenital anomalies are seen more commonly in multiple pregnancies. MZ twins have an additional two- to threefold higher incidence of congenital anomalies as compared with DZ twins, including neural tube defect (NTD), holoprosencephaly, vertebral, abdominal, thoracic, esophageal, and renal malformations (VATER) syndrome, cloacal malformations, and sacrococcygeal teratoma. Maternal serum alpha-fetoprotein (MS-AFP) screening for NTD has been validated for twin gestations but not for higher-order multiple pregnancies. Conjoined twins and twin reversed arterial perfusion (TRAP) sequence are rare complications of MZ twinning.

Fetal Aneuploidy

In DZ twins, the risk of aneuploidy is independent for each fetus. As such, the chance that one or both fetuses have a karyotypic abnormality is greater than for a singleton pregnancy at the same maternal age. This is not true of MZ twins. The risk of trisomy 21 (Down syndrome) in at least one fetus of a DZ twin gestation is similar at maternal age 32 to that of a 35-year-old woman with a singleton pregnancy. Women with multiple pregnancies should therefore be offered genetic counseling and prenatal diagnosis at a younger age. Serum analyte screening for fetal aneuploidy has been validated for twin pregnancies using separate cutoffs for each of the analytes, but the detection rate is lower than for singletons (e.g., for trisomy 21, detection rate is 43% in DZ twins compared with 70% in singleton pregnancies, with a false-positive rate of 5%). Serum analyte screening for fetal aneuploidy is not reliable in higher-order multiple pregnancies or in pregnancies complicated by a fetal demise or multifetal pregnancy reduction (MFPR). Sonographic measurement of nuchal translucency (NT) thickness at 11 to 14 weeks' gestation is a reliable screening test for fetal aneuploidy in multiple pregnancies, although the specificity of this test is lower in twins because NT measurements also are increased in chromosomally normal MZ twins. In the hands of an experienced operator, the risks of amniocentesis and chorionic villus sampling (CVS) do not appear to be increased in women with multiple pregnancies.

Twin-to-Twin Transfusion Syndrome (TTTS)

DZ twins do not share a circulation and, as such, do not develop TTTS, which is a disorder specific to MZ twins. TTTS is not seen in MZ twins with monochorionic/monoamniotic placentation. TTTS complicates approximately 15% (range, 4%-35%) of MZ twins and is responsible for 15% of perinatal deaths in twins. It is an ultrasound diagnosis with evidence of discrepancy in amniotic fluid volume (polyhydramnios/oligohydramnios sequence) and fetal growth in a MZ twin pregnancy with monochorionic/diamniotic placentation. Some degree of placental vascular anastomoses (artery-to-artery, vein-to-vein, or artery-to-vein) can be demonstrated in almost all MZ twin placentae. TTTS results from an imbalance in blood flow to the twins through one or more of these placental vascular anastomoses, resulting in a donor twin (which is typically smaller and anemic) and a recipient twin (which is larger and plethoric). The net direction of blood flow appears to be determined by the nature rather than the number of vascular anastomoses and the discordance in arterial pressure. Both fetuses are at risk of fetal hydrops, neurologic injury, and IUFD. It can develop as early as 14 to 16 weeks' gestation.

The management of TTTS depends on the severity of the disorder and gestational age. TTS that develops early in gestation (<20 weeks) and is associated with a severe discordance in amniotic fluid volume and fetal growth is associated with poor prognosis and a mortality rate in excess of 90%. Management options include elective pregnancy termination (if <24 weeks), intentional septostomy (which converts a monochorionic/diamniotic to a monochorionic/monoamniotic placentation), serial amnioreduction, and/or in utero laser ablation of the offending placental vascular communications. Because all are invasive techniques, they are associated with significant complications. Management algorithms for such pregnancies are still being developed.

TRAP Sequence

TRAP sequence results from abnormal vascular communications in the umbilical cord of MZ twin pregnancies such that deoxygenated blood returning from twin no. 1 travels first to twin no. 2 before returning to the placenta.

The end result is that blood travels in the reverse direction through the rudimentary heart of twin no. 2 and the low oxygen content leads to abnormal development or lack of development of the upper extremities and head in this "acardiac" recipient twin. This is a rare complication, with an overall incidence of 1 in 35,000 pregnancies or 1% of MZ twin gestations. The acardiac twin is not salvageable. As such, the management of such pregnancies should be focused on the donor twin. In the absence of obstetric intervention, the mortality rate of the donor twin is 50% to 75% primarily because of cardiac failure (hydrops fetalis). Interruption of the vascular anastomoses between the two fetuses can salvage the donor twin. This can be achieved by surgical ligation, endoscopic laser coagulation, or radiofrequency ablation of the recipient umbilical cord. Although effective, the procedure-related pregnancy loss rate of such techniques may be as high as 20%.

Long-Term Neurologic Outcome

Although overall survival in multiple pregnancies has improved, such fetuses are at greater risk for CP than singleton fetuses. CP is characterized by abnormal control of movement or posture that is cerebral in origin, arises early in development, and is permanent and non-progressive. It may be associated with seizures, sensory impairment, and/or cognitive limitations. Twins make up 10% of all children with CP. This is due in part to fetal birth weight because low birth weight (<2500 g [LBW]) and very low birth weight (<1500 g [VLBW]) are strongly associated with CP in both twins and singletons and a disproportionate number of LBW babies are delivered of multiple pregnancies. However, birth weight alone does not account for the high prevalence of CP in twins. Even among normal birth-weight babies, twins are three- to fourfold more likely to develop CP. Risk factors for CP in multiple pregnancies include MZ twinning and death of a co-twin.

MANAGEMENT

Management of multiple pregnancies depends on the number of fetuses, zygosity, chorionicity, the presence of maternal and/or fetal complications, gestational age, and the obstetric and medical history of the pregnant woman. A few selected management issues are reviewed in detail in the following.

Multifetal Pregnancy Reduction

As discussed previously, a proportion of higher-order multiple pregnancies (around 14%) will reduce spontaneously by the end of the first trimester. For those that do not reduce spontaneously, nonselective MFPR to twins has been recommended. Although the techniques are similar, this should be distinguished from *selective reduction*, which refers to targeted termination of a specific fetus in the setting of a multiple pregnancy because of major structural or karyotypic abnormalities. These procedures, which aim to improve the outcome for the remaining fetus(es), represent an alternative to either expectant management or termination of the entire pregnancy. The medical and ethical implications of such procedures remain controversial.

MFPR is typically carried out at 10 to 15 weeks' gestation. Several techniques are described, but the most commonly used method is intrathoracic injection of potassium chloride into the most accessible fetus(es) under ultrasound guidance until asystole is confirmed. Following MFPR, the risk of losing the entire pregnancy before 20 weeks is around 17% (range, 6%-35%). The risk is higher if more than one fetus or if the presenting fetus is terminated. Reduction of a monochorionic twin will lead almost invariably to the death of its co-twin.

The benefits of multifetal reduction in higher-order multiple gestations are numerous, including reduction in prematurity, increased birth weight, and reduced neonatal mortality and morbidity. For every additional fetus present in the first trimester, the duration of pregnancy is reduced by approximately 3.6 weeks. For each fetus reduced (either spontaneously or selectively), gestation is prolonged by approximately 3.0 weeks. Given the high rates of neonatal mortality and morbidity for quadruplet pregnancies and upward, the advantages of MFPR in this population clearly outweigh the risks. Although twin pregnancies are at increased risk of adverse outcome compared with singletons, there is no clear benefit for reduction to a singleton in the absence of a fetal anomaly. As to whether triplet pregnancies benefit from MFPR to twins remains controversial. The majority of studies suggest that the perinatal outcome of triplet pregnancies reduced to twins is better than that of nonreduced triplet pregnancies as evidenced by a lower incidence of premature birth (54% vs. 87%-92%), increase in birth weight (on average, 380-450 g per fetus), reduced stay in the neonatal intensive care (21 vs. 8 days), and reduced perinatal mortality (33 vs. 51-93 per 1000 births) (Table 15-5). Multiple pregnancies reduced to twins are still at increased risk of premature birth compared with spontaneous twin

Table 15-5

Outcome of Triplet Pregnancies With and Without Multifetal Pregnancy Reduction (MFPR) to Twins

Outcome	MFPR to twins (n = 185)	No MFPR (n = 70)	p Value
Birth weight ≤1000 g	5.6%	6.6%	NS
Birth weight ≤1500 g	11.0%	28.4%	<.0001
Birth weight ≤2500 g	68.6%	92.9%	<.0001
Birth weight (mean ± SEM)	2300 ± 467 g	1760 ± 480 g	<.05
Miscarriage before 24 weeks	8.1%	2.9%	NS
Premature birth before 28 weeks	6.0%	10.0%	NS
Premature birth before 32 weeks	11.2%	36.8%	<.0001
Premature birth before 35 weeks	40.6%	83.8%	<.0001
Gestational age at delivery (median)	36 weeks	33 weeks	<.05
Total fetal losses	15.4%	4.8%	<.0001
Chance of taking home at least one live baby per pregnancy	97.2%	87.6%	<.05
Expected severe handicap because of extreme prematurity	0.6%	1.6%	—

Data from Antsaklis A et al: Embryo reduction versus expectant management in triplet pregnancies. *J Matern Fetal Neonatal Med* 16:219, 2004.

pregnancies. Whether reduced pregnancies are at increased risk for IUGR remains unclear.

Timing of Delivery

In most cases, the timing of delivery will be determined by the natural history of the pregnancy. For example, 40% of twin pregnancies are complicated by preterm labor and birth. In the absence of spontaneous preterm labor or medically indicated preterm delivery, delivery of twins should be affected by 40 weeks' gestation. According to the American College of Obstetricians and Gynecologists (ACOG), fetal lung maturity should be confirmed (typically in the nonpresenting twin) if an elective delivery is planned before 39 weeks' gestation.

Although rare (1 in 10,000 of all pregnancies and <1% of MZ twins), monochorionic/mono-amniotic MZ twin pregnancies comprise a specific subset of twins. Because both fetuses are present in a single sac, cord entanglement is seen in almost all cases. The perinatal mortality rate in such pregnancies is approximately 25% primarily because of cord accident. If one fetus does survive a cord accident, it is at high risk of severe neurologic morbidity. The management of such pregnancies is controversial. Although regular fetal monitoring starting in mid-pregnancy is often recommended, there is no evidence that it can reliably predict or prevent cord accident. Delivery of such pregnancies is usually achieved by elective cesarean at 32 to 34 weeks' gestation.

Route of Delivery

The optimal route of delivery depends on chorionicity, gestational age, fetal presentation, the patient's prior obstetric history, and the experience of the obstetric care provider. Elective cesarean delivery is recommended for the usual obstetric indications including, among others, nonvertex presentation (20% of twins), prior cesarean delivery, nonreassuring fetal testing, and placenta previa. Vertex-vertex twins (42% of twins) are ideal candidates for attempted vaginal delivery, although the patient should be aware of the possibility (although rare) of a vaginal delivery for the first twin followed by cesarean for the second twin. In 38% of twin gestations, the fetal presentation is vertex-nonvertex. Options for delivery include elective cesarean, vaginal delivery with external cephalic version of the second twin, or vaginal delivery with breech extraction of the second twin. Breech extraction of the second twin is best performed after 32 weeks with an estimated fetal weight of 1550 to 3500 g by an experienced accoucheur in a woman with a proven pelvis. The risk of perinatal death resulting from intrapartum hypoxia of a second twin delivered at term is approximately 1 in 350.

Intrapartum Management

Epidural analgesia is generally recommended for women attempting vaginal delivery of a multiple pregnancy. This is because of the increased risk of cesarean delivery and the possible need to manipulate the second twin. As for singletons, amniotomy and oxytocin augmentation can be used if labor dystocia is encountered. The heart rate of both fetuses should be monitored throughout labor and delivery. After vaginal delivery of the first twin, the presentation, position, and station of the second twin should be determined immediately by vaginal examination with or without ultrasound. Ultrasound can also be used to assist external cephalic version, breech extraction, or internal podalic version of the second twin. Entrapment of the aftercoming head of the breech can occur and is seen most commonly in preterm deliveries. Release of the head can be achieved by administering intravenous nitroglycerin or inhalational anesthesia to relax the cervix. Alternatively, Dührson's incisions may need to be made in the cervix to release the head.

Initial studies suggested that a prolonged time interval between delivery of the first and second twins was associated with poor outcomes. However, more recent data show no association between delivery interval and pregnancy outcome. So long as the fetal heart rate tracing of the second twin is reassuring, it is not necessary to set a time limit for delivery. Amniotomy and oxytocin augmentation may be required to facilitate delivery of the second twin.

KEY POINTS

- The incidence of multiple pregnancies in developed countries is increasing primarily because of the expanded use of fertility treatments and older maternal age at childbirth.
- Multiple pregnancies constitute significant risk to both mother and fetuses. Antepartum complications (preterm labor, PPROM, IUGR, IUFD, gestational diabetes, preeclampsia) develop in more than 80% of multiple pregnancies, compared with approximately 25% of singleton gestations.
- Both zygosity (the genetic composition of the pregnancy) and chorionicity (the number and arrangements of the fetal membranes) are important determinants of perinatal outcome in multiple pregnancies.
- The death of one twin after the first trimester confers an increased risk of major morbidity to the surviving twin, including IUFD, neurologic injury, multiorgan system failure, thrombosis, distal limb necrosis, placental abruption, and premature labor and birth.
- Because of the increased number of fetuses, congenital anomalies and fetal aneuploidy are seen more commonly in multiple pregnancies.
- Although overall survival in multiple pregnancies has improved, such fetuses are at greater risk for long-term neurologic injury and CP than singleton fetuses.
- Antepartum and intrapartum management of multiple pregnancy should be individualized depending on the number of fetuses, zygosity, chorionicity, the presence of maternal and/or fetal complications, gestational age, and the obstetric and medical history of the pregnant woman.

SUGGESTED READINGS

American College of Obstetricians and Gynecologists: Multiple gestation: complicated twin, triplet, and high-order multifetal pregnancy. Practice Bulletin No. 56. *Obstet Gynecol* 104:869, 2004.

Ballabh P et al: Neonatal outcome of triplet versus twin and singleton pregnancies: a matched case control study. *Eur J Obstet Gynecol Reprod Biol* 107:28, 2003.

Bianco AT et al: The clinical outcome of preterm premature rupture of membranes in twin versus singleton pregnancies. *Am J Perinatol* 13:135, 1996.

Blickstein I, Keith LG: Neonatal mortality rates among growth-discordant twins, classified according to the birth weight of the smaller twin. *Am J Obstet Gynecol* 190:170, 2004.

Donovan EF et al: Outcomes of very low birth weight twins cared for in the National Institute of Child Health and Human Development Neonatal Research Network's intensive care units. *Am J Obstet Gynecol* 179:742, 1998.

Hogle KL et al: Cesarean delivery for twins: a systematic review and meta-analysis. *Am J Obstet Gynecol* 188:220, 2003.

Newman RB et al: Effect of cerclage on obstetrical outcome in twin gestations with a shortened cervical length. *Am J Obstet Gynecol* 186:634, 2002.

Pharoah PO: Risk of cerebral palsy in multiple pregnancies. *Clin Perinatol* 33:301, 2006.

Russell RB et al: The changing epidemiology of multiple births in the United States. *Obstet Gynecol* 101:129, 2003.

Sibai BM, et al: Hypertensive disorders in twin versus singleton gestations. *Am J Obstet Gynecol* 182:938, 2000.

Smith GC, Pell JP, Dobbie R: Birth order, gestational age and risk of delivery-related perinatal death in twins: retrospective cohort study. *BMJ* 325:1004, 2002.

Stephen GM et al: Is zygosity or chorionicity the main determinant of fetal outcome in twin pregnancies? *Am J Obstet Gynecol* 193:757, 2005.

Yaron Y et al: Multifetal pregnancy reductions of triplets to twins. *Am J Obstet Gynecol* 180:1268, 1999.

16

PREECLAMPSIA
Edmund F. Funai

Preeclampsia, manifested by new-onset hypertension and proteinuria during pregnancy, is believed to complicate 5% to 7% of all deliveries in the United States. It is a multisystem disorder with profound derangements of renal, hepatic, cardiovascular, and central nervous systems. In 2002, eclampsia, defined as seizures in a woman with preeclampsia not attributable to other causes, occurred in 1 in 278 pregnancies. Worldwide, preeclampsia results in an estimated 75,000 maternal deaths annually.

PATHOGENESIS

The etiology of preeclampsia remains unclear. Many observations about this disease have been made, but none have yet resulted in a clear elucidation of pathogenesis.

Epidemiologic studies of preeclampsia are intriguing. Nearly two thirds of cases occur in nulliparas. Preeclampsia is more common at extremes of reproductive age, whereas smoking, which is clearly associated with other adverse pregnancy outcomes, has been found to be protective. Maternal, paternal, and fetal contributions to the pathogenesis of preeclampsia have been suggested because preeclampsia is more likely among sisters and if either parent is the result of a pregnancy complicated by preeclampsia, that parent is more likely to produce a pregnancy complicated likewise.

Three associated abnormalities consistently reported include the following:

1. Oxidative stress: Levels of hydroperoxides are higher in maternal blood than in fetal blood during pregnancy. Pregnancy results in a significant increase in free radical production. However, placental production of significant amounts of antioxidant enzymes such as glutathione peroxidase may serve as a barrier for transport of hydroperoxides to the fetus. Several investigators have found levels of lipid peroxides and thromboxane to be significantly higher in preeclamptic placentas than in placentas from normal pregnancies. Unchecked, hydroperoxides can damage the vascular endothelium, a rich source of nitric oxide, with resulting vasospasm.
2. Abnormal trophoblast invasion: A disturbance in embryonic implantation and trophoblast invasion has been demonstrated in preeclampsia, resulting in the failure of trophoblast to develop a vascular endothelial

phenotype, and, as a result, the failure to adequately invade the maternal spiral arteries. This process may be dependent on angiogenic proteins, such as vascular endothelial growth factor (VEGF). Preeclampsia is characterized by shallow trophoblast invasion and narrow spiral arteries, thereby potentially compromising uteroplacental blood flow. This phenomenon may also contribute to oxidative stress.

3. Endothelial cell dysfunction: The vascular endothelium has been increasingly recognized as playing a critical role in the normal regulation of peripheral vasomotor tone. Nitric oxide, endothelin-1, prostaglandins, and other vasodilating and vasoconstricting factors are released by the vascular endothelium in response to a diverse array of hormonal, pharmacologic, chemical, and physical stimuli. Thus abnormalities of vascular endothelial function may be directly relevant to the pathophysiology of hypertension and preeclampsia. There is a growing body of evidence that generalized systemic maternal endothelial cell dysfunction contributes to the pathogenesis of preeclampsia. However, it is not yet known if the endothelial cell dysfunction of preeclampsia persists in the months and years following delivery or whether it is a cause or effect of the disease. One study attempted to address this question by examining brachial artery Doppler waveforms in response to nitroglycerin but was flawed by failing to control for the differences in baseline blood pressure between the groups.

Soluble fms-like tyrosine kinase 1 (sFlt1), an antagonist of VEGF, and placental growth factor (PlGF), increases in the serum of patients with preeclampsia; however, levels rise relatively close (5 weeks) to the development of symptoms and its predictive accuracy appears to be low. Although sFlt1 may not be an optimal serum marker of preeclampsia, it is upregulated in the placentas and serum of patients with preeclampsia and may play a role in its pathogenesis, especially with regard to maternal signs and symptoms. Infusion of anti-VEGF in mice leads to proteinuria and glomerular lesions similar to those found in humans with preeclampsia, and bevacizumab, a neutralizing antibody against VEGF, causes hypertension and proteinuria when infused in patients with metastatic renal cell carcinoma. These findings suggest that preeclampsia may be associated with placental overexpression of sFlt1, with increased circulating levels leading to decreased circulating levels of free VEGF and PlGF, resulting in endothelial dysfunction. However, as is the case with the disease itself, it is unclear whether this phenomenon is a cause or an effect of preeclampsia.

CLINICAL PRESENTATION

Early detection of preeclampsia, usually a disease of late pregnancy, is virtually the sole rationale for the routine antepartum strategy of weekly prenatal visits beginning at 36 weeks. With milder disease, symptoms may not be present, and the diagnosis is made based on blood pressure and proteinuria criteria described subsequently. Many symptoms may be present, and some may mimic other disease processes. Some of the signs and symptoms of preeclampsia may include the following:

- Headache
- Epigastric pain
- Hyperreflexia
- Dizziness
- Tinnitus
- Tachycardia
- Fever
- Diplopia
- Scotoma
- Blurred vision
- Amaurosis
- Nausea/vomiting
- Hematemesis
- Oliguria/anuria
- Hematuria
- Hemoglobinuria

DIAGNOSIS

According to the most recent (2000) National Institutes of Health (NIH) Working Group Report on High Blood Pressure in Pregnancy, hypertensive disorders are classified as follows:

- Chronic hypertension: Present and observable before pregnancy or is diagnosed before the twentieth week of gestation. Hypertension is defined as a blood pressure equal to or greater than 140 mmHg systolic or 90 mmHg diastolic. Hypertension that is diagnosed for the first time during pregnancy and that does not resolve postpartum is also classified as chronic hypertension. Unfortunately, women with chronic hypertension have more than a 20% risk of developing preeclampsia, and even aggressive pharmacotherapy to lower blood pressure does not modify this risk.
- Preeclampsia-eclampsia: Usually occurs after 20 weeks of gestation (or earlier with trophoblastic diseases such as hydatidiform mole or hydrops). It is determined by increased blood pressure (140/90 mmHg or greater) and by proteinuria. Proteinuria is defined as the urinary excretion of 0.3 g protein or greater in a 24-hour specimen, and usually correlates with 1+ or greater by dipstick.
- Preeclampsia superimposed on chronic hypertension: As described in the previous criteria, this diagnosis is made when a patient with chronic hypertension develops new-onset proteinuria and blood pressure exacerbation. This diagnosis is usually made after new-onset proteinuria develops, but when proteinuria has long been present, a definitive diagnosis may be quite challenging. Often, blood pressure elevation or multisystem organ dysfunction (e.g., the HELLP syndrome *H*emolysis, *E*levated *L*iver enzymes, and *L*ow *P*latelets) suggests the diagnosis. Antithrombin

III is noted to be markedly lower in preeclamptic women, but often this test has a slow turnover time and, as a result, is rarely clinically useful.

- Gestational hypertension: The woman who has blood pressure elevation detected for the first time after midpregnancy (>20 weeks) without proteinuria is classified as having gestational hypertension.

Gestational hypertension has two subcategories:

1. Transient hypertension of pregnancy if preeclampsia is not present at the time of delivery and blood pressure returns to normal by 12 weeks postpartum (a retrospective diagnosis)
2. Chronic hypertension if the elevation persists up to 12 weeks postpartum

Note that gestational hypertension is a relatively new and strictly provisional term. At up to 12 weeks postpartum, the diagnosis must be revised to either transient hypertension or chronic hypertension, depending on the maternal blood pressure at the end of the puerperium.

PREDICTION

Because the etiology of preeclampsia remains obscure, efforts to predict its development have been unsuccessful. Previous efforts have focused on blood pressure changes in the supine and sitting position, but early blood pressure changes were ultimately found to be unreliable. Others have examined responses to angiotensin II infusion, changes in renal function, and changes in coagulation, but none of these findings have had clinical use. Sex hormone binding globulin has shown modest promise as an early predictor. The prognostic limitations of sFlt1 and PlGF have been discussed. Thus currently there is no simple, safe, or sensitive test to predict this disease, and no such screening tests are used by obstetricians in the United States outside of research protocols.

PREVENTION

Currently, there are no interventions in widespread clinical use that are efficacious in preventing preeclampsia. Several modalities have been investigated.

Calcium

Calcium supplementation may prevent high blood pressure through a number of mechanisms. The CPEP trial included 4589 healthy nulliparous women who were 13 to 21 weeks' pregnant and were randomized to therapy with either calcium (2000 mg/day) or placebo for the rest of their pregnancy. No benefit of calcium supplementation could be identified. A recent Cochrane Review suggests there may be some benefit in high-risk women who have low dietary calcium intake, but this therapy is not used routinely.

Aspirin

A multicenter trial sponsored by the National Institutes of Health randomly assigned over 3000 healthy nulliparous women to either aspirin (60 mg) or placebo therapy at 13 to 26 weeks of gestation. Aspirin appeared to reduce the incidence of preeclampsia slightly (4.6% vs. 6.3%, relative risk [RR] 0.7, 95% confidence interval [CI] 0.6 to 1). The greatest effect was among the 519 patients with higher initial systolic pressures (more than 120 mmHg) in whom the incidence of preeclampsia was 6% as compared with 12% in the placebo group. There were no differences in birth weight or incidence of growth restriction between groups. A similar study of women at high risk (secondary hypertension, diabetes, multiple gestation, and previous preeclampsia) also found no benefit. Again, a review from the Cochrane Database showed a modest 15% reduction in the risk of preeclampsia associated with the use of antiplatelet agents (32 trials with 29,331 women; RR 0.85, 95% CI [0.78, 0.92]). Because 89 subjects may require treatment to prevent one case of preeclampsia, this modality is also not in widespread use.

Antioxidants

Several previous studies have been performed in which antioxidants were given to women who already had severe preeclampsia, and no benefit was shown. When used prophylactically in high-risk women by starting vitamin C (1000 mg /day) and vitamin E (400 IU/day) supplementation at 16 to 20 weeks' gestation, antioxidant supplementation was associated with a significant reduction in the frequency of preeclampsia (8% vs. 17%). These results were based on a small number of patients and merit confirmation in a larger trial.

TREATMENT

The only curative therapy for preeclampsia is delivery. On removal of the placenta, most signs and symptoms of preeclampsia resolve within several days. To paraphrase the eminent preeclampsia researcher Jane Roberts, delivery is always in the best interest of the mother; however, depending on the gestational age, it is not always in the best interest of the fetus. In about 25% of affected patients, preeclampsia occurs remote from term and is the leading cause of indicated preterm birth in the United States. Fortunately, the use of magnesium sulfate for seizure prophylaxis and modern methods of hypertension management have dramatically decreased acute maternal mortality.

Magnesium sulfate is usually given as a bolus dose of 4 to 6 g intravenously over approximately 20 minutes. Maintenance dosing is usually 2 g/hour. The serum levels of this regimen correlate well with 5 g given intramuscularly (IM) every 4 hours. Magnesium sulfate is superior to phenytoin in preventing seizures, reducing the risk from 1% to 3% to about 0.2%.

A serum creatinine is recommended on all patients before magnesium therapy. If normal for pregnancy (less than 0.9 mg/dl), magnesium serum levels should not be required, but rather a careful neurologic and lung examination every 2 hours should be sufficient. Patellar reflexes usually disappear when serum levels approach 10 mEq/L. When there is evidence of renal impairment, especially with a serum creatinine greater than 1.2 mg/dl, consideration should be given to reducing the maintenance infusion and obtaining serum levels every 4 to 6 hours. In all patients, calcium gluconate (1 g intravenously) should be readily available.

Magnesium sulfate is *not* sufficient therapy to treat severe hypertension. When systolic pressures exceed 160 mmHg or diastolic pressures exceed 110 mmHg, antihypertensive therapy is indicated to prevent maternal stroke. Care must be taken not to lower blood pressure too quickly or too far because fetal bradycardia may result from relative hypotension and reduction of uteroplacental blood flow. Usually, 5 to 10 mg of hydralazine given every 20 minutes, or labetalol 10 to 20 mg every 10 minutes, is used reduce blood pressure to ideally about 140/90 mmHg.

It should also be noted that magnesium sulfate therapy does not prevent progression of disease unrelated to convulsions. Roughly 10% to 15% of women in mild preeclampsia will develop signs of severe preeclampsia (severe hypertension, headache, visual disturbance, epigastric pain, laboratory abnormalities) whether or not they receive magnesium therapy. As such, magnesium is purely a medication useful for seizure prophylaxis.

Treatment Remote from Term

Women who develop preeclampsia remote from term merit careful follow up. Often, the disease may initially present as mild, with creatinine, liver function tests, and platelets being in the normal range. Blood pressure may remain near 140/90 mmHg, and proteinuria, as measured by a 24-hour collection, may be stable and close to 0.3 g/L. If there is no evidence of multisystem organ involvement and no symptoms, and if the fetus is appropriately grown with reassuring testing, outpatient management may be considered. Office visits should take place two to three times weekly with liver function tests, urine collection, complete blood count, and fetal testing performed at least weekly. If less than 34 weeks' gestation, antenatal corticosteroids should be administered. In all cases, consultation with a maternal-fetal medicine specialist is suggested.

More severe, or worsening, disease merits hospitalization. The mother should be informed that delivery is the safest course of action to protect her health, but, depending on the gestational age and fetal status (i.e., growth, biophysical examination), continued observation may benefit the fetus. Potential maternal risks include eclampsia, subcapsular liver hematoma or liver rupture, severe hemorrhage, and renal failure.

Because fetal outcome is generally excellent at 32 to 34 weeks, expectant management of severe or worsening preeclampsia beyond this gestational age is not recommended. It is recommended that the decision to manage such patients expectantly be made in conjunction with a maternal-fetal medicine specialist.

After a careful and detailed discussion of the risks and benefits, if patient and physician choose expectant management, a prudent trial of observation includes the following:

1. Intravenous magnesium sulfate during the period of initial observation, which is usually not necessary for greater than 24 hours. When one is certain that the disease is not worsening, the magnesium may be discontinued. Prolonged magnesium therapy is *not* recommended because of the risks of toxicity and osteoporosis.

236

2. Antenatal corticosteroids.
3. 24-hour urine collection for protein and creatinine clearance, liver function tests, electrolytes, complete blood count, and strict recording of fluid intake and urine output and hourly blood pressures.

After this initial evaluation, blood pressure should be measured every 1 to 2 hours, and all laboratory tests other than the urine collection (which may be done one to two times per week) should be repeated daily. Nonstress testing should take place daily, assessment of amniotic fluid volume should be performed one to two times per week, and fetal growth measured every 2 weeks.

Delivery is recommended if *any* of the following are noted:

1. Hypertension (systolic pressures exceeding 160 mmHg or diastolic pressures exceeding 110 mmHg) not responsive to medical therapy
2. Persistent symptoms such as headache or epigastric pain
3. Eclampsia
4. Pulmonary edema
5. Laboratory abnormalities such as:

    a. Liver function tests greater than two times the upper limit of normal
    b. Platelets less than 100,000
    c. Marked rise in serum creatinine

6. Evidence of fetal compromise (nonreassuring testing, absence of interval growth based on serial ultrasound, oligohydramnios)

SEQUELAE

Until recently, most authorities have believed that preeclampsia, in and of itself, is not associated with health problems later in life. The National High Blood Pressure Education Program's Working Group on High Blood Pressure During Pregnancy has asserted that unusual circumstances, such as recurrent hypertension in pregnancy, preeclampsia in a multiparous woman, or early-onset disease in any pregnancy, may be associated with future health risks.

Current knowledge of any potential long-term sequelae is largely the result of the work of Leon Chesley, who followed a cohort of women with eclampsia in their first pregnancy and reported no increased risk of hypertension or death. However, he did show a two- to fivefold excess mortality over the next 35 years among women with eclampsia in any pregnancy after the first. Chesley's finding led to speculation that multiparous women with preeclampsia/eclampsia would be more likely to have the diagnosis confounded by underlying chronic hypertension and that this underlying disease, and not the preeclampsia per se, caused the subsequent increase in morbidity and mortality. In support of this hypothesis, Sibai et al. have shown that women with recurrence of preeclampsia (PE) are more likely to have chronic hypertension.

However, a recent report from Norway has suggested that, although nulliparous patients with preeclampsia at term suffered no long-term health risks, women with preterm preeclampsia were noted to have excess long-term mortality. Another report from Scotland found a link between preeclampsia and future maternal ischemic heart disease. Scottish investigators have shown that nulliparous women with preeclampsia are four times more likely to develop hypertension later in life (odds ratio [OR] = 3.98, 2.82-5.61).

Although much ignored in the United States, emerging evidence does indeed suggest a strong link between preeclampsia and future risk of cardiovascular disease. These observations may ultimately shed light on the pathogenesis of preeclampsia and may ultimately identify subgroups of women at highest risk of heart disease, whose risk may be favorably modified by appropriate preventive measures.

KEY POINTS

- Preeclampsia, manifested by new-onset hypertension and proteinuria during pregnancy, is believed to complicate 5% to 7% of all deliveries in the United States. It is determined by increased blood pressure (140/90 mmHg or greater) and by proteinuria.
- Preeclampsia is more common among nulliparas and at extremes of reproductive age. It has been associated with oxidative stress, abnormal trophoblast invasion, and endothelial cell dysfunction.
- Currently, there is no simple, safe, or sensitive test to predict this disease, and no such screening tests are used by obstetricians in the United States outside of research protocols.
- The only curative therapy for preeclampsia is delivery.
- The use of magnesium sulfate for seizure prophylaxis and modern methods of hypertension management have dramatically decreased acute maternal mortality. Magnesium sulfate is superior to phenytoin in preventing seizures, reducing the risk from 1% to 3% to about 0.2%. Magnesium sulfate is *not* efficacious to treat severe hypertension; antihypertensives should be used when systolic pressures exceed 160 mmHg or diastolic pressures exceed 110 mmHg.
- Expectant management of preeclampsia should be considered only in conjunction with a maternal-fetal medicine specialist and only when neither the mother nor fetus show signs of worsening disease.

SUGGESTED READINGS

Atallah AN, Hofmeyr GJ, Duley L: Calcium supplementation during pregnancy for preventing hypertensive disorders and related problems. *Cochrane Database Syst Rev* 3, 2000.

Chappell LC et al: Effect of antioxidants on the occurrence of pre-eclampsia in women at increased risk: a randomised trial. *Lancet* 354:810, 1999.

Chesley LC, Annitto JE, Cosgrove RA: The remote prognosis of eclamptic women. Sixth periodic report. *Am J Obstet Gynecol* 124:446, 1976.

Funai EF et al: Long-term mortality after preeclampsia. *Epidemiology* 16:206, 2005.

Gifford R: *Working Group Report on High Blood Pressure and Pregnancy.* Washington, DC, 2000, National Institutes of Health.

Knight M et al: Antiplatelet agents for preventing and treating pre-eclampsia. *Cochrane Database Syst Rev 2,* 2000.

Levine RJ et al: Trial of Calcium for Preeclampsia Prevention (CPEP): rationale, design, and methods. *Control Clin Trials* 17:442, 1996.

Roberts J: Pregnancy-related hypertension. In Creasy R, editor: *Maternal Fetal Medicine, Principles and Practice.* Philadelphia, 1994, WB Saunders.

Roberts JM, Cooper DW: Pathogenesis and genetics of pre-eclampsia. Lancet 357:53, 2001.

Sibai BM et al: Prevention of preeclampsia with low-dose aspirin in healthy, nulliparous pregnant women. The National Institute of Child Health and Human Development Network of Maternal-Fetal Medicine Units. *N Engl J Med* 329:1213, 1993.

Wilson BJ et al: Hypertensive diseases of pregnancy and risk of hypertension and stroke in later life: results from cohort study. *BMJ* 326:845, 2003.

24

17

CHRONIC HYPERTENSION IN PREGNANCY

Maria J. Small and John Paul Hayslett

Chronic hypertension affects 1% to 5% of pregnant women and is one of the most common medical complications of pregnancy. The prevalence varies between populations and increases with age. Because the incidence increases with advancing age and maternal obesity, chronic hypertension is likely to be encountered more often in pregnancy. The demographic changes in obstetrics, reflected by increasing numbers of older women and the epidemic of corpulence/obesity, fuel this association.

EPIDEMIOLOGY

The risk factors for chronic hypertension include advancing age, obesity, and ethnicity, with black women at increased risk. The prevalence of chronic hypertension for African Americans is among the highest in the world and disease onset is earlier. The incidence of hypertension in African Americans is approximately twice that of non-Hispanic whites. In women of reproductive age, the prevalence of chronic hypertension is approximately 10% by age 30, as compared with 5% of white, non-Hispanic women. Overall, the age-adjusted prevalence of hypertension in the U.S. population is as follows: in the non-Hispanic black, non-Hispanic white, and Mexican American populations the prevalence is 32.4%, 23.3%, and 22.6%, respectively.

Given the prevalence of this disease and the fact that approximately one third of the hypertensive population is unaware of their disease, obstetric providers are likely to treat both known and unknown pregestational hypertensive women in pregnancy.

In approximately 90% of individuals, the etiology of chronic hypertension is unknown or essential. In approximately 10%, however, hypertension is secondary to another condition. Essential hypertension is thought to arise from several mechanisms: sympathetic nervous system overactivity, renin-angiotensin overexpression/increased activity, hyperinsulinemia, decreased endothelium-derived vasodilators, or increased numbers of endothelium-derived vasoconstrictors. Many of these factors also contribute to the pathology of preeclampsia, the hypertensive proteinuric state unique to pregnancy. Chronic hypertension is one of the leading causes of superimposed preeclampsia. Although 5% to 7% of pregnant women develop preeclampsia, women with chronic hypertension have an approximately 10% to 25% risk of acquiring superimposed preeclampsia during pregnancy. Hypertensive disease is a leading cause of maternal mortality (Table 17-1).

DEFINITIONS

The National High Blood Pressure Education Program working group established the following definitions for hypertension in pregnancy:

Chronic hypertension—Elevated blood pressure that precedes pregnancy or is first detected before 20 weeks gestational or after 6 weeks postpartum. The condition may have been undetected before pregnancy and may have escaped medical management. In a woman first noted to have hypertension in pregnancy, failure of blood pressure to normalize within days or weeks postpartum suggests preexisting chronic hypertension.

Gestational hypertension—Blood pressure elevation appearing in the second half of pregnancy, in the absence of proteinuria or other signs of preeclampsia. If signs of proteinuria develop, the diagnosis changes to preeclampsia. If the blood pressure fails to normalize postpartum, the condition is characterized as chronic hypertension.

Preeclampsia—Pregnancy-associated syndrome occurring after 20 weeks of gestation with systolic blood pressure of 140 mmHg or higher and diastolic blood pressure of 90 mmHg or higher in combination with proteinuria (300 mg in 24 hours or 1+ on dipstick).

Eclampsia—Development of seizures or coma with no other identifiable cause in the woman with preeclampsia. Seizures typically occur after midgestation but may also occur in the postpartum period.

Preeclampsia superimposed on chronic hypertension—Development of preeclampsia/eclampsia in a woman with preexisting chronic hypertension. The risk is approximately 10% to 25% that a woman with chronic hypertension will develop superimposed preeclampsia.

One of the difficult diagnostic dilemmas in pregnancy is the distinction of preeclampsia from chronic hypertension in the patient who either was not prenatally diagnosed or who had borderline blood pressure elevations during pregnancy. In pregnancy, blood pressure physiologically nadirs in the second

Table 17-1

Maternal and Perinatal Risks in Mild and Severe Hypertensive Disease

Risk	Mild Disease/Low Risk (%)	Severe Hypertension/High Risk (%)
Superimposed preeclampsia	10-25	50
Abruption	0.7-1.5	5-10
Preterm birth <37 weeks	12-34	60-70
Intrauterine growth restriction	8-16	30-40

trimester and rises in the third trimester; therefore blood pressure elevation before 20 weeks may suggest preexisting chronic hypertension.

HYPERTENSION RISK ASSESSMENT

Women with chronic hypertension are at increased risk for preterm delivery, fetal growth restriction, intrauterine fetal demise, placental abruption, and heart and renal failure (Table 17-2). The baseline risk for abruption is approximately doubled in chronic hypertensives as compared with normotensive women. In the absence of superimposed preeclampsia, mildly hypertensive women have similar obstetric outcomes as normotensive women. Perinatal mortality is increased threefold in the hypertensive woman, largely secondary to complications resulting from iatrogenic preterm delivery and fetal growth restriction in the setting of preeclampsia. In the subset of women with severe early-onset hypertension, approximately 30% to 40% of these women have underlying chronic hypertension.

"High-risk" hypertension is characterized by severe blood pressure elevation in the woman 20 weeks' gestation or less with systolic blood pressure 160 mmHg or higher or diastolic blood pressure 110 mmHg or higher. The high-risk hypertensive may also characterize the woman with mild hypertension and associated end-organ disease. These patients are at risk for adverse maternal and perinatal outcomes, primarily in the setting of superimposed preeclampsia. Maternal risks include pulmonary edema, hypertensive crisis, encephalopathy, stroke, and renal failure. In contrast, women with mild hypertension generally have favorable pregnancies. Approximately 15% of all hypertensive women have uncomplicated pregnancies.

"Low-risk" hypertension is characterized by blood pressure elevation 140/90 mmHg before 20 weeks' gestation and absent end-organ dysfunction. Treatment is not routinely recommended for these women because antihypertensive therapy is not associated with improvement in perinatal outcomes and may result in uteroplacental insufficiency for the mildly hypertensive woman. Treatment is recommended for women with chronic hypertension in the

Table 17-2

Characteristics of High-Risk Chronic Hypertension

Severe hypertension	Hypertension with preexisting maternal or perinatal factors	**Hypertension and maternal comorbidity**
SBP ≥160 mmHg and or DBP ≥110 mmHg under 20 weeks' gestation	Previous perinatal loss	**Pregestational diabetes**
	Prior preeclampsia	**Cardiac disease**
	Age >40 yr	**Collagen vascular disease**
	Hypertension duration four years or longer	**Primary renal disease**
	End-organ damage: cardiomyopathy, retinopathy, renal insufficiency	

DBP, Diastolic blood pressure; *SBP,* systolic blood pressure.

setting of mild disease when systolic blood pressure is persistently greater than 160 mmHg or diastolic blood pressure is greater than 105 mmHg. In the setting of high-risk hypertension with end-organ damage, the threshold for treatment is lower and diastolic blood pressure should be maintained at less than 90 mmHg.

INVESTIGATIONS

In antenatal visits or early in pregnancy, assessment for end-organ damage is important secondary to the increased risk for superimposed preeclampsia in women with chronic hypertension. Baseline evaluation should include urinalysis, urine culture, blood urea nitrogen (BUN), creatinine, 24-hour urine for creatinine clearance, protein, complete blood count with platelets, and electrocardiogram (Box 17-1).

Women with long-standing disease or severe uncontrolled disease should have maternal cardiac echocardiograms. Echocardiography should be performed for the woman with disease duration greater than 4 years, severe disease, and those aged 40 years and older.

ANTENATAL FETAL SURVEILLANCE

Although there are no standard guidelines for antenatal surveillance, an ultrasound during midtrimester for confirmation of fetal gestational age and for evaluation of fetal anatomy will provide baseline dating confirmation in the event growth restriction develops. Sonographic surveillance for fetal growth should occur every 4 to 6 weeks in patients with severe hypertension and/or evidence of vascular disease. These patients are at high risk for growth restriction. Similar ultrasound surveillance is also warranted for the patient who is difficult to assess clinically for fetal size, such as the morbidly obese hypertensive woman.

Antenatal testing in the third trimester with NST and/or biophysical profile testing is recommended. Weekly surveillance for preeclampsia with urinary protein dipstick and blood pressure surveillance should also occur at weekly intervals in the third trimester, beginning at 32 to 34 weeks. If

---

Box 17-1   Baseline Laboratory Tests for Pregnant Chronic Hypertensive Patient

Urinalysis and urine culture
BUN
Creatinine
24-Hour urine for protein, creatinine clearance
Electrolytes
ECG
Early ultrasound for confirmation of gestational age in midtrimester
Maternal echocardiogram*

BUN, Blood urea nitrogen; *ECG*, electrocardiogram.
*If long-standing disease and/or at age 40 years.

preeclampsia and/or growth restriction occurs, surveillance will increase depending on the severity of the condition; it is typically performed at least twice weekly in those settings.

LABOR AND BIRTH

Mild hypertension is not an indication for change in labor management, and these patients can receive standard care and await spontaneous labor. In the setting of severe hypertension, preeclampsia, prior poor perinatal outcome, or superimposed preeclampsia, pregnancy may be induced with appropriate antenatal confirmation of lung maturity if before 39 weeks, or earlier, when maternal or infant health is of concern (e.g., severe superimposed pre-eclampsia or severe fetal growth restriction).

245

MEDICAL THERAPY

In pregnancy, medical treatment must focus on prevention of maternal morbidities such as stroke or myocardial dysfunction, avoidance of known teratogenic agents, and early discontinuation of agents associated with adverse perinatal outcome.

One concern in the setting of pregnancy is potential induction of uteroplacental insufficiency from aggressive antihypertensive treatment. Antihypertensive therapy for mild hypertension is not proven beneficial for prevention of pregnancy-related complications such as preeclampsia, abruption, or growth restriction. For this reason, the harm may outweigh the benefit, and universal treatment of the uncomplicated, mild hypertensive (low-risk hypertensive) woman is not indicated during pregnancy. Exceptions include women with evidence of end-organ dysfunction or other medical comorbidity. Women with normal blood pressures of 120/80 mmHg in early pregnancy may have a trial of observation without their antihypertensive agents. If the blood pressure remains below 140/90 mmHg, these patients may remain off medications. They should undergo continued close surveillance, with blood pressure evaluations every 2 to 3 weeks.

Generally, diuretic use is limited to patients who were on these agents before 20 weeks' gestation and desire to continue this therapy or patients with underlying renal disease and accompanying edema.

Medications with the most extensive experience in pregnancy and lactation include alpha methyldopa and hydralazine. Alpha methyldopa is a centrally acting agent, not associated with teratogenicity or adverse perinatal outcomes throughout gestation or during lactation. Follow-up studies on children up to age 7 years demonstrate no developmental problems resulting from alpha methyldopa exposure. Alpha methyldopa is a weak antihypertensive, and approximately 15% of women do not tolerate its side effects. Somnolence is the most common complaint. Despite these limitations, alpha methyldopa remains a first-line agent for treatment of hypertension in pregnancy, largely because of extensive experience and its safety profile.

Hydralazine is a vasodilator with extensive use in pregnancy. It is not associated with teratogenicity or adverse perinatal outcomes. Because of its variable oral metabolism, it is reserved primarily for the acute parenteral treatment of hypertensive crises in pregnancy.

Beta blockers are widely applied for hypertension therapy outside of pregnancy. In pregnancy, however, growth restriction is associated with long-term use after first-trimester administration. This complication is largely identified with Atenolol exposure. There is limited first-trimester experience with acebutolol, pindolol, oxprenolol, or metoprolol, although these agents have been used in the third trimester without evidence of negative fetal or neonatal outcomes. Although continued use of beta blockers, beginning in the first trimester, is associated with lower birth weights and growth restriction, third-trimester treatment does not present the same risk. Beta blockers may worsen bronchospasm in patients with lung disease and should be used with caution in diabetes because they may mask symptoms of hypoglycemia.

Labetalol, a combined alpha-beta adrenergic blocker, has been applied extensively in pregnancy and is not associated with first-trimester teratogenicity, adverse perinatal outcomes, or growth restriction. This medication is an effective, alternative first-line agent for the management of hypertension in pregnancy.

Calcium channel blockers are not associated with adverse perinatal outcomes or teratogenicity. Nifedipine is the agent with the most extensive use and experience in pregnancy. Verapamil and nifedipine are not associated with increased teratogenicity. Sublingual formations should be avoided secondary to reported myocardial infarction in pregnancy and severe maternal hypotension with resultant uteroplacental insufficiency. Calcium channel blockers may worsen heart failure or conduction system disease.

Diuretics such as thiazides and Lasix are rarely used in pregnancy but are used as second- or third-line agents. The concern associated with diuretic use is related to inhibition of plasma volume expansion because absent plasma volume expansion is a feature of preeclampsia pathogenesis. Thiazides are not associated with teratogenicity following first-trimester exposure, and some patients may elect to remain on these medications if they are already receiving them; however, they should be offered conversion to an alternative medication not associated with impairment of plasma volume expansion. Third-trimester exposure to thiazides is associated with rare cases of life-threatening neonatal thrombocytopenia. First-trimester furosemide exposure is associated with hypospadias but no other teratogenicity. Patients with generalized edema, such as that encountered in nephrotic syndrome, may require chronic diuretic treatment with Lasix during pregnancy. Close attention to volume status is warranted in these cases.

Angiotensin-converting enzyme (ACE) inhibitors and receptor blockers are contraindicated in pregnancy. First-trimester exposure is not associated with teratogenicity; however, exposure after 16 weeks' gestation is associated with hypocalvaria, oligohydramnios, poor kidney development, neonatal renal failure, pulmonary hypoplasia, and growth restriction. ACE inhibitors are excreted in the breast milk in small amounts and generally are considered safe for lactation by the American Academy of Pediatrics (AAP).

THERAPEUTIC GOALS

The target blood pressure in women without end-organ damage is systolic pressure of 140 to 150 mmHg and diastolic pressure 90 to 100 mmHg. In the setting of end-organ damage, however, the blood pressure should be maintained below 140/90 mmHg.

LACTATION

All the antihypertensive agents concentrate in breast milk; however, the milk/plasma ratio is an important determinant of neonatal exposure. General recommendations include use of medications with lower lipid solubility, use of the lowest doses possible, and use of agents with established neonatal applications. Alpha methyldopa is found in low concentrations in milk and appears safe, whereas beta blockers such as atenolol are present in higher concentrations and may adversely affect the neonate. Diuretics are present in low concentration and may decrease milk production, although low doses of thiazides (25 mg/day) are not associated with milk suppression.

Calcium channel blockers such as nifedipine and verapamil are considered compatible with breast feeding by the AAP. Levels of diltiazem are higher in breast milk than those of nifedipine and verapamil; however, diltiazem is considered compatible with lactation.

ACE inhibitors are excreted in low concentrations in breast milk. Captopril and enalapril have been reviewed in limited series and are generally considered safe according to the AAP. If possible, their use should be avoided in the first month of life secondary to the known neonatal susceptibility to renal effects of ACE inhibitors.

Beta blockers such as propranolol and metoprolol are excreted in low amounts and considered compatible with lactation. Atenolol, nadolol, and sotalol are excreted in higher concentrations and are associated with neonatal hypotension, bradycardia, and tachypnea secondary to higher secretion in breast milk.

Generally, alpha methyldopa or labetalol are optimal first-line agents for breast-feeding mothers. Hydralazine is excreted in small amounts and is compatible with breast feeding.

Additional maternal recommendations include breast feeding immediately before medication doses when multiple doses are used and, with once-daily dosing, administration of medication before infant's longest sleep cycle, typically following feeding (Table 17-3).

Table 17-3

Antihypertensive Therapy in Pregnancy

Drug	Class	Pregnancy Category	Special Indications	Dose	Side Effects	Lactation
Adrenergic receptor blockade						
Labetalol	Alpha and beta blockade	C	Effective initial agent for pregnancy	100 mg po bid Max: 2400 mg/day	Hypersensitivity, tremor, flushing, headache	Compatible
Meto-prolol	Beta blocker	C		50-400 mg po daily	May blunt sensation of hypoglycemia, avoid in asthma	Compatible
Proprano-lol	Beta blocker	C	Thyrotoxicosis/inhibits T4→T3 conversion		May blunt sensation of hypoglycemia, avoid in asthma	Compatible
Atenolol	Beta blocker	D		50-100 mg po daily	May blunt sensation of hypoglycemia, avoid in asthma	Compatible
Central acting						
Alpha methyl-dopa	Central-acting alpha-adrenergic inhibitor	B	Common first-line agent for pregnancy	250 mg po bid/tid Max: 4 g/day	Fatigue, liver disease, hemolytic anemia 15% of women do not tolerate because of side effects	Compatible
Clonidine	Central-acting alpha-adrenergic agonist	C	Third-line agent, offers little advantage over alpha methyldopa	0.1mg po bid Max: 2.4 mg/day	Abrupt cessation may result in rebound hypertension	Compatible
Diuretics—generally not recommended in pregnancy						
Thiazide	Diuretic	C	Second- or third-line agent	25-100 mg po daily Max: >200 mg/kg/day	Rare cases of neonatal thrombocytopenia, hemorrhagic pancreatitis	Compatible, rare association with neonatal thrombocytopenia Doses above 25 mg/day associated with milk volume suppression

Table 17-3—cont'd

Drug	Class	Pregnancy Category	Special Indications	Dose	Side Effects	Lactation
Furosemide	Loop diuretic	C	Acute treatment of pulmonary edema or management of edema resulting from renal failure/nephrotic syndrome	20-80 mg po daily Max: 600 mg/day		Compatible, but associated with milk volume suppression
Vasodilators						
Hydralazine	Arteriolar vasodilator	B—considered safe in pregnancy	Poor po metabolism during pregnancy—not optimal oral agent	10 mg po daily Max: 100 mg/day	More effective as parenteral agent for hypertensive crisis	Compatible
Nifedipine	Calcium channel blocker	C	Careful with dosing in addition to magnesium; may cause severe hypotension Rx calcium gluconate	10-30 mg tid, not to exceed 120-180 mg/day SR tab: 30-60 mg daily Increase every 7-14 days Max: 120 mg/day		Compatible
Enalapril, captopril	ACE inhibitors	D—unsafe after first trimester	Avoid in pregnancy, association with fetal renal failure, oligohydramnios, fetal demise, deformations First-trimester exposure not associated with teratogenicity		—	Compatible

ACE, Angiotensin-converting enzyme; *bid,* twice daily; *po,* per os; *Rx,* treatment; *tid,* three times a day.

CONTRACEPTION

The woman with chronic hypertension has several options for pregnancy prevention. Care should be taken to tailor therapy for specific indications, such as renal disease or other comorbidities. Barrier methods such as condoms, foam, and the diaphragm are safe but not reliable when suboptimally used. Intrauterine devices (IUDs) are optimal for women in monogamous relationships and at low risk for sexually transmitted infections. Hormonal therapy with combined estrogen is not contraindicated in the hypertensive woman but depends on the risk profile. Low-dose estrogen-containing contraceptives with less than 50 μg or less of estinyl estradiol are acceptable. Higher doses are associated with thromboembolism, blood pressure elevation, stroke, pulmonary embolism, and deep venous thrombosis. Women with diabetes and hypertension who do not have underlying vascular disease may benefit from low-dose oral contraceptives containing progestin only or combination pills containing 20 to 35 μg ethinyl estradiol. Long-acting progestins such as Depo-Provera are not associated with worsening hypertension; however, these agents are associated with increased insulin and weight gain. Those side effects may worsen insulin resistance in susceptible patients.

FOOD AND DRUG ADMINISTRATION CATEGORIES FOR DRUG USE IN PREGNANCY

Category A: Controlled studies in women fail to demonstrate a risk to the fetus in the first trimester, and the possibility of fetal harm appears remote.

Category B: Either animal studies do not indicate a risk to the fetus and there are no controlled studies in pregnant women or animal studies have indicated fetal risk but controlled studies in pregnant women failed to demonstrate a risk.

Category C: Either animal studies indicate a fetal risk and there are no controlled studies in women or there are no available studies in women or animals.

Category D: There is positive evidence of fetal risk, but there may be certain situations in which the benefit may outweigh the risk.

Category X: There is a definite fetal risk based on studies in animals or humans, or a fetal risk based on human experience, and the risk clearly outweighs any benefit to pregnant women.

HYPERTENSIVE CRISIS

The goal of treatment in hypertensive emergencies is to interrupt the life-threatening increase in blood pressure. Care should be taken to avoid a rapid, severe decrease in the blood pressure and have a goal of a 10-mmHg drop in diastolic blood pressure with acute therapy. Precipitous decreases in blood pressure may result in decreased uteroplacental perfusion and worsen ischemia of vital organs such as the heart, kidneys, and brain. The decline in blood pressure should occur over several minutes to an hour, with a mean arterial pressure decrease of 25% in the first 6 hours of treatment. Parenteral medications should be used in hypertensive emergencies. When blood pressure control is achieved, oral medications may be used to maintain control.

In severe preeclampsia, beta blockers are often used secondary to the increased beta-sympathomimetic activity associated with preeclampsia. The goals are to maintain systolic blood pressure 130 to 155 mm Hg and diastolic blood pressure 90 to 105 mmHg.

Calcium channel blockers may also be administered in oral preparations for acute therapy. Beta blockers are contraindicated in acute heart failure. Hydralazine has the advantage of both intramuscular and intravenous preparations and is an effective arteriolar vasodilator for treatment of severe preeclampsia.

Nitroprusside may be associated with cyanide buildup in the fetus, particularly at doses greater than 10 μg/kg/min and/or treatment longer than 4 hours. This agent is effective because of rapid onset and titratability (Table 17-4).

SPECIAL CONSIDERATIONS

Diabetes and Hypertension in Pregnancy

The overweight/obesity epidemic is fueling the rise of type 2 diabetes among women of reproductive age. The constellation of obesity, abnormal lipid profile, hypertension, and diabetes, or syndrome X, is more common in this setting. The mechanisms resulting in hypertension for the type 1 and type 2 diabetic differ, with type 1 patients typically normotensive until the onset of renal disease. As antecedent microalbinuria (protein range 30-300 mg/day) progresses, blood pressure elevations occur. With progressive microalbinuria, overt albuminuria occurs and is detected on routine dipsticks (300 mg/day). Hypertension typically accompanies nephropathy in type 1 diabetics. The lifetime risk of hypertension is 40% to 50% in these patients. Diabetes confers an approximately 15% to 20% risk of preeclampsia. This risk rises to 50% in the setting of underlying vascular disease.

The majority of hypertensive diabetic women are type 2 diabetics. Diabetic women are twice as likely to have chronic hypertension than are nondiabetic women. Older age, obesity, and ethnicity are risk factors. African American and Hispanic women demonstrate an approximately twofold increased risk of diabetes. Hypertension often accompanies insulin resistance and may precede the onset of overt diabetes. Approximately 50% of patients with hypertension manifest impaired glucose tolerance. These relationships highlight the importance of screening women for hypertension if they present with diabetes and for diabetes screening if they have chronic hypertension. This testing is an important component for the at-risk woman presenting for preconception counseling.

For nonpregnant women with pregestational diabetes, the presence of microalbuminuria may prompt treatment with angiotensin-converting

Table 17-4

Emergency Antihypertensive Therapy in Pregnancy

Drug	Dose	Onset	Duration	Special Indications	Adverse Effects
Hydralazine	5-10 mg IV every 20 min After test dose of 1 mg over 2 min 10-40 mg IM Max: 30 mg/hr Max bolus dose: 20 mg IV	10-20 min (IV) 20-30 min IM	3-6 hr(IV) 4-6 hr (IM)	Preeclampsia IM route available Can use in most emergencies— contraindicated in acute heart failure	Headache, tachycardia, hypotension, ischemia, worsening angina, emesis
Labetalol	20-80 mg IV q 10 min	5-10 min	3-6 hr		Worsening heart block, bronchoconstriction
Nitroprusside	0.25-20 μg/kg/min IV	Seconds	1-2 min	Severe refractory hypertension	Cyanide toxicity: increased risk at doses 10 μg/kg/min or greater than 4-hr treatment
Nifedipine	10 mg po q 30 min	10-20 min	4-5 hr		Hypotension—may be severe in conjunction with magnesium therapy—Rx calcium gluconate
Phentolamine	5-10 mg IV	1-2 min	10-30 min	Pheochromocytoma/catecholamine excess	Tachycardia, headache

IM, Intramuscular; *IV,* intravenous; *po,* per os; *Rx,* treatment.

enzyme inhibitor (ACEI) to retard progression to nephropathy. This treatment, although potentially effective for both hypertension and renal disease, is contraindicated in pregnancy. Preconception consultation should address cessation of this therapy before pregnancy and, if not discontinued before pregnancy, exposed women should be reassured that the risk of teratogenicity is not demonstrated beyond the first trimester (see Table 17-2).

Weight loss and initiation of an exercise program are recommended for nonpregnant obese patients with diabetes and hypertension to improve both insulin sensitivity and blood pressure. Although continuation of an existing preconception exercise plan is recommended, during pregnancy, initiation of an exercise and weight loss program is not recommended. This treatment approach highlights the importance of preconception counseling for optimization of medical status before pregnancy.

Beta blockers may decrease catecholamine release in response to hypoglycemia and therefore blunt the diabetic patient's self-awareness of hypoglycemia. They are also associated with worsening lipid and glucose metabolism and should be used with caution in the diabetic patient.

Calcium antagonists are not associated with adverse impact on lipid profiles, glycemic control, or insulin absorption and may be appropriate initial agents for the diabetic patient. Care should be taken in administering these agents to pregnant diabetic patients with preexisting autonomic dysfunction because they may worsen their orthostatic hypotension.

Nephropathy and Hypertension

The prognosis of pregnancy in women with underlying renal disease is largely affected by the etiology of the renal disease and the presence of hypertension. Women with mild intrinsic renal disease (creatinine less than 1.4 mg/dl) and absent hypertension preceding pregnancy typically do well. These women remain at increased risk for preeclampsia, however, and the presence of preeclampsia increases the risk for perinatal morbidity and mortality in the setting of chronic hypertension. The risk of perinatal mortality is approximately 0.3% and this risk climbs to 10% in the woman with hypertension and superimposed preeclampsia.

The compounded presence of nephropathy and chronic hypertension further compounds obstetric risk. Women with moderate to severe renal disease (baseline creatinine greater than 1.4 mg/dl) are at high risk for adverse perinatal outcomes. These women have an approximately 59% risk of preterm delivery and 37% risk of intrauterine growth restriction. The risk of superimposed preeclampsia is approximately 50%, and the disease occurs earlier in gestation. Pregnant women with nephropathy experience functional renal loss above baseline, with one third to one half experiencing more accelerated decline in renal function. In approximately 10% of women, these changes do not reverse following pregnancy. Although aggressive treatment of hypertension is important to protect against long-term decline in renal function, this treatment is not completely protective against the pregnancy-associated deterioration. Untreated severe hypertension beginning in the first trimester is associated with a 50% risk of perinatal mortality and 40% decline in renal function. In contrast, women with renal disease and absent hypertension throughout pregnancy experience a 6% perinatal mortality rate and 7% deterioration of renal function. With therapy, the risk of perinatal mortality is 10% to 12% if hypertension is managed and the decline in renal function is approximately 10% to 12%.

Women with renal insufficiency should be followed closely with monthly evaluation of renal function, close monitoring and treatment of blood pressure, close surveillance for superimposed preeclampsia, serial fetal growth assessments every 4 to 6 weeks, and antenatal testing for fetal well-being in the third trimester, or sooner, if growth restriction or preeclampsia develops.

The distinction between underlying superimposed preeclampsia and nephropathy may present a clinical challenge. The clinical presence of worsening proteinuria or its appearance in patients previously without significant proteinuria or blood pressure elevations refractory to treatment suggests superimposed preeclampsia. These signs are not absolute because the presence of worsening proteinuria occurs in 50% of all patients with renal disease. The clinical condition is closely guarded, particularly in the preterm patient, and typically inpatient observation and management is necessary to evaluate and treat the patient with renal disease and suspected preeclampsia. In a renal patient with worsening hypertension and edema, medical management with close attention to volume status (daily weights and clinical edema), diuretic use, and increase in antihypertensive treatment may be warranted.

SECONDARY DISEASE

Pheochromocytomas are rare catecholamine-producing tumors originating from the neural crest chromaffin cells. Although rare, they may present with life-threatening hypertensive crisis in pregnancy secondary to epinephrine secretion. Approximately 10% of pheochromocytomas are malignant, and the majority of these are extraadrenal. The clinical findings may include intermittent blood pressure elevation and the triad of headache, diaphoresis, and tachycardia. Patients may also manifest hyperglycemia. Extraadrenal pheochromocytomas produce norepinephrine, which results in hypertension without many associated symptoms. Diagnosis is through measurement of 24-hour vanillylmandelic acid, catecholamines, and metanephrine. These values are unchanged in pregnancy. Magnetic resonance imaging (MRI) or computed tomography (CT) will assist in tumor site identification. Treatment is surgical resection in the second trimester. If patients are unable to undergo resection, they may be treated with phenoxybenzamine (pregnancy category C), or phentolamine (pregnancy category C) for effective alpha-adrenergic blockade. Labetalol is also an effective agent for treatment of these patients. Affected patients should not be treated with beta blocker therapy initially because they may develop unopposed alpha-adrenergic–driven hypertensive crises.

Hyperaldosteronism should be suspected in the patient with underlying hypertension, hypokalemia, and metabolic alkalosis. The etiology is typically an adrenal adenoma, bilateral hyperplasia, or (rarely) adrenocortical carcinoma. This condition is rare in pregnancy but may result from diuretic use, Cushing's disease, or licorice ingestion. Renovascular disease may result in activation of the renin-angiotensin-aldosterone syndrome and secondary hyperaldosteronism. Diagnosis is through direct measurement of rennin activity and aldosterone concentration. Renin levels will be lower and aldosterone levels higher than normal for pregnancy. Lack of aldosterone suppression with salt loading is also diagnostic. MRI or CT will localize adenomas, and treatment is surgical resection in the second trimester or hypertensive control with medical therapy.

Aortic coarctation should be suspected in the hypertensive patient with lagging radial and femoral pulses.

Renal artery stenosis may result in secondary hypertension. Renal artery stenosis resulting from fibromuscular dysplasia is approximately 2 to 10 times more common in young women than men. This condition is diagnosed before age 50 years in the majority of cases, making the likelihood of diagnosis in the reproductive period higher. The clinical findings are typically severe refractory hypertension, age younger than 30 years, and epigastric bruit. The gold standard for diagnosis is angiography; however, ultrasound, CT, and MRI/magnetic resonance angiography (MRA) also may be used for diagnosis. ACE inhibitors are the primary therapy outside pregnancy to inhibit the activation of the renin-angiotensin-aldosterone syndrome, but thiazides may also be used for blood pressure control in pregnancy.

Hypertensive crisis and maintenance therapy for **thyrotoxicosis** during pregnancy is best achieved through use of beta blocker therapy. Propranolol inhibits peripheral conversion of T4 to T3 and has been extensively applied in the treatment of thyrotoxicosis in pregnancy.

25

CONCLUSIONS

Hypertension is a pervasive, common medical disorder during pregnancy. Primary care providers treating hypertensive women should address pregnancy plans in women of reproductive age and perform risk assessment. Ideally, women seen before pregnancy can plan dietary interventions, exercise programs, and change medical therapies. Hypertensive women with severe disease, medical comorbidities, or history of adverse perinatal outcomes should be referred to a maternal-fetal medicine specialist for evaluation and consultation.

KEY POINTS

- Chronic hypertension affects approximately 1% to 5% of pregnant women.
- Chronic hypertension increases the risk for superimposed preeclampsia, with a 10% to 25% risk of superimposed preeclampsia.
- Baseline evaluations for the hypertensive pregnant woman should include urinalysis, urine culture, BUN, creatinine, complete blood count and platelets, 24-hour urine for total protein and creatinine clearance, electrocardiogram (ECG), and maternal echocardiogram for women with long-standing disease or in women older than 40 years.
- The prognosis for pregnancy in the setting of chronic hypertension depends on the severity of the disease; women with mild hypertension without superimposed preeclampsia have pregnancy risks comparable to nonhypertensive women.

KEY POINTS—cont'd

- Mild hypertension does not require medical treatment in pregnancy.

- The presence of severe hypertension or mild hypertension and medical comorbidities increases the risk for placental abruption, perinatal morbidity, fetal growth restriction, and maternal morbidity and mortality.

- Patients with severe disease should be medically managed during pregnancy and should have close maternal and fetal surveillance during pregnancy.

- Medical therapy should be directed at minimization of fetal exposure to teratogens, use of agents with wide experience in pregnancy or pediatrics, and understanding side effects of particular agents.

- In hypertensive crisis, the goal of management is to prevent maternal cardiovascular or cerebral event with avoidance of precipitous decline that may compromise uteroplacental circulation.

- Patients presenting with refractory hypertension or those with diagnoses in pregnancy or other symptoms suggestive of secondary disease should have evaluation for underlying secondary causes of hypertension.

SUGGESTED READINGS

August P: *Treatment of Hypertension in Pregnancy*. In Rose BD, editor: UptoDate.com. Waltham MA, 2006.

Burt V et al: Prevalence of hypertension in the US adult population, results from the Third National Health and Nutrition Examination Survey, 1988-1991. *Hypertension* 25:305, 1995.

Chobanian AV et al: The Seventh Report of the Joint National Committee on Prevention, Detection, Evaluation, and Treatment of High Blood Pressure: the JNC 7 report. *JAMA* 289:2560, 2003.

Creasy R, Resnik R, Iams J: *Maternal Fetal Medicine Principles and Practice*, ed 5. Philadelphia, 2004, WB Saunders.

Joint National Committee: The Sixth Report of the Joint National Committee on Prevention, Detection, Evaluation, and Treatment of High Blood Pressure (JNC VI). *Arch Intern Med* 157:2413, 1997.

Jones DC, Hayslett JP: Outcome of pregnancy in women with moderate or severe renal insufficiency. *N Engl J Med* 335:226, 1996.

National high blood pressure education program working group report on high blood pressure in pregnancy. National Heart Lung and Blood Institute. *Am J Obstet Gynecol* 183:S1, 2000.

Sibai BM: Chronic hypertension in pregnancy. *Obstet Gynecol* 100:369, 2002.

Sibai BH, editor: *Hypertensive Disorders in Women*. Philadelphia, 2001, WB Saunders.

Spencer J, Gonzalez L, Barnhart DJ: Medications in the breast-feeding mother. *Am Fam Physician* 64:119, 2001.

18

RENAL DISEASE IN PREGNANCY

John Paul Hayslett

PHYSIOLOGIC CHANGES IN NORMAL PREGNANCY

To identify possible pathologic alterations in renal function during pregnancy it is important to understand the physiologic changes that occur in normal pregnancy. Pregnancy is characterized by marked peripheral vasodilatation that begins by the eighth week of gestation and continues until term. The vascular change is associated with a cumulative retention of 500 to 700 mEq of sodium and a 50% increase in plasma volume. Cardiac output increases 50%, with a similar rise in blood flow to other visceral organs. The cause of the vascular dilatation may result from the secretion of relaxin by the placenta; this is a hormone related to the insulin family of hormones that causes cardiovascular changes in experimental animals that simulates changes in human gestation.

Despite the increased expansion of the vascular system, blood pressure remains stable because of retention of sodium most likely resulting from the action of aldosterone, which rises during gestation four to six times above normal levels to achieve plasma levels of 80 to 100 ng/dl. Diastolic pressure falls slightly in the second trimester, likely because of enhanced vascular compliance. When sodium is perturbed by increases or decreases in sodium balance, plasma levels of aldosterone change proportionately. When a large sodium load is administered to gravid women, the level of aldosterone falls to levels found in nonpregnant adults, indicating that the concentration of aldosterone is under dynamic control.

Renal blood flow increases by about 80% from conception until term, and glomerular filtration rate (GFR) reaches an incremental increase of 30% to 50%, compared with normal values. Studies in experimental animals and in pregnant women demonstrate that this remarkable rise in filtration rate correlates with the increase in glomerular plasma flow. In one report, the GFR in the third trimester averaged 140 to 160 ml/min compared with the level of 105 ml/min in the same women when not pregnant. Because of the increase in GFR and expansion of extracellular fluid volume the concentration of plasma creatinine is reduced from the average of 0.67 ± 0.2 mg/dl in nonpregnant women to 0.5 ± 0.1 mg/dl in pregnancy. Some authorities suggest that a plasma concentration of creatinine greater than 0.8 mg/dl should raise suspicion for renal insufficiency.

Other physiologic changes in pregnancy include a fall in the osmotic threshold for vasopressin from 280 mOsm/kg to about 270 mOsm/kg, and, as a consequence, the level of serum sodium falls modestly below 140 mEq. Furthermore, studies showed that the metabolic clearance of vasopressin is accelerated many fold because of the production of vasopressinase, an enzyme produced in the placenta that rapidly cleaves and degrades circulating vasopressin. Plasma levels of vasopressin, however, are normal because of the compensatory production of vasopressin. Some women fail to fully compensate for the degradation of vasopressin or have excess levels of vasopressinase near term and consequently develop diabetes insipidus. The capacity to concentrate urine can be restored by the administration of desmopressin (dDAVP) that resists the action of vasopressinase. It should be noted, however, that the ability to concentrate urine and alternatively to excrete a water load during normal pregnancy is unchanged compared with the nongravid state.

Pregnancy also alters renal tubular function. Studies show that the fractional excretion of glucose, small peptides and amino acids is increased during pregnancy. In some women, glucosuria, in the absence of an elevation of blood glucose level, is observed transiently during pregnancy. In addition, protein excretion increases twofold above the nonpregnant levels and can reach values of 250 mg per 24 hours. Taken together, these observations indicate that there is a generalized reduction in the absorption of nonelectrolyte solutes by the proximal tubule during pregnancy.

These insights into the physiologic alterations that occur in normal pregnancy indicate that a different scale of values must be considered in determining normal renal function when renal insufficiency is suspected. In instances when the level of renal function requires monitoring during pregnancy, GFR should be measured. In early pregnancy, the filtration rate can be estimated from a 24-hour urine collection. Figure 18-1 illustrates the marked increase

Figure 18-1

Mean glomerular filtration rate measured by three methods in 10 healthy women at 15 to 18, 25 to 28, and 35 to 38 weeks of pregnancy, and again at 8 to 12 weeks postpartum.

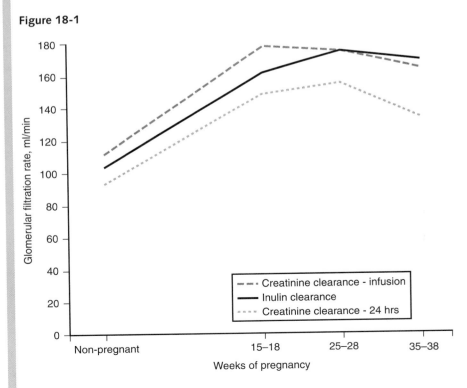

in GFR measured by the infusion of inulin or creatinine when the subject was lying on her side, compared with the urine collection method, when the filtration rate is sustained until delivery. This figure shows that the urine collection method underestimates the true GFR in the third trimester because of fluid accumulation in the lower extremities, when the subject is upright. In late pregnancy therefore the GFR should be measured with the gravida in a recumbent position.

PROTEINURIA IN PREGNANCY

Renal disease in pregnancy, as in nonpregnant individuals, can be caused by primary disease or secondarily by a systemic disease. In the evaluation of a patient with signs of renal disease, the first consideration is whether renal disease predates conception or occurs de novo during gestation. If there is no evidence of preexisting disease, the second consideration is whether renal disease began before or after the twentieth week of gestation because preeclampsia rarely occurs before that time. Regardless of the type of renal disease, the clinical signs of injury are recognized by two nonexclusive forms, namely proteinuria and renal insufficiency.

Proteinuria is a clinical term defined as the total protein excretion of more than 300 mg per 24 hours and usually denotes renal disease. Both diseases of the glomerulus and those involving the renal tubules and interstitium can result in proteinuria, but excretion rates more than 2.0 g per 24 hours usually indicate a glomerular disease. Patients with proteinuria excretion of less than 3.0 g per 24 hours are usually asymptomatic. In contrast, rates more than 3.0 g per 24 hours may cause the nephrotic syndrome that is symptomatic because of excess retention of sodium and water, resulting in dependent edema. The nephrotic syndrome is defined as proteinuria greater than 3.0 g per 24 hours and a serum albumin level of less than 3 g/dl. Edema does not occur in the absence of hypoalbuminemia, but in its presence patients exhibit a lower capacity to excrete sodium. Under that condition edema formation will occur if sodium intake exceeds the maximal capacity for sodium excretion.

The nephrotic syndrome in pregnancy may be caused by preexisting renal disease, renal disease that develops de novo, or preeclampsia. Several analyses have concluded that the presence of nephrotic syndrome attributable to renal diseases, in the absence of significant renal insufficiency and/or significant hypertension, does not seem to affect the natural course of renal disease or fetal survival. Regarding maternal complications, however, severe edema near term can cause or aggravate hypertension and complicate delivery because of vulva edema. It has been reported that preeclampsia is the most common cause for de novo nephrotic syndrome in pregnancy, and when that occurs the preeclampsia is regarded to be severe.

It should be emphasized that measures of urine protein before the twentieth week of gestation can be of great value in pregnancies complicated by the presence of proteinuria in the latter stages of gestation. In patients with established renal disease before conception or in whom proteinuria is documented before the twentieth week, the diagnosis of renal disease can be readily made because preeclampsia rarely occurs before that time. However, the onset of hypertension (often third trimester) and/or proteinuria after 20 weeks' gestation or when there is no information can present a diagnostic dilemma. It is important to distinguish underlying renal disease or chronic hypertension from preeclampsia because this distinction affects clinical management. In clinically stable patients with renal disease, the usual aim is term delivery with careful surveillance, whereas in preeclampsia the usual treatment is delivery. With preexisting hypertension or proteinuria, preeclampsia may manifest simply as an exacerbation of the chronic disease, posing the greatest diagnostic challenge. Decreased levels of antithrombin III, common in preeclampsia, may help to distinguish preeclampsia from an exacerbation of renal disease, but results are often not available in a timely fashion. Under that condition, most clinicians select preeclampsia as a working diagnosis.

The management of the nephrotic syndrome should aim to reduce edema formation to a level that allows comfort during ambulation. The dietary intake of sodium should be limited to 1.5 g of sodium per day (approximately 60 mEq) to reduce new edema formation. Often, bed rest in a recumbent position will suffice to mobilize preexisting edema by promoting an increase in the excretion of sodium. In general, the use of diuretic agents has been discouraged because of the possibility that reduction of extracellular fluid volume will decrease blood flow to the placenta. However, when diuretics are required to reduce intractable edema, therapy should aim only to reduce excessive edema at a slow rate of about 1 to 2 pounds per day with a loop diuretic, such as Lasix (Aventis Pharmaceuticals, Bridgewater, New Jersey), while a low-sodium diet is maintained. Because many patients with the nephrotic syndrome are resistant to low doses of the diuretic, the threshold dose capable of inducing a natriuresis can be determined by starting with an oral dose of 40 mg and then increasing the dose in a stepwise fashion until a natriuresis is achieved. If treatment on a chronic basis is needed, diuretic therapy should be administered on an alternating-day schedule to avoid a reduction of plasma volume and electrolyte disturbances. A written record of daily weights, taken by the patient, is highly recommended. Diuretics should not be administered to patients with preeclampsia because this condition is characterized by a reduction in circulating plasma volume.

RENAL INSUFFICIENCY RESULTING FROM PRIMARY RENAL DISEASE

The other sign of renal disease in pregnancy is a decrease in GFR. It should be noted that the use of serum creatinine as a surrogate marker of renal filtration rate is not a sensitive index for the early reduction in function because it may not rise above normal levels until the GFR is reduced by at least 50% of normal. The severity of renal insufficiency in pregnancy is usually classified as mild (>0.8 to < 1.4 mg/dl), moderate severe (>1.4 to < 2.5 mg/dl), and severe (>2.5 mg/dl).

The first large retrospective study of women with mild renal insufficiency was performed in the early 1960s. During pregnancy, hypertension increased or occurred de novo in about one fourth of pregnancies and a significant fall in GFR occurred in 16% of patients, shown in Table 18-1. In

Table 18-1

	Cr <1.4 mg/dl*	Cr >1.4 mg/dl†
Number pregnancies	121	82
Reduction in GFR (pregnancy and post partum)	16%	43%
Exacerbation or de novo onset of hypertension	28%	48%
Significant proteinuria	29%	41%

Cr, Creatinine; GFR, glomerular filtration rate.
*Kidney Int 18:192,1980.
†N Engl J Med 335:226,1996.

addition, urine protein excretion increased in 50% of patients, such that 68% exhibited the nephrotic syndrome by the third trimester. Long-term follow-up of these patients showed that the changes in blood pressure, renal function, and protein excretion were reversible after delivery in most cases and that the expected natural course was not altered.

Regarding pregnancy outcome, the birthrate was 93% and was associated with a perinatal morbidity of 10% (stillbirths and neonatal deaths), shown in Table 18-2. The incidence of preterm deliveries was 20% and growth restriction was 24%, substantially increased compared with that in the normal population. Subsequent reports published on pregnancies associated with mild renal insufficiency largely confirmed the initial report. All of these studies suggested that pregnancy did not alter the natural course of the underlying renal disease.

Women with moderate renal disease, reflected by a serum creatinine greater than 1.4 mg/dl but less than 2.5 mg/dl usually retain fertility. It is not uncommon therefore to encounter gravidas with preexisting renal disease resulting from primary renal disease or renal injury associated with systemic disorders. A recent retrospective study evaluated 82 pregnancies in 67 women with moderate and severe renal disease to assess maternal complications and pregnancy outcome during gestation and a 12-month

Table 18-2

	Cr <1.4 mg/dl*	Cr >1.4 mg/dl†	General Population in United States‡
Number pregnancies	121	82	
Preterm (<37 wk)	20%	59%	11%
Growth restriction (<10th percentile)	24%	37%	10%
Birth weight	2693 ± 878 g	2239 ± 839g	2800 g
Stillbirths	5%	5%	0.7%
Fetal deaths	2%	7%	0.7%
Neonatal deaths	4.9%	2%	0.7%
Infant survival	89%	91%	98.6%

*Kidney Int 18:192,1980.
†N Engl J Med 335:226, 1996.
‡Williams Obstetrics, ed 20. Stamford, CT, 1997, Appleton & Lange.

follow-up after delivery. Not surprisingly, adverse events were more commonly encountered when compared with women with mild renal disease. The incidence of hypertension in the third trimester (48% vs. 28%) and nephrotic syndrome (41% vs. 29%) are shown in Table 18-1 and were double the rate noted with mild renal disease. In addition, renal function was decreased during pregnancy and 6-weeks postpartum in nearly one half of this group and in many cases was irreversible. In 23% of this subgroup (10% of the total series) there was a rapid decline to end-stage renal failure within 6 months after delivery. The risk of a rapid decline in GFR was highest in patients with an initial antepartum serum creatinine of more than 2.0 mg/dl.

Obstetrical complications were also higher compared with women with mild renal disease, as shown in Table 18-2. Preterm delivery occurred in 59% of pregnancies and fetal growth restriction in 37%. Despite the high complication rate the overall fetal survival was 91%.

Most patients with renal insufficiency also exhibited hypertension. It has been difficult to determine whether the high rate of fetal growth restriction and preterm deliveries was related to hypertension per se or some factor specifically related to renal insufficiency. The National High Blood Pressure Education Program Working Group Report, published in 1990, indicated that women with chronic hypertension are at risk for preeclampsia, perinatal morbidity and death, and the possibility of deterioration of renal function and therefore suggested the continuation of antihypertensive agents if the diastolic pressure exceeds 100 mmHg, associated with systolic hypertension.

Since that report, however, new insights into the cause of the usual progressive loss in renal function in patients with renal insufficiency have markedly changed the attitude toward blood pressure control in patients with reduced renal function. Studies in experimental animals showed that in response to reduction in the number of surviving nephrons, there is a maladaptive hemodynamic change that results in glomerular capillary hypertension, which induces progressive renal injury. Subsequently, clinical trials in patients with chronic renal insufficiency demonstrated that the rate of decline of renal function can be markedly reduced by abolishing hypertension or attenuating its severity, suggesting that glomerular blood pressure can be modified by control of systemic blood pressure. Based on these findings in nonpregnant patients, it seems likely that gravidas with renal insufficiency and/or chronic hypertension would be at risk for accelerated renal injury if permitted to remain hypertensive during the course of pregnancy.

The Working Group Report also proposed continuation of successful antihypertensive therapy antedating pregnancy, except for angiotensin-converting enzyme (ACE) inhibitors and anti-receptor blockers (ARBs) because the latter are known teratogens. Methyldopa has been favored by the obstetrical community because of the proven demonstration of safety for the fetus. Unfortunately, this agent is not as potent as some of the newer categories of antihypertensive drugs. Although there is limited literature demonstrating safety, beta blocking agents, such as labetalol, and calcium channel blockers, such as nifedipine, are used widely and appear to be safe. Both categories of drugs can be used both orally and parenterally and therefore can be used for both outpatient management and for hypertensive crises.

Regarding mild or moderate transient hypertension in the third trimester, whether because of preeclampsia or some other condition, some latitude remains for individual decisions whether antihypertensive agents should be used. Recent reports, however, recall the observation that control of systolic blood pressure is important in patients with severe preeclampsia and eclampsia because of the risk of a hemorrhagic shock when systemic blood pressure exceeds 155 to 160 mmHg.

On the basis of these accounts of the course of pregnancy in women with preexisting primary renal disease, there is now better information on this group to assess risk for maternal complications and the likelihood of achieving a favorable pregnancy outcome. It should be remembered, however, that these data were derived from centers with high-risk pregnancy specialists and neonatal intensive care units. In women with mild renal insufficiency most complications were infrequent, except for the tendency for proteinuria to progress, then usually spontaneously remit after delivery. In addition, most pregnancy outcomes were successful, with a live birth rate of about 90%.

As could have been expected, the magnitude and frequency of significant maternal complications, often associated with severe hypertension, correlate with the severity of renal insufficiency in patients with moderate and severe renal disease. In most cases, the complications were not reversible. Although the infant survival was about 90%, the rate of preterm delivery and growth retardation was double the rate in women with mild renal disease and was associated with the well-known infant complications in infants born preterm and/or premature.

DIABETIC RENAL DISEASE

Type 1 diabetes begins in children and adolescents, and vascular complications often begin 8 to 12 years after the onset of disease. It is not surprising therefore that diabetic renal disease and other vascular complications are present in women during their reproductive years. Major recent advances have been made in diabetic pregnancies in general, at least in developed countries, such that there is now minimal maternal mortality, and fetal survival more closely approaches that of the general population, compared with the barely 50% survival in the early twentieth century. Obstetrical complications contribute to infant mortality and morbidity, however, in the forms of macrosomia, birth injuries related to shoulder dystocia, polyhydramnios, and major congenital anomalies. Because these complications are known to result from maternal hyperglycemia, which induces high levels of insulin, a growth hormone, efforts to control maternal blood glucose can prevent and/or reduce these metabolic-induced complications, especially if treatment begins in the early phase of gestation or ideally before conception.

The same success, however, has not extended to vascular complications that include retinopathy, nephropathy, and peripheral vascular disease. Several studies have been performed to delineate maternal complications and obstetrical outcome in women with diabetic renal disease. In two prominent reports involving about 60 patients, renal insufficiency was classified as mild or moderate severe. All patients had overt proteinuria and hypertension. Renal function worsened in approximately 40% during gestation and blood pressure increased in 30%. By the third trimester 70% of patients exhibited the nephrotic syndrome. Complications remitted in most patients after delivery and the long-term course was judged not to be different from the expected course if pregnancy had not occurred.

The perinatal outcome in women with diabetic renal disease is shown in Table 18-3, where it is compared with primary nondiabetic renal disease and the results from a large series of diabetic patients with nonproteinuric disease. Inspection of this table shows that the incidence of fetal death (6% to 7%), preterm delivery (24% to 26%), and growth-restricted infants (19% to 24%) was markedly different in the two groups with renal disease, compared with the group that had nondiabetic proteinuria, as with the incidence of perinatal survival (98% vs. 90%). In contrast, the presence of macrosomia, neonatal complications, and major genetic anomalies was largely confined to diabetic patients with or without renal disease.

Preconceptual evaluation of women with diabetes should stress the importance of normalization of blood glucose levels before conception and throughout gestation. In addition, optimal care requires facilities with a neonatal intensive care unit and a team of specialists to manage the obstetrical and medical complications in the mother.

Table 18-3

Comparison of Perinatal Outcome in Diabetics and Patients with Primary Renal Disease

	Diabetes	Diabetic Nephropathy	Nondiabetic Renal Disease
Number of pregnancies	232*	57[†]	121[‡]
Fetal death	0.4%	7%	6%
Preterm deliveries	4%	26%	20%
Small for gestational age	2%	19%	24%
Large for gestational age	40%	14%	5%
Major congenital anomalies	9%	9%	—
Neonatal Complications			
RDS	8%	23%	—
Death	3%	2%	5%
Perinatal survival	97%	91%	89%

RDS, Respiratory distress syndrome.
*Derived from *Am J Obstet Gynecol* 131:560, 1978.
[†]Derived from *Am J Obstet Gynecol* 141:741, 1981 and 159:56, 1988.
[‡]Derived from *Kidney Int* 181:192, 1980.

KEY POINTS

- Pregnancy induces major changes in the cardiovascular system. A different scale of values therefore should be used in determining normal renal function.
- The time when proteinuria is first noted, that is, before conception or before or after 20 weeks gestation, has critical importance in distinguishing renal disease from preeclampsia when proteinuria is present in the third trimester.
- In pregnancies associated with mild renal disease, maternal complications most often are mild and reversible, and pregnancy outcome is usually good. This is in contrast to patients with an initial serum creatinine greater than 2.0 mg/dl, who have a significantly worse prognosis.
- Complications in women with diabetic renal disease arise from the additive effects related to both renal disease and metabolic factors associated with diabetes.

SUGGESTED READINGS

Bader ME, Bader RA: Cardiovascular hemodynamics in pregnancy and labor. *Clin Obstet Gynecol* 11:924, 1968.

Baylis C: Relaxin may be the "elusive" renal vasodilatory agent of normal pregnancy. *Am J Kidney Dis* 34:1142; discussion 1144, 1999.

Davison JM, Hytten FE: Glomerular filtration during and after pregnancy. *J Obstet Gynaecol Br Commonw* 81:588, 1974.

Davison JM et al: Changes in the metabolic clearance of vasopressin and in plasma vasopressinase throughout human pregnancy. *J Clin Invest* 83:1313, 1989.

Fisher KA et al: Hypertension in pregnancy: clinical-pathological correlations and remote prognosis. *Medicine (Baltimore)* 60:267, 1981.

Fuhrmann K et al: Prevention of congenital malformations in infants of insulin-dependent diabetic mothers. *Diabetes Care* 6:219, 1983.

Katz AI et al: Pregnancy in women with kidney disease. *Kidney Int* 18:192, 1980.

Jones DC, Hayslett JP: Outcome of pregnancy in women with moderate or severe renal insufficiency [see comments] [published erratum appears in N Engl J Med 336:739, 1997]. *N Engl J Med* 335:226, 1996.

National High Blood Pressure Education Program Working Group report on high blood pressure in pregnancy. *Am J Obstet Gynecol* 163:1691, 1990.

Reece EA et al: Diabetic nephropathy: pregnancy performance and fetomaternal outcome. *Am J Obstet Gynecol* 159:56, 1988.

Sibai BM: Treatment of hypertension in pregnant women. *N Engl J Med* 335:257, 1996.

Studd JW, Blainey JD: Pregnancy and the nephrotic syndrome. *Br Med J* 1:276, 1969.

19

DIABETES AND PREGNANCY

Stephen F. Thung

Diabetes mellitus (DM), characterized by persistent hyperglycemia, is reaching concerning proportions in the United States. Seven percent of the population (20.8 million people) was diabetic in 2005; 3.3% of pregnancies are complicated by diabetes, and some high-risk populations have an incidence as high as 14%. With the increasing prevalence of obesity in the United States, the incidence of pregnancies complicated by diabetes has risen 40% from 1989 to 2002, highlighting the need for obstetricians experienced with diabetes care.

In the past, diabetes concurrent with pregnancy resulted in frequent miscarriage and stillbirth. Perinatal mortality exceeded 40% before insulin became available. Although care has progressed, these pregnancies remain at increased risk for both fetal and maternal adverse outcomes. Pregestational diabetes continues to be a significant risk factor for fetal congenital malformations. Persistent hyperglycemia during pregnancy remains an important contributor to the incidence of stillbirth, macrosomia, neonatal birth injury, and neonatal metabolic abnormalities. Fortunately, advances in diabetes management have made strict glycemic control possible and have significantly reduced the incidence of these adverse outcomes. A healthy mother and a healthy baby are now the expectation.

PHYSIOLOGY

Pregnancy is characterized by a multitude of changes that affect glucose homeostasis. On one hand, it is described as a state of *accelerated starvation* because of the increased metabolic needs of both fetus and mother. This results in a propensity to hypoglycemia in the fasting state. On the other hand, normal pregnancy is characterized by changes in the peripheral tissue response to insulin. Although pregnancy begins with a state of increased insulin sensitivity during the first trimester, the remainder of pregnancy is characterized as a *diabetogenic state* with reduced peripheral insulin sensitivity and compensatory hyperinsulinemia, a state similar to women with DM type 2. Increased insulin concentrations are observed with advancing gestation as a result of hyperplasia of the β-cells in the islets of Langerhans and in response to increasing peripheral insulin resistance. These changes are most pronounced in the third trimester. In normal pregnancy, glucose levels remain relatively unchanged.

In women with diabetes, a relative (gestational diabetes mellitus [GDM] or DM type 2) or absolute insulin deficiency (DM type 1) exists and available insulin is insufficient to compensate for the peripheral insulin resistance. The result is new-onset hyperglycemia in the previously euglycemic mother (GDM) or more profound hyperglycemia requiring increased insulin supplementation (DM types 1 and 2).

The control of maternal glucose metabolism shifts from the mother to the fetus/placenta. The mechanisms by which the placenta is able to reset the carbohydrate balance in the mother are unclear and involve the action of multiple placental- and fetal-derived hormones including human placental lactogen, progesterone, placental growth hormone, growth hormone, corticotropin-releasing hormone (CRH), cortisol, and leptin. These changes are likely designed to ensure a continuous supply of glucose for the developing fetus.

Glucose crosses the placenta to the fetus by facilitated diffusion. The Pedersen hypothesis implicates maternal hyperglycemia as responsible for subsequent fetal hyperglycemia. In turn, fetal pancreatic β cells secrete insulin and insulin-like growth factors. Fetal hyperinsulinemia ensues, resulting in an anabolic state and excessive fetal growth.

CLASSIFICATION

Diabetes may be classified as pregestational diabetes (DM) or gestational diabetes (GDM). The former is further classified as type 1 or type 2 depending on the absolute need for insulin therapy. Pregestational diabetes is present in 10% of pregnancies complicated by diabetes.

Gestational diabetes accounts for 90% of diabetes cases during pregnancy. It is diagnosed when hyperglycemia is identified for the first time during pregnancy and typically resolves after delivery, although 10% of cases may be undiagnosed pregestational diabetes. The prevalence is related to the population studied as well as the criteria used for defining the disease, ranging from 1% to 14%. Many features of GDM are similar to DM type 2, and the physiologic changes of pregnancy are thought to reveal an underlying predisposition for DM type 2. More than 50% of women with GDM will be diagnosed with overt diabetes within 20 years.

With respect to pregestational diabetes, DM type 2 is the more common, representing 90% to 95% of cases. It is commonly seen in older, obese, non-Caucasian women. The disease is familial. The disease is characterized by increased peripheral insulin resistance, a relative insulin deficiency, and serum insulin levels that are normal to high.

DM type 1 occurs less often and at a younger age. It is an autoimmune process resulting in the destruction of the insulin-producing β cells of Langerhans. Rather than a relative insulin deficiency with normal to high levels of insulin available (DM type 2), an absolute insulinopenia exists. Patients are dependent on exogenous insulin for survival and to prevent

White Classification

Table 19-1

Class	Age	Duration	Vascular Disease	Therapy
A	Any	During pregnancy	No	Diet
A2	Any	During pregnancy	No	Diet and hypoglycemic agents
B	>20yrs	<10 yr	No	Insulin
C	10-19 yr	10-19 yr	No	Insulin
D	Birth-10 yr	>20 yr	Benign retinopathy	Insulin
F	Any	Any	Nephropathy	Insulin
R	Any	Any	Proliferative retinopathy	Insulin
H	Any	Any	Heart disease	Insulin
T	Any	Any	Transplant	

diabetic ketoacidosis. Genetically predisposed individuals are at risk; however, monozygotic concordance for type 1 is less striking than type 2, less than 50%. Managing pregnant women with long-standing DM type 1 is the greatest challenge to the obstetrician because of a high prevalence of pre-existing medical disorders and the wide and less predictable changes in serum glucose throughout the day.

The White classification (Table 19-1), established by Priscilla White, often has been used to assess the severity of pregestational diabetes in pregnancy. Important prognostic factors such as the onset of diabetes, the duration of disease, and the degree of vasculopathy resulting from chronic hyperglycemia are used to assign a diabetes classification. A prospective study from Sweden demonstrated that perinatal morbidity risk increased with worsening diabetes according to the White classification. For example, preeclampsia occurred in 12% of pregnancies with class B DM and 54% with class F DM. In the days of suboptimal glycemic control, this system was useful because the duration of disease was closely related to vasculopathy, end-organ damage, and poor prognosis. Today the White classification is less commonly used. More relevant than disease onset and duration is the presence of vasculopathy and end-organ dysfunction such as hypertension, nephropathy, retinopathy, and coronary artery disease.

PREGESTATIONAL DIABETES

Diagnosis

The diagnosis is based on persistent hyperglycemia before or after pregnancy (Table 19-2). Screening for diabetes outside of pregnancy is accomplished by measuring either a fasting plasma glucose or glucose after a 2-hour, 75-g oral glucose tolerance test (2h-OGTT). It may also be diagnosed by a random plasma glucose level greater than 200 mg/dl when accompanied by signs and symptoms consistent with diabetes.

A fasting measurement greater than 126 mg/dl on two occasions is diagnostic for diabetes. Less than 100 mg/dl is considered normal, whereas a

Table 19-2

Classification	Normal (mg/dl)	Prediabetes (mg/dl)	Diabetes (mg/dl)
Random glucose with symptoms	—	—	>200
Fasting plasma glucose	<100	100-125	>126
2-hour, 75-g OGTT	<140	141-199	>200

From Diagnosis and classification of diabetes mellitus. American Diabetes Association 2007. *Diabetes Care* 30(Suppl 1):S42, 2007.
OGTT, Oral glucose tolerance test.

measurement between 100 and 125 mg/dl is considered "prediabetes" or impaired fasting glucose.

If using the 2h-OGTT, less than 140 mg/dl is considered a normal response, 141 to 199 mg/dl is "prediabetes" or impaired glucose tolerance, and more than 200 mg/dl is considered diagnostic for diabetes if confirmed on two occasions. Confirmatory testing may be deferred in women who have clear symptoms consistent with diabetes.

Women with "prediabetes" are at high risk for future diabetes and cardiovascular disease and should be screened annually. During pregnancy, these levels warrant further evaluation.

Maternal Considerations

Long-standing pregestational diabetes is associated with a host of concurrent maternal medical issues that may adversely affect the course of the pregnancy. Pregnancy rarely alters the long-term course of these conditions.

- *Diabetic retinopathy* is the most common cause of blindness in the United States and progresses from background disease to proliferative disease (neovascular changes on the retina), which ultimately results in blindness when untreated. Whether pregnancy accelerates this condition remains debated. Rapid glucose control, which commonly occurs after medical care is begun, may exacerbate disease in the short term. Therapy is managed with an ophthalmologist and consists of immediate laser photocoagulation when proliferative disease is present. It is important to impress on both patient and ophthalmologist that pregnancy is not a contraindication to therapy. All women who become pregnant with concurrent diabetes should have an ophthalmologic examination in the first trimester or before pregnancy if possible.
- *Nephropathy*, commonly defined as 500 mg/24 hours, exists in 5% to 10% of diabetic women who become pregnant. Mild to moderate disease has not been associated with permanent renal function decline. However, moderate to severe disease, a serum creatinine of more than 1.5mg/dl or proteinuria greater than 3 g per 24 hours has been associated with worsening renal dysfunction associated with pregnancy. Identifying nephropathy is important because of its association with adverse perinatal outcomes such as preeclampsia, fetal growth restriction, and worsening renal disease. Approximately 50% of women with class F diabetes develop preeclampsia. Renal function studies (serum creatinine, 24-hour urine protein) before pregnancy or at the first prenatal visit are warranted.

- *Chronic hypertension* is seen in 5% to 10% of women with diabetes. This finding is associated with an increased incidence of preeclampsia, growth restriction, and stillbirth. Methyldopa, calcium channel blockers, or beta blockers are typically used to control blood pressure. Angiotensin-converting enzyme (ACE) inhibitors are the ideal antihypertensive in the nonpregnant diabetic because of their renal protective effects. However, ACE inhibitors are contraindicated in pregnancy because of the increased risk for cardiovascular and central nervous system defects if exposure occurs in the first trimester and renal abnormalities in the second and third trimesters. They should be discontinued when conception is planned. A detailed anatomical survey may be performed if exposure to an ACE inhibitor has occurred in the first trimester.
- *Hypothyroidism* can be associated with DM type 1 in 5% to 40% of women. A thyroid-stimulating hormone (TSH) may be checked in all diabetic women who are pregnant or contemplating pregnancy.
- *Diabetes ketoacidosis* occurs in 1% to 3% of all diabetic pregnancies. Women with DM type 1 are at risk because of their insulin deficiency and increased insulin resistance during pregnancy. Risk factors include new infection, noncompliance with therapy, treatment with glycemic agents that cause hyperglycemia such as β-mimetic therapy (terbutaline), or corticosteroids (dexamethasone or betamethasone) for impending premature birth. Hyperglycemia resulting from these therapies may persist for as long as 5 days. Persistent acidemia may result in fetal compromise, and more than 20% of women will present with a fetal demise.

In general, the long-term prognosis of diabetes is unaffected by pregnancy. However, special attention should be paid to women with known moderate to severe diabetic nephropathy because renal dysfunction may be exacerbated by pregnancy and the decline in function may be permanent. A basic maternal evaluation for the first prenatal visit and follow-up visits is outlined (Box 19-1).

Box 19-1   **Assessment of the Pregestational Diabetic Mother**

First prenatal visit or preconception (pregestational diabetes)

- Baseline renal function assessment (serum creatinine, 24-hour urine protein, and creatinine clearance)
- Blood pressure
- Ophthalmologic consultation
- Baseline urine culture
- Hemoglobin A1c
- Electrocardiogram
- Thyroid-stimulating hormone
- Assessment of exercise tolerance and coronary heart disease

Second and third trimester
- Urine culture
- Hemoglobin A1c
- Reassessment of renal status
- Frequent blood pressure check every 1-2 weeks

Pregnancy Considerations

Managing pregestational diabetes during pregnancy is a tremendous undertaking. Adverse fetal, neonatal, and maternal outcomes are well established. These may be mitigated by preconception counseling and early glycemic control, strict glycemic control throughout the pregnancy and during delivery, and appropriate management of associated end-organ maternal disease. An understanding of these issues is critical for counseling and managing these pregnancies appropriately.

The adverse outcomes associated with pregestational diabetes were illustrated by Hanson and Persson, who evaluated a cohort of women with DM type 1. The study demonstrated an increased risk of preeclampsia, preterm birth, macrosomia, stillbirth, and perinatal mortality (Table 19-3) beyond baseline risks in a normal pregnancy.

- *Preeclampsia* is seen with increased frequency, especially in the presence of hypertension and nephropathy. The incidence has been estimated at 15% to 20% without and 40% to 50% with nephropathy. Proteinuria of more than 500 mg per 24 hours is clearly associated with an increased preeclampsia risk compared with women without proteinuria. Whether proteinuria between 190 and 499 mg per 24 hour poses an increased risk remains unclear.
- An increased *first trimester spontaneous abortion* risk has been attributed to hyperglycemia in multiple studies. This risk increases with higher levels of hemoglobin A1c (HbA1c) and may be reduced with periconceptional glycemic control. The risk of spontaneous abortion was 12.4% with first-trimester HbA1c less than or equal to 9.3% and 37.5% with HbA1c greater than 14.4%.
- The rate of *preterm birth* is increased in women with pregestational diabetes. Both medically indicated (21.9% vs. 3.4%) and spontaneous preterm births (16.1% vs. 10.5%) contribute to this observation. Increased risks of preeclampsia, comorbid medical problems, and poor glycemic control are factors for indicated preterm birth. The etiology for spontaneous preterm birth risk remains a mystery.
- *Congenital anomalies* are the leading contributor to perinatal mortality in pregestational diabetic pregnancies with an incidence of 6% to 12% and a mortality rate as high as 40%. Persistent hyperglycemia during organogenesis (weeks 5 to 8) is teratogenic, and glycosylated

Table 19-3

Outcomes in Percent of Pregnancies Complicated by Type 1 Diabetes Compared with National Data in Sweden (1983-1985)

Factor	Type 1 Diabetes (n = 491)	National Data (n = 279,000)	p Value
Preeclampsia	21%	5%	<0.001
Preterm birth	25%	6%	<0.001
Macrosomia	20%	4%	<0.001
Growth restriction	1%	3%	<0.05
Stillbirths	2%	0.4%	<0.01
Perinatal mortality	3%	0.7%	<0.0001

Adapted from Hanson U, Persson B: Outcome of pregnancies complicated by type 1 insulin dependent diabetes in Sweden: acute pregnancy complications, neonatal mortality and morbidity. *Am J Perinatol* 10(4): 330-3, 1993, with permission.

hemoglobin levels correlate with the incidence of congenital birth defects. A normal HbA1c is associated with a 2% to 3% risk, whereas an HbA1c level of 10% has been associated with a 20% to 25% risk. Cardiac, central nervous system, and musculoskeletal defects are the most common. Conditions such as caudal regression are highly associated with hyperglycemia but are vanishingly rare. Maternal serum alpha-fetoprotein (AFP) screening, a targeted anatomical survey by ultrasound, and fetal echocardiography may be used to identify many of these congenital birth defects. Preconception counseling and achieving euglycemia before conception and through the first trimester are the best methods of prevention.

- *Stillbirth* was a significant problem before the wide availability of insulin. Before modern antenatal surveillance, a strategy of preterm delivery was used because many of the stillbirths occurred late in the third trimester, after 36 weeks' gestation. The etiology of stillbirth remains unclear. Some losses are the result of maternal acidemia resulting from diabetic ketoacidosis (DKA). In cases without DKA, a combination of fetal hyperinsulinemia and chronic hypoxia has been implicated. Hyperinsulinemia may result in increased fetal metabolic rates and oxygen requirements. In the setting of vasculopathy and subsequent placental insufficiency, the ability to compensate for increased metabolic demands may be compromised and a state of chronic hypoxia results. Serial nonstress testing and/or biophysical profiles are performed beginning at 32 to 36 weeks' gestation depending on the severity of diabetes and the quality of glycemic control.

- The most common problem that diabetic women face is *excessive fetal growth (macrosomia)* and therapy for diabetes revolves around prevention. Various definitions of fetal macrosomia are used: birth weight greater than 4000 g, birth weight greater than 4500 g, or birth weight greater than 90%. Macrosomia rates are high in women with gestational and pregestational diabetes, approximately 20% to 50%, compared with 10% in nondiabetic pregnancies. Neonates of mothers with diabetes have increased fat proportions and proportionally larger shoulders and abdominal circumferences than in nondiabetics. This disproportion predisposes to *shoulder dystocia* and *birth injury.* Risk of shoulder dystocia is as high as 5% to 23.1% over 4000 to 4500 g and from 20% to 50% if greater than 4500 g. The American College of Obstetricians and Gynecologists (ACOG) suggests that a discussion about the mode of delivery be initiated when the fetal weight is estimated to be greater than 4500 g.

- *Polyhydramnios* is commonly associated with diabetes and is thought to be associated with fetal polyuria resulting from hyperglycemia. It may be associated with discomfort and preterm contractions.

- *Neonatal metabolic alterations* are often identified. Neonatal hypoglycemia occurs rapidly after delivery. Fetal hyperinsulinemia and maternal hyperglycemia at the time of delivery place the fetus at risk. Maternal euglycemia during labor minimizes this risk and the intrapartum goal is to maintain glucose levels at 80 to 100 mg/dl. Hypocalcemia and hypomagnesemia are also commonly noted neonatal complications of unknown etiology. Polycythemia, hyperbilirubinemia, and subsequent jaundice are frequent neonatal issues, possibly because of chronic hypoxia in utero.

A multitude of potential obstacles to a successful pregnancy are faced by women with diabetes during pregnancy. A suggested outline for the maternal surveillance of these pregnancies is found in Box 19-1 and a suggested outline for fetal surveillance is found in Box 19-2.

Management

Achieving Glycemic Control

The management of diabetes revolves around strict glycemic control. Lifestyle changes, attention and adherence to a judicious diet, and hypoglycemic therapy when diet fails to correct hyperglycemia are all integral to optimal care. The physiologic changes (see physiology section) during pregnancy make glycemic control difficult, with wide swings between hypoglycemia and hyperglycemia, especially in women with DM type I. Because insulin resistance increases with each trimester, there is greater potential for higher postprandial glucose excursions and an invariable need to increase insulin requirements.

Glucose Monitoring

Self-monitoring of blood glucose should be conducted before breakfast and 1 or 2 hours after breakfast, lunch, and dinner (postprandial). The use of postprandial levels rather than preprandial levels to guide therapy has been associated with improved outcomes including lower risk for macrosomia, neonatal hypoglycemia, and lower cesarean delivery for labor dystocia. Premeal glucose levels may be obtained in addition to postprandial levels in more difficult to control cases. The optimal level of glycemic control has not been established, though persistent fasting glucose levels greater than 105 mg/dl has been associated with an increased risk for third-trimester stillbirth.

Box 19-2 Antenatal Surveillance of Pregnancy Requiring Hypoglycemic Therapy

First trimester
- First-trimester ultrasound to establish reliable gestational age

Second trimester
- Maternal serum alpha-fetoprotein from 15-20 weeks because of increased risk of neural tube defects
- Targeted ultrasound at 18-20 weeks to identify congenital defects
- Fetal echocardiography (if available) to identify congenital heart defects

Third trimester
- Ultrasonography for fetal growth every 4-6 weeks after 24 weeks' gestation
- Antenatal surveillance (nonstress tests or biophysical profile) once or twice per week beginning at 32-36 weeks (depending on duration of disease and degree of control)

The following targets are recommended (ACOG):

Fasting goal	<95 mg/dl
Premeal goal (if used)	<100 mg/dl
1-hour postprandial goal	<130-140 mg/dl
2-hour postprandial goal	<120 mg/dl
Glycosylated A1c	<6%

The American Diabetes Association (ADA) agrees that glycemic control must be strict and suggests the following goals:

Preprandial	<105 mg/dl
1-hour postprandial	<155 mg/dl
2-hour postprandial	<130 mg/dl

Glycosylated hemoglobin, a marker of long-term glycemic control over 6 to 8 weeks, may be monitored. A hemoglobin A1c of 6% is roughly similar to an average glucose of 120 mg/dl, with each 1% increase associated with an average 30 mg/dl elevation. HbA1c levels may be measured intermittently at least once every trimester. The goal is to achieve levels less than 6%, especially in the periconception period, when elevations above 6% have been associated with an increased frequency of congenital birth defects.

Diet

The objective of dietary therapy is to control fasting and postprandial glucose levels, to support adequate maternal and fetal nutrition, and to prevent ketosis. There are increased calorie requirements during pregnancy, typically 300 kcal higher than prepregnancy. Average-weight women will require 30 to 35 kcal/kg/day. Women who are underweight may require 30 to 40 kcal/kg/day, whereas those who are overweight (>120% ideal body weight) may require fewer. Patients should be referred to a dietician familiar with the unique needs of pregnancy.

Caloric composition recommendations are as follows:

- 40% to 50% from complex carbohydrates
- 20% from protein
- 30% to 40% from unsaturated fats

Each meal should provide the following:

- Breakfast 10% to 20% of the daily calories
- Lunch 20% to 30%
- Dinner 30% to 40%
- Snacks distributed throughout the day (especially before bedtime) 30%

Pharmacologic Therapy

Women with pregestational diabetes typically require insulin to maintain euglycemia throughout pregnancy. Beginning and optimizing hypoglycemic therapy is based on fasting and postprandial glycemic control after an appropriate diet is established. Validated criteria for diet failure do not exist and most practitioners use a persistent elevated fasting more than 95 to 105 mg/dl, 1-hour postprandial more than 130 to 140 mg/dl, or 2-hour postprandial more than 120 mg/dl as indications for therapy.

Insulin is used to control hyperglycemia and maintain levels below goals. A combination of rapid-acting (Lispro) or short-acting (Regular) with an intermediate-acting insulin (NPH) accomplishes this in most cases (Table 19-4).

Rapid- or short-acting insulin given before meals reduces glucose excursions from meals. Although a rapid-acting insulin or short-acting insulin may both be used before meals, administration differs because of the onset of action. Regular insulin is given 30 minutes before a meal is planned and rapid-acting insulin is given at the commencement of a meal, a potential compliance advantage. Lispro is commonly used in place of regular insulin. It does not significantly cross the placenta.

Long-acting (glargine) and intermediate acting (NPH) insulins are intended to prevent hepatic gluconeogenesis between meals and during the fasting state. In the nonpregnant state, glargine is commonly given in conjunction with short- or rapid-acting insulin. However, there remains insufficient experience with glargine to demonstrate its safety during pregnancy. Increased mitogenic activity found during in vitro studies causes concern about potential fetal effects. Retrospective studies examining glargine demonstrate uncomplicated neonatal outcomes to date.

Insulin requirements vary considerably among women, although they predictably increase through gestation. Typical insulin needs are as follows:

First trimester: 0.7 to 0.8 U/kg/day
Second trimester: 0.8 to 1 U/kg/day
Third trimester: 0.9 to 1.2 U/kg/day

Many women with diabetes are using insulin before they become pregnant. For those not already taking insulin, a total insulin requirement may be estimated by weight. The greatest experience is with a combination of NPH and Regular insulin. Lispro may be substituted for Regular insulin, as long as attention is paid to the onset of action. Multiple regimens have been used, with no evidence available that any are superior. A three-injection regimen is easy and commonly used as a starting point. Two thirds of the total estimated dose is given before breakfast. This is divided into two thirds intermediate acting and one third short- or rapid-acting insulin. The evening dose is given before dinner and is one third of the total. NPH and

Table 19-4

Commonly Used Insulins

Type	Onset of Action	Peak Action	Duration of Action
Lispro	1-15 min	1-2 hr	4-5 hr
Aspart	1-15 min	1-2 hr	4-5 hr
Regular	30-60 min	2-4 hr	6-8 hr
NPH	2 hr	6-10 hr	18-28 hr
Glargine	1 hr	None	24 hr

Box 19-3 Example of Insulin Dosing

- 70-kg woman in second trimester
- 70 kg × 0.8 U/kg/day   56 units total per day
- Two-thirds (56) of total insulin in AM   38 units total for AM
  - NPH dose is two thirds of AM dose (38)   26 units NPH
  - Regular/Lispro dose is one third of AM dose (38)   12 units Regular/Lispro
- One third (56) of total insulin in PM   18 units total for PM
  - NPH dose is one half of total PM dose (18)   9 units NPH
  - Regular/Lispro dose is one half of PM dose (18)   9 units Regular/Lispro

---

short/rapid-acting insulins are given in equal parts. Commonly the NPH in the evening is delayed to bedtime to achieve euglycemia throughout the night and into the morning. See Box 19-3 for an example.

Because hypoglycemic episodes may result in significant untoward side effects, we use the weight-based insulin requirements as a guideline rather than a rule. We follow glucose measurements for 3 days to 1 week before initiation of insulin, identifying which portion of the day is associated with consistent hyperglycemic episodes. Insulins are begun at half the calculated weight-based dose and targeted to cover periods of hyperglycemia. Insulins are increased rapidly to obtain euglycemia.

Continuous subcutaneous insulin infusion (insulin pump) is an effective therapy typically used by endocrinologists in the management of highly motivated and knowledgeable patients with DM type 1. It may be used as an alternative to insulin injections and is dosed to mimic physiologic insulin. A basal insulin infusion is accompanied by boluses before meals. Experience with the pump suggests that excellent glucose control may be obtained with the insulin pump. However, there has been no demonstrated advantage during pregnancy over multiple insulin injections. Patients who reduce their oral intake are at risk of hypoglycemic episodes.

Antepartum Surveillance

The many potential effects of pregestational diabetes reviewed in detail throughout this chapter merit a comprehensive evaluation of both mother (Box 19-1) and fetus (Box 19-2). In most cases, recommendations are based on expert opinion rather than prospective studies.

GESTATIONAL DIABETES

Diagnosis   The optimal method for screening pregnant women for gestational diabetes is unclear and is based on committee opinions.

Who Should Be Screened?

Options include *universal screening* (all patients), which is thought to have the highest sensitivity and highest cost, versus *risk-based screening*, which defers screening for women who are at the lowest risk for GDM. In practice, more than 90% of clinicians use universal screening because risk-based screening adds a layer of complexity impractical for the typical busy obstetrical practice without significant cost savings.

The U.S. Preventive Services Task Force (USPSTF) has found insufficient evidence to make a recommendation. The ADA and ACOG support the choice of the practitioner to use either universal or risk-based screening.

The first prenatal visit should include a risk assessment for GDM to determine the extent of a patient's risk (Box 19-4).

Average Risk

These individuals have neither high- nor low-risk characteristics that are described later. In this group, routine screening should be offered at 24 to 28 weeks' gestation.

High Risk

These women are obese (body mass index [BMI] >30), have a personal history of previous GDM (33% to 50% recurrence), or a strong family history of first-degree relatives with diabetes. Because of the high risk of undiagnosed pregestational diabetes, screening before conception or at the first prenatal visit may be performed. This is particularly true if they have not recently been screened for diabetes. If screening is negative, it should be repeated between 24 and 28 weeks' gestation because gestational diabetes may develop later in pregnancy. Repeat screening may also be initiated if signs or symptoms consistent with hyperglycemia are identified.

Low Risk

Both ACOG and the ADA agree that universal screening for GDM is the most sensitive approach but also acknowledge that omitting GDM screening is acceptable in low-risk women. Interestingly, only 10% of women undergoing pregnancy satisfy these criteria in most obstetrical practices. A woman who is deemed low risk should have all the characteristics listed in Box 19-5.

How to Screen for Gestational Diabetes

The standard screening approach in the United States begins with a 50-g 1-hour glucose challenge test (GCT) at 24 to 28 weeks' gestation followed by a 100-g 3-hour oral glucose tolerance test (3h-OGTT) for women who test

---

Box 19-4 Risk Factors for Diabetes during Pregnancy

- Age >25 years
- Obesity
- History of impaired glucose tolerance or impaired fasting glucose
- Child with birth weight >9 or <6 pounds
- Family history of diabetes
- Member of higher-risk ethnic group
- Previous unexplained child with congenital malformation
- Use of medications such as corticosteroids or antiretroviral medications for human immunodeficiency virus (HIV) infection

> **Box 19-5**   Criteria for Women at Low Risk for Gestational Diabetes
>
> - Age < 25 years
> - Body mass index (BMI) <25
> - No history of gestational diabetes mellitus (GDM) or abnormal glucose homeostasis
> - No first-degree family history of diabetes
> - Not a member of a high-risk ethnic group
> - No history of poor obstetrical outcome

positive on the GCT. Timing of testing is arbitrary, balancing the increased identification of GDM with later testing and the time available for potential intervention.

There is no universally accepted standard for the diagnosis of GDM. The GCT and 3h-OGTT screening thresholds are somewhat arbitrary and were initially developed to identify women at risk of developing diabetes in later life rather than to diagnose GDM. Although all thresholds proposed are predictive of macrosomia, no randomized studies have demonstrated the superiority of any given threshold.

The GCT is a random test, and fasting is not required. Two thresholds have been recommended: a 130 mg/dl cutoff with 90% sensitivity and a 25% test positive rate or 140 mg/dl with 80% sensitivity and 15% test positive rate. Either threshold is acceptable.

Women who fail the 50-g GCT then undergo a 3-hour 100-g OGTT. A fasting glucose measurement followed by measurements at 1 hour, 2 hours, and 3 hours after ingesting the 100 g of glucose load is required. At least two values of the four must be exceeded to make the diagnosis of GDM. One should be aware that even one elevated value is associated with an increased incidence of macrosomia and birth injury. The ADA recommends use of the Fourth International Diabetes Data Group criteria (Carpenter and Coustan criteria) for diagnosing GDM, whereas ACOG states that either the Fourth International Diabetes Data Group or the National Diabetes Data Group criteria may be used (Table 19-5).

Pregnancy Implications

The clinical significance of gestational diabetes is debated, although GDM is associated clearly with *fetal macrosomia, birth injury,* and *neonatal metabolic alterations* when persistent hyperglycemia is present. These risks are similar to those of women with pregestational diabetes (see Pregestational Diabetes: Implications to Pregnancy). Furthermore, women may be predisposed to

Table 19-5

Alternative Criteria for Diagnosis of Gestational Diabetes

	Fourth International Diabetes Data Group	National Diabetes Data Group
Fasting	95 mg/dl	105 mg/dl
1 hour	180 mg/dl	190 mg/dl
2 hour	155 mg/dl	165 mg/dl
3 hour	140 mg/dl	145 mg/dl

develop hypertensive disorders and stillbirth, although these complications have not been well established. Congenital defects, miscarriage, and significant maternal vasculopathy are not significant risks. One should be aware that an estimated 10% of women with undiagnosed DM type 2 are diagnosed during pregnancy and erroneously receive the diagnosis of GDM. These women remain at risk for the fetal and maternal complications associated with pregestational diabetes.

Management

Achieving Glycemic Control

In most cases, women with GDM may be euglycemic with diet alteration alone. Fifteen percent require pharmacologic support. Insulin is considered the standard of care for glycemic control (see Pregestational Diabetes: Achieving Glycemic Control).

Rationale for Therapy

For gestational diabetes, a recent randomized trial (Crowther 2005) comparing women with diagnosed and treated GDM and women with untreated GDM demonstrated that glycemic control using dietary counseling, blood glucose monitoring, and insulin for persistent hyperglycemia improves neonatal outcomes. Care for the intervention group included blood glucose monitoring four times daily and maintaining fasting glucose less than 99 mg/dl and 2-hour postprandial levels less than 126 mg/dl. The primary outcome of the study (serious perinatal injury) was a composite of: death, shoulder dystocia, bone fracture, and nerve palsy. The intervention group had a lower incidence of this composite outcome than routine care (4% to 1%). There was a reduction in the diagnosis of macrosomia (21% to 10%) but an increase in intensive care unit (ICU) admissions (61% to 71%). Induction of labor was increased with a GDM diagnosis (from 29% to 39%) with no increase in the cesarean delivery rate.

Oral Hypoglycemic Agents: Glyburide

Although insulin has been the standard for gestational diabetes with persistent hyperglycemia, glyburide is becoming more widely accepted among obstetricians.

Glyburide, a second-generation sulfonylurea that does not significantly cross the placenta, bypasses the disadvantages of insulin treatment, which include patient discomfort, inconvenience, and expense. Glyburide enhances insulin secretion.

A randomized trial (Langer 2001) compared insulin with glyburide and found neonatal outcomes to be similar. There were no differences in mean maternal blood glucose, frequency of large-for-gestational-age infants, neonatal respiratory complications, neonatal hypoglycemia, and length of neonatal intensive care unit (NICU) stays. Glyburide was not identified in neonatal cord blood immediately after delivery. Approximately 82% of women who require treatment for hyperglycemia will achieve good control with glyburide, slightly lower than that of insulin (88%). Risk factors for failing glyburide include: pregestational diabetes, advancing maternal age, multiparity, obesity, and high fasting glucose measurements.

Current contraindications to glyburide therapy include DM type 1, significant hepatic or renal impairment, and warfarin (Coumadin; Bristol-Myers Squibb, Princeton, New Jersey) use. Women with a known adverse reaction to sulfonamides, sulfonylurea, carbonic anhydrase inhibitors, thiazides, or loop diuretics should not be prescribed glyburide. Pregestational DM type 2 may be a relative contraindication because failure seems to be more likely to occur in these women. For women who are not tolerating oral feeding, glyburide should be discontinued because of the risk for hypoglycemia.

After the patient fails diet modification to achieve euglycemia, glyburide is begun at starting dose of 2.5 mg orally every morning, 30 minutes before breakfast or with the meal. An additional 2.5 mg may be added if adequate control is not achieved within 3 to 7 days. If euglycemia is not achieved at 5 mg/day, increases of 5 mg may be made to a maximal dose of 20 mg/day. Many clinicians split the dose, every 12 hours. These additions may be added to an evening dose, rather than the morning dose, depending on the clinical scenario. The onset of action is between 15 and 60 minutes with peak action at 4 hours. Insulin is substituted for glyburide if control is not obtained with maximal glyburide dosing.

The ADA and the ACOG caution against glyburide use until more research is completed. Regardless, increasing numbers of physicians are using it as a first-line treatment in women who have mildly elevated glucose levels.

Oral Hypoglycemic Agents: Metformin

Unlike glyburide, metformin is known to cross the human placenta, which has reduced enthusiasm for its use during pregnancy. Metformin reduces peripheral insulin resistance. Insulin is a potent growth factor and there is theoretical concern that this action in the fetus may result in excessive fetal growth. Regardless of these concerns, metformin exposure during the first trimester is commonly witnessed because of its use in anovulatory women with polycystic ovarian syndrome (PCOS) who subsequently begin to ovulate and become pregnant. Multiple small retrospective studies have demonstrated no adverse outcomes with first-trimester metformin exposure. However, the ADA and ACOG recommend against its routine use during pregnancy and suggest switching patients to insulin when pregnancy is discovered and if hyperglycemia is a concern. There are no studies to demonstrate that metformin is as effective as insulin when managing GDM.

Antepartum Surveillance

Unlike pregestational diabetes, the risks to the fetus and mother in diet-controlled gestational diabetes (A1) are small. With the exception of a third-trimester evaluation of fetal growth, little additional evaluation is usually required. Antenatal surveillance is commonly initiated beyond 40 weeks' gestation.

The patient with gestational diabetes requiring insulin (A2) may be at an increased risk for adverse outcomes and stillbirth. Antenatal surveillance by nonstress testing or biophysical profile similar to women with pregestational diabetes is begun between 32 and 36 weeks' gestation, depending on the clinical scenario. Fetal growth is assessed at or near term (Box 19-2).

Postpartum Considerations

Unfortunately, postpartum diabetes screening is commonly overlooked in this high-risk group. More than 50% of women with GDM will subsequently develop type 2 diabetes over 20 years of follow-up. The highest-risk women are those with elevated fasting glucose levels throughout gestation and those that require insulin.

A 2-OGTT, 75-g glucose load is recommended at the time of the postpartum visit, 6 to 8 weeks after delivery. The criteria for postpartum diabetes testing are the same as screening the nonpregnant woman. A fasting glucose greater than 126 mg/dl or a 2-hour more than 200 mg/dl on two occasions is diagnostic for diabetes if confirmed at later date or if there are symptoms consistent with overt diabetes (Table 19-2). Those with persistent diabetes require ongoing care with a primary care physician or an endocrinologist.

The ADA suggests diabetes screening every 3 years in women with previous GDM and normal screening and annually for women with borderline testing consistent with "prediabetes."

INTRAPARTUM CARE

Macrosomia

Women with any form of diabetes are more likely to produce a fetus with excess central fat deposition, making shoulder dystocia more likely. Whether diabetes is gestational or pregestational, in light of increasing risk for shoulder dystocia with increasing fetal weight, cesarean may be offered if fetal weight is estimated beyond 4500 g. Induction for suspected macrosomia has not been demonstrated to reduce birth injury or cesarean delivery rate. *"Impending" or "suspected" macrosomia is not an indication for labor induction.*

Timing of Delivery

The optimal time for delivery is not clear. Because there is no increased risk of stillbirth in diet-controlled gestational diabetes, most experts will allow pregnancies to progress to 41 weeks' gestation with reassuring antenatal surveillance beginning at 40 weeks.

Insulin-requiring diabetic pregnancies may progress to their due date if good glycemic control is maintained. Most experts would recommend against expectant management beyond this time. Induction of labor at 39 weeks with a favorable cervix is common practice. In poorly controlled patients, delivery before 39 weeks may be considered after fetal lung maturity is assured by amniocentesis.

Intrapartum Care

During labor, maternal euglycemia is critical to prevent neonatal hypoglycemia. When the patient is made NPO for active labor, receives insulin, or when glucose measurements fall below 70 mg/dl, 5% dextrose at 100 to 150 ml/hour may be initiated to prevent hypoglycemia. Glucose levels are monitored every 1 to 2 hours and are controlled with short-acting insulin to keep physiologic levels at approximately 80 to 100 mg/dl.

Insulin should be given intravenously as boluses or by continuous insulin drip after maternal glucose levels exceed 140 mg/dl or earlier. An insulin drip is titrated based on glucose measurements and commonly is started at 1 to 2 units of short-acting insulin per hour. Insulin infusion rate is altered based on subsequent glucose levels. As an example, insulin infusion may be increased by 1 unit/hour if glucose is more than 140 mg/dl or decreased by 1 unit/hour if glucose is less than 80 mg/dl.

Elective Cesarean Section

For insulin/glyburide-requiring women undergoing elective cesarean section, NPH insulin/glyburide may be given the night before. Morning insulin or glyburide is held before admission. On arrival to the labor and delivery unit, a continuous infusion of insulin and glucose is used.

POSTPARTUM CARE

28.

Hypoglycemic Agents

Insulin requirements fall after the placenta is delivered. After the patient with pregestational diabetes has begun eating, insulin may be restarted at one half of the predelivery dose and titrated further as needed in subsequent days. For women with gestational diabetes, insulin or glyburide may not be required at all.

Contraception

In the woman with gestational or pregestational diabetes there are no absolute contraindications to any of the available contraceptive methods. Progestin-only contraception such as Depo-Provera (Pfizer, New York, New York) and the levonorgestrel intrauterine device (IUD) have little effect on glucose levels and may be offered. Although there is theoretical risk for increased infection with the intrauterine device and diabetes, this finding has yet to be demonstrated. Combined oral contraception is safe in most women with diabetes. However, it may not be appropriate in women with significant vasculopathy because of the risks for venous thrombosis and stroke.

Breast Feeding

Breast feeding is encouraged after delivery. Caloric intake should be increased by 500 kcal/day from prepregnancy levels.

PRECONCEPTION COUNSELING

Pregestational Diabetes

For women with pregestational diabetes, preconception counseling is the most effective prevention of diabetes-related congenital birth defects and spontaneous abortion. Counseling and euglycemia at conception reduces the risk of spontaneous abortion and congenital birth defects. Unfortunately, only one third of women take advantage of preconception counseling and 60% of pregestational diabetic women will have suboptimal glycemic control at conception. An insulin regimen that reduces HbA1c levels to a normal level and avoids hyperglycemia before and after meals should be the goal before conception (see Pregestational Diabetes: Achieving Glycemic Control).

A baseline evaluation for vasculopathy and end-organ dysfunction should be initiated before conception if not recently performed. The basic elements of preconception evaluation are similar to that of a first prenatal visit for a pregestational diabetic woman (Box 19-1). At least 400 μg/day of folate may be prescribed because of the increased risk for central nervous system defects in diabetic pregnancies.

History of Gestational Diabetes

For women with a history of GDM, the recurrence risk in subsequent pregnancies is 30% to 50% and the long-term risk for overt diabetes is more than 50%. These women may be screened for diabetes before conception if they did not receive postpartum screening, if that postpartum screening result was consistent with "prediabetes," or if a normal diabetes screen was more than 3 years ago. If found to have overt diabetes, these women should be treated as other women with pregestational diabetes (see previous).

KEY POINTS

- Diabetes mellitus (DM) is a condition characterized by persistent hyperglycemia.
- 3.3% of pregnancies are complicated by diabetes; 90% of these pregnancies are complicated by gestational diabetes.
- Normal pregnancy is a diabetogenic state characterized by increasing insulin resistance and hyperinsulinemia. Gestational diabetes is thought to be an unmasking of a predisposition to DM type 2. Greater than 50% of women with GDM will develop overt diabetes in 20 years.
- Pregestational diabetes
  a. Early hyperglycemia (pregestational diabetes) is teratogenic and is associated with an increased incidence of congenital fetal anomalies and first-trimester pregnancy loss. The risk may be reduced by preconception counseling and early glycemic control.
  b. Comorbid medical problems (hypertension, nephropathy, retinopathy) are commonly associated with pregestational diabetes and these should be assessed early in pregnancy.
  c. Pregestational diabetes during pregnancy is associated with multiple perinatal complications including preeclampsia, polyhydramnios, macrosomia, and stillbirth.
  d. Glycemic control using diet and insulin is associated with improved outcomes including reduced perinatal loss, macrosomia, and congenital abnormalities.
- Gestational diabetes
  a. Universal or risk-based screening for gestational diabetes is acceptable.
  b. Screening for gestational diabetes occurs between 24 and 28 weeks in average-risk women. Women who are at high risk for diabetes are screened at the first prenatal visit or a preconception visit. If negative, high-risk women are screened again at 24 to 28 weeks.

KEY POINTS—cont'd

    c. A 1-hour glucose challenge test (GCT) is the initial screening test. Using a threshold of 130 mg/dl or 140 mg/dl is acceptable.

    d. A 3-hour glucose tolerance test (OGTT) is the diagnostic test for gestational diabetes. Two values out of four must be above the predetermined thresholds.

    e. Macrosomia is the most common complication associated with hyperglycemia and the risk is reduced with strict glycemic control.

    f. Insulin is the standard therapy for women who fail diet control, although glyburide is becoming more often used.

    g. Postpartum diabetes screening is important to identify women who develop overt diabetes after pregnancy.

- Cesarean delivery may be considered if the estimated fetal weight is greater than 4500 g.
- Suspected macrosomia is not an indication for induction of labor.
- Intrapartum glycemic control is important to reduce the incidence of neonatal hypoglycemia.
- Peripheral insulin resistance drops after the delivery of the placenta and requirements for postpartum hypoglycemic therapy are reduced and sometimes eliminated.
- Postpartum screening for women with gestational diabetes will identify women with overt diabetes.

285

SUGGESTED READINGS

ACOG Committee on Practice Bulletins: ACOG Practice Bulletin. Clinical Management Guidelines for Obstetrician-Gynecologists. Number 30, 2001, Gestational diabetes. *Obstet Gynecol* 98:525, 2001.

ACOG Committee on Practice Bulletins: ACOG Practice Bulletin. Clinical Management Guidelines for Obstetrician-Gynecologists. Number 60, 2005. Pregestational diabetes mellitus. *Obstet Gynecol* 105:675, 2005.

Crowther CA et al: Australian Carbohydrate Intolerance Study in Pregnant Women (ACHOIS) Trial Group: Effect of treatment of gestational diabetes mellitus on pregnancy outcomes. *N Engl J Med* 352:2477, 2005.

Cunningham FG et al: *Williams Obstetrics*, ed 21. New York, 2006, McGraw-Hill.

Diagnosis and classification of diabetes mellitus. American Diabetes Association 2007. *Diabetes Care* 30:S42, 2007.

Gabbe SG, Graves CR: Management of diabetes mellitus complicating pregnancy. *Obstet Gynecol* 102:857, 2003.

Greene MF et al: First-trimester hemoglobin A1 and risk for major malformation and spontaneous abortion in diabetic pregnancy. *Teratology* 39:225, 1989.

Hanson U, Persson B: Outcome of pregnancies complicated by type 1 insulin-dependent diabetes in Sweden: acute pregnancy complications, neonatal mortality and morbidity. *Am J Perinatol* 10:330, 1993.

Langer O et al: A comparison of glyburide and insulin in women with gestational diabetes mellitus. *N Engl J Med* 343:1134, 2000.

U.S. Preventive Services Task Force. Screening for gestational diabetes. In: *Guide to Clinical Preventive Services*, ed 2. Washington, 1996, Office of Disease Prevention and Health Promotion, pp 193-208.

20

INFECTIOUS DISEASES IN PREGNANCY

Karlijn Woensdregt, Hee Joong Lee, and Errol R. Norwitz

Infectious diseases remain a leading cause of maternal and neonatal mortality during pregnancy, labor, and the puerperium. In the United States alone, despite a fivefold reduction in the last 50 years, pregnancy-related maternal mortality rate remains at approximately 9 per 100,000 live births, with infections still accounting for 3% to 10%.

Although profound changes are observed in the immune system during pregnancy, it remains unclear whether pregnant women are generally more susceptible to infection. Pregnancy does complicate the management of infectious diseases because of concerns regarding fetal well-being and the effect of pregnancy on antimicrobial agents. For example, pregnancy profoundly alters drug pharmacokinetics because of changes in drug absorption, volume of distribution, and metabolism and elimination of drugs. In addition, if the fetus is exposed during the critical period of embryogenesis (days 17-54 postconception), certain infections are teratogenic (Table 20-1).

The most common pregnancy and puerperal infections result from ascending contamination of the uterine cavity from the lower genital tract flora and include such conditions as intraamniotic infection (also referred to as chorioamnionitis), urinary tract infection and pyelonephritis, postpartum endometritis, and (rarely) pelvic inflammatory disease. Such infections are often polymicrobial in nature, involving both aerobic and anaerobic organisms. In addition to polymicrobial infectious conditions, specific infections occur in pregnant women as they do in their nonpregnant counterparts. Because of the overwhelming diversity of these infections, a discussion of the obstetric implications of every infection is not possible. As such, a series of tables summarizing the prevention (Table 20-2) and management (Tables 20-3 and 20-4) of infections in pregnancy have been included. Several infections have been singled out for further discussion, including a review of the causative organisms, modes of transmission, maternal and fetal effects, and recommendations for counseling and management.

Table 20-1

Infections with
Known Teratogenic
Effects

Infection	Effects	Comments
Cytomegalovirus	Hydrocephaly, microcephaly, chorioretinitis, microphthalmos, cerebral calcifications, intrauterine growth restriction, mental retardation, deafness.	Most common congenital infection. Congenital infection occurs in 40% of cases after primary infection during pregnancy and in 14% of cases after recurrent infection. Of infected infants, physical effects are present in 20% after primary infection and 8% after secondary infection. No effective therapy exists.
Rubella	Microcephaly, mental retardation, cataracts, deafness, congenital heart disease. All organ systems may be affected.	The rate of permanent organ damage is 50% if the infection is acquired during the first trimester; 6% if infection occurs in mid-pregnancy. Immunization of nonpregnant adults and children is necessary for prevention. Although the live attenuated virus vaccine has not been shown to cause the malformations of congenital rubella syndrome, immunization is not recommended during pregnancy.
Syphilis	Effects range from hydrops fetalis, fetal demise (if infection is severe) to detectable abnormalities of skin, teeth, and bones (if infection is mild).	Penicillin treatment is effective to prevent progression of damage. Severity of fetal damage depends on duration of fetal infection (damage is worse if infection is diagnosed >20 weeks). Prevalence is increasing.
Toxoplasmosis	All organ systems may be affected. Most common manifestations include chorioretinitis and other central nervous system effects (microcephaly, hydrocephaly, cerebral calcifications). Severity of manifestations depends on duration of disease.	Low prevalence during pregnancy (0.1%-0.5%). Initial maternal infection must occur during pregnancy to place fetus at risk. *Toxoplasma gondii* is transmitted to humans by raw meat or exposure to infected cat feces. The incidence of fetal infection increases as gestational age increases (9%-10% in first trimester; 60% in the third trimester). However, the severity of congenital infection is greater in the first trimester than at the end of gestation.
Varicella	May affect all organ systems. Common manifestations include skin scarring, chorioretinitis, cataracts, microcephaly, hypoplasia of the hands and feet, muscle atrophy.	Overall risk of congenital varicella is low (around 2%-3%) and occurs most commonly between 7 and 21 weeks' gestation. Varicella zoster immune globulin should be administered to newborns exposed in utero during the last 4 to 7 days of gestation. No adverse effect from herpes zoster.

Adapted from Norwitz ER, Schorge JO: *Obstetrics and gynecology at a glance,* 2nd ed. Oxford, 2006, Blackwell Science Ltd, p. 98.

Table 20-2

Infection (Causative Organism)	Primary Therapy	Alternative Therapy	Comments
Postpartum endometritis	Cefazolin 1 g IV × 1 dose OR Ampicillin 1-2 g IV × 1 dose OR Clindamycin 600-900 mg IV and gentamicin 1.5 mg/kg IV × 1 dose		Prophylaxis should be administered preoperatively to women at high risk. Once-daily dose of gentamicin has not been validated for efficacy or safety during pregnancy and in the puerperium. Other aminoglycosides may be substituted for gentamicin (Aztreonam is effective but is expensive and is therefore reserved for women with renal insufficiency). The American Heart Association does not recommend antibiotic prophylaxis for cesarean delivery or normal vaginal delivery, with the possible exception of high-risk women for whom it is optional.
Bacterial endocarditis (primary against enterococci)	Ampicillin 2 g IM/IV and gentamicin 1.5 mg/kg IM/IV within 30 min of delivery PLUS Ampicillin 1 g IM/IV or amoxicillin 1 g po × 1 dose within 6 hr of delivery	Vancomycin 1 g IV over 1-2 hr and gentamicin 1.5 mg/kg IM/IV within 30 min of delivery (no post-delivery dose)	
Pyelonephritis (mainly *Escherichia coli*)	Nitrofurantoin 50-100 mg po each night before bedtime OR Sulfisoxazole 500 mg po each night before bedtime		Consider antibiotic suppression after acute pyelonephritis or recurrent UTI in pregnancy, and in women at high-risk for UTI/pyelonephritis.
Group B streptococcus (GBS)	Penicillin G 5 million units IV loading dose, followed by 2.5 million units IV q4h	Ampicillin 2 g IV loading dose, followed by 1-2 g q4-6h OR Clindamycin 600 mg IV q6h or 900 mg IV q8h OR Erythromycin 500 mg IV q6h	Intrapartum—but not antepartum—chemoprophylaxis against GBS has been shown to decrease early-onset neonatal GBS sepsis.

Continued

Table 20-2—cont'd

Infection (Causative Organism)	Primary Therapy	Alternative Therapy	Comments
Genital herpes simplex virus (usually HSV-2)	Acyclovir 200 mg po qid from 35-36 weeks' gestation to delivery (not postpartum) OR Acyclovir 400 mg po bid from 35-36 weeks' gestation to delivery (not postpartum)	Famciclovir 250 mg po bid OR Valacyclovir 250 mg po bid OR Valacyclovir 500 mg po daily OR Valacyclovir 1 g po daily	Suppression therapy reduces the frequency of recurrences by ~75% in patients with ~6 recurrences/year. Goal of suppression is to decrease the incidence of HSV prodrome and/or genital lesion in labor that would necessitate cesarean delivery. Suppression may be offered to women with first-episode genital HSV infection during the index pregnancy or frequent recurrence.
Sexual assault (*Chlamydia trachomatis, Neisseria gonorrhoeae, Trichomonas vaginalis*)	Ceftriaxone 125 mg IM × 1 dose PLUS Metronidazole 2 g po × 1 dose PLUS Azithromycin 1 g po × 1 dose or doxycycline 100 mg po bid × 7 days	For alternative treatments, refer to sections in this table that specifically address alternative therapeutic options for each of the potential infectious agents under consideration.	Hepatitis B vaccine should be administered with follow-up at 1-2 and 4-6 months after first dose. Testing for HIV and possible antiretroviral prophylaxis should be considered.

Adapted from 1998 Recommendations by the Centers for Disease Control and Prevention.
bid, Twice daily; *HSV*, herpes simplex virus; *IM*, intramuscular; *IV*, intravenous; *po*, per os; *qid*, four times a day; *UTI*, urinary tract infection.

BACTERIAL INFECTIONS

Intraamniotic Infection (IAI)

IAI (chorioamnionitis) refers to the infection of amniotic fluid, fetal membranes, or placenta. The incidence of IAI varies from 0.5% to 10.5% of all deliveries depending on the definition used (histologic evidence of IAI, a positive amniotic fluid culture, or clinical criteria such the presence of fever and uterine tenderness). IAI is associated with one third of all cases of preterm labor with intact membranes and 40% to 75% of patients with preterm premature rupture of the fetal membranes (PPROM). The main cause of IAI is a bacterial infection with either aerobes (*Streptococcus agalactiae, Escherichia coli, Staphylococcus aureus*) or anaerobes (*Gardnerella vaginalis, Bacteroides fragilis*).

Treatment of Sexually
Transmitted Diseases
in Pregnancy*

Table 20-3

Infection (Causative Organism)	Primary Therapy	Alternative Therapy	Comments
Bacterial vaginosis (BV) (*Proteus* species, *Mobiluncus* species, *Mycoplasma hominis*, *Gardnerella vaginalis*)	Metronidazole 250 mg po tid × 7 days	Metronidazole 2 g po × 1 dose OR Clindamycin 300 mg po bid × 7 days OR Metronidazole gel (0.75%) one applicator full (5 g) intravaginally bid × 5 days (recommended for low-risk pregnant women only)	BV is associated with adverse perinatal outcome, including low birth weight and preterm birth. Pregnant women with symptomatic BV should be treated. It remains unclear whether screening/treatment of asymptomatic women improves perinatal outcome. Lower dose of metronidazole is recommended to reduce risk to fetus. Clindamycin vaginal gel is not recommended (may be associated with an increase in preterm delivery).
Chancroid (*Haemophilus ducreyi*)	Azithromycin 1 g po × 1 dose OR Ceftriaxone 250 mg IM × 1 dose OR Erythromycin base 500 mg po qid × 7 days		Exclude HSV, *T. pallidum*. Consider HIV screening (erythromycin is recommended for HIV+ women). Ciprofloxacin is an alternative treatment but is contraindicated in pregnancy.
Chlamydial infections (*Chlamydia trachomatis*)	Erythromycin base 500 mg po qid × 7 days OR Amoxicillin 500 mg po tid × 7 days	Erythromycin base 250 mg po qid × 14 days OR Erythromycin ethylsuccinate 800 mg po qid × 7 days OR Erythromycin ethylsuccinate 400 mg po qid × 14 days OR Azithromycin 1 g po × 1 dose	Erythromycin estolate, doxycycline, and ofloxacin are contraindicated in pregnancy. There is insufficient data to recommend the routine use of azithromycin in pregnancy. Repeat cultures 3 weeks after therapy has been completed because of the high rate of noncompliance and the lower efficacy of erythromycin treatment regimens.

Continued

Table 20-3—cont'd

Infection (Causative Organism)	Primary Therapy	Alternative Therapy	Comments
Gonococcal infections (Neisseria gonorrhoeae)	Cefixime 400 mg po × 1 dose OR Ceftriaxone 125 mg IM × 1 dose PLUS A regimen effective against possible concomitant infection with C. trachomatis: Erythromycin base 500 mg po qid × 7 days OR Amoxicillin 500 mg po tid × 7 days OR Azithromycin 1 g po × 1 dose OR Doxycycline 100 mg po × 7 days	Spectinomycin 2 g IM × 1 dose OR Ceftizoxime 500 mg IM × 1 dose OR Cefotaxime 500 mg IM × 1 dose OR Cefotetan 1 g IM × 1 dose OR Cefoxitin 2 g IM × 1 dose with probenecid 1 g po × 1 dose	Azithromycin 2 g po single dose is effective but expensive, and causes GI upset (1 g dose is ineffective). In pregnancy, quinolones (ofloxacin, ciprofloxacin, lomefloxacin, enoxacin, norfloxacin) and tetracycline are contraindicated. If cephalosporins cannot be tolerated, treat with spectinomycin 2 g IM × 1 dose. For disseminated gonococcal infection, treat in hospital setting with ceftriaxone 25-50 mg/kg/day IM/IV daily × 7 days OR cefotaxime 25 mg/kg IM/IV bid × 7 days (up to 10-14 days if meningitis is documented).
Genital herpes simplex virus (usually HSV-2)	**First Clinical Episode of Genital Herpes** Acyclovir 400 mg po tid × 7-10 days or until clinically resolved OR Acyclovir 200 mg po 5×/day × 7-10 days or until clinically resolved OR Famciclovir 250 mg po tid × 7-10 days or until clinically resolved OR Valacyclovir 1 g po bid × 7-10 days or until clinically resolved **Recurrent Clinical Episodes of Genital Herpes** Acyclovir 400 mg po tid × 5 days OR Acyclovir 200 mg po 5×/day × 5 days OR Acyclovir 800 mg po bid × 5 days OR Famciclovir 125 mg po bid × 5 days OR Valacyclovir 500 mg po bid × 5 days **Disseminated Herpes** Acyclovir 5-10 mg/kg IV q8h × 5-7 days		Topical acyclovir is less effective than oral treatment and is discouraged. First clinical episode during pregnancy may be treated with acyclovir. Safety of valacyclovir and famciclovir in pregnancy is not well established, but benefits may outweigh risks. Treatment must be initiated during prodrome or within 1 day of onset of lesions for patient to experience benefit from therapy.

Table 20-3—cont'd

Infection (Causative Organism)	Primary Therapy	Alternative Therapy	Comments
Genital warts (human papillomavirus [HPV])	Cryotherapy with cryoprobe or liquid nitrogen OR Trichloroacetic acid (TCA) 80%-90%, apply only to warts. Use powder with talc or baking soda to remove unreacted acid. Repeat weekly if necessary. OR Surgical removal	Intralesional interferon OR Laser surgery	Imiquimod, podofilox, and podophyllin are contraindicated in pregnancy. As such, therapy during pregnancy is severely limited. No therapy has been shown to eradicate or affect the natural history of HPV. If lesions persist after one type of treatment, other therapies should be considered. Genital warts are not a contraindication to vaginal birth but may bleed excessively at delivery.
Pubic lice (Pediculosis pubis)	Permethrin 1% cream rinse, applied to affected areas and wash off after 10 min OR Pyrethrins with piperonyl butoxide, applied to affected areas and washed off after 10 min		Lindane 1% shampoo is not recommended for use in pregnant or lactating women. Toxicity related to prolonged lindane exposure includes seizures and aplastic anemia. Decontaminate clothing and bedding or remove from body contact for at least 72 hours. Fumigation is not necessary. Evaluate and retreat in 1 week if symptoms persist or lice observed. Treat sexual partners.
Scabies (Sarcoptes scabiei)	Permethrin cream (5%), applied to all areas of the body from the neck down and washed off after 8-14 hr	Sulfur (6%) precipitated in ointment, applied thinly to all areas nightly for 3 consecutive nights; wash off previous application before applying new ones. Wash off thoroughly 24 hours after the last application.	Lindane is not recommended in pregnant or lactating women. Decontaminate clothing and bedding. Pruritus may persist for several weeks. Consider retreatment after 1 week if still symptomatic. Both sexual and close personal and household contacts within the preceding month should be examined and treated. Scabies among children is generally not sexually transmitted. Treatment of entire populations may be required to control scabies epidemics.

Continued

Table 20-3—cont'd

Infection (Causative Organism)	Primary Therapy	Alternative Therapy	Comments
Trichomonas (Trichomonas vaginalis)	Metronidazole 2 g po × 1 dose	Metronidazole 500 mg po bid × 7 days	Metronidazole is not recommended in the first trimester. If treatment fails, consider 375-500 mg bid × 7 day regimen. If repeated failure, consider 2 g daily × 3-5 days.
Syphilis† (Treponema pallidum)	**Primary/Secondary/Early Latent Syphilis** Benzathine penicillin G, 2.4 million units IM × 1 dose (usually administered as 1.2 million units into each buttock). Some experts recommend a second dose of penicillin for such women 1 week after the initial dose **Late Latent/Tertiary/Unknown Duration** Benzathine penicillin G, 2.4 million units IM/week × 3 weeks (7.2 million units total) **Neurosyphilis** Aqueous crystalline penicillin G, 12-24 million units IV daily (administered as 2-4 million units IV q4h) × 10-14 days OR Aqueous procaine penicillin G, 2.4 million units IM daily plus probenecid 500 mg po qid × 10-14 days		Routine screening for syphilis at first prenatal visit. High-risk women should be screened again at 28 weeks and at delivery. All women with syphilis should be offered HIV testing. Penicillin is effective in preventing transmission to and established infection in fetuses. Women treated in the second half of pregnancy are at risk for preterm labor, possibly because of Jarisch-Herxheimer reaction. If pregnant patient with syphilis is penicillin allergic, desensitize and treat with penicillin. Doxycycline and tetracycline are contraindicated in pregnancy. Erythromycin cannot be relied on to treat the infected fetus. Insufficient data on azithromycin or ceftriaxone.

*Adapted from 1998 Recommendations by the Centers for Disease Control and Prevention. (Rayburn WF: Treatment of sexually transmitted diseases. *J Reprod Med* 43:471-6, 1998.)
†Adapted from Centers for Disease Control: 1998 guidelines for treatment of sexually transmitted diseases. *MMWR* 47:28, 1998.
bid, Twice daily; *GI*, gastrointestinal; *HIV*, human immunodeficiency virus; *HSV*, herpes simplex virus; *IM*, intramuscular; *IV*, intravenous; *po*, per os; *qid*, four times a day; *tid*, three times a day.

The diagnosis of IAI relies most commonly on clinical features; specifically, the presence of maternal tachycardia, fetal tachycardia, maternal fever, and/or uterine tenderness or evidence of pus emanating from the cervix. Although several indirect diagnostic tests are available (e.g., amniotic fluid Gram stain, glucose concentration, white blood cell count, leukocyte esterase level, and cytokine measurements), such tests have relatively low sensitivity and specificity. The gold standard for the diagnosis of IAI remains an amniotic fluid culture obtained by amniocentesis. The association between amniotic fluid culture and histologic evidence of chorioamnionitis remains unclear.

Treatment of Other
Infections in
Pregnancy

Table 20-4

Infection (Causative Organism)	Primary Therapy	Alternative Therapy	Comments
Asymptomatic bacteriuria (primarily *Escherichia coli*; also *Klebsiella/Enterobacter* sp, *Proteus* sp, Group B streptococcus, enterococci)	Nitrofurantoin macrocrystals 50-100 mg po qid × 3 days OR Nitrofurantoin monohydrate 100 mg po bid × 3 days OR Cephalexin 250-500 mg po qid × 3 days	Ampicillin 250-500 mg po qid × 3 days OR Amoxicillin 250-500 mg po tid × 3 days OR Trimethoprim/sulfamethoxazole 160 mg/180 mg po bid × 3 days OR Trimethoprim 200 mg po bid × 3 days OR Sulfisoxazole 2 g loading dose po followed by 1 g po qid × 3 days	Complicates 2%-9% of pregnancies. Consider treatment when 25,000-100,000 colony-forming units/ml of a single pathogenic organism are found in a clean-catch midstream urine specimen. Single-dose treatment is effective but has a higher failure rate; a 3-day course is usually recommended. Obtain a follow-up culture 7-10 days after completion of treatment.
Pyelonephritis (mainly *E. coli*)	Ampicillin 1-2 g IV q6h and gentamicin 1.5 mg/kg q8h OR Ceftriaxone 1-2 g IM/IV q24h	Trimethoprim/sulfamethoxazole 160 mg/800 mg IV q12h OR Gentamicin 1.5 mg/kg q8h	Treat IV until asymptomatic and afebrile for 24-48 hours, followed by oral antibiotics to complete 10 days of therapy. After acute treatment, obtain a follow-up culture in 7-10 days, place on prophylactic therapy, and perform periodic screening.

Continued

295

Table 20-4—cont'd

Infection (Causative Organism)	Primary Therapy	Alternative Therapy	Comments
Intraamniotic infection (mainly Group B streptococcus, *E. coli*)	Ampicillin 2 g IV q4-6h and gentamicin 1.5 mg/kg IV q8h intrapartum OR Penicillin 2.5-5 million units q4-6h and gentamicin 1.5 mg/kg IV q8h intrapartum PLUS Clindamycin 900 IV q8h OR Metronidazole 500 mg IV q8h added after delivery only if delivery is by cesarean	Ampicillin/ sulbactam 3 g IV q6h OR Cefotetan 2 g IV q12h OR Cefoxitin 2 g IV q6h OR Cefotaxime 25 mg/kg IM/IV q12h PLUS Clindamycin 900 IV q8h OR Metronidazole 500 mg IV q8h added after delivery only if delivery is by cesarean	Intraamniotic infection remains a clinical diagnosis (fetal tachycardia, uterine tenderness and contractions, maternal tachycardia, and fever). Amniotic fluid culture remains the gold standard for diagnosis; Gram stain is only 50% sensitive. Delivery should be expedited, irrespective of gestational age. Following delivery, antibiotic coverage should probably be continued. If delivery is by cesarean, antibiotic coverage should also be broadened (clindamycin is preferred over metronidazole for lactating women).
Postpartum endometritis (polymicrobial infection with both anaerobes and aerobes)	Clindamycin 900 mg IV q8h and gentamicin 1.5 mg/kg IV q8h with or without ampicillin 1-2 g IV q4-6h or penicillin 2.5-5 million units IV q4-6h	Cefotetan 2 g IV q12h OR Cefoxitin 2 g IV q6h OR Cefotaxime 1-2 g IM/IV q6-8h OR Piperacillin 3-4 g IM/IV q4-6h OR Ampicillin/ sulbactam 3 g IV q6h	Treatment should be continued until the patient has been asymptomatic and afebrile for 24-48 hours. Around 10% of patients will not be cured with initial therapy. Approximately 20% of treatment failures are because of resistant organisms. Women who do not respond within 48-72 hours often have another source of fever (drug fever, wound infection, septic pelvic thrombophlebitis, infected hematoma, abscess, retained products of conception).

Table 20-4—cont'd

Infection (Causative Organism)	Primary Therapy	Alternative Therapy	Comments
Vulvovaginal candidiasis (*Candida albicans* and other *Candida* species, *Torulopsis* species, or other yeasts)	Butoconazole 2% cream 5 g intravaginally × 3 days OR Clotrimazole 1% cream 5 g intravaginally × 7-14 days OR Clotrimazole 100 mg vaginal tablet × 7 days OR Clotrimazole 100 mg vaginal tablet, two tabs × 3 days OR Clotrimazole 500 mg vaginal tablet × 1 dose OR Miconazole 2% cream 5 g intravaginally × 7 days OR Miconazole 200 mg vaginal suppository, 1 dose × 3 days OR Miconazole 100 mg vaginal suppository, 1 dose × 7 days OR Tioconazole 6.5% ointment 5 g intravaginally × 1 dose OR Terconazole 0.4% cream 5 g intravaginally × 7 days OR Terconazole 0.8% cream 5 g intravaginally × 3 days OR Terconazole 80 mg suppository, 1 dose × 3 days		In pregnancy, topical azole products should be used rather than nystatin. Most effective are butoconazole, clotrimazole, and terconazole; 7-day regimens are preferred. Oral agents such as ketoconazole (100 mg po single dose) and fluconazole (150 mg po single dose) may be as effective as topical agents, but potential toxicity and drug interactions must be considered. Treatment of sexual partners has not been shown to decrease frequency of recurrences.
Malaria (*Plasmodium falciparum, P. vivax, P. malariae, P. ovale*)	Chloroquine 1 g po × 1 dose; then 500 mg at 6, 24 and 48 hr; then weekly until delivery PLUS Proguanil 200 mg po qd	Quinine 650 mg po tid × 3-7 days PLUS Sulfadoxine/ pyrimethamine 3 tablets × 1 dose on day 3 of treatment	Malaria is the major cause of fetal growth restriction worldwide. Primaquine should not be used in pregnancy because the drug crosses the placenta and can cause hemolytic anemia in a glucose-6-phosphate dehydrogenase (G6PD) deficiency. Cerebral malaria should be treated with IV quinine gluconate.

Continued

Table 20-4—cont'd

Infection (Causative Organism)	Primary Therapy	Alternative Therapy	Comments
Listeriosis (*Listeria monocytogenes*)	Ampicillin 1-2 g IV q6h and gentamicin 1.5 mg/kg IV q8h	Trimethoprim/sulfamethoxazole 160 mg/800 mg IV q12h OR Erythromycin 500-2000 mg IV q6h	The best length of therapy is not known. Treat IV until asymptomatic and afebrile for 24-48 hours. Consider prompt delivery if listeria amnionitis is confirmed.
Pelvic inflammatory disease (PID) (*Neisseria gonorrhoeae, Chlamydia trachomatis, Gardnerella vaginalis,* etc.)	**Regimen A** Cefoxitin 2 g IV q6h OR Cefotetan 2 g IV q12h PLUS Doxycycline 100 mg po bid × 14 days total **Regimen B** Clindamycin 900 mg IV q8h PLUS Gentamicin 2 mg/kg IV/ IM loading dose then 1.5 mg/kg maintenance dose q8h PLUS Doxycycline 100 mg po bid × 14 days total or clindamycin 450 mg po qid × 14 days total	Ampicillin/sulbactam 3 g IV q6h and doxycycline 100 mg IV/po q12h OR Azithromycin 500 mg IV × 2 days followed by 500 mg po × 10 days	PID in pregnancy is very rare. All pregnant women with PID should be hospitalized and treated with IV therapy. Quinolones (ciprofloxacin, ofloxacin) are contraindicated in pregnancy. Treatment may be discontinued 24 hours after clinical improvement. When tubo-ovarian abscess is present, surgery may be required and clindamycin may be preferred for continued therapy. Other second- and third-generation cephalosporins may be effective, but clinical data are limited.

Table 20-4—cont'd

Infection (Causative Organism)	Primary Therapy	Alternative Therapy	Comments
Tuberculosis (*Mycobacterium tuberculosis*)	**Positive PPD/No Active Disease** Isoniazid 300 mg po daily after delivery for 6-9 months OR Isoniazid 300 mg po daily after first trimester for 6-9 months (for high-risk women, including recent seroconversion, recent immigrant, known recent TB contact, immunocompromised women, skin test >15 mm and not previously treated) **Active Disease** Isoniazid 300 mg po daily × 9-12 months PLUS Rifampin 600 mg po daily × 9-12 months PLUS/OR Ethambutol 2.5 g (15 mg/kg) po daily × 9-12 months or until sensitivity of the AFB culture returns PLUS Pyridoxine 50 mg po daily × 9-12 months		Isoniazid prophylaxis should be avoided in the puerperium because of the high incidence of hepatic toxicity. In pregnancy, drugs such as kanamycin, streptomycin, capreomycin (congenital deafness), ethionamide (teratogenic), and cycloserine (CNS side effects) are contraindicated in pregnancy. Pyrazinamide may be used in place of ethambutol, but this approach is not generally recommended because there are limited data on pyrazinamide use in pregnancy.

Adapted from 1998 Recommendations by the Centers for Disease Control and Prevention.
AFB, Acid-fast bacillus; *bid*, twice daily; *CNS*, central nervous system; *IM*, intramuscular; *IV*, intravenous; *po*, per os; *PPD*, purified protein derivative; *qid*, four times a day.

Treatment for IAI should be initiated immediately with administration of intravenous ampicillin and gentamicin or alternative antibiotics with a similar spectrum. If the causative organism is known, the spectrum can be narrowed. In addition to antibiotics, urgent delivery is usually indicated. Delay in delivery may lead to maternal sepsis.

Group B Streptococcus

Group B β-hemolytic streptococcus (GBS), or *Streptococcus agalactiae*, is a gram-positive commensal organism that intermittently colonizes the lower genital tract of 20% (range, 15%-40%) of women at any one time. Although most pregnant women with genital tract colonization are asymptomatic,

GBS can cause clinical infections such as urinary tract infections, amnionitis, endometritis, sepsis, or even meningitis. Intrapartum maternal GBS colonization poses a significant risk of early-onset GBS disease in the newborn, which remains one of the most common causes of life-threatening perinatal infections in the United States. Recent studies have shown a substantial decline in the incidence of early-onset GBS disease in term newborns to approximately 0.5 per 1000 live births.

GBS infection can be acquired in utero or, more commonly, during passage through the colonized birth canal. Half of all infants born to women colonized with GBS will themselves become colonized with GBS, but the vast majority will be asymptomatic. Early-onset neonatal GBS infection, which accounts for 80% to 85% of all cases, is characterized by neonatal respiratory distress, apnea, pneumonia, and septic shock within 1 week of life, although most cases are apparent within 12 hours of birth. Confirmed by a positive blood culture, the infection has an overall mortality rate of 5% (but may be as high as 25% among preterm infants) with surviving neonates often exhibiting significant long-term neurologic sequelae. By contrast, late-onset GBS infection usually results from community- or hospital-acquired (nosocomial) infections in preterm infants and presents as meningitis or sepsis after 1 week and up to 3 months after birth.

A number of strategies have been proposed to prevent early-onset GBS infection, including intrapartum maternal and postpartum neonatal antibiotic regimens. However, such antibiotic use has been associated with the emergence of antibiotic resistance and with maternal anaphylaxis (estimated as 1:60,000 for penicillin). Because of these limitations, routine administration of GBS chemoprophylaxis is not recommended for all women in labor. Instead, the American College of Obstetricians and Gynecologists (ACOG) and the Centers for Disease Control and Prevention (CDC) in the United States suggest that a culture-based protocol be followed. This involves intrapartum prophylaxis of women who are known GBS carriers. To predict carrier status in labor, GBS cultures should be sent as late as possible during pregnancy, but before the onset of labor (ideally, 35-37 weeks' gestation), to accurately reflect GBS carrier status at delivery. GBS status should not be determined at the first prenatal visit because of an estimated 8% to 10% crossover of GBS carrier status during each trimester. The culture-based protocol results in treatment of 15% to 20% of pregnant women and prevention of 70% to 80% of GBS disease.

If a woman presents in labor with an unknown GBS carrier status, it is recommended that a *risk factor-based protocol* be used. Such a patient should receive intrapartum GBS chemoprophylaxis if one or more risk factors are present, including preterm labor, PPROM, prolonged rupture of membranes (≥18 hours regardless of gestational age), a prior GBS-infected infant, maternal fever in labor (≥100.4° F), and GBS bacteriuria or urinary tract infection at any time during the index pregnancy.

Should the decision to proceed with intrapartum GBS chemoprophylaxis be made, a number of general guidelines should be followed. Intravenous penicillin G, instead of ampicillin, is the antibiotic of choice because of a narrower spectrum and reduced likelihood of leading to antibiotic resistance. A minimum of 4 hours of antibiotic prophylaxis is recommended, with discontinuance at delivery.

Listeria

Listeria monocytogenes is a facultative anaerobic, gram-positive rod that can cause listeriosis, an alimentary infection resulting from the ingestion of contaminated food such as unpasteurized milk, uncooked meat, soft cheeses, and uncooked vegetables. Listeriosis mostly affects newborns and the elderly; however, 25% of all infections occur during pregnancy. This may be due to a decrease in T-cell-mediated immunity, the major defense against listeriosis, during pregnancy.

Approximately two thirds of pregnant women with listeriosis will present with flulike symptoms, and one third will experience gastrointestinal symptoms, particularly diarrhea. Maternal fever followed by preterm labor (especially in the setting of an abnormal fetal heart rate tracing and "fetal distress" in labor) or in utero fetal demise has been associated with *Listeria*. Intrauterine infections during pregnancy are believed to occur through hematogenous dissemination at the time of maternal septicemia; however, ascending infection from the lower genital tract or perirectal area may also be responsible. Following transplacental infection, the amniotic fluid typically turns bright green and can easily be confused with meconium. The newborn may present with GBS-like symptoms, erythematous skin lesions, microabscesses in the liver or spleen, or meningitis. Confirmation of the diagnosis requires isolation of *L. monocytogenes* from maternal or neonatal blood, fetal membranes, gastric aspirates, amniotic fluid, and placental tissue. Placental histology with evidence of microabscesses and a distinct multifocal villitis can also suggest the diagnosis following delivery.

Adverse pregnancy outcomes from listeriosis may occur at any gestational age, and perinatal mortality has been estimated to range from 20% to 50%. In Europe, *Listeria* has been reported to account for 0.5% to 3% of all cases of spontaneous abortion and preterm labor. When *Listeria* infection is suspected, prompt initiation of antibiotic therapy may improve perinatal survival. Although the best antibiotic regimen has not been identified by clinical trials, parenteral ampicillin with gentamicin is usually given (see Table 20-4). Trimethoprim/sulfamethoxazole and erythromycin are also effective. Neonates should be treated aggressively with broad-spectrum antibiotics, although the ideal length of therapy is unknown. Perinatal outcome is determined primarily by the gestational age at delivery and complications related to prematurity.

Tuberculosis

Tuberculosis (TB) refers to infection with *Mycobacterium tuberculosis*. After declining steadily for three decades, the number of cases of maternal and fetal TB reported annually in the United States began to rise again in the 1980s because of increases in both human immunodeficiency virus (HIV) infections and multi-drug-resistant strains. Although there is no apparent increase in TB progression during or immediately after pregnancy, most infected parturients are symptomatic and convert to a positive response to purified protein derivative (PPD) skin testing.

Diagnosing TB can be difficult. Pregnant women considered to be at high-risk for TB (including women with symptoms suggestive of TB, known recent exposure, seroconversion within the past 1-2 years, immunocompromised patients, and recent immigrant status) should be skin tested. Skin testing involves intradermal injection of 5 tuberculin units of PPD and measurement of the induration (not erythema) in 48 to 72 hours. Interpretation of the PPD test depends on the risk status of the patient and is not affected by pregnancy. A positive reaction requires further investigation to exclude active disease, which includes a chest x-ray (usually a single anteroposterior view with abdominal shielding in pregnancy), submission of early morning sputum specimens for smear and culture if symptoms are present, and appropriate biopsy specimens if there is evidence of extrapulmonary disease. Although the demonstration of acid-fast bacilli (AFB) raises the possibility of TB, subsequent culture confirmation is mandatory because sputum may contain strains of nontuberculous *Mycobacterium*.

Therapy of active TB does not change in pregnancy. For latent (asymptomatic) TB, isoniazid is usually given with pyridoxine for nine months, and may be initiated during pregnancy. For active TB, a two-drug regimen, usually isoniazid (with pyridoxine) and rifampin, should be used for a minimum of 9 months. Isoniazid may be hepatotoxic, so the patient should be aware of signs of jaundice. Some experts suggest periodic liver function tests and assessment of baseline liver function before starting therapy. Ethambutol should be added if there is potential isoniazid resistance. Although rifampin crosses the placenta and may theoretically cause fetal injury through inhibition of DNA-dependent RNA polymerases, no such damage has been reported. Isoniazid and ethambutol have been shown to be safe as well. Streptomycin is contraindicated in pregnancy because of an association with eighth cranial nerve injury and hearing impairment in up to 17% of infants. Ethionamide and cycloserine have been known to cause fetal neurologic injuries and are best avoided. Mothers taking antituberculous medications can breast feed, although approximately 20% of isoniazid and 10% of other antituberculous drugs will cross into breast milk. Thus if an infected infant is also being independently treated, a dose reduction should be considered.

Congenital TB infection is believed to occur via ingestion or aspiration of infected amniotic fluid or direct seeding via the umbilical vein. The latter will lead to infection of the periportal lymph nodes (the primary complex with congenital infection), but, after passing through the liver, the lungs remain the most important target organ. Hematogenous infection may also affect bone marrow, skin, kidneys, adrenal glands, spleen, and intestines, and, in nearly 50% of cases, the brain will also be affected. Infants with congenital TB do not usually manifest symptoms or signs of the disease for several days to weeks after delivery, resulting in delayed treatment and a mortality rate approaching 50%. In the majority of cases, nonspecific signs, including respiratory distress, fever, lethargy, failure to thrive, lymphadenopathy, and hepatosplenomegaly, are the only clues. With early diagnosis and treatment, neonatal treatment is usually successful. Although daily isoniazid and rifampin are the usual neonatal therapy, a four-drug regimen (including isoniazid, rifampin, streptomycin, and pyrazinamide) is used for drug-resistant strains. Ethambutol is avoided because of its potential for causing retrobulbar neuritis.

VIRAL INFECTIONS

Cytomegalovirus

Cytomegalovirus (CMV) is a double-stranded DNA herpesvirus transmitted by contact with infected blood, saliva, urine, or breast milk or through sexual contact. The mean incubation period is 40 days (range, 28-60 days). Although a brief, self-limited, flulike illness with fever, chills, malaise, myalgia with leukocytosis, and elevated liver function tests may be experienced, the majority of infected adults are asymptomatic. After the initial infection, CMV, like other herpesviruses, remains latent in host cells and may reactivate. In rare cases, recurrent disease may be caused by infection with a different strain of the virus.

The prevalence of CMV infection in pregnant women varies from 0.7% to 4% for primary infections and up to 13.5% for recurrent infections. For both types of infection, vertical transmission may occur via the transplacental route, during vaginal delivery, or through breast feeding. Fetal infections occur most commonly during the third trimester; however, more serious sequelae typically result following first trimester transmission. Compared with recurrent maternal CMV infection, primary infection has a much higher risk of vertical transmission (30%-40% vs. 0.15%-2%) and causes more severe fetal neurologic morbidity.

CMV is the most common congenital infection, occurring in 0.2%-2.2% of all neonates and is the leading cause of congenital hearing loss. Prenatally, CMV infection can be suspected following a documented maternal primary infection or suggestive ultrasound findings. These include abdominal, liver, and lateral brain ventricle calcifications; ventriculomegaly; hydrops fetalis; echogenic bowel; ascites; and hepatosplenomegaly. Structural anomalies, especially within the central nervous system (CNS), dictate a much poorer fetal prognosis. Diagnostic confirmation can usually be made through detection of CMV in amniotic fluid by culture or polymerase chain reaction (PCR). Fetal blood sampling for antibody response is less sensitive because of the immaturity of the fetal immune system, and alterations of platelet count and liver function tests are nonspecific. Although most infants with congenital CMV are asymptomatic at birth, evidence of the previously mentioned ultrasound findings and growth restriction, jaundice, petechiae, and thrombocytopenia may be observed.

No therapies are currently available for maternal or fetal CMV infection, and thus routine serologic screening for CMV during pregnancy is not recommended. Because ganciclovir can cause severe side effects and has not been shown to prevent long-term neurologic sequelae, it is only used in life-threatening cases. A vaccine is under development but is not currently available. As such, patient education efforts should focus on preventive measures, including careful handling of potentially infected articles (such as diapers) and thorough hand-washing when around young children or immunocompromised individuals.

Hepatitis

One of the most serious infections that can occur during pregnancy, viral hepatitis can be caused by a diverse collection of viruses, including CMV, Epstein-Barr, varicella zoster, coxsackie B, herpes simplex, and rubella. However, a family of seven hepatitis viruses, designated by the letters A through E, G, and TT are the predominant sources of the disease process, and although distinct, similarities in clinical manifestations, diagnosis, management, and obstetric and anesthetic implications can be observed (Table 20-5). The following information concerns this family of hepatitis viruses.

Malaise, fatigue, anorexia, nausea, and right upper quadrant or epigastric pain are the most common symptoms of acute viral hepatitis and are often accompanied by signs of jaundice, upper abdominal tenderness, and hepatomegaly. Although hepatitis A and E are usually self-limited, hepatitis B, C, and D often progress to a chronic carrier state. Hepatitis G and TT may also result in a carrier state; however, their ability to exist independent of other hepatitis forms as acute or chronic hepatitis has yet to be established. Although the majority of chronic carriers are asymptomatic, up to one third eventually develop chronic active or persistent hepatitis.

Hepatitis B is the most relevant virus type in causing neonatal infection because transmission of hepatitis A and E seldom cause symptomatic disease of the newborn, and vertical transmission of hepatitis C is relatively rare in itself (unless the mother is coinfected with HIV). The risk of transmission from mother to child is greatest during acute infection in pregnancy and with maternal HBeAg-positive carrier status. In 95% of these pregnancies transmission occurs, and without intervention 90% of these newborns will develop chronic carrier status. In HBeAg-negative pregnancies, however, the risk of transmission is only 25%, of which 12.5% becomes a carrier. Although it is likely that most transmissions occur during labor and delivery, the exact mechanism and time frame of transmission has not been revealed yet. Current data suggest that elective cesarean delivery does not prevent

Table 20-5

Details of Viral
Hepatitis Serotypes

Type	Virus	Incidence*	Transmission	Vertical Transmission	Perinatal Transmission
A	RNA	1 per 1000	Fecal-oral	No	No
B	DNA	Acute:1-2 per 1000 Chronic: 5-15 per 1000	Parenteral-sexual	Yes	Yes
C	RNA	6 per 1000	Parenteral-sexual?	Rare	Yes
D	RNA	Unknown	Parenteral-sexual	Yes	Yes
E	RNA	Unknown	Fecal-oral	Yes	Not reported
G	RNA	Unknown	Parenteral-sexual	Yes	Not reported
TT	DNA	Unknown	Parenteral-sexual?	Yes	Not reported

*Incidence in the United States during pregnancy.

vertical transmission, which suggests that infection may occur at an earlier gestational stage. Transmission can also occur through breast feeding.

Confirming a diagnosis of viral hepatitis during pregnancy does not differ substantially from nonpregnant patients. However, therapeutic recommendations are different. Management of women infected with viral hepatitis should begin with avoidance of activities that can result in upper abdominal trauma, maintenance of good nutrition, and avoidance of intimate contact until the involved parties have received appropriate prophylaxis. In the setting of severe illness, the patient should be hospitalized with correction of nutritional, fluid, electrolyte, and coagulation dysfunction. Interferon alpha therapy is known to alter the natural course of acute hepatitis and is recommended in symptomatic nonpregnant women. However, because of its possible abortifacient effect, interferon alpha therapy is contraindicated in pregnancy.

Because treatment is not completely curative, the emphasis has been placed on the prevention of viral hepatitis through education and immunization. Passive immunization with antibody immune globulin (IG) preparations purified from the plasma of normal donors is active against hepatitis A, B, and D (through immunization against B). A specific immune globulin against hepatitis B (HBIG) is also available and has been demonstrated to be more efficacious than standard IG preparations. Of note, plasma-derived IG preparations are considered to be of no infectious risk because of an ethanol fractionation process that inactivates viral (including HIV) and other blood-borne infectious diseases. IG can be given during pregnancy and does not pose a risk to the woman or her fetus. Two active immunizations, Recombivax HB and Engerix-B, have been developed against hepatitis B and, because they are produced via yeast cultures with recombinant DNA technologies, pose no infectious risk. Should exposure to hepatitis A or B (before immunization) occur, passive IGs should be administered as soon as possible. With hepatitis B, the more specific HBIG should be given and an immunization series of three vaccinations should be commenced. These regimens are approximately 75% effective in preventing hepatitis A and B (and thus D). Currently no immunoprophylaxis is available for hepatitis C or E, and there is insufficient evidence regarding the effects of IGs on hepatitis G or TT.

The CDC and the ACOG recommend hepatitis B virus screening (HbsAg) for all pregnant women. Seropositive women should have serum transaminases measured and be encouraged to inform their sexual partners and children of the need for testing and vaccination. Universal active hepatitis immunization is recommended for all infants born in the United States. In seronegative women, infant immunization should commence preferably before discharge and no later than 2 months of age. In seropositive women (HBsAg positive) or unknown status, infants should receive both passive and active immunization treatments, starting within 12 hours after birth.

Herpes Simplex Virus

A member of the DNA Herpesviridae family, herpes simplex virus (HSV) has two major types designated HSV-1 and HSV-2, which are primarily responsible for nongenital (gingivostomatitis, keratoconjunctivitis) and genital lesions, respectively. HSV is one of the most common viral pathogens; an estimated 500,000 new cases of genital herpes are diagnosed each year, with more than 45 million Americans infected. HSV-2 infections are more common in women, perhaps reflecting a more effective transmission rate, and approximately 30% of the female American population has antibodies to HSV-2.

Three stages of HSV infection have been identified, based on clinical presentation and serology. First-episode primary genital HSV occurs when herpes antibodies are absent at the time of infection. First-episode nonprimary genital HSV occurs when the acquisition of one type of HSV occurs when antibodies to the other type exist. Recurrent infection occurs when reactivation of genital HSV occurs when antibodies of the same type are present.

Initial HSV genital infections and recurrences may be with or without symptoms. When symptomatic, primary infections appear 2 to 14 days following exposure as ruptured vesicles on the vulva, vagina, and or cervix. Lesions usually resolve within 3 weeks without treatment; however, they may persist up to 6 weeks with secondary bacterial or mycotic infections. Commonly accompanied with localized pain, HSV infections may also present with systemic symptoms (malaise, myalgia, and fever) in up to two thirds of cases. Recurrent disease is generally accompanied with less severe symptoms. Viral shedding presents an infectious risk and may occur in the absence of symptoms; individuals with so-called subclinical shedding are a major source of infection because they are not aware of being a carrier and therefore will not take precautions to prevent transmission. Although significant variation in the frequency, severity, and duration of shedding exists, shedding occurs less often with recurrent herpes. When primary genital herpes occurs during pregnancy, an increased frequency of viral shedding occurs.

Approximately 1500 to 2000 newborns contract herpes each year, mostly from contact with infected maternal secretions during the perinatal period. Although thought to be an infrequent occurrence, in utero transmission can also occur and may result in a variety of anomalies or the onset of preterm labor and delivery. With recurrent maternal infection, the risk of neonatal infection is relatively small (5% risk of disease) because of passive immunization of the fetus through the placenta. However, the risk of neonatal disease increases substantially with primary infection of the mother, because in that case the newborn does not have protective immunoglobulins. Neonatal disease may result in localized (skin, eyes, mouth, and CNS) or disseminated disease. Neonatal mortality increases dramatically with the disseminated disease to 15% to 57%.

Diagnosis of HSV is dependent on virus isolation; however, specimen sampling and transporting difficulties limit test sensitivity even with overt infections to 60% to 70%. A positive test is strongly suggestive of a nonprimary first or recurrent episode. More sensitive techniques are under investigation, and serologic tests should soon be able to reliably identify and even distinguish the two HSV forms. Because of the low yield of viral cultures and the presence of asymptomatic viral shedding, virologic monitoring or screening is not recommended.

Primary HSV infection presents the highest vertical transmission risk, and antiviral therapy with acyclovir has been demonstrated to reduce viral shedding, pain, and duration of the primary lesions. Recurrent HSV infections may benefit from acyclovir therapy as well, although smaller reductions in viral shedding are believed to occur. Acyclovir, which can cross the placenta, concentrate in the amniotic fluid and breast milk, and reach therapeutic levels in the fetus, has been safely used during pregnancy, although the improved bioavailability of valacyclovir and famciclovir may provide greater benefit. Because of their beneficial effects, antiviral agent prophylaxis has been recommended for those parturients closer to term (>35 weeks' gestation), experiencing first episode primary or nonprimary genital infections or having frequent (>12 per year) recurrences. Cesarean delivery should be performed on women with first episode or recurrent HSV who have active genital lesions or prodromal symptoms at time of delivery.

Human Immunodeficiency Virus

An RNA virus that possesses a unique reverse transcriptase enzyme that encodes proviral DNA into the nucleus of the host cells, HIV currently affects an estimated 13.8 million women worldwide. Delays in diagnosis and treatment of the female gender and the ease of fetal transfer represent significant parturient concerns. A multisystem disease, HIV primarily attacks cells positive for the CD4 surface antigen, especially helper T lymphocytes, which play an integral role in cell-mediated immunity, B-cell activation, and antibody production. Associated alterations in macrophage activation and neutrophil function lead to an overall increased vulnerability to bacterial, viral, fungal, parasitic, and mycobacterial infections and certain malignancies. Patients may present with a mononucleosis-like illness with symptoms of headache, meningism (neck stiffness), fever, altered mental status, and isolated cranial nerve palsies at any time during the disease's course, but it is most common within a month of the primary infection. These symptoms result from early involvement of the brain and CSF. Indeed, even in the early course of the disease, the viral titer in the brain is typically higher than in any other organ. Although the combined effect of HIV and pregnancy on the immunologic system remains unclear, an increase in acquired immunodeficiency syndrome (AIDS) or AIDS-related complex has been observed in the postpartum period.

On a population basis, pregnancy rates among women with HIV infection are comparable with uninfected women until the onset of AIDS opportunistic infections, when the rates fall considerably. During pregnancy, with advanced disease (CD4 counts below 30% or progression to AIDS), an increase in adverse outcomes, including miscarriage, premature rupture of membranes, preterm delivery, and low birth weight, has been observed.

The transfer of HIV from mother to infant accounts for nearly all of the cases of HIV infection in children and depends on a number of maternal, fetal, and viral factors. HIV transmission may occur at any time, and with early gestational infection, fetal loss occurs often. Recent randomized and observational trials in both developing and developed nations have indicated that shorter antenatal regimens, and even postpartum neonatal treatments, are successful in dramatically reducing the transmission rate.

Two particular interventions deserve attention: reducing antepartum maternal plasma HIV RNA levels and limiting intrapartum and postpartum neonate exposure to maternal blood and genital and breast secretions. The first intervention, using antiviral medications in therapy-naïve parturients to reduce their viral load, was validated by the AIDS Clinical Trials Group (ACTG) Protocol 076, in which zidovudine (ZDV) therapy reduced the rate of vertical transmission of HIV infection from 25.5% to 8.3%. In this trial, ZDV was administered orally and intravenously to parturients before and during delivery, respectively, and orally to their infants for 6 weeks after birth. Further study will be needed to identify the optimal medications, time period, and long-term impact for this and other therapies; one potential concern is the creation of multi-drug-resistant strains of HIV and other comorbid infections later in the course of the parturient's disease process.

The second intervention, elective cesarean delivery before onset of labor or membrane rupture, was evaluated by the International Perinatal HIV Group via a meta-analysis of 15 prospective cohort studies (5 European and 10 North American) conducted between 1982 and 1996. The HIV transmission rate associated with elective cesarean delivery before onset of labor and membrane rupture was compared with either vaginal or cesarean delivery performed after these events. With the restriction of the primary analysis to 8533 mother-infant pairs for whom the route, circumstances of delivery, and neonatal HIV status were known, a strongly protective effect of elective cesarean delivery was discovered (odds ratio [OR] 0.43; 95% confidence interval [CI] 0.33 to 0.56). These results suggest that either labor or membrane rupture could potentially increase the risk of vertical HIV transmission. However, the indiscriminate use of cesarean delivery may not necessarily be beneficial because an increase in maternal morbidity and mortality from an operative delivery, particularly in third world countries, has been observed in this population. ACOG recommends cesarean delivery if viral load is 1000 copies/ml.

Additional fetal concerns may lead to the use of a cesarean delivery. Because IgG antiplatelet antibodies have been detected in HIV-infected patients, transplacental passage with resultant fetal thrombocytopenia and systemic or intracranial hemorrhage may occur. Thus, in addition to the inoculation risk, procedures involving the puncture of fetal skin or epithelium, including funipuncture and scalp sampling, are avoided to decrease the risk of fetal bleeding. This may offer another indication, in the scenario of nonreassuring external fetal monitoring with the inability to do fetal scalp pH samples or intrauterine monitoring, to perform an operative delivery.

Collectively these concerns have shaped the components of an "optimal approach" for limiting maternal fetal transmission, which includes promoting earlier HIV detection, using antiretroviral therapy during pregnancy, selecting obstetrical interventions, including elective cesarean delivery, and using neonatal antiretroviral therapy.

Parvovirus B19

Composed of a single-stranded DNA virus, parvovirus B19 is responsible for childhood exanthem erythema infectiosum (fifth disease) and transient aplastic crisis in patients with underlying hemoglobinopathy. Even in immunocompromised individuals, parvovirus B19 infections are usually mild, requiring only supportive care.

A disease transmitted most commonly through respiratory secretions and hand-to-mouth contact, infected persons remain infectious for 5 to 10 days following exposure. Household members of infected persons have an approximately 50% risk of infection. With the onset of a reticular rash on the trunk or other symptoms such as peripheral arthropathy, a loss of infectious risk occurs. Maternal diagnosis can be made through enzyme-linked immunosorbent assay (ELISA) or Western blot tests of parvovirus B19 antibodies or through direct visualization of viral particles in infected tissues. IgM and IgG antibodies are produced in response to an infection and last a few months and indefinitely, respectively. When only IgG is detected, this represents both a prior infection and immunity. Seropositivity to parvovirus B19 increases with age, and more than 60% of adolescents and adults have antibodies.

Transplacental transmission of parvovirus B19 has been reported to be as high as 33%, although the risk of serious fetal morbidity, such as hydrops fetalis, spontaneous abortion, and stillbirth, is low. Serious sequelae occur with infections before 20 weeks' gestational age; however, should the fetus survive, long-term development tends to be normal. Fetal parvovirus B19 can be diagnosed through the detection of viral particles or DNA in fetal specimens, including serum, amniotic fluid, placenta, or autopsy tissues. Ultrasonography looking for the presence of hydrops for up to 10 weeks following maternal infection has also been advocated.

Treatment for parvovirus B19 is primarily supportive. Should hydrops fetalis occur, treatment is unfortunately limited to performing percutaneous umbilical blood sampling for transfusion preparation if anemia is present.

Rubella

Rubella is caused by a single-stranded RNA virus belonging to the togavirus family, for which humans are the only natural host. Extremely contagious, with an attack rate within closed populations close to 100%, rubella is infectious from 7 days before and 14 days following the associated rash, which typically lasts 2 days. With a peak incidence among children aged five to nine, and immunity for life once infected, only 6% to 8% of women of reproductive age remain susceptible to infection with rubella virus.

Rubella is a respiratory disease transmitted by airborne or direct contact. The incubation period varies from 14 to 21 days. Because of the usually mild presentation of the disease, clinical diagnosis may be difficult. When present, symptoms can include a maculopapular 3-day rash of the face, which can spread to the trunk and extremities, postauricular or occipital adenopathy, fever, transient arthralgias, and arthritis. Pregnancy does not affect the clinical manifestations. Diagnosis can occur through viral isolation from nasopharyngeal secretions; however, few laboratories provide the service and isolation takes 4 to 6 weeks. The more sensitive rubella-specific IgM antibody, which appears rapidly and remains detectable for up to 1 month or longer, is recommended. A fourfold increase in rubella-specific IgG may also be used for diagnostic confirmation.

Although transplacental infection may occur with primary maternal rubella infection, transmission rarely occurs with reinfection. Fetal infection can be confirmed through the detection of rubella-specific IgM or viral cultures from fetal blood or by rubella DNA isolation from chorionic villi. Such testing, however, is rarely used because the infection severity does not correlate accurately with viral presence. Congenital rubella syndrome results in a number of manifestations, including fetal growth restriction, ophthalmologic abnormalities (cataracts, microphthalmia, glaucoma, chorioretinitis), cardiac malformations, and neurologic manifestations (mental retardation, microcephaly, encephalitis). Sensorineural deafness is the most common consequence; however, thrombotic thrombocytopenic purpura, hepatosplenomegaly, myocarditis, pneumonitis, anemia, and jaundice may also be observed. Although fetal infection may occur at any stage of pregnancy, the gestational age affects the manifestations, with first-trimester maternal infection producing a high incidence (70%-90%) of developmental malformations. By contrast, although structural defects do not occur as a consequence of infection during the third trimester of pregnancy, deafness and mental retardation may result. Moreover, the absence of clinical signs at birth does not exclude the possibility of subclinical damage or subsequent impairment; manifestations of congenital rubella infection (including endocrinopathies, hearing or visual impairment, and progressive panencephalitis) may develop up to 10 to 20 years later in 70% of individuals. Consequently, offspring of women who have sustained rubella infections during pregnancy should undergo long-term follow-up.

There is no effective treatment for rubella. Rubella vaccines produce seroconversion and long-term immunity from infection in 95% of cases. Complications of rubella vaccination include mild and self-limiting flulike symptoms, fever, lymphadenopathy, and rash. Rubella vaccination is not recommended during pregnancy because of theoretic concerns of fetal damage. Despite this recommendation, the risk of congenital rubella syndrome from vaccination within 3 months of conception is considered negligible. Clinicians should routinely offer the rubella vaccine to all potentially susceptible nonpregnant women lacking contraindications for vaccination.

Varicella Zoster

Varicella zoster virus (VZV) is a DNA herpesvirus. Primary infection (chickenpox) is seen most commonly in children, whereas reactivation of the latent virus (herpes zoster) is a disease of older patients. The virus is transmitted by respiratory droplets or close contact. Because of its highly contagious nature, only 5% of adults do not have protective immunity. Consequently, varicella infection is uncommon in pregnancy, occurring in only 0.4 to 0.7 per 1000 live births. Although primary infection in children is usually benign and self-limited, it results in significant maternal, fetal, and neonatal effects when occurring during pregnancy, especially during the first 16 weeks of gestation. Fetal skin scarring, limb hypoplasia, chorioretinitis, and microcephaly may occur. The mortality rate of neonatal VZV infection is especially high when maternal disease develops from 5 days before to 48 hours after delivery because of the relative immaturity of the neonatal immune system and the lack of protective maternal antibodies.

The diagnosis of the primary infection is based on clinical findings. Although not required, identification within skin lesions and vesicular fluid of antigens or antibodies by immunofluorescence or ELISA, respectively, can be performed. However, fetal infection is difficult to diagnose. Ultrasound findings (including hydrops fetalis, echogenic foci in the liver and bowel, cardiac malformations, limb deformities, microcephaly, and/or intrauterine growth restriction [IUGR]) are nonspecific, and identification of the virus by antibodies, cultures, or viral DNA identification is difficult and does not accurately predict the severity of fetal infection.

Oral acyclovir has been shown to reduce symptoms in healthy adults but does not appear to prevent fetal sequelae. Because mortality rates are high among infants born to women who develop varicella between 5 days before and 2 days after delivery, these newborns should receive varicella immune globulin (VZIG), although this does not universally prevent neonatal varicella.

Because treatment options are limited, efforts should be made to identify and vaccinate nonpregnant women of childbearing age who are nonimmune. Because the vaccine is a live attenuated strain, it is not approved for use during pregnancy, and conception should be delayed until 1 month after the second vaccination dose is given. Nonimmune women should also be counseled to avoid contact with individuals who have chickenpox; however, if exposure occurs, administration of VZIG should occur as soon as possible up to 72 hours after exposure to prevent or attenuate the maternal disease. Unfortunately, should VZIG fail to prevent the disease, no alterations of fetal infection occur as the result of its administration.

PARASITIC INFECTIONS

Lyme Disease

A disease caused by the spirochete *Borrelia burgdorferi*, Lyme disease is the most common vector-borne disease in the United States. Its incidence has increased about twenty-fivefold since national surveillance began in 1982, with approximately 12,500 new cases annually. Lyme disease is most likely transmitted to humans during the tick nymph stage, when the ticks are most likely to feed and their small size prevents them from being noticed. The transmission of the infection most likely takes place after approximately 2 or more days of feeding. Lyme disease spirochetes can spread from the site of the tick bite by cutaneous, lymphatic, and blood-borne routes and have been identified in spinal, synovial, and amniotic fluids.

The most common presentation of Lyme disease is a characteristic "bull's-eye" rash called erythema migrans, accompanied by nonspecific symptoms such as fever, malaise, fatigue, headache, myalgias, and arthralgias. Although most individuals present with symptoms after an incubation period of 7 to 14 days, some infected individuals are asymptomatic or only experience nonspecific symptoms. Rarely, cardiac and neurologic manifestations may occur. During pregnancy, *B. burgdorferi* can infect both the placenta and fetus; however, the risk for and timing of infection is unknown. Although maternal infection has been associated with preterm delivery, stillbirths, fetal neurologic abnormalities, and delayed neonatal effects (respiratory distress and sudden infant death syndrome [SIDS]), the overall risk of adverse outcomes appears low. Recent prospective and case control studies have demonstrated no association between maternal Lyme disease and fetal cardiac defects.

Diagnosis of Lyme disease is based primarily on clinical findings, and treatment is often commenced based on symptoms or known exposure. Serologic testing may provide valuable diagnostic information; however, the tests are of variable sensitivity and specificity. A number of serologic tests are available, and the CDC recommends testing initially with an ELISA or an indirect fluorescent antibody (IFA) test, with the more specific Western immunoblot (WB) test should equivocal results be obtained.

Treatment with doxycycline or amoxicillin (cefuroxime or erythromycin in persons allergic to the first two regimens) for 3 to 4 weeks is generally effective in early disease. With more advanced disease, particularly with neurologic manifestations, intravenous ceftriaxone or penicillin should be administered for at least 4 weeks, noting that treatment failures may occur and, even with successful treatment, some symptoms may persist. Aggressive treatment of Lyme disease during pregnancy may be warranted with the belief that a reduction in fetal/neonatal infection may occur, although the efficacy of this therapy is unknown.

Antibiotic treatment in early disease may blunt an antibody response; however, patients with disseminated or late-stage disease usually have strong serologic reactivity and demonstrate expanded WB immunoglobulin G (IgG) banding. Antibodies, which often persist for months or years even after successful treatment, do not confer immunity from reinfection. A recombinant outer-surface protein A vaccine (LYMErix) for the prevention of Lyme disease has been developed, although it is not recommended during pregnancy. Unfortunately, the vaccine does not protect all recipients against infection with *B. burgdorferi* and offers no protection against other tick-borne diseases.

Syphilis

An indolent systemic infection caused by the spirochete *Treponema pallidum*, syphilis has undergone a dramatic resurgence in the 1980s because of an increase in intravenous drug abuse and HIV. After a decade of continuous decline (1990-2000), rates started to rise again in 2001. Currently, the incidence of syphilis is 2 to 3 per 100,000 in the United States. Whereas efforts to reduce syphilis among women have been effective, the incidence among men continues to rise, and the male-to-female ratio now approaches 3.5. Much of the increase in syphilis among men can be attributed to a rise in homosexual contacts. Of women with syphilis, 80% are of reproductive age, potentially risking fetal transmission.

Transmitted most commonly through sexual contact, the risk of transmission after sexual contact with a person with primary or secondary syphilis is estimated at 30% to 50%. This high transmission rate is because of the ability of *T. pallidum* to pass across abraded skin and intact mucous membranes. During pregnancy, no alterations occur in the characteristic clinical stages of the disease.

Because *T. pallidum* cannot be cultured, the diagnosis of syphilis requires either direct visualization of the organism (by dark-field microscopy or fluorescent antibody staining) or, more commonly, serologic testing. Newer diagnostic techniques (i.e., PCR) are currently being developed. Lumbar puncture is often performed, even during pregnancy, to assist in the evaluation of CNS symptoms, evaluation of syphilis of unknown or advanced stages, and when concurrent immunosuppression exists. CSF abnormalities suggestive of syphilis infection include elevated counts of white cells (≥ 5 cells/mm^3) and total proteins (≥ 45mg/dl), normal glucose concentrations, and a positive syphilis serologic test. Antenatal syphilis poses a significant threat to the pregnancy and fetus and, if untreated, is associated with IUGR, stillbirth (30%), preterm birth, neonatal death (10%), and congenital infection (>60%). Only 20% of children born to mothers with untreated syphilis will be unaffected. *T. pallidum* readily crosses the placenta and transmission can occur at any time during pregnancy and at any stage of the disease. However, both the disease stage and fetal gestational age influence the rate of perinatal transmission. Vertical transmission is more common with primary (50%) and secondary syphilis (50%), as compared with early latent (40%), late latent (10%), and even tertiary syphilis (10%). Universal antepartum screening and treatment with appropriate antibiotics could virtually eliminate syphilis during pregnancy.

Serologic screening should occur at the first prenatal visit and, in high-risk populations, again during the third trimester and at delivery. Mothers properly treated have a 1% to 2% risk of fetal transmission versus 70% to 100% in untreated mothers.

Penicillin is the treatment of choice for syphilis in both pregnant and non-pregnant individuals because of its efficacy and lack of resistant strains. Treatment is directed according to the stage of disease. Following treatment, nontreponemal antibody serologic titers should be checked at 1, 3, 6, 12, and 24 months. Titers should decrease fourfold by 6 months and become nonreactive by 12 to 24 months. Titers that do not decrease appropriately suggest either treatment failure or reinfection, and treatment should be repeated. Treatment failure should be further evaluated by a lumbar puncture to evaluate CNS involvement and HIV testing. In pregnant individuals with a history of penicillin allergy, the only satisfactory treatment is penicillin desensitization, because erythromycin, doxycycline, and tetracycline cannot be used safely and effectively to treat syphilis during pregnancy. Desensitization can be achieved either orally (simpler and safer) or intravenously. It involves exposing the patient to a small amount of penicillin and gradually increasing the dose until an effective level is reached. This procedure can be accomplished in approximately 4 hours and requires close inpatient monitoring.

Toxoplasmosis

Caused by the intracellular parasite *Toxoplasma gondii*, toxoplasmosis infects more than 60 million people in the United States alone. Contact with infected materials such as animal feces or soil and ingestion of infected undercooked meats are common routes of infection. Rarely, infected blood transfusions or organ transplants may result in the disease.

Infection usually presents as asymptomatic cervical lymphadenopathy, but after an incubation period of 5 to 18 days, nonspecific symptoms such as night sweats, fever, malaise, myalgias, and hepatosplenomegaly may occur. An intact immune system usually allows for a benign and self-limited course. By contrast, infection in immunosuppressed individuals and fetuses in utero can result in chorioretinitis, hearing loss, metal retardation, seizures, and hepatosplenomegaly. Vertical transmission risk is dependent on the timing of maternal infection, increasing from 10% to 60% from the first to third trimesters. Earlier fetal transmission results in more severe disease, which is revealed in 55% to 85% of infected neonates not at birth but at later stages of life.

Although the isolation of *T. gondii* from bodily fluids establishes an acute infection, serologic testing for antibodies is the primary method of diagnosis. IgM antibodies appear first, reach maximum levels in 1 month, and are followed by the immunity-conferring IgG antibodies. Because high titers of both IgM and IgG may persist for years, both tests should be used for the initial evaluation. Although the Sabin-Feldman IgG test is the gold standard, it is performed in only a few laboratories; consequently, indirect fluorescent antibody, indirect hemagglutination, and ELISA testing are often used. Unfortunately, serologic assays for toxoplasmosis are not well standardized and have high false-positive rates. Therefore, serial testing 3 weeks apart, with specimen saving for repeat testing in recognized reference laboratories, has been recommended. In the United States, routine screening during pregnancy is currently not recommended. In countries with a high prevalence of seropositivity, such as France and Austria, however, serologic screening has had a favorable impact and is routinely performed.

Prior infection and treatment of toxoplasmosis before pregnancy does not confer a congenital transmission risk. However, should the disease be diagnosed and treatment initiated during pregnancy, a risk of congenital infection exists. Spiramycin, a drug available only through the U.S. Food and Drug Administration, may reduce fetal transmission by 60% and should be started immediately. Fetal ultrasonography (looking for ventriculomegaly, intracranial calcifications, microcephaly, ascites, hepatosplenomegaly, and IUGR) and fetal blood sampling for IgM after 20 weeks' gestation has been recommended. Should fetal infection be established, pyrimethamine, sulfonamides, and folinic acid are added to increase the efficacy against placental and fetal parasites. Infants with congenital toxoplasmosis should continue treatment of pyrimethamine and sulfadiazine, alternating monthly with spiramycin, for a year. Treatment may diminish intracranial calcifications and improve neurologic function.

KEY POINTS

- Infectious diseases are a major cause of maternal and neonatal mortality during pregnancy, labor, and the puerperium.
- Perinatal infections generally have more serious fetal outcome when they occur early in gestation because they may disrupt organogenesis.
- Second- and third-trimester infections are more likely to cause neurologic impairment or growth disturbance.
- For most infectious diseases, primary infection is more likely to cause adverse neonatal outcome than recurrent infection.
- The most common congenital infection is caused by CMV. Approximately 40,000 infants are born with congenital CMV annually in the United States, and it is the leading cause of congenital hearing loss. Unfortunately, there is as yet no effective therapy.
- Because effective treatment is not yet available or incompletely curative for many infectious diseases in pregnancy, patient education efforts should focus primarily on preventive measures.

SUGGESTED READING

Antimicrobial Therapy for Obstetric Patients. Educational Bulletin No. 245. Washington, DC, March 1998, American College of Obstetrics and Gynecology.

Baltimore RS et al: Early-onset neonatal sepsis in the era of group B streptococcal prevention. *Pediatrics* 108:1094, 2001.

Bizzarro MJ et al: Seventy-five years of neonatal sepsis and Yale: 1928-2003. *Pediatrics* 116:595, 2005.

Center for Disease Control: 1998 guidelines for treatment of sexually transmitted diseases. *MMWR* 47:28, 1998.

Centers for Disease Control and Prevention. Early-onset and late-onset neonatal group B streptococcal disease; United States 1996-2004. *MMWR Morb Mortal Wkly Rep* 54:1205, 2005.

Jones JL, Schulkin J, Maguire JH: Therapy for common parasitic diseases in pregnancy in the United States. *Obstet Gynecol Surv* 60:386, 2005.

Management of Herpes in Pregnancy. Practice Bulletin No. 8. Washington, DC, October 1999, American College of Obstetrics and Gynecology.

Moore MR, Schrag SJ, Schuchat A: Effects of intrapartum antimicrobial prophylaxis for prevention of group B streptococcal disease on the incidence and ecology of early-onset neonatal sepsis. *Lancet Infect Dis* 3:201, 2003.

Perinatal Viral and Parasitic Infections. Practice Bulletin No. 20. Washington, DC, September 2000, American College of Obstetrics and Gynecology.

Pinto NM et al: Neonatal early-onset Group B Streptococcal disease in the era of intrapartum chemoprophylaxis: residual problems. *J Perinatol* 23:265, 2003.

Prevention of early-onset group B streptococcal disease in newborns. Washington, DC, December 2002, American College of Obstetrics and Gynecology Committee Opinion No. 279.

Primary and secondary syphilis—United States, 2002. *MMWR* 52:1117, 2003.

Puopolo KM, Madoff LC, Eichenwald EC: Early-onset Group B Streptococcal disease in the era of maternal screening. *Pediatrics* 115:1240, 2005.

Schrag S, Gorwitz R, Fultz-Butts K, Schuchat A: Prevention of perinatal group B streptococcal disease. *MMWR Recomm Rep* 51:1, 2002.

Schrag SJ et al: Prenatal screening for infectious diseases and opportunities for prevention. *Obstet Gynecol* 102:753, 2003.

Schrag SJ et al: Risk factors for invasive, early-onset *Escherichia coli* infections in the era of widespread intrapartum antibiotic use. *Pediatrics* 118:570, 2006.

Schrag SJ et al: Group B streptococcal disease in the era of intrapartum antibiotic prophylaxis. *N Engl J Med* 342:15, 2000.

21

HUMAN IMMUNODEFICIENCY VIRUS

Urania Magriples

DEFINITION

Human immunodeficiency virus (HIV) belongs to the family of human retroviruses (Retroviridae). The most common cause of HIV disease throughout the world is HIV-1. HIV-2 is predominantly limited to West Africa. HIV-1 contains a single-stranded RNA genome that is nine kilobases long and contains nine genes that encode 15 different proteins. Three major viral classes have emerged: M (Main), N (New), and O (Outlier). The M group accounts for 90% of HIV infections worldwide and has nine subtypes or clades. Clade B is the subtype found most commonly in the Americas and Western Europe and differs from subtypes found in Asia and Africa, where most HIV-infected persons reside. Most drug testing and treatments have been targeted to Clade B, which may hinder the use and efficacy of tested regimens in other countries. Variations among subtypes are also seen as a result of mutations and are a significant obstacle to the development of effective worldwide therapies and vaccines.

EPIDEMIOLOGY

The first U.S. cases of acquired immunodeficiency syndrome (AIDS) were reported in 1981 as case reports of homosexual men with atypical infections. By 2002, more than 40 million people were infected worldwide. Almost half of infected persons are women. The vast majority of infected individuals (95%) live in the developing world. The disease has reached epidemic proportions in developing countries, accounting for a significant decrease in life expectancy and an increase in orphaned children. In sub-Saharan Africa, women represent almost 60% of existing HIV infections. According to UNAIDS, the Joint United Nations Programme on HIV/AIDS, up to 40% of women attending antenatal clinics in many areas of sub-Saharan Africa are HIV positive.

The United States is the industrialized country most heavily affected by HIV. There are approximately 100,000 infected women of childbearing age in the United States, with an estimated 7000 infants born to HIV-positive mothers per year. The new HIV infection rate is increasing more rapidly among women than men, with 25% of AIDS cases in 1999 reported among women as compared with 7% in 1985. HIV is the fourth leading cause of death in women aged 25 to 44 years. Almost 80% of U.S. cases are among African-American and Hispanic women, although they represent only 25% of all U.S. women.

In the United States, perinatal transmission accounts for 90% of AIDS cases in children, with 85% of cases in African Americans or Hispanics. A variety of factors affect perinatal transmission, including stage of disease, viral load, low CD4 count (also correlates with disease stage), treatment, prolonged rupture of membranes, prolonged labor, invasive monitoring in labor, and hemorrhage in labor. Breast feeding in the setting of acute versus chronic HIV infection has a 30% and 15% transmission rate, respectively. In developing countries, where access to clean water and food significantly affect pediatric mortality, regimens of maternal antiretroviral treatment in conjunction with breast feeding may represent the most viable option.

MECHANISM

HIV has a predilection for T4 cells (helper/inducer), macrophages, and neural cells. The infection of a cell is initiated by binding to the CD4 receptor, which activates a cascade of events leading to fusion of the viral and host cell membranes and entry of the viral contents into the host cell cytoplasm. Reverse transcription (copying of viral genetic material from RNA to DNA) occurs and the virus proliferates. The integrated virus may remain latent for hours to years before becoming active through transcription. Full-length viral RNA may be transported out of the cell or it may leave the cell as smaller spliced versions. The viral RNA acts on ribosomes for the creation of different proteins, which affect both viral and cell function, host immunity, and replication.

The initial infection induces both cellular and antibody-mediated responses. Cytotoxic T lymphocytes (CTL or CD8 cells) inhibit HIV replication directly by killing infected cells and by producing cytokines to attract other host factors. CD4 cells also respond to the infection but are decreased by the destruction of infected cells. After the initial viremia, an equilibrium between the virus and CD4+ cells occurs and the virus is maintained at a certain level ("set point") with relatively preserved T-cell function but significant T-cell turnover. Eventually, a reduction in the T4 population occurs, and in the presence of a normal T8 population (suppressor), a reversal of the T4/T8 ratio occurs. Also, impairment of lymphokine production occurs and defective cytotoxic activity by natural killer cells is observed. There is poor antibody response to new antigens and inappropriate polyclonal activation, with resultant elevated level of serum immunoglobulins, circulating immune complexes, and various autoimmune phenomena such as positive anticardiolipin, antinuclear antibodies, and immune thrombocytopenia. Infection alters the ability of cells to perform their usual functions and ultimately causes cell death. Thus, individuals become susceptible to opportunistic infections as T cells are depleted.

Primary infection may be characterized by flulike symptoms with fever, lymphadenopathy, fatigue, maculopapular rash, pharyngitis, and headache. It is defined as the time of infection until an antibody response is detectable. At the onset of infection, the CD4 counts initially drop then rise back to normal levels. Viral RNA levels (viral load) are initially high and then decrease as the virus becomes incorporated into cells and T cells respond to the infection. Antibody is detectable within a few months. A more severe clinical syndrome of primary infection has been reported with a more rapid progression of HIV disease. This phenomenon has also been correlated with higher "set points." The nonspecific viral or flulike symptoms make diagnosis of HIV at this stage without a known exposure unlikely.

Early-stage HIV is usually asymptomatic and has an extended latency. It is characterized by an equilibrium of HIV replication and host destruction of virus. The latency period and rate of progression varies widely. It is not until CD4 cells decrease and viral load increases that symptoms begin. On average CD4 counts will drop by 50 to 90 cells per year in asymptomatic individuals.

Middle-stage HIV (characterized by T cells between 200 and 500 cells/mm^3) is usually asymptomatic but characterized by an increased risk of infections (Table 21-1). The Centers for Disease Control and Prevention (CDC) defines AIDS as T cells less than 200 cells/mm^3 or the presence of an opportunistic infection. Clinical criteria tend to be a late sequelae and the median survival after a single AIDS-defining condition ranges from 3 to 51 months.

Table 21-1

Centers for Disease Control and Prevention Classification System

Category A	Asymptomatic human immunodeficiency virus (HIV) infection Persistent generalized lymphadenopathy Acute infection
Category B	Bacillary angiomatosis Candidiasis oral (thrush) Candidiasis vulvovaginal Cervical dysplasia (moderate/severe) Constitutional symptoms greater than 1 month (fever or diarrhea) Hairy leukoplakia Herpes zoster (2 distinct episodes or more than 1 dermatome) Idiopathic thrombocytopenic purpura Listeriosis Pelvic inflammatory disease Peripheral neuropathy
Category C	Opportunistic infection (toxoplasmosis, cryptosporidia, coccidioidomycosis, *Cryptococcus*, toxoplasmosis, histoplasmosis, *Pneumocystis*) Non-Hodgkin's lymphoma Encephalopathy Esophageal candidiasis Invasive cervical cancer Pulmonary tuberculosis Two occurrences of bacterial pneumonia within a 12-month period CD4 count less than 200 cell/mm^3

Before the availability of treatment in the United States, the mean survival time after the diagnosis of AIDS was less than 1 year.

RISK FACTORS

The primary method of transmission of HIV is sexual contact. In developing countries, heterosexual contact accounts for the majority of transmission. Even in the United States and Europe, homosexual contact currently accounts for less than half of the new cases. HIV-1 has been isolated from blood, semen, vaginal secretions, breast milk, spinal fluid, saliva, and tears, although the amount of virus in tears and saliva is low. The average risks of transmission from one HIV exposure are listed in Box 21-1. Transmission occurs most often through penile-anal and penile-vaginal sex, although cases have been reported with oral sex. Transmission is greatest in the receptive partner in anal intercourse (probably because the rectal mucosa is thinner and more subject to trauma than vaginal mucosa) and in the female partner in vaginal intercourse. Increased risks of female-to-male transmission have been associated with intercourse during menses and postcoital bleeding. Other factors that affect transmission include advanced disease state (including high viral load, low CD4 count, and certain viral subtypes), lack of condom use, number of sexual contacts, genital trauma and ulcerations, and the presence of other sexually transmitted infections. Transmission among intravenous drug abusers (IVDAs) occurs through contamination of shared needles and because of the increase in high-risk sexual behaviors, prostitution, and polysubstance abuse (particularly crack/cocaine). Needle sharing prevalence highly correlates with seroprevalence rates, and needle exchange programs have been demonstrated to be effective in reducing transmission of both HIV and hepatitis.

Nonsexual transmission through transfusion and needle sticks is now less common in the United States. Almost all the transfusion cases were caused by blood transfusion before 1985, when testing for blood products became available. Ninety percent of patients transfused with HIV-positive blood before 1985 became infected. Other measures such as screening the blood pool with p24 antigen, voluntary deferral of at-risk donors, and techniques to deactivate the virus in pooled plasma products have further decreased the risk. Postexposure prophylaxis (PEP) after recent exposures (<72 hours) has been associated with a reduction of transmission of 80%.

Box 21-1   Transmission Risk of Encounter with Known Human Immunodeficiency Virus Source

- Following blood transfusion: 95%
- Perinatal exposure (untreated): 25%
- Receptive anal-penile sex: 0.1 to 3%
- Intravenous needle: 0.67%
- Occupational exposure: 0.4%
- Receptive vaginal-penile sex: 0.1%-0.2%

In the absence of antiretroviral treatment, perinatal transmission occurs in approximately 25% of live births to HIV-infected mothers. Risk factors associated with an increased risk of perinatal transmission include maternal stage of disease, the presence of opportunistic infections, prolonged rupture of membranes, prolonged length of labor, antepartum and intrapartum bleeding, and invasive monitoring in labor. Treatment with antiretroviral medications is effective in significantly decreasing this risk. In several studies performed before viral load testing and highly active antiretroviral therapy (HAART), cesarean delivery before the onset of labor or rupture of membranes was associated with a significant decrease in transmission by approximately 50%. Treatment with zidovudine (AZT) showed less of a dramatic effect but was still significant. Nonelective cesareans (performed after onset of labor or rupture of membranes) were not associated with a protective effect. However, monotherapy with AZT does not represent standard treatment in Western countries. Transmission rates of less than 1% have been reported with the use of HAART, therefore elective cesarean delivery is unlikely to further reduce this low rate. Consideration should be given to a scheduled cesarean delivery with viral load greater than 1000 copies/ml and inadequate antenatal treatment, including treatment initiated late in pregnancy. A discussion of risk and benefits of cesarean delivery should include the increased risk of endometritis and wound infection that has been noted in HIV-positive women.

Breast feeding accounts for up to 30% of perinatal transmission, and the risk increases with duration of breast feeding, recent infection, and level of viremia. Women with safe alternatives to breast feeding are counseled to not breast feed.

A number of host factors also influence disease progression. Older age is associated with more rapid disease, as are certain HLA alleles. Certain subtypes seem to progress at varying rates. Concomitant substance abuse, smoking, poor nutrition, and depression have been associated with more rapid progression of disease but may also represent comorbid socioeconomic factors that demonstrate the effects of poor access to care, noncompliance with treatment regimens, and overall poor health on outcome.

HIV also seems to affect the course with other viral diseases. Hepatitis C has a more rapid progression in the presence of HIV and is associated with poorer response to antiretrovirals and a faster progression to AIDS. Immunosuppression also seems to predispose to the acquisition and retention of oncogenic strains of human papillomavirus (HPV), the causative virus in cervical cancer. This manifests itself as more aggressive progressive of intraepithelial cervical neoplasia and necessitates close follow-up of Papanicolaou smears, colposcopy, and treatment in HIV-positive women.

HIV TESTING

HIV testing is strongly recommended in pregnancy and in at-risk populations. Different states have adopted laws to improve testing through mandatory maternal or neonatal HIV testing. Basics in pretesting and posttest counseling are outlined in Box 21-2.

Box 21-2 Human Immunodeficiency Virus (HIV) Counseling

Information at pretest counseling should include the following:

1. What HIV and AIDS means
2. Modes of transmission
3. What the antibody test is and the personal implications of a positive or negative test (how an individual would react to positive result and support systems)
4. Importance of knowing one's HIV status with regard to pregnancy and perinatal transmission
5. Risk-reduction behaviors

Information at posttest counseling should include the following:

1. Implications of positive test
2. Review HIV infection and transmission
3. Implications of HIV infection in pregnancy
4. Risk reduction behaviors (i.e., discuss safer sex, safer needle use)

AIDS, Acquired immunodeficiency syndrome.

Initial screening for HIV is done with enzyme-linked immunosorbent assay (ELISA) or enzyme immunoassay (EIA). A colorimetric change is noted from the antigen-antibody reaction. Reactive results are rescreened and repeatedly reactive results are confirmed by Western blot. Confirmatory tests tend to be more expensive and labor-intensive; therefore, they are not appropriate to be used as screening tests. The Western blot identifies antibodies against specific portions of the virus. It is considered positive if the patient has antibodies to multiple virus specific bands—p24, p31, and either gp41 or gp160. If fewer bands are identified, the test is indeterminate. A small number (15%-20%) of tests from low-risk patients will be indeterminate and remain so even if repeated over many months. This is likely caused as a result of nonspecific reactions, hypergammaglobulinemia, the presence of cross-reactive antibodies, and potentially pregnancy. Recently infected individuals may also have indeterminate results, but repeat testing in 3 to 6 months will usually reveal a positive Western blot. Published sensitivity and specificity of combined tests are 99%. In most cases, antibody will be detected by 6 to 12 weeks after infection. Interpretation of results is shown in Box 21-3.

Box 21-3 Interpretation of Human Immunodeficiency Virus (HIV) Testing Results

- Negative ELISA in a patient with significant risk factors and high suspicion of primary infection
  - Viral load negative—HIV negative
  - Viral load positive—seroconverting HIV positive
- Positive ELISA/negative Western blot—HIV negative (false-positive ELISA)
- Positive ELISA/indeterminate Western blot
  - Viral load negative—repeat tests in 1-2 months; if still negative—false-positive ELISA
  - Viral load positive—seroconverting: HIV positive
- Positive ELISA/positive Western blot—HIV positive

ELISA, Enzyme-linked immunosorbent assay.

Rapid testing has become available in the United States as OraQuick and SUDS. Both are Food and Drug Administration (FDA) approved. Urine and saliva tests and home testing kits are available but are not currently FDA approved. Rapid testing has been proposed for use in pregnancy in cases of late registration and at the time of delivery in women who have not been tested in pregnancy. A colorimetric reading is available within 10 to 15 minutes of adding two drops of serum to the cartridge and the results are easily reproducible. The false-positive rate to rapid testing is 0.4% to 1% (similar to ELISA in pregnancy). In 1998, the CDC changed its recommendations and advocated giving out results of a positive rapid test before confirmation because it is seen as an opportunity for counseling and intervention.

HIV antigen (p24 antigen) testing is not routinely used to test individuals but can be used to screen blood products and to test for recently infected cases. p24 antigen assay measures the viral capsid, which is present before the development of antibody. It may have some use in testing in primary infection, although it is less sensitive than viral load testing in this setting.

Testing recently infected individuals with viral RNA can identify the recent seroconverters before the development of detectable antibody. It is also a useful measurement in determining disease progression and treatment efficacy. Three different assays are available for viral load testing: reverse transcription–polymerase chain reaction (RT-PCR), branched DNA (bDNA), and nucleic acid sequence–based amplification assay (NASBA). Results may vary between types of test; therefore, it is important to be consistent in using the same test over time. Samples are also significantly affected by collection, storage, and processing times. Results of viral load testing are often expressed in log units, in which each increase of 1 log is a factor of 10. Less than 0.5 log variation is expected normally because of assay variation and diurnal change and greater than 0.5 log variation is considered clinically relevant. Lower limits of detection vary by assay but tend to be around 500 cells/ml. Ultrasensitive assays are now available for viral detection between 50 and 500 cells/ml. Levels of less than 500 cells/ml are "undetectable" by the standard assay but do not indicate the absence of virus. In general, less than 5000 copies/ml indicates a lower risk of progression, whereas a value above 50,000 copies/ml indicates a high risk. Tables are available to estimate the risk and timing of the progression to AIDS based on CD4 count and viral load.

CD4 counts are a mainstay of therapeutic monitoring. They are useful in determining stage of disease, initiation of therapy, and timing of prophylaxis against opportunistic infections (Box 21-4). The CDC recommends CD4 testing every 3 to 6 months in all HIV-infected persons. Testing is performed more often in pregnancy because decreases in CD4 counts are helpful markers for drug adherence and resistance and the increased risk of vertical transmission. Normal CD4 counts are in the range of 500 to 1300 cells/mm^3. CD4 counts do not physiologically decrease in pregnancy in the setting of adequate treatment.

HIV resistance testing is a useful adjunct in treated patients who have decreasing CD4 counts or increasing viral loads on a specific regimen. It can also be used in previously untreated individuals to guide therapy. There are two types of resistance testing available. Genotypic assays detect genetic

---

Box 21-4 Primary Care Recommendations

- Treatment of positive PPD >5 mm
- Pneumococcal vaccine
- Hepatitis B vaccination if susceptible
- Influenza vaccine
- Prophylaxis
- Pneumocystis if CD4 count <200 cells/mm^3
- Toxoplasma if CD4 count <100 cells/mm^3 and toxoplasma IgG +
- *Mycobacterium avium* if CD4 count <50 cells/mm^3

PPD, Purified protein derivative.

---

mutations in the coding regions of protease and reverse transcriptase enzymes and the results are used to predict resistance to various antiretrovirals. Phenotypic assays are more like bacterial culture and sensitivity, in which a certain amount of infected serum is used and its activity against specific antiretrovirals is tested. Genotype testing identifies only dominant strains representing 10%-20% of the circulating virus and requires a minimum of 1000 viral copies/ml to be performed. They are cheaper, more readily available, and easier to perform than phenotypic assays. A phenotype assay has the advantage of reporting results in an easier format for clinicians to interpret (similar to bacterial culture and sensitivity) and to recognize that degrees of resistance occur. It only tests the virus for the effects of one drug at a time and it may be difficult to extrapolate the effects of multiple drugs on the virus, but it has clinical relevance in a highly resistant virus that has failed multiple regimens. All resistance testing must be reviewed with the patient's prior and current medication history because prior resistance may not be accounted for.

TREATMENT

Guidelines for treatment are available through the CDC (www.hivatis.org). The term HAART refers to any regimen that includes three or more antiretroviral agents known to suppress HIV. Before initiation of treatment, an assessment of risks and benefits and potential factors affecting adherence to a regimen should be addressed. A complete history and physical examination and blood work should be performed. Baseline evaluations are shown in Box 21-5. Treatment should be offered to all symptomatic persons, all pregnant women, and asymptomatic persons with a CD4 count of less than 350 cells/mm^3 or viral load greater than 55,000 copies/ml. There is still debate on whether early initiation of treatment in the setting of a normal CD4 count prolongs life or leads to the development of early resistance and the need for more complicated drug regimens. Treatment should be individualized and should include an assessment of adherence, lifestyle, and support systems before initiation. Regimens with the smallest amount of pill burden and least side effects should be used and the patient should be closely monitored for toxicity and therapeutic efficacy.

Box 21-5   Baseline Evaluation before Initiation of Antiretroviral Therapy

- Complete history and physical
- CD4 count
- Viral load
- Complete blood and platelet count
- Electrolytes, BUN, creatinine
- Liver function tests
- Lipid profile (if not pregnant)
- STD cultures
- Pap smear
- VDRL
- Hepatitis B surface Ag and antibody
- Hepatitis C
- PPD

Ag, Antigen; *BUN,* blood urea nitrogen; *Pap,* Papanicolaou; *PPD,* purified protein derivative; *STD,* sexually transmitted disease; *VDRL,* Venereal Disease Research Laboratory.

There are four classes of drugs approved by the FDA for the treatment of HIV: nucleoside reverse transcriptase inhibitors (NRTIs), nonnucleoside reverse transcriptase inhibitors (NNRTIs), protease inhibitors (PIs), and fusion inhibitors (FIs) (Table 21-2). Each class affects a different aspect of replication of the virus; therefore certain combinations have been shown to be more effective than others. The reverse transcriptase enzyme is used by the virus to convert its RNA to DNA after entry into the cell. NRTIs mimic nucleotides and undergo intracellular phosphorylation to an active triphosphate metabolite, which competes with host nucleotides and interrupts DNA chain elongation. NNRTIs bind to a site adjacent to the reverse transcriptase enzyme, which leads to a structural change and decreased enzyme activity. NNRTIs affect cytochrome P450 function; therefore, they can require dose adjustments if administered with a drug that also is metabolized by the cytochrome system. They may also affect the efficacy of other medications. With NNRTIs, there is the potential for cross-resistance because they all bind at the same site of the reverse transcriptase enzyme.

PIs interfere with protease, the enzyme that is responsible for cleavage of the HIV polyproteins into functional units, and cause the creation of nonfunctional viral particles. Although they have similar chemical structures, their side effects and resistance patterns differ. FIs prevent HIV entry into cells.

Treatment with single or double agents should be avoided as it leads to the development of viral resistance. All agents should be initiated and stopped simultaneously with close monitoring of therapeutic efficacy and toxicity. The goal of treatment is to prolong and improve the quality of life and prevent both disease progression and viral resistance. Resistance exists before initiation of treatment and can occur with a single mutation, which replicates at a rate of 10 billion copies per day. Incomplete suppression hastens the predominance of resistant strains.

The CDC recommends one of three categories of regimens for initiating treatment- 1-NNRTI and 2-NRTIs, 1 or 2-PIs and 2 NRTIs, or 3 NRTIs. These

Antiretroviral
Medications

Table 21-2

	Medication	Trade Name	Type	Pregnancy Category*	Dose†	Side Effects
1	Abacavir (ABC)	Ziagen	NRTI	C	300 mg bid	Hypersensitivity reaction. Limited studies in pregnancy/use not recommended
2	Zidovudine (AZT)	Retrovir	NRTI	C	300 mg bid	Bone marrow suppression, anemia, neutropenia, headache, nausea, malaise, myopathy, lactic acidosis
3	Didanosine (ddl)	Videx	NRTI	B	400 mg qd	Pancreatitis, peripheral neuropathy, nausea, diarrhea, lactic acidosis (rare)
4	Emtricitabine (FTC)	Emtriva	NRTI	B	200 mg qd	No studies in pregnancy/minimal toxicity, lactic acidosis, hepatic steatosis
5	Lamivudine (3TC)	Epivir	NRTI	C	150 mg bid or 300 mg qd	Minimal toxicity, diarrhea, lactic acidosis, hepatic steatosis (rare)
6	Stavudine (d4T)	Zerit Zerit-XR	NRTI	C	40 mg bid 100 mg qd	Not to be used with AZT. Peripheral neuropathy, lipodystrophy, pancreatitis, lactic acidosis
7	Tenofovir	Viread	NRTI	B	300 mg qd	No studies in pregnancy/use not recommended, asthenia, headache, nausea, vomiting, lactic acidosis, hepatic steatosis
8	Zalcitabine (ddC)	Hivid	NRTI	C	0.75 mg tid	No studies in pregnancy/use not recommended, peripheral neuropathy, stomatitis, lactic acidosis, hepatic steatosis
9	1 and 5	Epzicom	NRTI	C	1 tablet bid	
10	1, 2, and 5	Trizivir	NRTI	C	1 tablet bid	
11	4 and 7	Truvada	NRTI	B	1 tablet qd	
12	2 and 5	Combivir	NRTI	C	1 tablet bid	
13	Delavirdine	RescriptorR	NNRTI	C	400 mg tid	No studies in pregnancy/use not recommended, rash, transaminitis, headaches
14	Efavirenz	Sustiva	NNRTI	C	600 mg qd	Avoid in the first trimester (teratogenic in monkeys), rash, transaminitis, false-positive cannaboid test
15	Nevirapine	Viramune	NNRTI	C	200 mg qd × 2 weeks then increase to bid	Rash, hepatitis, hepatic failure

Table 21-2—cont'd

Medication	Trade Name	Type	Pregnancy Category	Dose†	Side Effects
16 Amprenavir	Agenerase	PI	C	1200 mg bid	No studies in pregnancy/ use not recommended, nausea, vomiting, rash, paresthesias, transaminitis, hyperglycemia, lipodystrophy, oral solution contains large amount of propylene glycol
17 Atazanavir	Reyataz	PI	B	400 mg qd	No studies in pregnancy/ use not recommended, indirect hyperbilirubinemia, prolonged PR interval (asymptomatic first degree AV block), hyperglycemia, lipodystrophy
18 Fosamprenavir (f-APV)	Lexiva	PI	C	1400 mg bid	No studies in pregnancy/ use not recommended Skin rash, diarrhea, nausea, hyperglycemia, transaminitis, hyperglycemia, lipodystrophy
19 Indinavir	Crixivan	PI	C	800 mg tid	Nephrolithiasis, GI intolerance, nausea, indirect hyperbilirubinemia, headache, thrombocytopenia, hyperglycemia, lipodystrophy
20 Lopinavir and ritonavir	Kaletra	PI	C	3 capsules (400 mg/100 mg) bid	GI intolerance, nausea, transaminitis, hyperglycemia, lipodystrophy, oral solution contains 42% alcohol
21 Nelfinavir	Viracept	PI	B	750 mg tid or 1250 mg bid	GI intolerance, nausea, transaminitis, hyperglycemia, lipodystrophy
22 Ritonavir	Norvir	PI	B	600 mg bid	GI intolerance, nausea, transaminitis, hyperglycemia, lipodystrophy
23 Saquinavir	Fortovase	PI	B	1200 mg tid	GI intolerance, nausea, transaminitis, hyperglycemia, lipodystrophy
24 Enfuvirtide	Fuzeon	FI	B	90 mg sq bid	No studies in pregnancy/ use not recommended, increased risk of bacterial pneumonia, hypersensitivity

AV, Atrioventricular; *bid,* twice daily; *FI,* fusion inhibitor; *GI,* gastrointestinal; *NNRTI,* nonnucleoside reverse transcriptase inhibitor; *NRTI,* nucleoside reverse transcriptase inhibitor; *PI,* protease inhibitor; *qd,* daily; *sq,* subcutaneous; *tid,* three times a day.

*FDA Pregnancy categories: A, adequate, well-controlled human studies fail to demonstrate fetal teratogenicity; B, animal studies fail to demonstrate fetal teratogenicity; adequate, well-controlled human studies have not been performed; C, safety in human studies has not been confirmed; drug should be used only if benefits outweigh risks; D, positive evidence of human fetal risk based on investigational or clinical experience, but potential benefits may be acceptable despite risk; X, animal studies or reports of adverse reactions in humans have demonstrated that the risk outweighs the benefits.

†Oral doses (unless specified) based on weight >60 kg. Adjustments of doses necessary with some medications based on weight and with renal or hepatic insufficiency.

regimens are preferred secondary to proven efficacy, tolerability, and minimal side effects. By not using all categories of drugs simultaneously, other drugs are available for use when resistance occurs. The latest recommendations outside of pregnancy are efavirenz (NNRTI) and AZT and lamudivine (3TC) (combination NRTI) as the preferred initial therapy. The CDC also recommends that a 3-NRTI regimen consisting of abacavir (ABC), AZT, and 3TC should only be used when an alternative therapy is contraindicated and that regimens of ABC, tenovir and 3TC or ddI, and tenovir and 3TC should not be used at all because of decreased efficacy. In general, the 3-NRTI regimens have been shown to be less effective than NNRTI or PI-based regimens and should not be used as first-line therapy. As a combination of the 2 NRTIs, AZT and 3TC (Combivir) are recommended as first-line treatment with either a NNRTI or PI because of ease of administration (one dose twice a day) and minimal toxicity. Combination of abacavir and 3TC (Epzicom) may be used as an alternative.

After initiation of treatment, close monitoring of physical symptoms and laboratory results for the prompt evaluation of side effects is necessary. Once patients are clinically stable (outside of pregnancy), evaluation can be limited to 3 to 6 months and should include CD4 count and viral load testing and monitoring of complete blood count, electrolytes, liver function tests, and lipid profiles. Recommendations for follow-up care and prophylaxis have also been established. In pregnancy, closer evaluation is warranted.

HIV IN PREGNANCY

In 1994, the Pediatric AIDS Clinical Trial Group (PACTG 076) demonstrated that oral antenatal, intravenous intrapartum, and oral neonatal treatment with AZT was effective in decreasing the risk of transmission of HIV by almost 70% (from a baseline of 25% to 8%). The trial did not distinguish which arm was most effective in reducing transmission. Subsequent trials have looked at shorter therapies out of practical necessity. In a trial from Thailand, a 4-week antenatal course of AZT and oral intrapartum dosing was effective in reducing transmission by 50% in non–breast feeding women. A subsequent trial comparing 4- and 12-week antenatal course, intrapartum treatment and short (3-day) or long (6-week) courses of neonatal therapy revealed higher transmission rates correlated with shorter periods of antenatal treatment. Prolonging neonatal therapy with this combination did not improve outcomes. The PETRA trial investigated the effects of treatment in breast feeding Ugandan women. Combination therapy of AZT and 3TC from 36 weeks, oral intrapartum medication, and treatment for 1 week postpartum of the mother and infant with the regimen reduced transmission at 6 weeks by 63%. In this study, treatment with AZT and 3TC initiated in labor was only effective if combined with the postpartum and neonatal therapies (reduction of 42%). In landmark studies, a single dose (200 mg) intrapartum treatment with nevirapine followed by neonatal treatment at 48 to 72 hours was effective in reducing transmission when compared with both intrapartum and neonatal AZT and to AZT and 3TC. The decrease of

HIV transmission with this therapy has been noted in both breast feeding and non–breast feeding women, making it a more viable option in developing countries without a reliable water supply and limited nutritional alternatives to breast feeding. Combination of nevirapine and AZT has also been shown to be more effective than AZT alone in women naïve to medication though the addition of intrapartum Nevirapine has not significantly changed rates of transmission in Western countries in women already receiving HAART.

Transmission rates of less than 5% have been reported with the use of HAART in the United States and Europe. This low rate of vertical transmission relates to the decrease in risk associated with a decrease in viremia. Unfortunately, there is no absolute number that can be used as a predictor of transmission, and transmission has occurred with undetectable viral levels. This may be secondary to other obstetric factors and discordance in the amount of virus in the genital tract compared with peripheral blood and host and viral factors. Regardless of the antenatal therapy used, AZT prophylaxis is still recommended in the intrapartum and neonatal period unless there is a history of maternal hypersensitivity or allergy. In those cases, neonatal therapy is still recommended. Interventions to minimize the risk of transmission and shorten the course of labor such as avoidance of invasive procedures, artificial rupture of membranes, and judicious use of Pitocin should be strongly considered. In cases of undetectable viral load, there are no data available that cesarean delivery further diminishes the risk of transmission. In cases of inadequate therapy, elective cesarean before labor has been shown to significantly decrease the risk of transmission. For a scheduled cesarean section, intravenous AZT should be begun 3 hours before surgery, according to standard dosing regimens (Table 21-3). Other antiretroviral medications should be continued regardless of the mode of delivery.

Although the use of AZT has been accepted as the standard of care in the obstetric management of HIV-positive women, there is still considerable controversy about the initiation of HAART in pregnancy in medication-naïve patients and about which medications to begin. The CDC recommends that standard combination antiretrovirals regimens should be offered to all pregnant women regardless of viral load. Some women may choose to initiate therapy after the first trimester to decrease the potential risk of teratogenicity. After 10 weeks' gestation, the risk of teratogen exposure is negligible. Also, consideration for initiating medication in the setting of nausea and vomiting of pregnancy (hyperemesis) must be given

Table 21-3

Pediatric AIDS Clinical Trial Group (PACTG) 076 AZT Regimen

Time of Administration	Regimen
Intrapartum	Intravenous AZT in 1 hr initial bolus of 2 mg/kg, followed by infusion of 1 mg/kg/hr until delivery
Postpartum	Neonatal oral AZT (syrup) 2 mg/kg/dose every 6 hours for first 6 weeks of life beginning 8-12 hr after birth

AZT, zidovudine.

because this can affect drug adherence and absorption and therefore may enhance the development of viral resistance.

For women already on a well-tolerated, effective antiretroviral therapy, their medications should not be stopped preconceptually or with pregnancy testing. This may hasten the development of resistance. Consideration should always be taken to adding AZT to a pregnancy regimen and its use in initial therapy in medication-naïve pregnant women. D4T-containing regimens are not recommended as initial regimens because of known antagonism with AZT. ddI and D4T should not be used in combination because of reports of maternal mortality from lactic acidosis with this combination. Also, AZT should not be used in cases of known drug resistance or allergy despite pregnancy. Aggressive follow-up of increasing viral load and decreasing CD4 counts is necessary in pregnancy to avoid drug changes in the third trimester (during which side effects may be potentiated by the pregnant state) and inadequate therapy conferring an increased risk of transmission.

Pregnancy does not alter the long-term consequences or progression of HIV disease, but an increase in toxicities may be related to the pregnancy. There does not seem to be an increased risk of prematurity, preterm labor, or growth restriction associated with HIV or HAART therapy in the absence of other risk factors. Several toxicities have been reported. Hyperglycemia is a known side effect of PI therapy. Gestational diabetes complicates 5% of all pregnancies. It is not known whether the use of PIs accentuates the risk of gestational diabetes or increases the need for insulin therapy. Early glucose tolerance testing should be considered in patients receiving PIs in pregnancy.

Short- or long-term use of nucleoside analogs is known to cause mitochondrial dysfunction. Clinical disorders linked to mitochondrial toxicity include neuropathy, myopathy, hepatitic steatosis, symptomatic lactic acidosis, and pancreatitis. There may be a female predisposition to the development of lactic acidosis and hepatic steatosis, which may also be accentuated by pregnancy. The syndromes have characteristics similar to acute fatty liver of pregnancy, severe preeclampsia, and hemolysis, elevated liver functions, low platelets (HEELP) syndrome. These syndromes have also been linked to carriers of gene defects involved in mitochondrial fatty acid oxidation. The risk in pregnancy theoretically would be exacerbated by the inability to metabolize both maternal and fetal fatty acids and by the increased metabolic demands of the pregnancy itself. There are currently no available tests to distinguish which women would be at increased risk in pregnancy, although women who are overweight may be at increased risk. These factors and similarities in presentation with typical pregnancy symptoms warrant close monitoring in pregnancy. Typical initial symptoms include nausea, vomiting and abdominal pain, dyspnea, and weakness. Metabolic acidosis and transaminitis are seen. Prompt discontinuation of medication is necessary.

All PIs and NNRTIs have been associated with transaminitis. Among the NNRTIs, nevirapine is the most likely to cause significant transaminitis. A twelvefold higher incidence of hepatotoxicity has been observed in women with pre-nevirapine CD4 count greater than 250 cells/mm^3. The reports included both pregnant and nonpregnant women. The toxicity is seen at higher CD4 counts in men. This toxicity is generally seen in the first 4 months of therapy, and unfortunately symptoms do not necessarily regress with discontinuation of the medication. Patients with underlying hepatic disease from hepatitis B or C may be at higher risk for its development. Almost half of patients present with a rash; therefore, all patients should be counseled on symptoms and instructed to seek medical attention and discontinue medication if a rash or jaundice appear. Close monitoring of liver function tests are warranted with the initiation of medication and dosing should be initiated daily, with an increase in the dose to twice daily after evaluation of the patient in 2 weeks. PIs can demonstrate liver toxicity at any time during treatment.

Tremendous advances in the knowledge and treatment of HIV have occurred in the last 20 years. Research in the development of new medications and vaccines is necessary to stop the epidemic, as is widespread availability of cost-effective treatment modalities for developing countries.

KEY POINTS

- Antiretroviral therapies should be initiated simultaneously to avoid development of drug resistance.
- Close monitoring is necessary in pregnancy as hepatotoxicity from medications may be more common.
- PACTG 076 demonstrated a 70% reduction in vertical transmission with AZT monotherapy in the antenatal, intrapartum, and neonatal periods. HAART with complete suppression of viral load has less than a 5% vertical transmission rate.

SUGGESTED READINGS

Centers for Disease Control and Prevention: Management of possible sexual, injecting drug use, or other nonoccupational exposure to HIV, including considerations related to antiretroviral therapy. Public Health Service Statement. *MMWR* 47(no RR-17), 1998.

Centers for Disease Control and Prevention: *Guidelines for the Use of Antiretroviral Agents in HIV-1-infected Adults and Adolescents.* March 23, 2004.

Centers for Disease Control and Prevention: *Recommendations for use of Anti-Retroviral Drugs in Pregnant HIV-1 Infected Women for Maternal Health and Interventions to Reduce Perinatal HIV-1 Transmission in the United States, June 23, 2004.*

Cohen PT, Sande MA, Voberding PA: *The AIDS Knowledge Base,* ed 3. Philadelphia, 1999, Lippincott Williams and Wilkins.

http://hivinsite.ucsf.edu/

http://www.hivatis.org

22

CARDIAC DISEASE
D. Yvette LaCoursiere and Michael Varner

Pregnancy is associated with substantial maternal cardiovascular adaptations (Table 22-1). Increases in stroke volume and heart rate begin early in the first trimester. The combination of increased cardiac output and decreased systemic vascular resistance (SVR) results in characteristic blood pressure changes. Mid-trimester systolic blood pressure decreases by 5 to 10 mmHg in uncomplicated pregnancy, and diastolic pressures decrease by 10 to 15 mmHg at the same time point. Whereas blood volume and cardiac output increase by 30% to 50% in a normal singleton pregnancy, vascular resistance (defined by the ratio of cardiac output and mean arterial pressure) declines. In fact, decreased SVR is one of the earliest changes in the pregnant woman's vasculature. These adaptations ensure optimal perfusion of the developing fetoplacental unit. These changes essentially resolve by 2 weeks postpartum.

The pregnant woman with normal cardiovascular function adapts to these physiologic changes without difficulty. However, the presence of maternal cardiac disease, be it known preconceptionally or diagnosed only during the pregnancy, can lead to serious maternal and/or perinatal morbidity or mortality. Although overall maternal mortality rates in developed countries have dropped by several orders of magnitude during the preceding century, the relative decrease in deaths attributable to maternal cardiac disease has been less, resulting in a progressive increase in the percent of maternal deaths resulting from cardiac disease and its complications. Most current American reviews place the percentage of maternal deaths resulting from cardiac disease between 10% and 25%.

Cardiac disease is a common medical problem among women of reproductive age. Heart disease ranks as the third leading cause of death of women aged 15 to 44 years behind cancer and unintentional injuries. Recent Centers for Disease Control and Prevention (CDC) reports reveal a 30% increase in sudden cardiac death among American women aged 15 to 34 years from 1989 to 1996. Current estimates suggest approximately 0.5% to 1% of pregnant women have cardiac disease.

The second half of the twentieth century documented a dramatic reversal of the types of heart disease seen among women of reproductive age, and thus of maternal heart disease during pregnancy. Before the mid-twentieth century, the majority of maternal heart disease in pregnancy was rheumatic in etiology. Early in the twentieth century, the ratio of rheumatic to congenital heart disease (CHD) seen during pregnancy was at least 10:1.

Table 22-1

Arterial blood pressure	Decreases by 5-10 mmHg systolic and 10-15 mmHg diastolic during mid-trimester, returns to normal by term
Heart rate	Increases by 10-15 beats per minute
Blood volume	30%-50% increase by term in a singleton pregnancy; 50%-70% increase in twin pregnancy
Arterial media	Thickening and fragmentation of reticular fibers, mild hyperplasia of smooth muscle cells

This ratio has now reversed itself, with all recent reports from the developed world reporting more cases of CHD than rheumatic heart disease.

CHD is the single most common birth defect seen at the time of delivery, affecting 8 of every 1000 live births. These defects are equally distributed between boys and girls. The advent of neonatal intensive care plus improved medical and surgical treatments has resulted in an ever-increasing number of women reaching childbearing age who themselves were born with congenital heart defects.

Contemporary references to cardiovascular disease in the nonobstetric literature emphasize hypertension, coronary vascular disease, and stroke as the dominant causes of morbidity and mortality. Of these, hypertensive heart disease has remained the third most common cause of heart disease in pregnancy, with a gradual shift from chronic hypertension seen in older gravidas toward obesity-associated heart disease. Beyond these three major subgroups of cardiac disease, other cardiac complications that can be encountered in the pregnant woman include myocardiopathy, arrhythmias, and cardiac disease resulting from various metabolic and/or infectious etiologies. It is the intent of this chapter to review the epidemiology, etiology, clinical presentation, differential diagnosis, treatment, and expected outcomes of cardiac disease during pregnancy.

DEFINITION

Normal function of the human heart requires an appropriately contractile myocardium, a functional electromechanical conduction system that coordinates myocardial activity and rate, and functional valves that allow forward flow of adequate blood volumes at appropriate time yet prevent reflux of blood at other appropriate times in the cardiac cycle (Box 22-1).

Box 22-1   Requirements for Normal Function

Normal function of the human heart requires the following:
1. Appropriately contractile myocardium
2. Functional electromechanical conduction system
3. Functional valves
   Given the physiologic cardiovascular changes in pregnancy, abnormalities of any of these three essential elements may either exacerbate known heart disease or unmask previous unrecognized heart disease.

Abnormalities of any of these functions can result in clinically apparent cardiac disease.

EPIDEMIOLOGY

The three most common cardiac diseases are CHD, rheumatic heart disease, and cardiovascular disease (hypertension, coronary heart disease, and stroke). Nearly one million Americans are affected by CHD. Although CHD rates are quoted to be approximately 8 per 1000 live births, the actual rate is likely much higher. The rates that range between 8 and 9 per 1000 live births do not include several of the most commonly experienced cardiac defects such as bicommissural aortic valves, which often present late in life, abnormalities in the leaflets, which lead to mitral valve prolapse (MVP), and the patent ductus arteriosus (PDA) experienced by many preterm neonates. Also, the aforementioned rates are calculated using live births. The inclusion of stillborn fetuses with cardiac defects would increase these rates because stillborn fetuses are tenfold more likely to exhibit cardiac abnormalities compared with their live-born counterparts.

Although rheumatic heart disease is the most common cause of acquired heart disease among the young worldwide, it has significantly decreased in developed countries as a result of improved antibiotic treatment of Group A streptococcal pharyngitis, improved living conditions, and access to medical care. The rates of rheumatic fever in the United States are less than 2 per 100,000 annually with a parallel decrease in rheumatic heart disease rates.

ETIOLOGY

The causes of CHD are a multifactorial interplay of genetic and environmental factors that remain poorly understood. Less than 1 in 6 of congenital cardiac malformations result from known genetic aberrations. Some environmental and infectious agents have been identified as cardiac teratogens, including thalidomide, isotretinoin, lithium, excessive alcohol use, and gestational rubella infection. Parents who themselves have survived CHD are more likely to have children with CHD, generally estimated at 2% to 5% risk of having an affected child. Future efforts to identify etiologies are warranted given the increasing rates of CHD over the past several decades.

Rheumatic heart disease occurs after pharyngeal infection with group A streptococcus. During the acute phase an inflammatory response occurs in connective tissue and collagen throughout the body. The cardiac valves and chordae tendineae experience edema and cellular infiltration, which leads to hyaline degeneration. This forms verrucae at the valve leaflets that impair its ability to close. With chronic inflammation, fibrosis and calcification occur, leading to stenosis.

Cardiovascular disease—including hypertension, coronary heart disease, and stroke—affects more than 4% of women aged 20 to 34 years and this rate increases to 13.6% in women aged 35 to 44 years. Risk factors include cigarette smoking, elevated cholesterol, obesity, diabetes, family history, and nonwhite race/ethnicity.

CLINICAL PRESENTATION

Many women with heart disease are asymptomatic. Pregnancy may exacerbate underlying cardiovascular pathophysiology and produce symptoms for the first time. To provide appropriate care clinicians must have a low threshold of suspicion for cardiac disease and liberal use of echocardiography. Cardiovascular symptoms include fatigue, dyspnea (on exertion, at rest, or paroxysmal nocturnal), orthopnea, hemoptysis, pulmonary or systemic emboli, progressive edema, syncope, and chest pain. Some of these symptoms, including dyspnea, edema, sensations of hyperdynamism/palpitations, and fatigue are common to normal pregnancy. Physical examination findings can likewise obscure the clinical scenario given the physiologic mild tachycardia, mid-systolic ejection murmur, pronounced S_1 and S_2 splitting, and edema from the physiologic changes of pregnancy. Symptoms of chest pain, worsening dyspnea, hemoptysis or syncope, or the findings of diastolic murmurs, continuous murmurs, 3/6 or greater systolic murmurs, irregular rhythm, clubbing, cyanosis, and early-onset or progressive severe edema warrant evaluation.

The New York Heart Association (NYHA) classification system (Box 22-2) has proven to be a useful prognostic classification of cardiac symptomatology during pregnancy.

Electrocardiographic changes occur in normal pregnancy. Some of these changes result from the diaphragmatic elevation and subsequent cardiac deviation. Changes seen may include mild tachycardia, shifting of the QRS axis, inverse T waves in lead III, and q waves in lead III and aVF (Box 22-3).

Box 22-2 New York Heart Association Classification–Functional Capacity

Class I. Patients with cardiac disease but without resulting limitation of physical activity. Ordinary physical activity does not cause undue fatigue, palpitation, dyspnea, or anginal pain.
Objective Assessment: No objective evidence of cardiovascular disease.
Class II. Patients with cardiac disease resulting in slight limitation of physical activity. They are comfortable at rest. Ordinary physical activity results in fatigue, palpitation, dyspnea, or anginal pain.
Objective Assessment: Objective evidence of minimal cardiovascular disease.
Class III. Patients with cardiac disease resulting in marked limitation of physical activity. They are comfortable at rest. Less than ordinary activity causes fatigue, palpitation, dyspnea, or anginal pain.
Objective Assessment: Objective evidence of moderately severe cardiovascular disease.
Class IV. Patients with cardiac disease resulting in inability to carry on any physical activity without discomfort. Symptoms of heart failure or the anginal syndrome may be present even at rest. If any physical activity is undertaken, discomfort is increased.
Objective Assessment: Objective evidence of severe cardiovascular disease.

> **Box 22-3** Electrocardiographic Changes during Normal Pregnancy
>
> Mild tachycardia
> Shifting of the QRS axis
> Inverse T waves in lead III
> q waves in lead III and aVF

Recent reports indicate that oxytocin administration can prolong the QT interval. Echocardiographic changes in normal pregnancy have been reported: cardiac chamber enlargement between 5% and 20%, dilation of the tricuspid, pulmonary, and mitral valve, and ensuing minimal regurgitation. Maternal mortality risks for various cardiac lesions has been estimated and categorized. The American College of Obstetricians and Gynecologists (ACOG) classification of cardiac lesions by maternal mortality risk is shown in Box 22-4. This system is useful when specific lesions are known or categorized. Other classification systems use clinical signs/symptoms to predict a patient's likelihood of having an adverse cardiac event. Siu et al. describe four predictors of cardiac events: prior cardiac events such as congestive heart failure (CHF), transient ischemic attack (TIA), or cerebrovascular accident (CVA) before pregnancy or arrhythmia; NYHA class greater than II (see Box 22-2) or cyanosis; left heart obstruction; and systemic ventricular dysfunction. Patients without any of the aforementioned predictors had an estimated risk of cardiac events of 5%, those with one predictor had a 27% chance, and 75% of those with more than one of the four risk factors experienced a cardiac event.

The clinical presentation, intrapartum management, and outcomes of parturients with cardiac disease depends on not only the severity of disease

> **Box 22-4** The American College of Obstetricians and Gynecologists (ACOG) Classification of Cardiac Lesions by Maternal Mortality Risk
>
> **Low-risk lesions (<1% mortality):**
> Left to right shunts
> Pulmonic or tricuspid disease
> Corrected tetralogy of Fallot
> Bioprosthetic valve
> Mitral stenosis (class NYHA class I or II)
>
> **Moderate-risk lesions (5%-15% mortality):**
> Mitral stenosis (class III and IV or atrial fibrillation)
> Aortic stenosis
> Coarctation (without valvular disease)
> Prior myocardial infarction
> Marfan's (normal aortic root)
> Mechanical valves
>
> **High-risk lesions (25%-50% mortality):**
> Pulmonary hypertension
> Coarctation with valvular disease
> Critical mitral or aortic stenosis
> Marfan's (dilated aortic root)
>
> Dildy III GA, Belfort MA, Saade G, et al: *Critical Care Obstetrics*, 4th ed. Wiley-Blackwell, 2003. *NYHA*, New York Heart Association.

but also the location and type of lesion (stenotic or regurgitant). A conceptual framework based on the location and type of lesion can aid in the understanding of the management of these women. This discussion groups diagnoses by the functional impairment they impose, specifically left heart functional impairment, right heart functional impairment, multifocal or diffuse involvement, and arrhythmias. In general, regurgitant valvular lesions are better tolerated in pregnancy as a result of the physiologic decrease in SVR, subsequent improvement in forward flow, and overall decrease in the regurgitation. Contrarily, the functional effects of valvular stenosis are worsened by the physiologic increase in blood volume, heart rate, and resultant stroke volume. As a result of these functional perturbations, an array of cardiac drugs has been developed. See Table 22-2 for a listing of common cardiac medications and their effects in pregnancy.

Left Heart Functional Impairment

Mitral Valve Disease

Mitral Stenosis

Mitral stenosis (MS) results from progressive fibrosis, scarring, and calcification of the mitral valve. Normal valve area in women is 4 cm^2. Once the valve area decreases to 2 cm^2, an audible murmur becomes apparent, and as the valve area nears 1 cm^2 the lesion is deemed severe. In the developing world, MS results primarily from rheumatic fever; in the developed world CHD accounts for a greater etiologic fraction with lesions uncommonly also resulting from endomyocardial fibroelastosis and systemic lupus erythematosus. Initially MS presents with dyspnea on exertion and then, as edema occurs progressively in the pulmonary vascular tree, orthopnea and paroxysmal nocturnal dyspnea develop. Physical findings may include significant jugular A waves, an apical systolic nonradiating rumble, an early diastolic rumble at the left sternal border (if pulmonary hypertension has developed), right ventricular heave, edema, hepatomegaly, ascites, and/or evidence of systemic emboli. The fixed valve area of MS may allow acceptable function outside of pregnancy. However, the increased heart rate and blood volume of pregnancy may unmask this limitation and thus MS may initially present in pregnancy as CHF. To avoid cardiac decompensation, careful observation for evidence of volume overload and pulmonary edema is needed. Treatment includes exercise limitation and/or bed rest, beta blockade to avoid tachycardia, observation for development of atrial fibrillation (AF), acute arrhythmia treatment with calcium channel blockade or electrocardioversion, chronic arrhythmia therapy with beta blockade, digoxin, and/or anticoagulation, and surveillance for CHF. Surgical treatment such as valve replacement or percutaneous valvuloplasty may be necessary. Intrapartum management should avoid tachycardia, sudden increases in volume, and decreases in SVR. Limiting pain and anxiety and avoiding fluid overload during delivery are crucial.

Mitral Regurgitation

Mitral regurgitation (MR) occurs when a significant portion of left ventricular outflow returns to the left atrium, resulting in increases of left atrial volume and pulmonary pressure and ultimately right heart failure. It has been classified in three categories: acute, chronic compensated, and chronic

Common Cardiac Medications—Use in Pregnancy

Table 22-2

Drug	Use	Maternal Side Effects	Fetal Adverse Outcomes	Pregnancy Category/ Acceptability	Breast Feeding
ACE Inhibitors					
Captopril, Enalapril	Competitive inhibitors of angiotensin I converting enzyme; HTN/CHF	Cough, angioedema, rash, hypotension	Compromise of fetal renal system and resultant severe and possibly fatal oligohydramnios	C first Δ; D second Δ NOT acceptable	+
Angiotensin Receptor Blockers					
Losartan, Valsartan	Inhibitors of angiotensin II receptor; HTN, ± CHF	Headaches, dizziness	Similar to ACE inhibitors	C first Δ; D second Δ NOT acceptable	Avoid, safety not established
Antiadrenergics					
Clonidine	Stimulates adrenergic receptors at CNS; HTN narcotic withdrawal	Fatigue, dizziness, constipation, dry mouth, severe rebound HTN (sudden withdrawal)	Limited first-trimester use, but no teratogenicity reported, no neonatal hypotension	C	Found in breast milk, minimal data without neonatal hypotension, no long-term data
Methyldopa	Metabolite—alpha methylnorepinephrine replaces NE, decreased adrenergic outflow and decreased total peripheral resistance; HTN	Drowsiness, headache, weakness, GI upset, dry mouth, rash; Iron decreases availability	Fetal levels attained, no teratogenicity reported	B	+
Antiarrythmics					
Adenosine	Purine based nucleoside, slows AV node conduction; PSVT	Facial flushing, headache, dyspnea, dizziness, CP, nausea	No adverse effects reported in fetus with maternal administration, fetal administration—death 2 week following	C	NA

Continued

33

Table 22-2—cont'd

Drug	Use	Maternal Side Effects	Fetal Adverse Outcomes	Pregnancy Category/ Acceptability	Breast Feeding
Amiodarone	Multiple effects, delayed conduction and repolarization, prolonged action potential	Pulmonary, hepatic and neurologic toxicity, thyroid abnormalities	Growth restriction, hypothyroidism, transient bradycardia and prolonged QT after birth	D	−, not recommended if used in past several months
Atropine	Anticholinergic			C	+, passage − controversial
Digoxin	Atrial fibrillation, atrial flutter, PAT; direct inotropic effect	Arrhythmias, nausea/vomiting, blurred vision, gynecomastia, headache	Preterm labor?	C	+
Flecainide	Maternal and fetal arrhythmias	Blurred vision, dizziness, chest pain, dyspnea, edema, shakiness	Fetal death reported but cause difficult to interpret, ?conjugated hyperbilirubinemia	C	+
Lidocaine	Ventricular arrhythmias	Dizziness, hypotension, anxiety, delirium	Possible CNS depression, seizures	B-C	+
Quinidine	Maternal and fetal arrhythmias	Nausea, vomiting, lightheadedness, headache, abdominal pain	?IUGR, high doses—oxytocic properties	C	+
Sotalol	Ventricular arrhythmias, fetal arrhythmias, HTN	Fatigue, bradycardia, dyspnea, asthma, dizziness, torsades de pointes	IUGR	B	−
Anticoagulants					
Enoxaparin	Low molecular weight heparin with increased antifactor Xa to antifactor IIa activity (3:1)	Hematoma, hemorrhage, thrombocytopenia, osteopenia, mechanical valves—reports		B	?

Table 22-2—cont'd

Drug	Use	Maternal Side Effects	Fetal Adverse Outcomes	Pregnancy Category/ Acceptability	Breast Feeding
Heparin	Binds ATIII, accelerates rate ATIII neutralizes activated forms of factors II, VII, IX, X, XI, XII (Xa:IIa 1:1)	Hemorrhage, thrombocyto-penia, osteopenia		B-C	+
Warfarin	Inhibits hepatic synthesis of coagulation factors (II, VII, IX, X)	Hemorrhage	Fetal warfarin syndrome 6-9 weeks gestation (nasal hypoplasia/ IUGR/eye defects, hypoplastic extremities, MR, seizures, deafness, scoliosis, CHD), SAB, FD, prematurity hemorrhage	X—first Δ, use 12-35 weeks common	+
Beta Blockers					
Atenolol	Beta 1 adrenergic blocker (cardioselective at low doses only); HTN	Dizziness, bradycardia, fatigue, hypotension, wheezing	IUGR (time dependent)	D	–, may accumulate in breast milk, safer beta blockers are available
Labetalol	Beta adrenergic blocker and alpha 1 vasodilator; HTN	Dizziness, headache, nausea, fatigue, hypotension, dyspepsia	IUGR—one study, mild transient hypotension 24-48 hr	C	+
Metoprolol	Beta adrenergic blocker; HTN, MI, angina	Fatigue, dizziness, hypotension, bradycardia, dyspnea	IUGR	C	+
Propranolol	Beta adrenergic blocker; HTN, angina, arrhythmias, IHSS, post MI	Fatigue, bradycardia, hypotension, bronchospasm	IUGR	C	+

341

Continued

Table 22-2—cont'd

Drug	Use	Maternal Side Effects	Fetal Adverse Outcomes	Pregnancy Category/ Acceptability	Breast Feeding
Calcium Channel Blockers					
Diltiazem	HTN, angina, Arrhythmias	Hypotension, edema, headache, dizziness, bradycardia	No documented abnormalities	C	+
Nifedipine	HTN, angina	Edema, headache, flushing, dizziness, gingival hyperplasia	Commonly used, data limited, hypotension mediated fetal hypoxia	C	+
Verapamil	HTN, angina, arrhythmias	Constipation, dizziness, headache, bradycardia, hypotension	Fetal hypoxia secondary to maternal hypotension	C	+
Diuretics					
Furosemide	Acts at loop of Henle and distal tubules; preload reduction; HTN, edema, acute pulmonary edema	Granulocytopenia, thrombocytopenia, anemia, rash, liver function abnormalities, headache, confusion	Possible association with hypospadias with first-trimester use, decrease placental perfusion, yet no reports of adverse outcomes	C	No adverse reports
Spironolactone	Aldosterone agonist; HTN, edema, hypokalemia, hypoaldosteronism	Hyponatremia, GI complaints, gynecomastia	Not clear given antiandrogenic and estrogenic effects	D	+
Hydrochlorothiazide	Interferes with resorption of sodium and water at cortical diluting HTN, edema	Mild diabetogenic,	Possible first-trimester teratogenesis, may decrease placental perfusion, potential neonatal hypoglycemia, thrombocytopenia?	D	+
Miscellaneous					
Hydralazine	Direct vascular smooth muscle relaxation; HTN	Headache, GI complaints, hypotension, angina, tachycardia	Isolated lupus-like syndrome case reported	C	+

Table 22-2—cont'd

Drug	Use	Maternal Side Effects	Fetal Adverse Outcomes	Pregnancy Category/ Acceptability	Breast Feeding
Aspirin	Inhibiting prostaglandin production; MI	Hemorrhage	High dose—teratogenicity, IUGR, mortality, premature closure of ductus arteriosus	C-D	Cautious use recommended
Nitroglycerin	Vascular smooth muscle relaxation; angina, CHF associated with MI	Headache, lightheadedness, hypotension	Transient hypotension	C/B	No data available

ACE, Angiotensin-converting enzyme; *ATIII*, antithrombin III; *AV*, atrioventricular; *CHD*, congenital heart disease; *CHF*, congestive heart failure; *CNS*, central nervous system; *CP*, chest pain; *FD*, fetal distress; *GI*, gastrointestinal; *HTN*, hypertension; *IHSS*, idiopathic hypertrophic subaortic stenosis; *MI*, myocardial infarction; *MR*, mental retardation; *NA*, not available; *PAT*, paroxysmal atrial tachycardia; *PSVT*, paroxysmal supraventricular tachycardia; *SAB*, spontaneous abortion; +, positive; −, negative; ?, unknown.

decompensated. Although it was most often associated with rheumatic heart disease, MR now results most often as a sequel of MVP, Ehlers-Danlos syndrome, Marfan's syndrome, osteogenesis imperfecta, or systemic lupus erythematosus. Women typically present with symptoms of fatigue, dyspnea, orthopnea, and hemoptysis, or, in the setting of concomitant MVP, they may present with atypical chest pain and palpitations. In severe cases, CHF may develop. On examination, women may demonstrate apical lift and thrill as well as a high-pitched holosystolic murmur that radiates to the axilla. MR is usually well tolerated in pregnancy because the decrease in SVR and associated afterload reduction typically decrease the regurgitant flow. In moderate and severe cases, medical and/or surgical interventions may be required. Medical therapy includes salt restriction and diuretics, and digitalis for inotropic effect (or rate control if AF is present). Nifedipine and hydralazine can decrease afterload and improve forward flow. Anticoagulation is used in the presence of AF. In severe cases with insufficient response to medical treatment, definitive treatment remains surgical (i.e., valve replacement or repair). Intrapartum management objectives include avoidance of increases in systemic and pulmonic vascular resistance, myocardial depressants, and bradycardia. Isometric activity should be avoided by shortening the second stage of labor and/or adding hydralazine to decrease afterload.

Mitral Valve Prolapse

MVP is often identified incidentally in young women. It is seen more commonly in connective tissue disorders. It may be associated with septal defects, Marfan's syndrome, Ebstein's anomalies, or hypertrophic cardiomyopathy (CM). Most women are asymptomatic. However, symptoms may be present and include chest pain and/or palpitations. Affected women may develop MR, arrhythmia, or embolic events. On auscultation, an apical click and a mid to late systolic murmur may be heard. The diagnosis is confirmed with echocardiography. Women with severe symptoms may require further evaluation including exercise testing and Holter monitoring to exclude other underlying cardiac disease. Therapies are typically not indicated and reassurance is often adequate. When palpitations or pain oblige treatment, beta blockade may be useful (decreases heart rate and stretch on valve leaflets). Surgical remedy with valve replacement may rarely be required if patients exhibit NYHA class II-IV disease (see Box 22-2) or significant left ventricular function impairment. Pregnancy is typically well tolerated. Efforts to maintain preload, watch for development of arrhythmias, and avoid vasoconstriction are important intrapartum.

Aortic Valve Disease

Aortic Stenosis

Aortic stenosis (AS) stems from several etiologies including rheumatic heart disease, stenosis at a congenitally acquired lesion such as a unicuspid or bicuspid aortic valve, and calcific changes. Normally the aortic valve area is approximately 3 to 4 cm^2 and severe disease occurs when the area decreases to less than 1 cm^2 or the pressure gradient is 50 mmHg or greater across the valve. The stenotic aortic valve leads to increased volume and pressure in the left ventricle (LV). This results in hypertrophy with decreased compliance and impaired left ventricular systolic function (i.e., CHF) and potentially a decrease in coronary artery filling. Most common complaints include palpitations, fatigue, dyspnea, angina, syncope, and ultimately CHF symptoms. On physical examination a loud crescendo-decrescendo systolic murmur is audible at the apex or base with radiation to the neck and is accompanied by a decreased slope and intensity of carotid upstroke and strong apical impulse. In pregnancy, the increased heart rate and blood volume can adversely affect the relatively fixed cardiac output across a stenotic valve. Previously asymptomatic patients should still be observed closely. Medical treatment of symptomatic women includes restriction of activity. If CHF develops, sodium restriction and diuretics should be used. Calcium channel blockers or digoxin should be used if AF occurs. Given the poor 5-year survival with symptomatic AS, valve replacement may be recommended for such patients during pregnancy. Despite a predisposition to restenosis, balloon valvuloplasty is a temporizing procedure that can be used in pregnancy and also as a palliative measure for poor surgical candidates. Women with severe disease do not tolerate hypotension (blood loss, fluid depletion, and medication side effects), tachycardia, or caval compression. For these patients, care should be taken to maintain ventricular preload and a normal heart rate. Even previously asymptomatic patients require close monitoring.

Aortic Regurgitation

Aortic regurgitation (AR) may result from infective endocarditis, rheumatic heart disease, trauma, congenital bicuspid aorta, syphilitic aortitis, spondylitis, or systemic lupus erythematosus. It leads to an increased filling pressure and volume overload in the LV and progresses to dilation and hypertrophy of the LV with eventual systolic dysfunction. Symptoms of fatigue, dyspnea on exertion, syncope, and chest pain occur. Physical findings may include widened pulse pressure, "water hammer" pulses, a decrescendo blowing diastolic murmur at left sternal border, and an apical diastolic rumble. Pregnancy in women with AS is generally well tolerated secondary to the decrease in SVR and improvement of forward flow. Hydralazine can be used to further left ventricular afterload reduction when necessary. Medical therapy with vasodilators may slow disease progression by improving forward flow. Additionally, bradycardia and agents that depress the myometrium should be avoided. In AR patients with CHF, digitalis, diuretics, and salt restriction are commonly used. Surgical intervention is reserved for women with chronic disease who remain symptomatic despite optimal medical management or who have acute-onset regurgitation with concomitant left ventricular failure.

Coarctation of the Aorta

Coarctation of the aorta is an aortic stricture that is classified as simple if it is an isolated lesion or complex if other cardiac defects co-occur. Patients with coarctation of the aorta are at increased risk of having a bicuspid aortic valve, circle of Willis aneurysms, aortic dissections, and AS. They may be completely asymptomatic but can present with complaints of headaches, epistaxis, lower extremity weakness, and chest pain. Complex coarctation of the aorta has been associated with maternal mortality rates as high as 8%. Findings in such cases may include a temporal delay in pulses from the radial to the femoral artery, crescendo-decrescendo murmur throughout the precordium and upper extremity hypertension with a differential of 10 mmHg between the blood pressures in the upper and lower extremities. Significant lesions warrant intervention and may prompt consideration of pregnancy termination if signs and symptoms are progressive during early pregnancy. Surgical treatment is predominantly the standard of care in adults. Balloon dilation is being used, but long-term follow-up data are needed. Repaired lesions should be evaluated for persistent vascular turbulence that would necessitate endocarditis prophylaxis (Table 22-3). Clinical surveillance for hypertension, CHF, and severe headaches is essential in pregnancy. Close fetal growth surveillance is warranted given the increased rate of intrauterine growth restriction. During delivery, SVR and preload must be maintained, tachycardia avoided, and arrhythmias aggressively treated.

Right Heart Functional Impairment

Tricuspid Valve Disease

Tricuspid Regurgitation

Tricuspid regurgitation may result from a primary valvular lesion, from right ventricular dysfunction secondary to mitral valve abnormalities, from long-standing pulmonary disease, or from pulmonic stenosis (PS). It is associated with increased right ventricular volume and pressures. Primary etiologies include congenital anomalies such as Ebstein anomaly (apical displacement of the valve leaflets), prolapse (in association with mitral prolapse), and lesions of rheumatic heart disease, endocarditis, carcinoid syndrome, and connective tissue disorders. Affected women may be asymptomatic or may experience weakness, fatigue, pulsations in the neck and/or right upper quadrant pain. An S_3 gallop is usually present; some will develop jugular venous distention (JVD) with a prominent v wave, a right ventricular heave and gallop, a high-pitched pansystolic murmur with a diastolic rumble, ascites, and edema. If right atrial enlargement is present, AF can

Table 22-3

	Prophylaxis Indicated	
	Uncomplicated Delivery	**Suspected Bacteremia**
High-Risk Lesions Prosthetic valves, prior bacterial endocarditis, complex congenital heart disease (transposition), surgically constructed systemic pulmonary shunts or conduits	Optional	Recommended
Moderate-Risk Lesions Congenital cardiac malformations (except repaired ASD, VSD, PDA, or isolated secundum ASD), tetralogy of Fallot, acquired valvular dysfunction (RHD), hypertrophic cardiomyopathy, MVP with regurgitation and/or thickened leaflets	Not recommended	Recommended
Negligible-Risk Lesions MVP without regurgitation, physiologic murmurs, previous Kawasaki disease without valvular dysfunction, previous rheumatic fever without valvular dysfunction, cardiac pacemakers or defibrillators, prior CABG	Not recommended	Not recommended

From American College of Obstetricians and Gynecologists: ACOG Practice Bulletin # 47: *Prophylactic Antibiotics in Labor and Delivery. Obstet Gynecol* 102:875-882, 2003.
ASD, Atrial septal defect; *CABG*, coronary artery bypass grafting; *MVP*, mitral valve prolapse; *PDA*, patent ductus arteriosus; *RHD*, rheumatic heart disease; *VSD*, ventricular septal defect.

occur. Salt restriction and diuretics are initiated to control fluid overload. In the setting of AF, digoxin is useful to increase myocardial contractility and rate control. Hydralazine is used for afterload reduction to decrease right ventricular volume. For primary tricuspid regurgitation with severe symptoms, surgical treatment such as annuloplasty or valve replacement is indicated. There is a high rate of valve thrombosis at this valve and porcine valves are commonly used. Anticoagulants may be used to decrease the risk of thrombus formation after surgical intervention.

Pulmonic Valve Disease

Pulmonic Stenosis

PS refers to an obstruction in the pulmonary vascular system. This typically occurs at the valve itself but may occur in the subvalvular region or the main pulmonary artery. It can occur as a result of rheumatic heart disease, CHD, and myxomatous lesions from carcinoid syndrome. The normal pulmonic valve area is approximately 2 cm^2, with mild disease occurring from 1 to 2 cm^2 (valve gradient <50 mmHg), moderate disease 0.5 to 1 cm^2 (valve gradient 50-75 mmHg), and severe disease with valve area of less than 0.5 cm^2 (gradient >75 mmHg). PS may be asymptomatic in low-grade lesions and these are often well tolerated in pregnancy, but in higher-grade obstructions patients may complain of dyspnea, fatigue, angina, and/or syncope. As the obstruction impedes flow from the right ventricle, right-sided CHF may develop, with associated symptoms. A crescendo-decrescendo systolic murmur may be heard at the left upper sternal border with radiation throughout the precordium. In mild cases of PS it may be difficult to differentiate the murmur from that of the physiologic flow murmur of pregnancy. However, PS is also associated with prominent jugular venous a waves, a right ventricular lift, and/or pulmonic thrill. The physiologic changes of pregnancy can exacerbate PS. Percutaneous balloon valvuloplasty has been successful in treating PS during pregnancy and should be considered in patients with a gradient greater than 50 mmHg.

Primary Pulmonary Hypertension

Primary pulmonary hypertension (PPH) is a rare disease whose etiology is unknown but that results in vascular injury, endothelial dysfunction and smooth muscle proliferation (medial thickening and intimal fibrosis). These changes are thought to be mediated through decreased vascular nitric oxide and prostacyclin with resultant increases in endothelin and thromboxane. Ultimately this cascade leads to right-sided heart failure. Although the disease entity is rare (4/1,000,000), it has a predilection for women of reproductive age. Secondary pulmonary hypertension can result from cardiac diseases, pulmonary diseases, hemoglobinopathies, cocaine use, human immunodeficiency virus (HIV), or appetite suppressants. Both the maternal and fetal outcomes with PPH are guarded. PPH has a 50% maternal mortality in pregnancies continuing beyond the first trimester and the clinician must discuss these genuine risks and broach the subject of pregnancy termination. Pregnancy can facilitate right ventricular failure resulting from increased cardiac output and increased blood volume. Right ventricular decompensation symptoms include dyspnea, cyanosis, chronic cough ± hemoptysis, syncope, and fatigue. Physical findings may include a prominent S_2, pulmonic or tricuspid regurgitant murmur, right ventricular heave, increased JVD, hepatomegaly, and edema. Pulmonary artery pressures of greater than 25 mmHg at rest are used to make the diagnosis. Medical therapy is aimed at limiting activity, anticoagulation, digoxin in the setting of impaired right ventricular function, diuretics, calcium channel blockers, and pulmonary vasodilators such as nitric oxide and prostacyclins. Curative surgical treatment is limited to single or double lung transplantation, yet palliation of symptoms may be achieved by an atrial septostomy to create right to left shunting. Although antepartum changes contribute to decompensation, the transient augmentation in blood volume (± 500 ml) with uterine contractions and particularly the postpartum fluid shifts place these women at greater risk. Most maternal mortalities occur in the week following delivery. Intrapartum management includes avoidance of increased pulmonary vascular resistance (specifically avoid hypothermia, acidosis, hypercarbia, hypoxemia, and sympathomimetics) and decreases in preload and afterload (specifically, minimization of blood loss, avoidance of anesthetic-induced hypotension). Side effects of the prostacyclin can include platelet dysfunction, tachyphylaxis, and methemoglobinemia. Oxytocic agents should be administered carefully because they can increase pain and increase contraction-related blood volume changes.

Multifocal or Diffuse Impairment

Tetralogy of Fallot

Four lesions comprise the tetralogy of Fallot (TOF)—ventricular septal defect (VSD), right ventricular obstruction, overriding aorta, and right ventricular hypertrophy—and result from the anterior displacement of the insertion of the infundibular ventricular septum. The basic pathophysiology is the obstruction of pulmonary blood flow from the right ventricle and resultant shunting of unoxygenated blood through the VSD. This pathologic change results in hypoxemia and cyanosis. As a result, the great majority of cases are diagnosed in infancy, and most lesions are corrected early by total surgical repair. Women with successfully corrected lesions typically tolerate pregnancy well. Palliative procedures are reserved for patients with significant hypoplasia of pulmonary vasculature. Uncorrected lesions confer considerable risk during pregnancy because the decrease in SVR may increase the right to left shunting with resultant increased hypoxemia and cyanosis.

Transposition of the Great Vessels

This cardiac anomaly results in an aorta that originates from the right ventricle and the pulmonary artery from the LV. As a result the pulmonary and systemic circulations run in parallel and oxygenation occurs only via a communicative lesion, usually a PDA or VSD. Like TOF, the severity of the lesion promotes its identification in early infancy. Definitive surgical treatment is associated with an excellent prognosis during pregnancy.

Coronary Heart Disease

Although less common in women of reproductive age because of the increasing numbers of women who delay pregnancy into the fourth or fifth decade (now more than 100,000 women older than 40 years delivering each year in the United States) and the increase in obesity (a 40% increase in obesity in women of reproductive age in the preceding decade) coronary heart disease is an ever more important disease to understand in pregnancy. Currently 1 per 10,000 women experience an acute myocardial infarction (AMI) in pregnancy. The predominant cause of myocardial ischemia and infarction in pregnancy is the same as that in the general population, namely, atherosis. Other etiologies include coronary dissection, coronary arteritis, sickle crisis, preeclampsia, hemorrhage, embolism, congenital coronary abnormalities, ventricular hypertrophy, hypoxia secondary to pulmonary disease, cocaine abuse, and use of ergot derivatives. Women with coronary heart disease are more likely to be older, use tobacco, have hyperlipidemia, be physically inactive, overweight, or obese, have diabetes or chronic hypertension, and have a positive family history. Coronary heart disease may be asymptomatic (found incidentally in the course of unrelated evaluations) or present as angina pectoris or acute coronary syndrome (unstable angina or myocardial infarction [MI]). Symptoms of angina may be substernal chest pain (pressure, heaviness, or tightness) or vague discomforts that are reproduced by activities that increase myocardial oxygen demand. Other complaints may include palpitations, exertional dyspnea, and decreased exercise tolerance. The pain may be associated with nausea, diaphoresis, shortness of breath, and/or pain that radiates down the arms or to the neck/jaw. These symptoms also exist during an AMI; however, in AMI, they are unrelenting (lasting greater than 30 minutes) and do not completely respond to rest or nitroglycerin. Both angina and AMI result from similar underlying mechanisms, namely an alteration in blood flow resulting in inadequate myocardial oxygenation. During pregnancy, the physiologic tachycardia, increased blood volume, anemia, and the physical strain of labor place women with underlying atherosis at risk for coronary syndromes. Unlike angina, AMI results in myocardial necrosis and irreversible damage. Although there may be no physical findings associated with angina or AMI, patients with AMI may exhibit pale diaphoretic skin, a new-onset murmur of MR, and/or rales. Electrocardiogram (ECG) and serum enzyme studies are used to identify AMI. Troponin I and muscle band creatinine kinase (CK-MB) are the standard laboratory criteria used to diagnose MI in nonpregnant patients. However, CK-MB has been identified in the uterus and placenta, and some evidence suggests it may be elevated in the peripartum period. In pregnancy, troponin I is a reliable enzymatic maker of AMI. However, there are data that suggest that it may be elevated in women with preeclampsia. Thus in women without preeclampsia troponin I is the best marker for acute myocardial injury, yet if coexistent preeclampsia is present, troponin I in concert with ECG changes may be more reliable.

Treatment is aimed to decrease the amount of myocardial injury by reperfusion of the affected tissue. This is accomplished in several manners: beta adrenergic blockade, vasodilators, angioplasty, coronary stenting, coronary artery bypass grafting, and possibly thrombolysis. Acute therapy includes bed rest, oxygen, morphine for pain relief, nitroglycerin, beta blockade, lidocaine (to prevent arrhythmias), and possible anticoagulation. Reported safe administration of tissue plasminogen activator (TPA) during pregnancy is limited to case reports. TPA may be considered only if delivery is not imminent because of the increased risk of hemorrhage. Complications of AMI include arrhythmias, MR and insufficiency, cardiogenic shock, right ventricular infarction, pulmonary congestion, coronary artery dissection, VSD after weeks (from septal necrosis), and emboli (systemic and pulmonary). Intrapartum management should include measures to decrease myocardial oxygen demand.

Cardiomyopathy

CM is a syndrome characterized by cardiac muscle dysfunction. There are three defined categories of CM: dilated, hypertrophic, and restrictive. To diagnose a patient with CM, the cardiac abnormality cannot be the secondary result of congenital, valvular, ischemic diseases, pericardial, or hypertensive disease.

In dilated CM, the heart is enlarged and there is biventricular contractile dysfunction with congestion. Women with peripartum CM develop this pattern of disease. Symptoms include fatigue, dyspnea (at rest or with exertion), orthopnea, paroxysmal nocturnal dyspnea, palpitations, and/or emboli. Women may demonstrate tachypnea, tachycardia, increased JVP, rales, S_3, S_4, murmurs of mitral or tricuspid regurgitation, peripheral edema, and/or hepatomegaly. If there is a remediable underlying causative process, treatment begins with correcting the aberrancy. Otherwise treatment is supportive with bed rest, sodium restriction, diuretics, hydralazine (in lieu of angiotensin-converting enzyme [ACE] inhibitors), digoxin (if arrhythmias are present), anticoagulants, and/or beta adrenergic blockade. Intrapartum management requires strict observance of fluid balance. Although ACE inhibitors are more effective than hydralazine, their use should be restricted until after delivery because of their deleterious effects on fetal renal function. Heart transplant is often required at some point postpartum.

Peripartum CM is an idiopathic form of dilated CM with its onset between 1 month antepartum and 5 months postpartum. It is generally considered as a diagnosis only after other causes of CM have been excluded. This often requires an endomyocardial biopsy. In clinically "idiopathic" cases, an underlying diagnosis (such as hypertensive heart disease, obesity, or viral myocarditis) will be found in at least 50% of cases. It similarly presents with CHF, arrhythmia, and embolism. Although some women die or require transplantation from peripartum CM, a substantial proportion may regain normal left ventricular function. Unfortunately, subsequent pregnancies in women with a history of peripartum CM appear to confer risk of worsening left ventricular dysfunction and death even among women who had regained normal cardiac function. Hypertrophic CM typically occurs in elderly patients, with the exception of a familial form that is typically inherited and is transmitted with an autosomal dominant pattern. Interestingly, the hypertrophic change exhibits a propensity for the intraventricular septum leading to an obstructive phenomenon in the LV (idiopathic hypertrophic subaortic stenosis). Although the increased vascular volume of pregnancy may improve function, tachycardia and hypovolemia may cause a clinical deterioration. Thus affected women required careful attention during labor and delivery. Some of these patients may be asymptomatic but others complain of dyspnea, presyncope/syncope, palpitations, dizziness, chest pain, orthopnea, and/or paroxysmal nocturnal dyspnea. They will have a significant crescendo-decrescendo systolic murmur best heard between the apex and left sternal border and may have an S_3 or S_4. They may present with arrhythmia. Therapeutic goals are to increase ventricular stroke volume and improve contractility. Options to accomplish this include beta blockade and calcium channel blockers. Affected women should also be on activity restriction. Holter monitoring is useful to evaluate the presence of arrhythmias. Severe symptoms that are refractory to medical management may require left ventricular myomectomy or catheter septal ablation. Pacemakers and implantable defibrillators have also been used. Intrapartum management aims to minimize preload and afterload declines. As with dilated CM, cesarean delivery is reserved for obstetric indications. Spinal anesthesia should be avoided given the potential for significant hypotension. If hypotension occurs, phenylephrine has been used successfully. If the lesion is symptomatic or there is outflow obstruction, an assisted delivery to shorten the second stage may be helpful. Oxytocin is better tolerated than prostaglandins for induction given the latter's vasodilatory properties.

Restrictive CM is more commonly seen in children and is the least common form of CM encountered during pregnancy. Ventricular filling is restricted and typically limited to the first phase of diastole. Systolic function is typically spared, but the decreased compliance of the ventricle results in decreased cardiac output. Patients may be asymptomatic or present with syncope, fatigue, dyspnea, orthopnea, paroxysmal nocturnal dyspnea, peripheral edema, and ascites. No physical findings may be present with mild disease, but as the diastolic dysfunction increases patients may develop tachypnea, crackles, hepatomegaly, JVD, edema, and ascites. Medical care is symptomatic and includes diuretics and anticoagulation. Surgical care is limited to cardiac transplantation.

Congestive Heart Failure

CHF is one of the common final pathways of progressive cardiac disease. Although it affects only 1 to 5 per 1000 women between 20 and 35 years, it results in significant morbidity and mortality. CHF occurs when the heart fails to maintain an adequate forward flow. This results in pulmonary or systemic vascular congestion. CHF may result from dysfunction of either the left or right ventricle or both and may occur during systole (low ejection fraction [EF]) or diastole (normal or high EF). Clinical symptoms include dyspnea on exertion or at rest, orthopnea, paroxysmal nocturnal dyspnea, nocturnal angina, Cheyne-Stokes respiration, and fatigue or lethargy. The locality of the cardiac dysfunction will determine the resultant physical findings. Left heart failure may present with rales, tachypnea, murmurs, split S_2, and right-sided dysfunction will result in peripheral edema, JVD, ascites, hepatomegaly, and cyanosis. Except for identifying and correcting remediable conditions that cause or exacerbate CHF (i.e., anemia, thyroid disease, infection), treatment is based on the locality of the dysfunction. Systolic dysfunction is treated by two main pathways: (1) afterload reduction and (2) inotropic effects. To decrease afterload, sodium restriction, diuretics, hydralazine, and isosorbide are used. For moderate or severe disease, the addition of inotropic support may be necessary. In an outpatient setting, digoxin is helpful, whereas dobutamine, nitroprusside, and amrinone can be given intravenously in an inpatient venue. Treatment of diastolic dysfunction is etiology dependent. For women with CHF resulting from hypertension, calcium channel blockers are preferred. Beta blockers may be added if tachycardia is still present. For women with AS or MS, diuretics represent the mainstay of therapy. For AI or MI, diuretics, hydralazine and nitrates are helpful. For women with idiopathic hypertrophic subaortic stenosis (IHSS), beta blockers are indicated.

Arrhythmias

Atrial Fibrillation

AF is an aberration in electrical conduction from multiple atrial foci producing irregular ventricular contractions. It is the most common sustained arrhythmia and predominantly affects individuals beyond the childbearing age. However, it does occur in pregnancy and is often seen as a comorbidity with other conditions such as hyperthyroidism or other underlying cardiac conditions such as MS. When AF coexists with MS, patients are at risk for pulmonary edema, particularly in the setting of ventricular tachycardia. Patients may complain of palpitations, lethargy, dyspnea, syncope, and/or chest pain. They should be encouraged to avoid alcohol, tobacco, and caffeine. Physical examination will reveal an irregularly irregular pulse and some patients may demonstrate evidence of decreased perfusion, embolization, or CHF. Useful laboratory studies include cardiac enzymes, arterial blood gas, thyroid function tests, electrolytes, and hemoglobin. An ECG can show irregular QRS complexes and a lack of P waves. New-onset AF should warrant an echocardiogram. The mainstay of treatment is rate control. Digoxin, quinidine, beta blockade, and calcium channel blockade have been successful in pregnancy. Flecainide, procainamide, and disopyramide are all category C in pregnancy but have been used for rate control. Likewise amiodarone has been successful but has been reported to cause neonatal hypothyroidism. Consideration of anticoagulation in patients with AF and MS or MI, AS or AI, or history of embolic events is warranted. Isolated AF in pregnancy does not require anticoagulation. In women who do not respond to medical therapy or are unstable, electrocardioversion is very successful and acceptable in pregnancy. Cardioversion can result in thromboembolic events, particularly if the fibrillation is of long duration.

Atrial Flutter

Atrial flutter is an arrhythmia with regular atrial rates between 240 and 400 beats per minute. It results when ectopic or multiple reentrant atrial electrical pulses stimulate the atrioventricular (AV) node. It occurs in approximately 3 per 10,000 individuals in their thirties, although rates in the obstetric population may be lower given the propensity for males to be affected. This arrhythmia often co-occurs with other diseases such as thyrotoxicosis, hypertension, diabetes, coronary artery disease, or valvular lesions. Patients may present with palpitations, lethargy, dyspnea, syncope, and/or chest pain. The degree of ventricular tachycardia, if present, is dependent on the degree of AV block. Many patients exhibit a heart rate of approximately 150 beats per minute, but they may have an irregular heart rate. ECG findings include a sawtooth pattern with an AV conduction block (often 2:1 or 3:1). Assessment of etiology is important, and thyroid function tests, electrolytes, and hemoglobin should be obtained.

Atrial flutter can result in thromboembolic cerebrovascular accidents and/or CHF and its treatment is therefore warranted. Unstable patients may require direct current cardioversion. Rate control can sometimes be achieved with calcium channel blockers, beta blockers, or adenosine. Digoxin can be added if indicated. Many new drugs such as dofetilide are being used in nonpregnant patients. However, their safety in pregnancy is unknown. Up to 50% of patients will have a sufficient therapeutic response to the previous regimens. In those women who do not respond to medical therapy, radiofrequency ablation may be required. There is as yet very little published experience with this procedure during pregnancy.

Paroxysmal Supraventricular Tachycardia

Paroxysmal supraventricular tachycardias (SVTs) are reentrant arrhythmias, generated by the AV node, that are transient, lasting a few minutes to hours. They tend to occur in young patients and can be associated with reentry tachycardia such as Wolff-Parkinson-White (W-P-W) syndrome. Risk factors include use of caffeine, tobacco, and alcohol. Presenting symptoms are palpitations, anxiety, dyspnea, dizziness, and occasionally syncope. There may not be any physical findings besides tachycardia, but some patients demonstrate evidence of poor perfusion. Electrocardiographic findings are a regular rhythm at 150 to 250 beats per minute; P waves may or may not be present, and in the case of W-P-W syndrome wide QRS complexes are present. Nonpharmacologic treatment modalities include Valsalva maneuver, application of ice to the face, and carotid massage (physician monitored secondary to potential for resultant bradycardia). Patients with persistent disease or underlying cardiac disease can be treated with electrocardioversion, verapamil, adenosine, or metoprolol. Long-term treatment to prevent recurrence may include flecainide and sotalol, which have been used in pregnancy, and amiodarone, which may produce neonatal hypothyroidism. Radiofrequency catheter ablation has also been successful, but experience with this intervention in pregnancy is limited.

Shunting Lesions (Left to Right)

Septal Defects

Septal defects are the most common congenital lesions in women of reproductive age. VSDs are seen more often than atrial defects.

Atrial Septal Defects

The degree of shunting is proportional to the aperture of the defect. Patients with symptoms may experience fatigue and dyspnea. Arrhythmias, pulmonary hypertension, and CHF can result as more pronounced hemodynamic changes result. Findings include a pronounced right ventricular impulse, a fixed split S_2, and a mid-systolic ejection murmur in the pulmonary region. Large lesions can produce a diastolic rumble at the left sternal border. Auscultation often results in identification in early infancy. Although atrial septal defects (ASDs) may be asymptomatic, they are typically repaired in childhood. Normal myocardial function is preserved in patients who have their defect repaired. ASDs are generally well tolerated in pregnancy unless pulmonary hypertension coexists. Fetal echocardiography should be considered given that approximately 5% of such women will have a baby with a congenital heart defect.

Ventricular Septal Defects

VSDs are often classified by the anatomic location of the lesion in relation to the four compartments of the ventricular septum: membranous, inlet, trabecular, and outlet septa. However, the impairment caused by the lesion is less related to the anatomic location of the lesion and more related to the size of the lesion and the resultant increase in pulmonary vascular resistance. Like ASDs, most VSDs are asymptomatic in early life and are solely identified by auscultation. VSDs can result in a harsh systolic murmur at the left sternal border; larger lesions can have an accompanying thrill and diastolic rumble. Although nearly half of newborns with VSDs will experience spontaneous closure of their lesions in early childhood, others with moderate or severe defects require surgical repair. Unidentified, unrepaired lesions can result in an irreversible increase in pulmonary vascular resistance and pulmonary hypertension. This eventually reverses the direction of the shunt, creating a right to left cyanotic lesion (see Eisenmenger's syndrome). Smaller lesions are usually well tolerated in pregnancy. Hypotension intrapartum may cause shunt reversal and should be avoided.

Persistent Patent Ductus Arteriosus

Persistent PDA is a physiologic adaptation to shunt blood away from the pulmonary circulation in fetal life and the immediate neonatal period. Functional persistence of this structure accounts for 5% to 10% of congenital cardiac anomalies and is more common in females. Although small PDAs are often asymptomatic, lesions with medium or large left to right shunts typically present in infancy with hoarse cry, lower respiratory infections, dyspnea, and failure to thrive. Persistent PDAs are more common in babies born prematurely and many of these require surgical repair in early postnatal life. Untreated lesions may result in obstruction of the pulmonary vasculature as a result of chronic volume overload. Physical findings may include tachycardia, tachypnea, cyanosis, continuous machinery murmur at the left sternal border, and an apical diastolic rumble. Operative intervention (open ductal ligation, coil embolization, or thorascopic ligation) is typically performed at 1 to 2 years of age unless there are significant symptoms or cardiovascular compromise sooner. Surgically corrected PDAs do not typically compromise maternal or fetal well-being unless associated with persistent pre-repair pulmonary vascular damage. In pregnancy, women with uncorrected lesions can experience a change in the direction of the flow, increasing right to left shunting and hypoxia. The avoidance of hypotension is crucial.

Shunting Lesions (Right to Left)

Eisenmenger's Syndrome

When pulmonary hypertension results from large left to right shunts (congenital such as large VSD, nonrestricted PDA, and AV septal defect or postsurgical defects created to palliate other congenital lesions), patients develop a reversal or bidirectional flow that shunts blood flow away from the pulmonary vascular bed; this is called Eisenmenger's syndrome. This diminution of flow results in symptoms of impaired activity tolerance, breathlessness, fatigue, and (pre)syncope. These women also develop symptoms of heart failure, bleeding diatheses, erythrocytosis, emboli, nephrolithiasis, and cholelithiasis. This disorder is poorly tolerated in pregnancy and is associated with high maternal (50%) and fetal mortality (25%). Maternal mortality is related to the severity of the pulmonary hypertension. Most deaths result from cardiogenic shock after right ventricular failure and are most common in the first week after delivery. At intake, these risks need to be addressed frankly with the patient and appropriate counseling regarding the possibility of termination performed. Cardiovascular findings include a right ventricular heave, distinct P2, high-pitched early diastolic murmur, pulmonary ejection click, and fixed, wide split S_2. Laboratory studies should include complete blood count (CBC), bleeding time, blood urea nitrogen (BUN) and creatinine (Cr), chemistry panel with liver function analysis, iron studies, arterial blood gas (ABG), and urinalysis. CHD occurs in 10% of offspring, and 80% of fetuses are born preterm. Medical interventions are aimed at avoiding sudden volume changes. Hypotension should be avoided throughout pregnancy. During labor, shortening of the second stage is advantageous when possible. Acute bleeding requires prompt replacement with fresh frozen plasma, cryoprecipitate and platelets in addition to red blood cells. Therapy consists of diuretics, digoxin, pulmonary vasodilators (Flolan

[GlaxoSmithKline, Research Triangle Park, North Carolina]—category B) and vitamin/FeSO$_4$ supplementation to avoid symptomatic iron deficiency and hematocrit (HCT) less than 65. Surgical treatment consists of heart-lung transplantation or, in the case of an uncomplicated cardiac anomaly, bilateral lung transplant with correction of the underlying cardiac lesion.

Marfan's Syndrome

Marfan's syndrome is an autosomal dominantly transmitted connective tissue disease affecting 4 to 6 per 10,000 people. The defect has been localized to chromosome 15q12 and results in mutations to the gene (FIBN1) that codes for fibrillin I. Fibrillin I is extracellular matrix glycoprotein, which is a major component in elastic tissue and in the lens. This mutation can result in cardiovascular abnormalities such as aortic dilatation, regurgitation, and dissection. Associated defects include tricuspid and MVP and MR. The increase in pulse pressure and stroke volume during pregnancy increases the risk of adverse outcomes. Cardiac examination findings include a decrescendo diastolic murmur, ejection clicks, and a high-pitched holosystolic murmur. Dysrhythmias may be present. Women with an aortic root of less than 4 cm in diameter typically tolerate pregnancy well. Women with an aortic arch larger than 4 cm or those with associated mitral valve dysfunction may carry significant risk, and these findings should prompt a discussion of pregnancy termination. Antepartum management includes beta blockade, avoidance of isometric activity, surveillance for chest pain, echocardiogram every 6 to 10 weeks, and fetal echo with limb measurements. Intrapartum consideration should be given to continuation of beta blockade and continuous lumbar epidural to decrease vascular wall stress and shortening of the second stage. Aortic dissection is a real concern. It presents as severe chest or scapular pain and is diagnosed with ultrasound or computed tomography.

355

MANAGEMENT

Preconceptional Counseling

Women of reproductive age with underlying cardiac disease should be encouraged to seek preconceptional counseling. This message must be emphasized not only to women and obstetric care providers but also to those who provide ongoing care to these women as well. All of the previously mentioned individuals must remember that 50% of all pregnancies are unplanned.

Appropriate counseling includes risk of maternal morbidity and mortality, inheritance risks of genetically transmitted lesions, and fetal morbidity and mortality. Additionally, women with heart disease should be presented with appropriate birth control methods and if the maternal outcomes are significantly hazardous, surgical sterilization methods should be advised.

Antepartum Management

Many women with cardiac lesions present for care after conception. Again maternal and neonatal risks should be discussed. Women with severe cardiac lesions (pulmonary hypertension, critical valvular stenosis, coarctation of the aorta, or Marfan's syndrome) must be informed of the significant maternal mortality rates (Box 22-4) and should be offered termination of pregnancy. All pregnant women with heart disease should be educated regarding strict surveillance for sudden changes in functional status, dyspnea on exertion, edema, tachycardia, hemoptysis, and development of CHF. Preventive measures to avoid infection (including strict hand washing plus Pneumovax (Merck, Whitehouse Station, New Jersey) and influenza vaccinations) and elimination of tobacco or recreational drug use are imperative. A review of the patient's medicine regimen should be performed and alternatives to teratogenic medications should be substituted when possible. Baseline laboratory test and studies may include CBC, ABG, chest x-ray, ECG, and echocardiogram. Monitoring for disease progression may require additional ECGs and echocardiograms throughout pregnancy. Most women do not require invasive hemodynamic monitoring for evaluation of lesions and for assessment of cardiac function. Consideration to fetal echocardiography should be given to those patients whose heart disease is the result of either congenital structural or inherited metabolic origins. Given the propensity of decreased placental perfusion with cardiac disease, biophysical fetal monitoring should be considered. A clear written plan for cardiac, obstetric, and anesthetic care should be prepared for use during the intrapartum period, with all involved parties being in agreement.

Anticoagulation

Anticoagulation is most likely to be encountered in the settings of prior valve replacement, supraventricular tachyarrhythmias, or significant myocardial dysfunction. Women on long-term oral anticoagulants who are attempting pregnancy should check pregnancy tests often. When they have a positive pregnancy test, unfractionated heparin (UFH) or low molecular weight heparin (LMWH) should be initiated because these medications do not cross the placenta and are not associated with increased teratogenic or fetal hemorrhage risks. Warfarin, however, crosses the placenta and, when administered between 6 and 12 gestational weeks, can cause an embryopathy in 5% to 30% of fetuses known as warfarin syndrome (nasal hypoplasia and epiphyseal stippling). For this reason, women of reproductive age who are taking warfarin should be counseled to switch to heparin anticoagulation before pursuing a pregnancy and also to make this switch as soon as possible should an unplanned pregnancy occur. All agents can cause maternal hemorrhage at a rate estimated to be approximately 2%. UFH and LMWH have been associated with osteoporosis and immunoglobulin G (IgG)-mediated thrombocytopenia (1%-2% for UFH versus <0.1% with LMWH). Thrombotic events have been reported with UFH and LMWH, but it is suggested that inadequate dosing is often responsible. Given maternal changes in weight, volume of distribution and renal clearance adjustment in dosing should be made to ensure therapeutic levels. Therapeutic levels vary depending on indication for anticoagulation. Valvular disease and arrhythmias require lower levels of anticoagulation than mechanical heart valves. Mechanical valves require higher levels of anticoagulation. The management of mechanical cardiac valves poses an interesting clinical dilemma in pregnancy. Although porcine valves require no anticoagulation, they are limited in their longevity. Thus many women of reproductive age with cardiac valves have mechanical valves, and so the risk of maternal mortality resulting from thromboembolism has been estimated to be 1% to 4% despite anticoagulation. The field is further complicated by reports of valvular thromboembolic events with UFH and manufacturer-generated reports of similar events with LMWH. The American College of Chest Physicians (ACCP) has recently provided recommendations for the management of heart valves in pregnancy. Their recommendations are listed as part of Table 22-4 (ACCP Conference: Use of Antithrombotic Agents in Pregnancy). All anticoagulants have potential risks and patients should be carefully counseled regarding the possible options.

Intrapartum Management

Hemodynamic changes occur during labor mediated by anxiety, pain, and uterine contractions. Oxygen consumption rises as a function of increased cardiac output and increased muscle work. Pain relief can decrease oxygen demand and continuous epidurals are recommended for women with most types of cardiac lesions. Tachycardia, dyspnea, hypotension, pulmonary edema, and hypoxia are typical presentations of decompensation in the intrapartum period. Interventions that improve and confirm adequate oxygen supply to the maternal fetal unit are warranted. These include lateral positioning, oxygen, and continuous pulse oximetry. Given the increased incidence of arrhythmia and ischemia in women with cardiac lesions, continuous electrocardiography is helpful. Arterial monitors should be considered in women at risk for sudden decompensation or women with significant cardiac disease and superimposed preeclampsia, obstetric hemorrhage, or sepsis. The criteria published by the

Table 22-4

Use of Antithrombotic Agents in Pregnancy

Treatments	Medication	Therapeutic Goal
Option 1	Adjusted dose LMWH subq q 12 hours, throughout pregnancy (i.e., Lovenox 1 mg/kg q 12 hours)	Valve disease/arrhythmias/ mechanical valves* antifactor Xa levels 1-1.2 U/ml (4 hr after dose) or by weight
Option 2	Adjusted dose UFH subq q 12 hours, throughout pregnancy	Valve disease/arrhythmias/ mechanical valves aPTT 2× control (6 hr after dose) or Xa 0.35-0.70 U/ml (4 hr after dose)
Option 3	UFH or LMWH as above until thirteenth week then warfarin until mid third trimester then restart UFH/LMWH	Valve disease /arrhythmias/ mechanical valves INR 3 (range 2.5-3.5) INR 2.5 (range 2-3) if bileaflet aortic valve without atrial fibrillation or left ventricular dysfunction)
High risk PP	Add ASA 75-162 mg/day Long-term anticoagulant agent	

Modified from ACCP Conference.
aPTT, Activatated partial thromboplastin time; *ASA*, aspirin; *INR*, international normalized ratio; *LMWH*, low molecular weight heparin; *UFH*, unfractionated heparin.
*See discussion regarding literature.

American Heart Association and the ACOG state that bacterial endocarditis prophylaxis is recommended for women with moderate- or high-risk lesion if bacteremia (chorioamnionitis) is suspected but not recommended in the setting of an uncomplicated vaginal delivery in the case of negligible or moderate-risk lesion and merely optional for high-risk lesions (see Table 22-3). Nonetheless, the dire consequences of bacterial endocarditis in the untreated woman commonly prompt treatment despite these guidelines. Regimens for treatment are listed in Table 22-5. Vaginal delivery is generally the preferred mode of delivery. Inductions may be planned to facilitate interdisciplinary medical care. Heparin therapy should be discontinued 12 hours before planned inductions and reinstituted 6 to 12 hours after delivery. Shortening of second stage is often preferable to decrease maternal Valsalva and cardiac output. Women incur less systemic hypotension than spinal anesthesia that is of particular concern in preload dependent lesions such as pulmonary hypertension and AS. Cesarean delivery generally should be reserved for obstetric indications, although prolonged inductions should be avoided. Cesarean delivery is indicated for women with aortic dissection or significant aortic root dilatation. Hypotension, via hemorrhage or medications, should be avoided, particularly in lesions with preload dependent ventricular function. Oxytocin, misoprostol, Methergine (Novartis, East Hanover, New Jersey), Hemabate (Pfizer, New York), and blood products should be readily available. Reports have suggested that oxytocin prolongs the QT interval and thus awareness of this possibility should be considered in women predisposed to QT prolongation. Common contraindications to Methergine (hypertension, coronary heart disease) and Hemabate (asthma, pulmonary hypertension) may be even more concerning with underlying cardiac disease. See Table 22-6 for a summary of intrapartum management by cardiac lesion.

Postpartum Management

The puerperium can be a particularly morbid period during pregnancy. Despite the acute blood loss at delivery, an increase in venous return that occurs as caval compression resolves and uterine blood supply returns to the systemic circulation, possibly contributing to maternal decompensation. As a result of these fluid shifts, women should be observed 72 hours postpartum, although women predisposed to left-to-right shunting may experience sudden decompensation for up to several weeks following delivery.

Table 22-5

Bacterial Endocarditis Prophylaxis: Antibiotics and Dosage Recommendation

High risk	Ampicillin 2 g + gentamicin 1.5 mg/kg (≤120 mg) IM or IV within 30 min of procedure; then ampicillin 1 g IM/IV or amoxicillin 1 g PO 6 hr after later
High risk with allergy	Vancomycin 1 g IV over 1-2 hr + gentamicin 1.5 mg/kg IV or IM (≤120 mg) complete infusion 30 min before procedure
Moderate risk	Amoxicillin 2 g PO 1 hr before procedure or ampicillin 2 g IM/IV within 30 min of procedure
Moderate risk with allergy	Vancomycin 1 g IV over 1-2 hr complete 30 min before procedure

IM, Intramuscular; *IV*, intravenous; *PO*, per os.

Intrapartum Management Guide

Table 22-6

Diagnosis	Supplemental O$_2$ and Left Lateral Positioning	Continuous ECG	Arterial Line	CVP/ Invasive Monitoring	Preferred Anesthetic	Preferred Delivery Mode	Parameters to Monitor
Mitral stenosis	X	X	Consider if symptomatic	Consider moderate-severe	Epidural	V	Avoid ↑ HR, ↑ central blood volume, ↓ SVR, and ↑ PAP
Mitral regurgitation	X	X	Consider if symptomatic		Epidural	V	Avoid peripheral vasoconstriction and myocardial depressants; maintain normal to slight ↑ HR
Mitral valve prolapse (isolated)	X	-	-	-	-	-	Avoid ↓ preload; if moderate MR see MR row above
Aortic stenosis	X	X	Severe		General; if vaginal delivery—systemic, inhaled, pudendal	CD	Avoid ↓ SVR and ↓/↑ HR; maintain venous return and LV filling pressure
Aortic regurgitation	X	-	Consider if CHF		Epidural	V	Avoid ↑ SVR; maintain normal to slight ↑ HR; avoid myocardial depressants
Coarctation of the aorta	X		Consider if symptomatic			V	Avoid ↑ SVR and ↑ HR; maintain LV filling

Continued

Table 22-6—cont'd

Diagnosis	Supplemental O_2 and Left Lateral Positioning	Continuous ECG	Arterial Line	CVP/ Invasive Monitoring	Preferred Anesthetic	Preferred Delivery Mode	Parameters to Monitor
Pulmonic stenosis	X			Consider if symptomatic or progressive RV compromise	If symptomatic or compromise—systemic, inhaled or pudendal	OB indications	Avoid ↑ intravascular volume, ↓ in venous return, ↓ HR and ↓ SVR; avoid myocardial depressants
Primary pulmonary hypertension	X	X		Consider if symptomatic	Systemic opioids, inhaled, pudendal; consider general if cesarean	V	Avoid ↑ PVR, ↓ in venous return and ↓ SVR; avoid myocardial depressants
Tetralogy of Fallot	X	X		If uncorrected, palliative correction, symptomatic or RV compromise	Systemic, inhaled NO, pudendal Consider general for CD	V	Avoid ↓ SVR, ↓ blood volume, and ↓ venous return
Transposition of the great vessels	X	X			Epidural	V	
Coronary heart disease	X	X		Consider if MI <6 wk, CHF, unstable angina, or poor LV function	Epidural	V, Consider VAVD or FAVD	Minimize pain and stress, avoid nitroglycerin when simultaneous sympathetic block used—may decrease preload and CO

Table 22-6—cont'd

Diagnosis	Supplemental O₂ and Left Lateral Positioning	Continuous ECG	Arterial Line	CVP/ Invasive Monitoring	Preferred Anesthetic	Preferred Delivery Mode	Parameters to Monitor
Cardiomyopathies	X	X	X	Severe		V	Peripartum: avoid ↑ afterload; IHSS: avoid ↓ blood volume, ↓ venous return, and ↓ SVR, avoid myocardial depressants, avoid or correct tachycardia, fibrillation or flutter
Congestive heart failure	X	X	X			V	Avoid ↑ SVR and ↑ HR
Atrial fibrillation/ flutter	X	X	-	-	-	-	Have cardioversion therapies immediately available during labor, delivery and postpartum
Atrial septal defect	X	X		Consider if symptomatic, pulmonary hypertension or RV failure	Epidural	V	Treat dysrhythmias, avoid ↑ SVR and ↓ PVR
Ventricular septal defect	X			Consider if symptomatic, LV dysfunction or large lesion	Epidural	V	Avoid ↑ SVR and ↑ HR

Continued

Table 22-6—cont'd

Diagnosis	Supplemental O_2 and Left Lateral Positioning	Continuous ECG	Arterial Line	CVP/ Invasive Monitoring	Preferred Anesthetic	Preferred Delivery Mode	Parameters to Monitor
Patent ductus arteriosus	X			Consider if LV/RV failure, pulmonary hypertension or shunt reversal	Epidural	OB indication	Avoid ↑ SVR and marked ↑ blood volume
Eisenmenger's syndrome	X	X		Consider CVP—OK, but PA catheter is controversial and not routine secondary to arrhythmias	Systemic inhaled, pudendal, cautious epidural	V, planned CD since fetal distress	Avoid ↑ PVR, ↓ SVR and ↓ venous return
Marfan's syndrome	X	X		Consider if aneurysm or symptomatic	Epidural	CD if dilated root, dissection, compromise	Avoid ↑ HR or ↑ pulse pressure

CD, Cesarean delivery; CHF, congestive heart failure; CO, cardiac output; CVP, central venous pressure; ECG, electrocardiogram; FAVD, forceps-assisted vaginal delivery; HR, heart rate; IHSS, idiopathic hypertrophic subaortic stenosis; IUGR, intrauterine growth restriction; LV, left ventricular; MI, myocardial infarction; MR, mitral regurgitation; NO, nitric oxide; OB, obstetrics; PA, pulmonary artery; PAP, pulmonary artery pressure; PVR, peripheral vascular resistance; RV, right ventricular; SVR, systemic vascular resistance; V, vaginal; VAVD, vacuum-assisted vaginal delivery.

KEY POINTS

- There are marked physiologic cardiovascular adaptations to pregnancy that include a 30% to 50% increase in maternal blood volume and cardiac output and an equivalent increase in pulmonary blood flow that is accompanied by a decrease in pulmonary vascular resistance. Significant structural changes to the heart during the third trimester include myocardial hypertrophy and chamber enlargement plus mild multivalvular regurgitation. There are rapid intravascular volume shifts in the first 2 weeks postpartum.
- Women with stenotic lesions or myocardial dysfunction have difficulty adapting to the physiologic changes of pregnancy, whereas women with regurgitant lesions are more likely to do well.
- Pulmonary hypertension is a particularly ominous condition during pregnancy, with maternal mortality rates as high as 50% in pregnancies that continue beyond the first trimester.

KEY POINTS—cont'd

- Patients who themselves have congenital heart disease are more likely to have children with congenital heart disease. A fetal echocardiogram should be performed in such pregnancies and also in pregnancies where there is a strong family history of congenital heart disease.
- Current recommendations for bacterial endocarditis antibiotic prophylaxis are considerably less aggressive than in previous decades (see Table 22-3).
- Coronary artery disease is increasing in frequency during pregnancy in the United States, primarily in association with advanced maternal age and obesity-associated heart disease.
- Women with cardiac disease deserve thorough and accurate counseling about their potential risks during pregnancy. This requires knowledge and active provider participation, not only by obstetric care providers but also by those individuals who care for such women during their reproductive years.

SUGGESTED READINGS

American Heart Association: *American Heart Association. Heart Disease and Stroke Statistics–2004 Update.* Dallas, TX, 2003, American Heart Association.

Bates SM et al: Use of antithrombotic agents during pregnancy: the Seventh ACCP Conference on Antithrombotic and Thrombolytic Therapy. *Chest* 126:627S, 2004.

Bonow RO et al: Guidelines for the management of patients with valvular heart disease: executive summary. A report of the American College of Cardiology/American Heart Association Task Force on Practice Guidelines (Committee on Management of Patients with Valvular Heart Disease). *Circulation* 98:1949, 1998.

Botto LD, Correa A, Erickson JD: Racial and temporal variations in the prevalence of heart defects. *Pediatrics* 107:E32, 2001.

Briggs G, Freeman R, Jaffe S: *Drugs in Pregnancy and Lactation: A Reference Guide to Fetal and Neonatal Risk*, ed 7. Baltimore, MD, 2005, Lippincott, Williams, & Wilkins.

Dajani AS et al: Prevention of bacterial endocarditis. Recommendations by the American Heart Association. *JAMA* 277:1794, 1997.

Elkayam U. Pregnancy and cardiovascular disease. In Braunwald, editor: *Heart Disease: A Textbook of Cardiovascular Medicine*, ed 6. Philadelphia, 2001, WB Saunders.

eMedicine. eMedicine, Topics 31, 40, 46, 47, 80, 314, 327, 358, 642, 671, 1102, 1372, 1662, 1965, 2314, 2494, 2503, 2534; Accessed February 2005.

Fleming SM et al: Cardiac troponin I in pre-eclampsia and gestational hypertension. *BJOG* 107:1417, 2000.

Ginsberg JS et al: Anticoagulation of pregnant women with mechanical heart valves. *Arch Intern Med* 163:694, 2003.

Green S: *Tarascon Pocket Pharmacopoeia*. Loma Linda, CA, 2004, Tarascon.

Gynecology ACoOa: *Compendium of Selected Publications*. Washington, DC, 2005, American College of Obstetrics and Gynecology.

Hughes S, Levinson G, Rosen M: *Shnider and Levinson's Anesthesia for Obstetrics*, ed 4. Philadelphia, 2002, Lippincott, Williams & Wilkins.

Kuczkowski KM: Labor analgesia for the parturient with cardiac disease: what does an obstetrician need to know? *Acta Obstet Gynecol Scand* 83:223, 2004.

Leiserowitz GS et al: Creatinine kinase and its MB isoenzyme in the third trimester and the peripartum period. *J Reprod Med* 37:910, 1992.

Lupton M et al: Cardiac disease in pregnancy. *Curr Opin Obstet Gynecol* 14:137, 2002.

Ray P, Murphy GJ, Shutt LE: Recognition and management of maternal cardiac disease in pregnancy. *Br J Anaesth* 93:428, 2004.

Sermer M, Colman J, Siu S: Pregnancy complicated by heart disease: a review of Canadian experience. *J Obstet Gynaecol* 23:540, 2003.

Siu S, Colman JM: Cardiovascular problems and pregnancy: an approach to management. *Cleve Clin J Med* 71:977, 2004.

Siu SC et al: Prospective multicenter study of pregnancy outcomes in women with heart disease. *Circulation* 104:515, 2001.

23

PULMONARY COMPLICATIONS IN PREGNANCY

Stephanie R. Martin and Michael R. Foley

PHYSIOLOGIC CHANGES

Substantial anatomic and physiologic changes occur over the course of pregnancy that affect respiratory function. As early as the first trimester, up to 70% of women complain of dyspnea. Rising progesterone levels affect the respiratory center, leading to an increase in minute ventilation (MV). MV is determined by respiratory rate and tidal volume. The 40% increase in tidal volume (the amount of air exchanged during a cycle of inspiration and expiration) primarily drives the increase in MV. As these changes evolve, the levels of CO_2 decline, creating an alkalosis of pregnancy. To accommodate for the decrease in CO_2, the kidneys excrete HCO_3^-. An arterial blood gas in a normal pregnant woman, therefore will reflect a slightly increased pH, decreased PCO_2, and decreased serum HCO_3^- (Table 23-1). As the pregnancy progresses, increasing abdominal girth leads to a 4 cm upward displacement of the diaphragm, widening of the subcostal angle by 50%, and increase in the chest circumference. The end result is a decrease in the functional residual capacity (FRC) by 20%. FRC reflects the amount of air remaining in the alveoli at the completion of expiration. As FRC decreases, alveoli collapse and gas exchange decreases. This contributes to the sense of dyspnea that pregnant women often experience.

Pulmonary Edema

Pregnant women are predisposed to developing pulmonary edema because of the increase in plasma volume and cardiac output and decreased colloid oncotic pressure (COP), which occurs normally over the course of pregnancy. In the normal lung, the hydrostatic and colloid oncotic pressures are almost equivalent to the hydrostatic and oncotic pressures of the interstitial space. Alterations in the balance of pressure between the pulmonary vessels and the interstitial spaces can lead to pulmonary edema. The presence of fluid in the interstitium prevents normal gas exchange and leads to hypoxia. Patients with pulmonary edema will complain of shortness of breath, which generally worsens when supine. Evaluation of a patient with suspected pulmonary edema will reveal oxygen saturation less than 95%, tachypnea, and

Table 23-1

	Pregnant	Nonpregnant
pH	7.4-7.45	7.38-7.42
pCO_2	27-32 mmHg	38-45 mmHg
PO_2	70-100 mmHg	70-100 mmHg
HCO_3^-	18-21 meq/L	24-31 meq/L
O_2 saturation	95%-100%	95%-100%

crackles audible on auscultation of the lungs. Chest x-ray confirms the diagnosis.

The management of patients with pulmonary edema is focused on establishing the diagnosis, determining the etiology of the pulmonary edema, and improving oxygenation (Box 23-1).

Hydrostatic (Cardiogenic) Pulmonary Edema

This category includes pulmonary edema resulting from primary cardiac issues (cardiogenic) as well as alterations in colloid oncotic pressure.

The heart controls cardiac output through adjustments in heart rate and stroke volume. As venous return to the heart (preload) increases, the heart will compensate by pumping more blood with each stroke and by increasing the heart rate. According to Starling's laws, however, the ability of the heart to increase output is limited. At some point, the heart will no longer be able to compensate, either because of intrinsic cardiac abnormalities or excessive venous return. If blood is no longer being moved forward, an overflow results. If the left side of the heart is obstructed (as discussed later), then blood emptying from the lungs into the left atrium will remain in the pulmonary vasculature. This is reflected by an increased pulmonary capillary wedge pressure and pulmonary artery pressure. The net result is an increase in the intravascular hydrostatic pressure. When this pressure exceeds the interstitial pressures, fluid will be forced out of the pulmonary vasculature into the interstitial spaces, resulting in pulmonary edema.

Echocardiogram will help distinguish whether pulmonary edema is cardiogenic in origin. Evidence of poor ventricular systolic function will be identified by a decreased ejection fraction. Diastolic dysfunction is more difficult to evaluate but may be present in patients without pulmonary edema

---

Box 23-1   Management of Pulmonary Edema

1. Elevate head of the bed
2. Administer oxygen
3. Continuous pulse oximetry (goal >95% saturation)
4. Administer diuretics (furosemide 20-40 mg IV initial dose)
5. Control blood pressure
6. Evaluate and address precipitating factors
   Limit IV fluids
   Treat infections
   Consider discontinuing tocolytic drugs
7. Continuous fetal monitoring if a viable gestational age

IV, Intravenous.

in the absence of systolic impairment. This phenomenon is more commonly seen in patients with chronic hypertension. Lastly, valvular abnormalities may lead to compromised cardiac function and predispose patients to pulmonary edema.

Select Cardiogenic Causes of Pulmonary Edema

Peripartum Cardiomyopathy

Peripartum cardiomyopathy (PPCM) occurs in only 1 in 3000 to 4000 live births but is associated with mortality rates between 18% and 56%. Patients who develop pulmonary edema and who demonstrate systolic dysfunction on echocardiogram in the last month of pregnancy or within 5 months postpartum in the absence of an identifiable cause or preexisting heart disease may be suffering from PPCM. Risk factors for PPCM include multiparity, advanced maternal age, multifetal gestation, preeclampsia, hypertension, and African-American race.

The etiology of PPCM has not been definitively determined but may be the result of a viral myocarditis. Management of these patients is aimed at reducing preload with diuretic therapy, reducing afterload with vasodilators (i.e., hydralazine, nitroglycerin, nitroprusside), and improving contractility with inotropic agents (i.e., dopamine, digoxin). Dietary sodium restriction is also important. Approximately half of patients will demonstrate significant improvement following delivery. The prognosis for patients with PPCM is poor if left ventricular function does not normalize within 6 months postpartum. In this group of patients, mortality rates approach 85% by 5 years. Death usually results from arrhythmias, thromboembolic phenomena, or progressive heart failure. Cardiac transplantation is an option for patients who do not improve within 6 months postpartum.

Mitral Stenosis

Obstruction to outflow on the left side of the heart is a primary contributor to pulmonary edema. Mitral stenosis may be unrecognized before pregnancy but is the most common rheumatic heart lesion. Pulmonary edema in pregnancy may be the initial presentation. Mitral stenosis is defined as a valve area less than 1.5 cm^2 on echocardiogram. When the mitral valve area is diminished, filling of the left ventricle during diastole is limited. As the heart rate and fluid volumes increase, the left atrium may become progressively distended. Ultimately, pulmonary edema and atrial arrhythmias may develop. Treatment should focus on adequate diuresis, treatment of arrhythmias and control of heart rate through activity restriction, pain control, and beta blockers.

Aortic Stenosis

Aortic stenosis is also typically rheumatic in origin. The major issue for patients with aortic stenosis is maintaining adequate cardiac output. The hypervolemia of pregnancy is well tolerated by patients with mild disease (valve area $>1.5 \text{ cm}^2$, peak gradient <50 mmHg). As the orifice becomes progressively more stenotic, cardiac output is more fixed. These patients may be unable to maintain coronary or cerebral perfusion and can develop angina, myocardial infarction, syncope or sudden death. Patients with a valve area less than 1 cm², peak gradient greater than 75 mmHg, or an ejection fraction less than 55% have severe disease and are candidates for surgical correction.

The time surrounding labor and delivery is particularly risky for these patients. The goal is to maintain adequate cardiac output; therefore maintenance of adequate venous return to the heart is crucial. Decreased venous return can result from blood loss, hypotension, and ganglionic blockade from a regional anesthetic or vena caval occlusion in the supine position. Inadequate return can negatively affect coronary artery perfusion and lead to myocardial ischemia. The fixed cardiac output resulting from the stenotic aortic valve limits the ability of the heart to accommodate additional fluid that may be administered in efforts to avoid potentially disastrous inadequate venous return. Pulmonary artery catheterization may be indicated to accurately estimate intravascular volume and avoid hypovolemia. Historically the risk of death in pregnant patients with aortic stenosis is as high as 17%. Fortunately, more recent data indicate that patients with aortic stenosis (without coronary artery disease) who receive adequate care have a minimal risk of dying.

Colloid Oncotic Pressure Abnormalities

The presence of albumin and other proteins is the primary contributor to the intravascular COP. Hydrostatic forces exert the opposite effect and are present within the vessel and the interstitium. The normal COP in pregnancy is 22 mmHg. This is approximately 3 mmHg lower than prepregnancy values and is a dilutional effect from plasma expansion. Conditions that lead to further decreases in albumin, particularly nephrotic syndrome and preeclampsia, create a situation in which patients are predisposed to develop pulmonary edema. Excessive intravenous (IV) fluids, blood loss, and the postpartum autotransfusion effect all place patients at risk for pulmonary edema.

Other Causes of Pulmonary Edema

Preeclampsia

Pulmonary edema develops in approximately 3% of patients with preeclampsia. The etiologies are not completely understood but likely result from a combination of problems. Impaired left ventricular function may be a result of chronic hypertension, particularly if it develops in the antepartum period. Substantially increased systemic vascular resistance may also impair left ventricular function and lead to pulmonary edema, especially in the setting of iatrogenic fluid overload.

Preeclampsia is expected to lead to loss of albumin and decreased albumin production, which will lower COP. Endothelial damage may lead to increased capillary permeability.

In patients with preeclampsia, central venous pressure monitoring may not accurately reflect the pulmonary capillary wedge pressure (left ventricular preload) and should not be used alone to guide fluid replacement. Preeclamptic patients with pulmonary edema that fails to respond to oxygen, diuresis, and fluid restriction may require pulmonary artery catheterization to guide further therapy.

Box 23-2   Risk Factors for Developing Pulmonary Edema

Underlying cardiac disease
Mitral or aortic valve stenosis
Cardiomyopathy
Decreased oncotic pressure
   Preeclampsia
   Nephrotic syndrome
   Excessive IV fluid administration
   Blood loss
Increased vascular permeability
   Preeclampsia
   Infection
IV magnesium sulfate
Tocolytic use
Multiple gestation

IV, Intravenous.

Tocolytic-Induced Pulmonary Edema

In the past, the use of IV beta agonists such as terbutaline and ritodrine was more common and became associated with the development of pulmonary edema. Several mechanisms have been proposed to explain this observation. Beta agonists cause cardiac stimulation, which may lead to ischemia or unmask preexisting cardiac disease such as mitral stenosis. Underlying undiagnosed infection, particularly occult chorioamnionitis with resultant premature labor, may also increase the patient's risk for pulmonary edema. These agents also appear to stimulate the release of antidiuretic hormone, which leads to water retention. IV fluid administration may contribute to this effect, leading to increased hydrostatic pressure and development of pulmonary edema.

Magnesium sulfate IV has supplanted the use of IV beta agonists for tocolysis and is typically used for a short duration. The incidence of pulmonary edema related to tocolytic use appears to have diminished. Most instances occur in patients with multiple gestations, infection, anemia, preeclampsia, and significant imbalance of fluid intake and output. Box 23-2 lists risk factors for pulmonary edema in pregnant patients.

PULMONARY VASCULAR DISEASE

Pulmonary Embolus

Pulmonary embolism (PE) complicates 1 in 2500 pregnancies and is the leading cause of maternal death. Pulmonary embolus usually originates from a thrombus in the deep veins of the legs and pelvis (internal iliac, femoral, and popliteal veins). Approximately 15% to 25% of deep venous thrombosis (DVT) will embolize to the pulmonary circulation if not recognized and treated. Pregnant women are at particular risk for developing a deep venous thrombosis and subsequent PE resulting from the increase in factors II, VII, VIII, X, and fibrinogen and a decrease in protein S, which creates a propensity for clot formation. Physical obstruction by the gravid uterus leads to stasis, and delivery causes endothelial damage, both of which increase the risk of DVT formation. In fact, the risk for PE is at least five times more likely during pregnancy and increases three to fivefold postpartum. If a pregnant patient requires bed rest, smokes, is obese, or is diagnosed with a thrombophilia, her risk for DVT and PE increases considerably.

Recognition and treatment of PE decrease mortality from 18.4% to 2.5%. However, diagnosis of PE can be challenging and is missed often. Any patient who presents with the "classic" complaints of pleuritic chest pain, dyspnea, hemoptysis, or syncope must be evaluated for PE. However, patients will commonly experience more subtle and nonspecific signs such as tachypnea, tachycardia, and dyspnea. The key is to consider the diagnosis as a possibility and pursue an evaluation.

Diagnosis of Pulmonary Embolus

When PE is suspected, evaluation should begin immediately. Pregnancy should not change the indications for or the type of evaluation performed. If the clinical suspicion is high, treatment should be initiated until the evaluation is completed and the diagnosis excluded. Initial evaluation consists of a ventilation/perfusion (V/Q) scan or spiral volumetric computed tomography pulmonary angiography (spiral CT). A V/Q scan is composed of two parts. First, the pulmonary perfusion is assessed by injecting ^{99m}Tc labeled albumin. This is distributed to the pulmonary vascular bed and an image is taken. If a clot is blocking flow, a "defect" is noted where there is no perfusion. Next, the patient breathes ^{133}Xe and an image is taken. The images are then compared and areas of missing perfusion matched to areas of poor ventilation. If there are areas of absent perfusion with adequate ventilation, a PE is possible. However, V/Q scans are time-consuming, and sensitivity varies widely depending on degree of clinical suspicion. Radiation exposure to the fetus is minimal. If the V/Q scan is normal, no further evaluation is required. Conversely, if the scan is interpreted as high probability in a patient with a moderate to high clinical suspicion for PE, treatment can be instituted without further evaluation. Unfortunately, 40% to 70% of the time the V/Q scan is interpreted as low or moderate probability and further evaluation must be considered.

Spiral CT is becoming more accepted as a tool for diagnosing PE. It requires the use of IV contrast but the radiation exposure to the fetus is also minimal and spiral CT can be performed in a pregnant patient. Spiral CT can detect 88% to 100% of pulmonary emboli. A negative test excludes the possibility of PE at least 89% of the time. Spiral CT will not diagnose all PEs, however. Smaller, more peripheral clots may be missed by spiral CT; therefore if suspicion is high, further workup using pulmonary angiography should be considered. A significant advantage to spiral CT in the evaluation of these patients is the opportunity to evaluate other potential diagnoses (infiltrates, effusions, etc.) that may explain the patient's symptoms.

Pulmonary angiography is considered the "gold standard" for diagnosing PE. It involves IV contrast and minimal radiation exposure to the fetus. It is quite invasive, however, and carries approximately 5% risk of complications. Despite its high sensitivity, pulmonary angiography is not performed as a first-line test for PE. Refer to Figure 23-1 for a suggested approach to the workup of a patient with symptoms suggestive of a PE.

Treatment of Pulmonary Embolus

The mainstay of the treatment for PE is systemic anticoagulation. Supportive therapy such as oxygen, mechanical ventilation, and blood pressure and fluid support may also be indicated. Anticoagulation does not dissolve clots—it stops the progression of the clot so that the body's inherent fibrinolytic mechanisms predominate, thereby hastening dissolution. Anticoagulation with unfractionated heparin is initially administered intravenously for 7 to 10 days before converting to an outpatient subcutaneous or oral regimen. Although the use of low molecular weight heparin (LMWH) has been advocated as an initial therapy in the hemodynamically stable nonpregnant population, there is insufficient literature support regarding the safety of this approach during pregnancy. In general, treatment should continue for 3 to 6 months. If PE is diagnosed during pregnancy, treatment should continue throughout gestation and 6 to 8 weeks postpartum because of the high risk of recurrence.

371

Options for anticoagulant therapy consist of unfractionated heparin or LMWH. LMWH offers several advantages over unfractionated heparin. LMWH has better subcutaneous absorption and has a longer biologic half-life. It has greater bioavailability and more specific action; therefore it is also less likely to cause thrombocytopenia, bleeding complications, or osteoporosis. LMWH is significantly more expensive than heparin, however. Because of the pregnancy-induced changes in clotting factors (particularly the marked increase in factor VIII) the activated partial thromboplastin time (aPTT) may not accurately reflect anticoagulation status. It is our opinion that monitoring of the anti-Xa levels directly may provide a more accurate assessment of anticoagulation and minimize bleeding complications. Neither heparin nor LMWH crosses the placenta or into breast milk. Postpartum, patients may be maintained on heparin or LMWH or switched to warfarin (Coumadin; Bristol-Myers Squibb, Princeton, New Jersey). Coumadin is compatible with breast feeding

Figure 23-1

A suggested approach to the workup of a patient with symptoms suggestive of a pulmonary embolus. *CT,* Computed tomography; *PE,* pulmonary embolus; *V/Q,* ventilation perfusion; *U/S,* ultrasound.

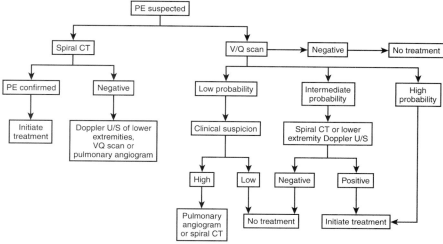

but should generally be avoided in pregnant women. Refer to Table 23-2 for treatment regimens. Contraindications to anticoagulation include active bleeding, a history of heparin-induced thrombocytopenia, recent spinal surgery, recent trauma, or inability or unwillingness to be compliant with therapy. Because of the reported increased risk of spinal hematoma with the use of a conduction anesthetic in patients on LMWH, most authorities recommend converting patients to unfractionated heparin before the peripartum period.

Alternatives to Anticoagulation
If the patient is hemodynamically unstable with a large PE, systemic thrombolytic therapy in the form of streptokinase, urokinase, or tissue-type plasminogen activator (tPA) may be required to achieve rapid lysis of the clot. Hemorrhagic complications are reported to occur in 8% of pregnant women requiring systemic thrombolytic therapy. Pulmonary thrombectomy is an option in select unstable patients requiring immediate therapy who may not receive thrombolytics.

Inferior vena cava filters have been used to capture emboli and prevent PE for decades in patients in whom anticoagulation is contraindicated. Historically these filters have been considered permanent, and physicians have demonstrated reluctance to use them in pregnant women. Retrievable inferior vena cava filters are now available and may prove beneficial in this group of patients.

Pulmonary Hypertension

Pulmonary artery hypertension (PAH) may arise as a primary lesion or develop secondary to underlying cardiac abnormality. Primary pulmonary hypertension is characterized by an unexplained elevation in pulmonary artery pressures (>25-30 mmHg). Prognosis is grim in patients with primary pulmonary hypertension; mean survival is 2.8 years from diagnosis. Accordingly, pregnancies are rare and the diagnosis is even less likely to be made de novo during pregnancy. Nevertheless, the physiologic demands during pregnancy are considerable and patients should be advised to terminate the pregnancy because of a high maternal mortality rate from PAH that in most reports exceeds 30%.

Eisenmenger's syndrome involves pulmonary hypertension that develops as a result of shunting of blood away from the lungs to the systemic circulation

Table 23-2

Anticoagulant Medications for Treatment of Pulmonary Embolus

Medication	Dose	Monitoring Goal
Unfractionated heparin	80 u/kg IV bolus then 18 u/kg/day IV infusion	aPTT 50-70 anti Xa .6-1.0 heparin assay 0.2-0.4
Low molecular weight heparin Enoxaparin (Lovenox [Sanofi-Aventis US, Bridgewater, New Jersey])	1 mg/kg subcutaneously twice daily	Anti Xa 0.6-1.0
Warfarin (Coumadin [Bristol-Myers Squibb, New York, New York])	5-10 mg PO daily initially then titrate	INR 2-3

aPTT, Activated partial thromboplastin time; *INR,* international normalized ratio; *IV,* intravenous; *PO,* per os.

across a defect within the cardiac circulation. For example, in a patient with an unrepaired ventricular septal defect, with each heart beat blood will flow across the opening from the left side of the heart to the right. Over many years, this leads to high resistance in the pulmonary vessels. Eventually the pressure in the pulmonary system may exceed systemic pressures. When this occurs, blood will follow the path of least resistance and flow in the opposite direction across the opening. When the flow is primarily right to left, the blood is not adequately oxygenated and the patient becomes cyanotic. Echocardiography is helpful in establishing the presence and direction of shunt flow. However, in pregnant patients, echocardiography may overestimate pulmonary artery pressures. This is most likely to be clinically relevant in those with mild degrees of pulmonary hypertension.

Eisenmenger's syndrome usually does not emerge until the third decade of life. Pregnancy is associated with high mortality rates in patients with Eisenmenger's syndrome (30%-40%). The decrease in systemic vascular resistance that occurs normally during pregnancy may precipitate a reversal in shunt direction. As with primary pulmonary hypertension, patients should be advised to avoid pregnancy and consider termination of pregnancy, recommended if early enough in gestation.

Therapy for patients with pulmonary hypertension is directed toward providing adequate oxygenation, dilating pulmonary vasculature, and avoiding decrease in systemic vascular resistance. Calcium channel blockers are commonly used in nonpregnant patients but may cause an unacceptable drop in systemic pressures for patients with Eisenmenger's syndrome. Selective pulmonary vasodilators such as inhaled nitric oxide or prostacyclin may be required in severe cases. Both have been used with success in pregnant patients.

OBSTRUCTIVE LUNG DISEASE

Asthma

Asthma is the result of chronic inflammation and hyperreactivity of the airways that results in airway obstruction and can be triggered by a variety of stimuli. Untreated asthma can lead to significant symptomatology such as wheezing, cough, and shortness of breath and is potentially life-threatening. Asthma is the most common pulmonary complication affecting pregnant women; approximately 4% of pregnancies are complicated by asthma. One third of pregnant asthmatics will improve during pregnancy, one third will worsen, and one third observe no change. Status asthmaticus occurs in 0.2% of pregnant asthmatics.

Asthma severity can be successfully assessed in a variety of ways. The frequency of symptoms such as shortness of breath, wheezing, and cough may be recorded with observed responses to therapy. Objective measurements such as peak expiratory flow rate (PEFR or peak flow) are also quite helpful in assessing the severity of the exacerbation. This measurement correlates well with forced expiratory volumes (forced expiratory volume at 1 second [FEV_1]). Diminishing peak flow measurements indicate worsening bronchoconstriction. These measurements are unchanged during pregnancy; typical values range from 380 to 550 L/min. Table 23-3 summarizes

Global Initiative for Asthma: Stepwise Management Approach

Table 23-3

Asthma Severity	Symptom Frequency	PEFR	Treatment
Intermittent	Less than once a week Brief episodes Symptoms at night less than once a month	≥80% predicted	No daily medication Inhaled beta agonists as needed
Mild persistent	Few episodes per week May limit activity Symptoms at night more than twice a month	≥80% predicted	Daily inhaled corticosteroid Or cromolyn sodium leukotriene antagonist sustained-release theophylline
Moderate persistent	Daily symptoms May limit activity Symptoms at night more than once a week Daily use of inhaled beta agonists	60%-80% predicted	Inhaled corticosteroid Plus Long-acting inhaled beta agonist twice daily Or Leukotriene modifier sustained-relief theophylline
Severe persistent	Daily symptoms Frequent episodes Frequent nightly symptoms Activities limited	<60% predicted	High-dose inhaled corticosteroid Plus Long-acting inhaled beta agonist twice daily And/or Leukotriene modifier oral beta agonist oral glucocorticoid sustained-release theophylline

PEFR, Peak expiratory flow rate. Normal range 380-550.

the classification of asthma severity with a suggested treatment approach as recommended by the Global Initiative for Asthma.

The treatment of asthma during pregnancy is essentially unchanged from the nonpregnant population. The goals of treatment are to minimize airway inflammation, prevent exacerbations, and effectively treat acute airway obstructions. A successful approach should emphasize the avoidance of triggers such as smoking, second-hand smoke, and known environmental allergens such as pets and dust. Often, medications may be required for the successful care of the pregnant asthmatic. The type and frequency will depend on the severity of the asthma. Both acute and chronic therapy should be considered in a step-wise fashion as suggested by the Global Initiative for Asthma (see Table 23-3). Therapy is initiated with inhaled beta agonists on an as-needed basis. If symptoms worsen, inhaled corticosteroids, cromolyn sodium, or a leukotriene receptor agonist may be added. If the exacerbation is pronounced, a week-long course of oral corticosteroids may be considered. If patients do not experience improvement in asthma symptoms and an improved peak flow (>60% of personal best) after appropriate outpatient treatment, then evaluation in the emergency department is warranted. Boxes 23-3 and 23-4 outline acute management of asthma. Antibiotics are not routinely indicated for

---

Box 23-3 Asthma Management

Asthma exacerbation requires immediate evaluation if:

1. Initial PEFR <50% predicted
2. PEFR <60% predicted after inhaled β-agonist use
3. Symptom relief not immediate and sustained for 3 hours
4. No improvement 2-6 hours after starting oral glucocorticoid
5. Worsening condition

Admission recommended if:

1. History of near-fatal asthma
2. Previous hospitalization or ED visit for asthma in past year
3. Recent oral steroid requirement
4. Overuse of short-acting beta agonists
5. Significant psychosocial issues
6. Noncompliance
7. Evidence of fetal compromise

ED, Emergency department; *PEFR,* peak expiratory flow rate.

---

the management of acute asthma. Their use should be restricted to patients with evidence of pneumonia, sinusitis, or other bacterial infection. Sedatives are considered contraindicated for the asthmatic suffering an exacerbation and may increase the risk of death. Stress doses of steroids are recommended during labor and delivery if systemic corticosteroids have been used in a dose exceeding 20 mg/day for 3 weeks during the preceding 6 months. IV Solu-Medrol (methylprednisolone sodium succinate [Pfizer, New York, New York]) or hydrocortisone 100 mg IV is administered every 6 to 8 hours during labor and for 24 hours postpartum. Medications available for use in controlling asthma, suggested doses, and Food and Drug Administration (FDA) categories are listed in Table 23-4.

Cystic Fibrosis

Approximately 1 in 29 Caucasians carry the gene for cystic fibrosis (4% of the population), making it the most common autosomal recessive disorder in Caucasians. The disease primarily manifests as chronic obstructive pulmonary

---

Box 23-4 Management of Acute Asthma Exacerbation in Pregnancy

1. Continuous pulse oximetry
2. Administer supplemental O_2 to maintain saturation >95% (pO_2 >60)
3. Perform baseline PEFR, arterial blood gas
4. Continuous fetal heart rate monitoring if >24 weeks' gestation
5. Administer high-dose beta agonist
   Albuterol 2.5 mg in 3 ml saline nebulized q 20 minutes × 3
   or
   Terbutaline 0.25 mg subcutaneous q 15 minutes × 3
6. Add methylprednisolone 80 mg IV every 6 hours if PEFR remains 40%-60% of baseline
7. PEFR remains <60%, admit for continued management
8. PEFR <25% or pCO_2 >35 mmHg, admit to ICU, intubation may be necessary if no improvement

ICU, Intensive care unit; *IV,* intravenous; *PEFR,* peak expiratory flow rate.

Classification of Common Asthma Medications

TABLE 23-4

Drug	Typical Dose	FDA Category in Pregnancy
Beta 2-Agonists–Short Acting		
Albuterol (Ventolin [GlaxoSmithKline, Research Triangle Park, North Carolina), Proventil [3M Pharmaceuticals, Northridge, California])	2 puffs tid-qid	C
Metaproterenol (Alupent [Boehringer Ingelheim, Ridgefield, Connecticut])	2 puffs every 4 hr	C
Pirbuterol (Maxair [3M Pharmaceuticals Northridge, California])	1-2 puffs every 4-6 hr	C
Levalbuterol (Xopenex [Sepracor, Marlborough, Massachusetts])	.63mg nebulized tid	C
Beta 2-Agonists–Long Acting		
Formoterol (Foradil Aerolizer [Novartis, East Hanover, New Jersey])	1 puff bid	C
Salmeterol (Serevent [GlaxoSmithKline])	2 puffs bid	C
Anticholinergic		
Ipratropium bromide (Atrovent [Boehringer Ingelheim])	1 puff tid-qid	B
Inhaled Corticosteroids		
Beclomethasone (QVAR [Teva Pharmaceuticals, North Wales, Pennsylvania])	2-5 puffs bid-qid	C
Budesonide (Pulmicort [AstraZeneca, Wilmington, Delaware])	1-2 puffs bid	B
Flunisolide (AeroBid [Forest Pharmaceuticals, St. Louis, Missouri])	2-4 puffs bid	C
Fluticasone (Flovent [GlaxoSmithKline])	88-220 µg bid	C
Triamcinolone (Azmacort [Abbott Laboratories, Abbott Park, Illinois])	2 puffs tid-qid	C
Oral Corticosteroids		
Prednisone, prednisolone, methylprednisolone	40-60 mg/day × 1 week taper over 1 week	C
Leukotriene Receptor Antagonists		
Zafirlukast (Accolate [AstraZeneca, Wilmington, Delaware])	20 mg po bid	B
Montelukast (Singulair [Merck, Whitehouse Station, New Jersey])	10 mg po every PM	B
Antiinflammatories		
Cromolyn sodium (Intal [King Pharmaceuticals, Bristol, Tennessee])	2 puffs qid	B
Nedocromil sodium (Tilade [King Pharmaceuticals])		
Other Bronchodilators		
Theophylline	100-200 mg po tid goal serum level 8-12 µg/mL	C
Combination Medications		
Fluticasone/salmeterol (Advair [GlaxoSmithKline])	1 dose bid	C
Albuterol/Ipratropium bromide (Combivent [Boehringer Ingelheim])	2 puffs qid	C

bid, Twice daily; *po,* by mouth; *qid,* four times daily; *tid,* three times daily.

disease and pancreatic insufficiency. Survival has improved steadily; women with cystic fibrosis have a median survival of 27 years. With improvement in long-term survival, and survivors reaching reproductive age, pregnancies have become more common.

Pregnancy is associated with several substantial physiologic changes that may negatively affect maternal and fetal well-being in the patient with advanced disease. Increased oxygen consumption, increased CO_2 production, and diminished functional residual capacity are tolerated poorly and may lead to decompensation. Other risk factors for adverse outcome include poor nutritional status, FEV_1 less than 60%, pulmonary hypertension, and diabetes. The presence of one or more of these risk factors warrants a thorough discussion with the patient regarding the option of pregnancy termination. In contrast, patients with mild disease generally tolerate pregnancy well. Pregnancy does not appear to adversely affect course of the disease; however, women with cystic fibrosis who become pregnant may experience pregnancy complications such as intrauterine growth restriction and premature delivery.

377

INFECTIOUS PULMONARY DISEASES

Pneumonia

Pneumonia in pregnancy is most commonly secondary to *Streptococcus pneumoniae* and varicella. Pneumonia develops in the second and third trimesters in the majority of cases and will lead to death in 4% of afflicted pregnant patients. Significant complications can occur including bacteremia, emphysema, respiratory failure, fetal distress, preterm delivery, and poor fetal growth. Risk of complications is increased if the patient is a smoker, abuses alcohol or illicit drugs, is on chronic corticosteroids, or has other medical diseases including diabetes, human immunodeficiency virus (HIV), and cystic fibrosis. Delivery does not appear to improve the course of pneumonia and is not recommended. In fact, in patients with respiratory failure the labor and delivery process or cesarean section will increase oxygen demand and may be detrimental. Because of the increased metabolic demands and cardiac output associated with infection, tocolysis should be undertaken only with extreme caution in patients with pneumonia and preterm labor. Regular fetal assessment is essential in these patients. The frequency of monitoring will be dictated by the gestational age of the fetus and the severity of maternal respiratory compromise.

Community-Acquired (Bacterial) Pneumonia
Patients with community-acquired pneumonia typically present with fever, chills, and cough and may have a recent history of an upper respiratory infection. Workup should include complete physical examination, complete blood count (CBC) with differential, blood cultures, sputum Gram stain and cultures, HIV testing, arterial blood gases, and chest x-ray. Chest x-ray should reveal a consolidation and may also demonstrate air bronchograms or a pleural effusion.

The advent of broad-spectrum antibiotic therapy has dramatically reduced the morbidity and mortality associated with bacterial pneumonia in pregnant women. *S. pneumoniae* is the etiologic agent in at least 50% of cases of community-acquired pneumonia in pregnancy. The next most likely agent is *Haemophilus influenzae*.

Therapy is initially empirical and broad spectrum in nature until an etiologic agent is confirmed. In the low-risk pregnant patient, a macrolide such as azithromycin will provide adequate coverage for the most common pathogens (*S. pneumoniae, H. influenzae*). In pregnant patients with risk factors such as a child in day care, chronic corticosteroid use, alcoholism, or serious medical diseases, cefuroxime, cefpodoxime, ceftriaxone, high-dose amoxicillin, or amoxicillin/clavulanate should be given in addition to a macrolide. If an atypical bacterium such as *Legionella* or *Chlamydia* is suspected, therapy should be adjusted accordingly. *Mycoplasma pneumoniae* is the most common cause of atypical pneumonia in young patients. Chest x-ray reveals patchy lower lobe infiltrates. The diagnosis is confirmed by serial increase in cold agglutinins in 50% to 70% of patients. These patients generally appear less compromised and may be managed as an outpatient with erythromycin or a macrolide antibiotic. Box 23-5 summarizes management of community-acquired pneumonia in pregnancy.

Viral Pneumonia

The two most serious causes of viral pneumonia in the pregnant patient are the influenza virus and varicella zoster virus. The Centers for Disease Control and Prevention recommend that all women who will be pregnant during influenza season receive the influenza vaccination. Administration of the vaccine can be performed safely in all trimesters. Varicella zoster infection in pregnancy is rare because of the high prevalence of immunity in the population. Even without a clear recollection of previous varicella infection, more than 90% of patients will be immune by serologic testing. Patients exposed to

---

Box 23-5 Management of Community-Acquired Pneumonia in Pregnant Patients

Physical examination
Assess fetal well-being if indicated
Chest x-ray
Sputum cultures
Exclude HIV infection
PPD skin testing
Exclude coccidioidomycosis if history of recent travel to southwest United States
History of any of the following:
    Cardiovascular disease
    Alcoholism
    Tobacco use
    Lung disease
    Drug abuse
If no: initial therapy with macrolide (e.g., azithromycin or clarithromycin)
If yes: give beta lactam plus macrolide (e.g., cefuroxime, high-dose amoxicillin, or amoxicillin/clavulanate plus azithromycin)
Patients in other situations may be at higher risk for unusual pathogens and require more specific therapy (e.g., ICU patients, HIV positive)

HIV, Human immunodeficiency virus; *ICU,* intensive care unit; *PPD,* purified protein derivative.

varicella while pregnant who cannot recall a previous infection should have varicella immunoglobulin G (IgG) titers drawn. If immune, no further action is necessary. If not immune, varicella zoster immune globulin (VZIG) is recommended within 96 hours following exposure. Varicella vaccine is not recommended during pregnancy because of the low risk of in utero transmission and development of congenital varicella syndrome. A pregnant woman who becomes infected with the varicella virus before 20 weeks gestation carries a 0.4% to 2% risk of congenital varicella syndrome in the fetus, a devastating complication consisting of limb deformities, skin scarring, and central nervous system and eye abnormalities. The vaccine can be administered immediately postpartum in a patient known to be nonimmune.

Of those who become infected with varicella during pregnancy, pneumonia is a common complication. Women who smoke or exhibit more than 100 skin lesions are more likely to develop varicella pneumonia. The availability of antiviral therapy (acyclovir) has decreased maternal mortality associated with varicella pneumonia from 41% to 14%. The diagnosis of varicella pneumonia should be suspected in patients with skin lesions consistent with varicella who develop shortness of breath or hypoxia and can be confirmed with chest x-ray. Once the diagnosis is established, patients should be admitted and acyclovir administered intravenously.

Tuberculosis

Screening for tuberculosis (TB) is safe in pregnancy. A purified protein derivative (PPD) skin test should be placed on any pregnant patient considered to be at high risk. According to the Centers for Disease Control and Prevention, this includes anyone who is a close contact of or living with someone with confirmed TB; HIV infection; IV drug use; medically underserved or low income; alcohol abuse; or coexisting medical risk factors that increase risk of infection such as diabetes, chronic renal failure, or chronic corticosteroid use. Patients born in a foreign country with high rate of TB and relocated to the United States within 5 years should also be screened. This includes patients from Mexico, South America, the Caribbean, Asia, Eastern Europe, Russia, and much of Africa. Many of these patients will have been vaccinated with bacille Camille-Guerin (BCG); however, screening is still recommended.

A positive skin test is defined as more than 10 mm induration (>5 mm if HIV+). Patients are at greatest risk for developing active tuberculosis within 2 years of conversion. A positive PPD skin test should be followed by a chest x-ray. If the chest x-ray is negative for active disease and the patient is asymptomatic, prophylactic therapy in the form of isoniazid (INH) 300 mg/day and pyridoxine (vitamin B_6) 50 mg/day for 6 months may be warranted. Treatment may be delayed until the postpartum period unless conversion is known to have occurred within the past 2 years in a patient younger than 35 years. INH may lead to a peripheral neuropathy, which can be prevented by the administration of pyridoxine. Hepatotoxicity can also occur in patients taking INH. This is more likely in patients older than 35 years; therefore these patients should not receive INH unless evidence exists for active disease. Liver function tests should be monitored on a monthly basis.

If active TB is confirmed, treatment should be initiated immediately with INH, rifampin, and ethambutol and continued for 9 months. Each of these drugs is considered safe during pregnancy.

ACUTE LUNG INJURY

Acute Respiratory Distress Syndrome

Acute respiratory distress syndrome (ARDS) is characterized by rapid onset of progressive respiratory distress. Evaluation reveals bilateral pulmonary infiltrates without evidence of cardiac failure or increased hydrostatic pressure (pulmonary capillary wedge pressure <18 mmHg). These patients require high concentrations of oxygen and often need intubation. ARDS is also defined as an abnormal ratio of the partial pressure of oxygen to the fraction of inspired oxygen ($PaO_2/FiO^2 \leq 200$). If the ratio falls between 200 and 300, then acute lung injury is present that is not yet severe enough to be called ARDS.

In pregnant women, infection, preeclampsia, eclampsia, and hemorrhage most commonly precipitate ARDS. Patients with sepsis are at greatest risk for developing acute pulmonary injury and ARDS. As a result of infection, pulmonary vascular damage occurs, facilitating the leakage of fluid into the pulmonary interstitial spaces. One striking feature in this process is the degree of pulmonary edema that occurs in the absence of fluid overload or cardiac failure. At this stage in the disease, substantial damage occurs to lung tissue. If the patient survives the initial phase of ARDS, then the lung tissue will begin to heal, creating fibrosis and scarring. Mortality rates are quite high and those patients who survive often have compromised pulmonary function.

ARDS cannot be treated by any specific therapy. Obviously if a precipitating factor is identified, such as infection, it should be treated aggressively. The goal of caring for these critically ill patients is to maintain adequate oxygen delivery and minimize lung trauma in an effort to facilitate healing of the lungs.

Aspiration Pneumonitis

Aspiration of gastric contents can create profound damage to lung parenchyma. The greatest damage occurs with the introduction of food matter into the lungs, higher volume of aspirate (>25 ml) and more acidic stomach contents (pH < 2.5). Pregnant and laboring women are at particular risk for aspiration because of the increased abdominal pressure from the gravid uterus, decreased tone of the lower esophageal sphincter to prevent reflux, and delayed gastric emptying. This delay is more pronounced in patients receiving narcotic agents during labor. Aspiration occurs predominantly in patients requiring general endotracheal anesthesia or during a tonic clonic seizure.

Depending on the volume and type of aspirate, the consequences can be severe, potentially resulting in death. Limiting oral intake during labor and using regional anesthesia will minimize risk. Patients requiring cesarean section should be premedicated with an H2-receptor blocker or sodium citrate to raise pH, and medication such as metoclopramide to promote gastric emptying in the event general anesthesia is necessary.

Anaphylactoid Syndrome of Pregnancy (Amniotic Fluid Embolus)

Amniotic fluid embolism is a rare but devastating complication of pregnancy characterized by acute onset of hypoxia, hypotension or cardiac arrest, and coagulopathy occurring during labor, delivery, or within 30 minutes postpartum. This same constellation of findings may be caused by other etiologies such as hemorrhage, uterine rupture, or sepsis, and these should be excluded before assigning a diagnosis of amniotic fluid embolism. The combination of sudden cardiovascular and respiratory collapse with a coagulopathy is quite similar to that observed in patients with anaphylactic or septic shock. In each of these settings, a foreign substance (e.g., endotoxin) is introduced into the circulation. This incites a cascade of events resulting in activation and release of mediators such as histamines, thromboxane, and prostaglandins that lead to disseminated coagulation, hypotension, and hypoxia. In this scenario, the inciting factor is presumed to be present in amniotic fluid, which is introduced into the maternal circulation. The precise factor(s) that initiate the sequence have yet to be identified. It is a commonly held misconception that the presence of fetal debris in the pulmonary circulation is diagnostic of an amniotic fluid embolus. In fact, fetal debris can be found in the pulmonary circulation in a predominance of normal laboring patients and is only identified in 78% of those patients who meet criteria for the diagnosis of amniotic fluid embolism.

Management of amniotic fluid embolism is entirely supportive. Replacement of blood and clotting factors, adequate hydration and blood pressure support, ventilatory support, and invasive cardiac monitoring in addition to resuscitation efforts are all generally required for these patients. Recent data suggest mortality rates approach 61% or greater. The majority of patients will not survive the initial course and die within 5 days. Of those who survive, neurologic impairment is common.

KEY POINTS

- Significant changes in pulmonary physiology occur during pregnancy that result in a respiratory alkalosis.
- Pregnant women are predisposed to developing pulmonary edema because of increased plasma volume and cardiac output and decreased oncotic pressure.
- Pregnancy should not alter the management approach to the asthmatic patient. The goals of the treatment of asthma are to minimize airway inflammation, prevent exacerbations, and effectively treat acute airway obstructions.
- Pregnancy increases the risk of developing deep venous thrombosis and pulmonary embolus. Spiral CT and V/Q scans are considered safe to perform in pregnant women suspected of having a pulmonary embolus.
- Community-acquired pneumonia is usually due to *Streptococcus pneumoniae, Haemophilus influenzae* or *Mycoplasma pneumoniae.*

KEY POINTS—cont'd

- Varicella pneumonia is associated with a greater risk of serious complications such as pneumonia in pregnant women. Maternal varicella infection occurring before 20 weeks' gestation is associated with up to a 2% risk of congenital varicella syndrome in the fetus.
- Influenza vaccine is recommended for all women who will be pregnant during influenza season.
- Women at high risk for having tuberculosis should be screened with a PPD skin test. Patients with a positive test and a negative chest x-ray require therapy with isoniazid and pyridoxine for 6 months.
- Acute respiratory distress syndrome (ARDS) most commonly develops in pregnant patients with infection, hemorrhage, and preeclampsia/eclampsia.
- Anaphylactoid syndrome of pregnancy (amniotic fluid embolus) is characterized by sudden onset of hypotension or cardiac arrest, hypoxia, and coagulopathy. Fetal debris in the maternal circulation is not specific to this group of patients and in fact can be commonly identified in normal laboring patients.

SUGGESTED READINGS

Gei A, Suarez V: Respiratory emergencies during pregnancy. In Foley MR, Strong TH, Garite TJ, editors: *Obstetric Intensive Care Manual*, ed 2. 2004, McGraw-Hill, pp xx-xx.

Global Strategy for Asthma Management and Prevention. Global Initiative for Asthma, updated October 2004. NIH Publication No. 02-3659.

Miller KS, Miller JM: Tuberculosis in pregnancy: interactions, diagnosis, and management. *Clin Obstet Gynecol* 39(1):120, 1996.

Ramsey PS, Ramin KD: Pneumonia in pregnancy. *Obstet Gynecol Clin* 28(3), 2001.

Sadosty AT, Boie ET, Stead LG: Pulmonary embolism. *Emerg Med Clin North Am* 21(2), 2003.

Zlatnick MG: Pulmonary edema: etiology and treatment. *Semin Perinatol* 21(4), 1997.

24

INHERITED AND ACQUIRED THROMBOPHILIAS IN PREGNANCY

Michael J. Paidas, De-Hui W. Ku, and Yale S. Arkel

Venous thromboembolism (VTE) poses significant maternal and fetal risks in pregnancy. Although it is estimated that VTE complicates approximately 1 in 1000 pregnancies, the actual frequency of thromboembolism is probably higher given the reluctance to perform diagnostic tests that pose some risk to the fetus. Pregnancy is associated with a sixfold higher incidence of VTE compared with age-matched non-pregnant women. Compared with combined oral contraceptive use, pregnancy has approximately a threefold higher risk for thrombosis. Table 24-1 describes the thromboembolic risks associated with pregnancy and hormonal therapy for comparison. In the United States, death secondary to pulmonary embolism (PE) occurs in 2 in 100,000 deliveries, accounting for 11% of maternal deaths. Deep venous thrombosis (DVT) is more common in the postpartum than the antepartum period, with reported rates of 0.61 in 1000 and 0.13 in 1000, respectively. Expedient diagnosis, followed by appropriate treatment of DVT is essential because one fourth of patients with DVT develop PE, with a 15% mortality rate. About two thirds of these deaths occur within 30 minutes of the PE. Anticoagulation treatment instituted on diagnosis significantly reduces both the risk of PE (5%), and the mortality rate (<1%). Inherited thrombophilias are a heterogeneous group of disorders associated with varying degrees of increased thrombotic risk and adverse pregnancy outcome (APO). At the present time, the predominant thrombophilic mutations include the factor V Leiden (FVL) mutation, prothrombin gene mutation G20210A (PGM), methylenetetrahydrofolate reductase (MTHFR) C667T, and deficiencies of the natural anticoagulants protein C (PC), protein S (PS), and antithrombin. Acquired thrombophilic conditions consist of the well-characterized antiphospholipid antibody syndrome (APAS) and hyperhomocysteinemia.

Risk of Venous
Thromboembolic
Disease in Women

Table 24-1

Risk Factor	Risk per 1000 Women/Year
Pregnancy	1.23
Puerperium	3.2
Pregnancy with known thrombophilia	40
Pregnancy and history of VTE	110
Third-generation oral contraception	0.3
Postcoital pill	No risk
Hormone replacement	0.2-5.9
Tamoxifen	3.6-12
Raloxifene	9.5

VTE, Venous thromboembolism.

HEMOSTATIC CHANGES IN PREGNANCY

Pregnancy is associated with significant elevations of a number of clotting factors. Fibrinogen concentration is doubled; there are 20% to 1000% increases in factors VII, VIII, IX, X, XII; and von Willebrand factor increases 20% to 1000%, with maximal levels reached at term. Prothrombin and factor V levels remain unchanged, whereas levels of factors XIII and XI decline modestly. The overall effect of these changes is to increase thrombin-generating potential. Coagulation activation markers in normal pregnancy are elevated, as evidenced by increased thrombin activity, increased soluble fibrin levels (9.2-13.4 nmol/L) and increased thrombin-antithrombin (TAT) complexes (3.1-7.1 μg/L), and increased levels of fibrin D-dimer (91-198 μg/L).

During pregnancy, significant changes occur in the natural anticoagulant and fibrinolytic systems. PS levels significantly decrease in normal pregnancy. Mean PS free antigen levels have been reported to be 38.9% ± 10.3 and 31.2% ± 7.4 in the second and third trimesters respectively. The PS carrier molecule, complement 4B-binding protein is increased in pregnancy and is one explanation for the diminished PS levels in pregnancy. Levels of plasminogen activator inhibitor-1 (PAI-1) increase three- to fourfold during pregnancy; plasma PAI-2 values are low before pregnancy and reach concentrations of 160 μg/L at term. Table 24-2 summarizes the relevant pregnancy-associated changes in the hemostatic system. The prothrombotic hemostatic changes are exacerbated by pregnancy-associated venous stasis in the lower extremities resulting from compression of the inferior vena cava and pelvic veins by the enlarging uterus and a hormone-mediated increase in deep vein capacitance secondary to increased circulating levels of estrogen and local production of prostacyclin and nitric oxide.

Substantial changes must occur in local decidual, and systemic coagulation, anticoagulant and fibrinolytic systems to meet the hemostatic challenges of pregnancy, including avoidance of hemorrhage at implantation, placentation, and third stage of labor. In addition to the systemic prothrombotic, anticoagulant, and fibrinolytic changes, there are potent

Table 24-2

Hemostatic Changes in Pregnancy

Variables (mean ± SD)	First Tri*	Second Tri*	Third Tri*	Normal Range
Platelet ($\times 10^9$ L^{-1})	275 ± 64	256 ± 49	244 ± 52	150-400
Fibrinogen (g/L)	3.7 ± 0.6	4.4 ± 1.2	5.4 ± 0.8	2.1-4.2
Prothrombin complex (%)	120 ± 27	140 ± 27	130 ± 27	70-30
Antithrombin (U/ml)	1.02 ± 0.10	1.07 ± 0.14	1.07 ± 0.11	0.85-1.25
Protein C (U/ml)	0.92 ± 0.13	1.06 ± 0.17	0.94 ± 0.2	0.68-1.25
Protein S, total (U/ml)	0.83 ± 0.11	0.73 ± 0.11	0.77 ± 0.10	0.70-1.70
Protein S, free (U/ml)	0.26 ± 0.07	0.17 ± 0.04	0.14 ± 0.04	0.20-0.50
Soluble fibrin (nmol/L)	9.2 ± 8.6	11.8 ± 7.7	13.4 ± 5.2	<15
Thrombin-antithrombin (µg/L)	3.1 ± 1.4	5.9 ± 2.6	7.1 ± 2.4	<2.7
D-dimers (µg/L)	91 ± 24	128 ± 49	198 ± 59	<80
Plasminogen activator inhibitor-1 (AU/ml)	7.4 ± 4.9	14.9 ± 5.2	37.8 ± 19.4	<15
Plasminogen activator inhibitor-2 (µg/L)	31 ± 14	84 ± 16	160 ± 31	<5
Cardiolipin antibodies positive	2/25	2/25	3/23	0
Protein Z (µg ml^{-1})†	2.01 ± 0.76	1.47 ± 0.45	1.55 ± 0.48	
Protein S (%)†		34.4 ± 11.8	27.5 ± 8.4	

*First Tri, wk 12-15, Second Tri, wk 24, Third Tri, wk 35.
†First trimester: 0-14 wk; second trimester: 14-27 wk; third trimester ≥ 27 wk.
Table modified from Bremme K: *Best Pract Res Clin Haematol* 16:153, 2003, Table 3, p. 157 Haemostatic changes in pregnancy; and Paidas MJ et al: Protein Z, protein S levels are lower in patients with thrombophilia and subsequent pregnancy complications. *J Thromb Haemost* 3:497, 2005.

local hemostatic effects in the decidua that occur during pregnancy. Progesterone augments perivascular decidual cell tissue factor and PAI-1 expression. Decidual tissue factor is critical in maintaining hemostasis, as evidenced by experiments with transgenic tissue factor knockout mice that have a significant risk of fatal postpartum hemorrhage. It is worthwhile to note that obstetrical conditions associated with impaired decidualization (e.g., ectopic and cesarean scar pregnancy, placenta previa and accreta) are associated with potential lethal hemorrhage.

INHERITED THROMBOPHILIAS

In 1965, a Norwegian physician, Egberg, reported a family with a partial antithrombin deficiency, and in his classic article he suggested the term thrombophilia, referring to hereditary or acquired conditions that predispose individuals to thromboembolic events. After the description of antithrombin deficiency, deficiencies of PC and PS were described in the 1980s.

Factor V Leiden

Interest in the thrombophilias significantly grew following the discovery of a relatively common genetic predisposition to clotting. In 1994, Dahlback, reporting on an association between a mutation in the factor V gene and increased thrombotic risk, termed the FVL mutation. The FVL mutation results from a substitution of adenine for guanine at the 1691 position of the factor V gene's tenth exon, causing an amino acid substitution, namely glutamine for arginine at position 506 in the factor V polypeptide (FV Q506). Factor V then is rendered resistant to cleavage by activated protein C (APC). The frequency of the FVL mutation varies among different ethnic groups. The mutation is present in 5.2% of Caucasians, 1.2% of African Americans, and 5% to 9% of Europeans, and it is rare in Asian and African populations. The FVL mutation and is primarily inherited in an autosomal dominant fashion. Heterozygosity for the FVL mutation is present in 20% to 40% of nonpregnant patients with thromboembolic disease, and homozygosity, the rarer condition, is associated with a significantly higher (>100-fold) risk of thromboembolism. However, in a large prospective observational study conducted by the Maternal Fetal Medicine Network, 5188 women were enrolled before 15 weeks' gestation: 134 women who were carriers for FVL mutation were compared with 4750 women who were not carriers. There were no significant differences in the rates of either preeclampsia, intrauterine growth restriction (IUGR), fetal deaths, or abruptio placentae between the two groups. The study evaluated only FVL, and it was not designed to evaluate the association of FVL and APO.

Prothrombin Gene Mutation G20210A

A mutation in the prothrombin gene, PGM was discovered in 1996, following the identification of the FVL mutation, and was associated with a significantly increased risk of thrombosis and, later on, pregnancy complications. The presence of heterozygosity of the PGM mutation is present in 2% to 3% of Europeans and leads to increased (150%-200%) circulating levels of prothrombin. It has accounted for 17% of thromboembolism in pregnancy in one large case-control study. The actual risk of clotting in an asymptomatic pregnant carrier is approximately 1 in 200 or 0.5%. The rarer condition, homozygosity for PGM, likewise confers a high risk of thrombosis, equal to that of homozygosity of FVL.

Protein S

PS is a vitamin K-dependent 69,000 molecular weight glycoprotein that has several anticoagulant functions, including its activity as a nonenzymatic cofactor to the anticoagulant serine protease APC. PS has a plasma half-life of 42 hours, longer than PC, the half-life of which is approximately 6 to 8 hours. Circulating PS exists in both free (40%) and bound (60%) forms. Plasma PS is reversibly bound (60%) to (C4BP) C4b-binding protein, which serves as a carrier protein for PS. PS also has an APC-independent anticoagulant function in the direct inhibition of the prothrombinase complex. PS also inhibits thrombin activatable fibrinolysis inhibitor (TAFI). PS deficiency occurs in 0.03% to 1.3% of the population, and inheritance is autosomal dominant. PS deficiency presents with one of three phenotypes: Type I, marked by reduced total and free forms; Type II, characterized by normal free PS levels but reduced APC cofactor activity; and Type III, in which there are normal total but reduced free PS levels. Of note, different mutations have highly variable procoagulant sequelae making it extremely difficult to predict which patients with PS deficiencies will develop thrombotic sequelae.

Pregnancy is associated with decreased levels of PS activity and free PS antigen in the majority of patients. Most normal pregnancies acquire some degree of resistance to APC, when measured by the first-generation global assays and tests that measure endogenous thrombin potential. Factor X, with its activation to FXa and involvement in the activation of prothrombin, is a central element in the generation of thrombin. It is possible that derangements in the control of factor Xa contribute to adverse prothrombotic sequelae in pregnancy.

Until recently, the significance and degree of the decrease in PS levels commonly seen in pregnancy had not been adequately evaluated. Paidas et al. compared second- and third-trimester PS levels in 51 healthy women with a normal pregnancy outcome with 51 healthy women with a poor pregnancy outcome. PS levels were significantly lower in the second and third trimesters among patients with adverse pregnancy outcome. A small case control study performed with subjects from the larger, multicenter, prospective study also found lower levels of PS activity and free antigen in the second and third trimesters.

Protein C deficiency

PC is a vitamin K-dependent 62,000 molecular weight glycoprotein substrate that is a precursor to a serine protease APC. PC is activated to APC by thrombin in the presence of thrombomodulin (TM) on the surface of endothelial cells. APC with PS and factor V as cofactors inactivate factor Va and factor VIIIa. The inactivation of factors Va and VIIIa decreases the generation of thrombin. Deficiencies of PC result from numerous mutations, although two primary types are recognized: Type I, in which both immunoreactive and functionally active PC levels are reduced; and Type II, in which immunoreactive levels are normal but activity is reduced. The prevalence of PC deficiency is 0.2% to 0.5%, and its inheritance is autosomal dominant.

The reported pregnancy and puerperal risks of thromboembolism with PC and PS deficiencies appear modest, 5% to 20%, and may be overstated because of ascertainment biases. Preston and associates have reported that the risk of stillbirth is modestly increased with adjusted odds ratios (ORs) (95% confidence interval [CI]) of 2.3 (0.6-8.3). The risk of miscarriage appears to be minimal with PC deficiencies (1.4 [0.9-2.2]) or not significant.

Antithrombin

Antithrombin, a vitamin K-independent glycoprotein, is a pivotal component of the natural anticoagulant system, acting as a major inhibitor of thrombin and other serine proteases. Heparin's anticoagulant effect occurs via increase of antithrombin's inhibitory activity of thrombin. Deficiency of antithrombin is the most thrombogenic of the inherited thrombophilias with a 70% to 90% lifetime risk of thromboembolism. In addition to its thrombin inhibitory properties, AT can also inactivate factors Xa, IXa, VIIa, and plasmin. The anticoagulant activity of AT is increased 5000- to 40,000-fold by heparin. Deficiencies in AT result from numerous point mutations, deletions, and insertions and are usually inherited in an autosomal dominant fashion. The two classes of AT deficiency are as follows: (1) Type I, the most common deficiency, is characterized by concomitant reductions in both antigenic protein levels and activity; and (2) Type II deficiency, which is characterized by normal antigenic AT levels but decreased activity. Type II deficiency is further classified by the site of the mutation (e.g., RS- reactive site; HBS-heparin binding site; PE-pleiotropic functional defects). The type II-HBS variant appears to have the least clinical significance. Because the prevalence of AT deficiency is low, 1 in 1000 to 1 in 5000, it is present in only 1% of patients with thromboembolism. The risk of thrombosis among affected patients is up to 60% during pregnancy and 33% during the puerperium. Preston et al. reported adjusted ORs (95% CI) for miscarriage and stillbirth of 1.7 (1.0-2.8) and 5.2 (1.5-18.1), respectively. However, because of its low prevalence compared with that of fetal loss, preeclampsia, IUGR, and abruption, AT deficiency is rarely the cause of these disorders.

Protein Z

Protein Z (PZ) is a 62-kDa vitamin K-dependent plasma protein that serves as a cofactor for a PZ-dependent protease inhibitor of factor Xa. PZ is critical for regulation of factor Xa activity in addition to tissue factor pathway inhibitor. PZ increases rapidly during the first months of life followed by slow increases during childhood, with adult levels reached during puberty. PZ deficiency influences the prothrombotic phenotype in FVL patients, and low plasma PZ levels have been reported in patients with antiphospholipid antibodies (APAs). There is a high prevalence of PZ deficiency in patients with unexplained early fetal loss (tenth to nineteenth weeks). Gris et al. found an increased risk of fetal loss associated with PZ deficiency (OR of 6.7, 95% CI 3.1-14.8, $p < .001$) and noted that the patients with late fetal loss and recurrent miscarriages had lower PZ levels.

Paidas et al. found that there was a significant decrease in the PZ levels in patients ($n = 51$) with a variety of adverse pregnancy outcomes, including IUGR, preeclampsia, preterm delivery, and bleeding in pregnancy compared with women ($n = 51$) with normal pregnancy outcomes (second trimester 1.5 ± 0.4 vs. 2.0 ± 0.5 µg/ml, $p < .0001$; and third trimester 1.6 ± 0.5 vs. 1.9 ± 0.5 µg/ml, $p < .0002$). PZ levels at the 20th percentile (1.30 µg/ml) were associated with an increased risk of adverse pregnancy outcome (OR 4.25 [1.536-11.759], with a sensitivity of 93%, specificity 32%). Mean first TRI PZ level was significantly lower among patients with adverse pregnancy outcomes, compared with pregnant controls (1.81 ± 0.7 vs. 2.21 ± 0.8 µg/ml, respectively, $p < .001$).

Gris et al. carried out a prospective randomized trial comparing the low molecular weight heparin (LMWH) enoxaparin (40 mg/day) with low-dose aspirin (100 mg/day) in 160 women with one unexplained fetal loss ($\geq$ tenth week of gestation) and either FVL, prothrombin 20210, or PS deficiency. Treatments were started at 8 weeks' gestation. The live birth rate was 86% in the enoxaparin-treated women versus 29% in the aspirin-treated group (OR for live birth with LMWH 15.5, 95% CI 7-34). Birth weights were higher and there were fewer small-for-gestational-age infants in the enoxa-parin group. Both groups of patients received folic acid 5 mg/day. Gris et al. found that the presence of PZ deficiency or the presence of PZ antibodies was more often present in cases of treatment failures (respectively, $p = .20$ and $p = .019$) as was the complex of PZ deficiency positive anti-PZ antibodies ($p = .004$); 15 of the 20 cases led to pregnancy failure, 9 being treated with aspirin and 6 with enoxaparin.

Hyperhomocysteinemia and Methylenetetrahydrofolate Reductase Thermolabile Mutant Gene Mutation (MTHFR C677T)

Homocysteine is generated from the metabolism of the amino acid methionine. It normally circulates in the plasma at concentrations of 5 to 16 μmol/L. Deficiencies in vitamins B6, B12, and folic acid can result in elevated levels of homocysteine in the setting of inherited hyperhomocysteinemia. Homocysteine levels can vary with diet, however, and normal levels in pregnancy are slightly lower than nonpregnant values.

Hyperhomocysteinemia can be diagnosed by measuring fasting homocysteine levels by gas-chromatography-mass spectrometry or other sensitive biochemical means. The disorder is classified into three categories according the extent of the fasting homocysteine elevation: severe (>100 μmol/L); moderate (25-100 μmol/L), or mild (16-24 μmol/L). Methionine loading can improve diagnostic sensitivity. Severe hyperhomocysteinemia results from an autosomal recessive homozygous deficiency in either cystathionine β-synthase (CBS), a prevalence of 1 in 200,000 or MTHFR. Clinical manifestations of hyperhomocysteinemia include neurologic abnormalities, premature atherosclerosis, and recurrent thromboembolism.

The mild and moderate forms can result from autosomal dominant (heterozygote) deficiencies in CBS (0.3-1.4% of population) or from homozygosity for the 667C-T MTHFR thermolabile mutant, present in 11% of white European populations. Patients with mild and moderate hyperhomocysteinemia are at risk for atherosclerosis, thromboembolism, fetal neural tube defects, and recurrent abortion. There are conflicting data on the link between hyperhomocysteinemia and recurrent spontaneous abortions. An older meta-analysis of the association between hyperhomocysteinemia and pregnancy loss before 16 weeks suggested a weak association with an OR of 1.4 (1.0-2.0). The natural history of the MTHFR mutation in pregnancy has not been well documented. The meta-analysis by Rey concluded that MTHFR was not associated with an increased risk of fetal loss.

Another recent meta-analysis concluded that, although FVL and PGM were modestly associated with an increased risk of early pregnancy loss, there was no such association with the MTHFR C677T mutation.

ACQUIRED THROMBOPHILIA

The well-characterized APAS is defined by the combination of VTE, obstetric complications, and APAs. By definition APA-related thrombosis can occur in any tissue or organ except superficial venous thrombosis, and accepted associated obstetric complications include at least one fetal death at or beyond the tenth week of gestation or at least one premature birth at or before the thirty-fourth week or at least three consecutive spontaneous abortions before the tenth week. All other causes of pregnancy morbidity must be excluded. APAs must be present on two or more occasions at least 6 weeks apart and are immunoglobulins directed against proteins bound to negatively charged surfaces, usually anionic phospholipids. Thus APAs can be detected by screening for antibodies that:

- Directly bind these protein epitopes (e.g., anti-β-2-glycoprotein-1, prothrombin, annexin V, APC, PS, PZ, ZPI, high- and low-molecular-weight kininogens, tissue type plasminogen activator, factor VII(a), and XII, the complement cascade constituents, C4, and CH, and oxidized low-density lipoproteins antibodies)
- Are bound to proteins present in an anionic phospholipid matrix (e.g., anti-cardiolipin and phosphatidylserine antibodies)
- Exert downstream effects on prothrombin activation in a phospholipid milieu (i.e., lupus anticoagulants)

Venous thrombotic events associated with APA include DVT with or without APE, and the most common arterial events include cerebral vascular accidents and transient ischemic attacks. At least half of patients with APA have systemic lupus erythematosus (SLE). Anti-cardiolipin antibodies were associated with an OR of 2.17 (1.51-3.11; 14 studies) for any thrombosis, 2.50 (1.51-4.14) for DVT and APE, and 3.91 (1.14-13.38) for recurrent VTE. Patients with SLE and lupus anticoagulants were at a sixfold greater risk for VTE compared with SLE patients without lupus anticoagulants, whereas SLE patients with anti-cardiolipin antibodies had a twofold greater risk of VTE compared with SLE patients without these antibodies. The lifetime prevalence of arterial or venous thrombosis in affected patients with APAs is about 30% with an event rate of 1% per year. These antibodies are present in up to 20% of individuals with VTE . A review of 25 prospective, cohort and case-control studies involving more than 7000 patients observed an OR range for arterial and venous thromboses in patients with lupus anticoagulants of 8.65 to 10.84 and 4.09 to 16.2, respectively, and 1 to 18 and 1 to 2.51 for anti-cardiolipin antibodies (Table 24-3).

There is a 5% risk of VTE during pregnancy and the puerperium among patients with APA despite treatment. Recurrence risks of up to 30% have been reported in APA-positive patients with a prior VTE; thus long-term prophylaxis is required in these patients. A severe form of APAS is termed "catastrophic antiphospholipid syndrome" (catastrophic APS, or CAPS), which is defined by potential life-threatening variant with multiple vessel thromboses leading to multiorgan failure. In the Euro-Phospholipid Project Group (13 countries included), DVT, thrombocytopenia, stroke, PE, and transient ischemic attacks were found in 31.7%, 21.9%, 13.1%, 9.0% and 7.0%, respectively.

APAs are associated with obstetric complications in about 15% to 20% including fetal loss after 9 weeks' gestation, abruption, severe preeclampsia, and IUGR. Reported ORs for lupus anticoagulant-associated fetal loss range from 3.0 to 4.8, whereas anticardiolipin antibodies display a wider range of reported ORs of 0.86 to 20.0. It is unclear whether APAs are also

Table 24-3

Thrombophilia	Inheritance	Prevalence in European Pop. (From Large Cohort Studies)	Prevalence in Patients with VTE (range)	Relative Risk or Odds Ratio VTE [95%CI] (lifetime)
Factor V Leiden (FVL) (homozygote)	AD	0.07%*	< 1%*	80 [22-289]
FVL (heterozygote)	AD	5.3%	6.6%-50%	2.7 [1.3-5.6]
Prothrombin G20201A (PGM) (homozygote)	AD	0.02%†	< 1%	> 80-fold*
PGM (heterozygote)	AD	2.9%	7.5%	3.8 [3.0-4.9]
FVL/PGM (compound heterozygote)	AD	0.17%*	2.0%	20.0 [11.1-36.1].
Hyperhomocystein-emia	AR	5%	< 5%	3.3(1.1-10.0)†
Antithrombin deficiency (<60% activity)	AD	0.2%	1-8%	17.5 [9.1-33.8]
Protein S deficiency Heerlen S460P mutation or free S antigen <55%	AD	0.2%	3.1%	2.4 [0.8-7.9]
Protein C (<60% activity)	AD	0.2%	3-5%	11.3 [5.7-22.3]

AD, Autosomal dominant; AR, autosomal recessive; VTE, venous thromboembolism.
*Calculated based on a Hardy-Weinberg equilibrium.
†OR adjusted for renal disease, folate and B12 deficiency, and odds ratios are adjusted for these confounders.

associated with recurrent (> 3) early spontaneous abortion in the absence of stillbirth. Fifty percent or more of pregnancy losses in APA patients occur after the tenth week. Patients with APAs more often display initial fetal cardiac activity as compared with patients with unexplained first-trimester spontaneous abortions without APAs (86% vs. 43%; $p < .01$). APAs have been commonly found in the general obstetric population, with one survey demonstrating that 2.2% of such patients have either IgM or IgG anticardiolipin antibodies, with most such women having relatively uncomplicated pregnancies. Other factors may play a role in the pathogenesis of APAs. Potential mechanism(s) by which APAs induce arterial and venous thrombosis and adverse pregnancy outcomes include APA-mediated impairment of endothelial thrombomodulin and APC-mediated anticoagulation, induction of endothelial tissue factor expression, impairment of fibrinolysis and antithrombin activity, augmented platelet activation and/or adhesion, and impairment of the anticoagulant effects of the anionic phospholipid binding proteins β-2-glycoprotein-I and annexin V. APA-induction of complement activation has been suggested to play a role in fetal loss, with heparin preventing such aberrant activation.

INHERITED THROMBOPHILIA AND PREGNANCY COMPLICATIONS

Inherited thrombophilic conditions have been implicated in a variety of obstetrical complications, including preeclampsia and related conditions, early and late fetal loss, IUGR, and abruptio placentae.

Preeclampsia

Several studies (mostly case controlled) have evaluated the relationship between heterozygous FVL and severe preeclampsia. FVL was identified in 4.5% to 26% of patients with severe preeclampsia, eclampsia or HELLP syndrome (i.e., **H**emolysis, **E**levated **l**iver enzyme levels and a **L**ow **P**latelet count). The systematic review by Alfirevic et al. suggested a positive association between FVL and preeclampsia/eclampsia (OR 1.6, 95% CI 1.2-2.1). FVL occurred in 11.4% (95/830) patients with severe preeclampsia, with an OR 2.84 (95% CI 1.95-4.14) in the study by Morrison. The PGM was identified in up to 9.1% of cases, whereas PS deficiency was reported in 5% to 25% of cases. Although the preponderance of the studies evaluating severe preeclampsia shows a positive association with inherited thrombophilias, there is evidence demonstrating no association. Maternal and fetal genetic thrombophilias (FVL, MTHFR, PGM) were compared between 110 patients with severe preeclampsia and 97 normotensive patients with healthy outcomes in Livingston et al. There were no differences in the rate of FVL (4.4% vs. 4.3%), MTHFR (9.6% vs. 6.3%), PGM (0% vs. 1.1%) between the two groups. Similar findings were noted among white ($n = 47$) and African American ($n = 63$) women and between those with early- or late-onset severe preeclampsia. In addition there were no differences in the frequency of the studied genetic thrombophilias in cord blood between severe preeclampsia and normotensive groups.

Paidas et al. found that there was a significant decrease in the PZ levels in patients ($n = 51$) with a variety of APOs, including IUGR, preeclampsia, preterm delivery, and bleeding in pregnancy compared with women ($n = 51$) with normal pregnancy outcomes (NPO) (second trimester 1.5 ± 0.4 vs. $2.0 \pm\pm 0.5$ μg/ml, $p < .0001$; and third trimester 1.6 ± 0.5 vs. 1.9 ± 0.5 μg/ml, $p < .0002$). PZ levels at the 20th percentile (1.30 μg/ml) were associated with an increased risk of adverse pregnancy outcome (OR 4.25 [1.536-11.759], with a sensitivity of 93%, specificity 32%).

Intrauterine Growth Restriction

Infante-Rivard found rates of 4.5% and 2.5% for FVL and PGM, respectively, when IUGR was defined as less than the 10th percentile. In a recent systematic review, FVL and PGM were associated an increased risk of IUGR: OR 2.7 (1.3-5.5), and OR 2.5 (1.3-5.0), respectively, in 10 case-control studies. However, in five cohort studies (three prospective; two retrospective), the relative risk (RR) was 0.99 (0.5-1.9). The authors concluded that both FVL and PG confer an increased risk of giving birth to an IUGR infant, although this may be driven by small, poor-quality studies that demonstrated extreme associations. Prevalence rates ranging from 5% to 35%, 2.5% to 15%, and 11% to 23% were reported for FVL, PGM, and PS deficiency, respectively.

Alfirevic found a significant association between PS deficiency and IUGR (OR 10.2, 95% CI 1.1-91).

Abruptio Placentae and Thrombophilia

The determination of the relationship between thrombophilias and abruptio placentae (decidual hemorrhage) is difficult secondary to the limited number of studies, confounding variables, including chronic hypertension, and cigarette and cocaine use. De Vries et al. found that 9 of 31 (29%) patients with abruption had a PS deficiency, compared with their general population prevalence of 0.2% to 2%. The prevalence of FVL, PGM, and PS deficiency ranged from 22% to 30%, 18% to 20%, and 0% to 29%, respectively.

Fetal Loss

In a meta-analysis of 31 studies, Rey et al. found that FVL was associated with increased risk of late fetal loss (OR 3.26, 95% CI 1.82-5.83). Gris et al. found a positive correlation between the number of stillbirths and the prevalence of thrombophilias among 232 women with previous late fetal loss (22 weeks) and 464 controls. PS deficiency was found in 9 of 84 (10.7%) with at least two stillbirths, and the presence of FVL was associated with a high risk of fetal loss at more than 22 weeks (OR 7.83, 95% CI 2.83-21.67). Martinelli et al. found that the risk of late fetal death (>20 weeks) was three times higher if the patient was a carrier of either FVL or PGM mutation. The RR of carriers (FVL, PGM) for late fetal loss was 3.2 (1.0-10.9) and 3.3 (1.1- 10.3), respectively. Martinelli et al. evaluated recurrent late loss and found that FVL was present in 28.6% of patients with recurrent late loss.

Rey et al. pooled data from nine studies (n = 2087) and found a significant association between fetal loss and the PGM. PGM was associated with recurrent fetal loss before 25 weeks (n = 690 women; OR 2.56, 95% CI 1.04- 6.29) and with nonrecurrent fetal loss after 20 weeks (five studies, n = 1299; OR 2.3, 95% CI 1.09-4.87). The prevalence of PGM ranges from 0% to 33% and for PS deficiency 29% to 92%. On the other hand, Hefler et al. did not find any significant association among FVL, PGM, or PS deficiency and fetal death (median gestational age 34 weeks, with range 20-42 weeks). Two studies that examined recurrent fetal loss and PS deficiency found a significant association (OR 14.7, 95% CI 0.99-218). Rey et al. found that PS deficiency was associated with nonrecurrent loss after 22 weeks in three studies (n = 565; OR 7.39, 95% CI 1.28-42.83).

Early Pregnancy Loss and Thrombophilia

The association between early pregnancy loss and thrombophilia also has yielded conflicting results. In three recent systematic reviews, the diversity among included studies implies that meta-analyses are performed including heterogeneous studies. Factors influencing results include inclusion of isolated or recurrent fetal loss, presence or absence of successful livebirth in obstetrical history, gestational age cut-off for evaluation, and inclusion of proper control groups. The typical OR for FVL is 1.67 (1.16-2.40) and for PGM the typical OR is 2.25 (1.20-4.21). There was no increased risk of loss and MTHFR C677T. Roque et al. reported that the odds for having thrombophilia was actually significantly lower in women with recurrent embryonic losses. The paternal or fetal genetic contribution has not been well studied to date. In a study of 357 couples with a history of three or more pregnancy losses under 12 weeks, the presence of multiple thrombophilic mutations in either partner was associated with a significantly increased risk of pregnancy loss (RR 1.9 [1.2-2.8]).

Thrombophilia, Prior History of Poor Pregnancy Outcome, and Recurrence

For patients who have had a prior adverse pregnancy outcome and harbor an inherited thrombophilic condition such as FVL, PGM or PS deficiency, the reported rate of recurrence of APO is high. Martinelli et al. found that of 82 women with late fetal loss, 7 had a recurrence, and 2 of 7 had FVL (28.6%). Kupferminc et al. have consistently reported very high rates of pregnancy complications in women with prior poor obstetrical outcomes, ranging from 83% of pregnancies in 18 women, 66% of pregnancies in 9 multiparous women with PGM, and 77% occurrence of complications in 9 multiparous women. In a cohort of 28 patients with thrombophilia (heterozygous PGM and prior APO), Kupferminc et al. reported that 7 of 62 pregnancies were normal. According to the meta-analysis by Rey, the presence of PGM was associated with recurrent fetal loss before 25 weeks ($n = 690$ women; OR 2.56, 95% CI 1.04-6.29) and with nonrecurrent fetal loss after 20 weeks (five studies, $n = 1299$; OR 2.3, 95% CI 1.09-4.87). Rey et al. also found that late fetal loss was associated with FVL mutation ($n = 1888$, OR 3.26, 95% CI 1.82-5.83), PGM ($n = 1299$, OR 2.30 [1.09-4.87]), PS deficiency ($n = 878$, OR 7.39 [1.28-42.83]) but not with MTHFR, PC deficiency, or AT deficiency. Several factors impact studies concerning thrombophilia and pregnancy complications, including the heterogeneity of the populations studied, the small sample size, the rarity of the endpoint evaluated, the number of thrombophilias assayed for, the detection methods used, the lack of consistent assessment of fetal thrombophilia status, and potential ascertainment biases. These limitations have been recently confirmed from two different independent studies on fetal genotype. Until more large population-based studies are performed, the debate regarding the association between inherited thrombophilias and adverse pregnancy outcomes will continue. For example, positive associations between pregnancy complications and thrombophilia may exist, but the association may be driven by small studies with extreme associations.

PREVENTION OF ADVERSE PREGNANCY OUTCOMES IN THE SETTING OF THROMBOPHILIA

Kupferminc et al. treated 33 women with a history of severe preeclampsia, abruptio placenta, IUGR, or fetal demise and a known thrombophilia with LMWH and low-dose aspirin (LDA). The babies of treated patients had a higher birth weight and a higher gestational age at delivery than in the previous pregnancy. Treated pregnancies were not associated with fetal losses or severe preeclampsia. Riyazi et al. found that treatment with LMWH and LDA in patients with previous early-onset preeclampsia and/or severe IUGR and a thrombophilic disorder resulted in a higher birth weight than patients with a comparable history not receiving this intervention. Paidas et al. evaluated a cohort of patients carrying either FVL or PGM who experienced at least one prior APO. A total of 41 patients (28 with FVL, 13 with PGM) had 158 pregnancies. Antenatal heparin administration was associated with an 80% reduction in adverse pregnancy outcome overall (OR 0.21, 95% CI 0.11, 0.39, $p < .05$). This relationship persisted if first-trimester losses were excluded ($n = 111$ total pregnancies, OR 0.46 95% CI 0.23, 0.94, $p < .05$). Brenner et al. reported on the LIVE-ENOX Study, a multicenter prospective randomized trial to evaluate the efficacy and safety of two doses of enoxaparin (40 mg/day or 40 mg twice a day) in 183 women with recurrent pregnancy loss and thrombophilia. Inclusion criteria were three or more losses in the first trimester, two or more losses in the second trimester, and one or more losses in the third trimester. Compared with the patient's historical rates of live birth and pregnancy complications, enoxaparin was significantly associated with an increased the rate of live birth rate, decreased rate of preeclampsia, and decreased the rate of abruption. Better outcomes were associated with higher dosing.

Gris et al. compared administration of LDA 100 mg/daily with enoxaparin 40 mg daily from the eighth week of gestation in a cohort of patients with a prior loss after 10 weeks and the presence of heterozygous FVL, PGM, or PS deficiency. The authors found that 23 of 80 patients treated with aspirin and 69 of 80 patients treated with enoxaparin had a successful pregnancy (OR 15.5, 95% CI 7-34, $p < .0001$). Birth weights were higher and there were fewer small-for-gestational-age infants in the enoxaparin group.

The small size and inadequate study designs of the published studies do not permit any firm recommendation regarding the antenatal administration of heparin for the sole indication of the prevention of adverse pregnancy outcome. These authors strongly recommended a randomized trial to address the use of anticoagulation for prevention. According to a recent Cochrane review, based on an extensive literature search from 1966 to 2004, for women with history of two or more spontaneous losses or one fetal demise without apparent cause other than inherited thrombophilia, only two trials were available for review. The other study besides the Gris trial was the trial reported by Tulppala et al. that involved 82 patients and compared aspirin 50 mg versus placebo from positive urine pregnancy test in women with three or more unexplained consecutive losses. No difference was noted in the aspirin group compared with the placebo group (RR 1.00 [0.78-1.29]). Table 24-4 summarizes the results of studies using anticoagulation to prevent adverse pregnancy outcome in the setting of thrombophilia.

Heparin and LDA administration is the best strategy for the treatment of recurrent pregnancy loss associated with APAS, according to the Cochrane review in 2002. This approach has been associated with a 54% reduction in pregnancy loss and is better than aspirin alone. Steroid administration is associated with an excessive risk of prematurity and therefore is not recommended as a first-line prevention strategy.

Anticoagulation to
Prevent Adverse
Pregnancy Outcome
in the Setting of
Thrombophilia

Table 24-4

Author	Year	No. of Patients	Drug	Patients Studied	Outcome
Riyazi	1998	26	Nadroparin + ASA 80 mg	Thrombophilia plus prior preeclampsia or IUGR	Treatment associated with lower rates of preeclampsia/IUGR compared with historical control
Brenner	2000	50	Enoxaparin	Thrombophilia plus recurrent fetal loss	Treatment associated with higher live birth (75% vs. 20%) compared with historical control
Ogueh	2001	24	Unfractionated heparin	Thrombophilia plus IUGR or abruption	No improvement compared with historical control
Kupferminc	2001	33	Enoxaparin + ASA 100 mg	Thrombophilia plus preeclampsia or IUGR	Higher birth weight and gestational age at delivery
Grandone	2002	25	Unfractionated heparin or enoxaparin	Thrombophilia + APO	Treatment was associated with lower rates of APO (10%) in treated vs. (93%) nontreated
Paidas	2004	41	Unfractionated or low molecular weight heparin	FVL or PGM plus history of fetal loss	Treatment was associated with an 80% reduction in fetal loss (OR 0.21, 95% CI 0.11−0.39)
Gris	2004	160	Enoxaparin or 100 mg aspirin; folic acid 5 mg	Thrombophilia + fetal loss	Enoxaparin was superior to aspirin. 29% patients treated with LDA. 86% treated with enoxaparin had healthy live birth (OR 15.55, 95% CI, 7-34)
Brenner	2004	183	Enoxaparin (40 mg/day or 40 mg bid)	Thrombophilia + ≥3 losses in the first trimester, or ≥2 losses in the second trimester, or ≥1 loss in the third trimester	Enoxaparin increased the rate of live birth (81.4% vs. 28.2%, $p < .01$ for 40 mg, 76.5% vs. 28.3%, $p < .01$ for 80 mg), decreased the rate of preeclampsia (3.4% vs. 7.1%, $p < .01$ for 40 mg; 4.5% vs. 15.7%, $p < .01$ for 80 mg), and decreased the rate of abruption (4.4% vs. 14.1%, $p < .01$ for 40 mg; 3.4% vs. 9.6%, $p < .1$ for 80 mg)

APO, Adverse pregnancy outcome; *ASA*, aspirin; *bid*, twice a day; *CI*, confidence interval; *FVL*, factor V Leiden; *IUGR*, intrauterine growth restriction; *LDA*, low-dose aspirin; *OR*, odds ratio; *PGM*, prothrombin gene mutation.

THROMBOPHILIA SCREENING: TESTING AND CANDIDATES

The selection of suitable patients for thrombophilia screening and the thrombophilia workup continues to evolve. At this time, suitable candidates for thrombophilia screening include history of unexplained fetal loss at 10 or more weeks, history of severe preeclampsia/HELLP at less than 36 weeks, history of abruption, history of IUGR (<5th percentile), personal history of thrombosis, and family history of thrombosis. Initial thrombophilia evaluation should include PC (functional level); PS (functional level, free antigen); ATIII (functional level); FVL (polymerase chain reaction [PCR]); prothrombin gene mutation 20210A (PCR); lupus anticoagulant; anticardiolipin antibody (ACA) IgG, IgM; β-II glycoprotein I IgG, IgM; platelet count; and fasting homocysteine levels. Other commonly ordered screens include ACA IgA; β-II glycoprotein I IgA; and MTHFR (not recommended). Large prospective studies are needed to address the role of the interaction of thrombophilic conditions in the causation of VTE and APO. A recent meta-analysis and cost-effectiveness study has concluded that universal thrombophilia screening in pregnancy is not useful, but a selective approach based on personal and family history is most advantageous.

397

PHARMACOLOGY OF ANTICOAGULATION IN PREGNANCY

Thromboembolism and adverse pregnancy outcome management continue to present clinical challenges. The available anticoagulant drugs for the prevention and treatment of VTE include warfarin, unfractionated heparin (UFH), LMWH, warfarin, factor-Xa inhibitors, and direct thrombin inhibitors. However, heparins are the mainstay of therapy in pregnancy. Unfractionated heparin enhances antithrombin activity, increases factor Xa inhibitor activity, and inhibits platelet aggregation. LMWH is generated by chemical or enzymatic manipulation of UFH from a molecular weight of 15,000 Daltons to 4000 to 6500 Daltons. The smaller size impedes its antithrombin but not anti-factor Xa effects. Both LMWH and UFH do cross the placenta, are considered safe for pregnancy, and are compatible with breast feeding. Complications associated with heparins include hemorrhage, osteoporosis, and thrombocytopenia. Heparin-induced thrombocytopenia (HIT) occurs in two forms: Type I HIT typically occurs within days of heparin exposure, is self-limited, and is not associated with significant risk of hemorrhage or thrombosis. Type II HIT is an immunoglobulin-mediated syndrome and occurs in the setting of venous or arterial thrombosis, usually 5 to 14 days following initiation of heparin therapy. Fortunately, it is quite rare in pregnancy. Type II HIT can be confirmed by serotonin release assays, heparin-induced platelet aggregation assays, flow cytometry, or solid phase immunoassay.

UFH has a short half-life and is administered subcutaneously or via continuous infusion. Usually patients receiving UFH require frequent laboratory monitoring and dosage adjustment. LMWH is administered subcutaneously either once or twice daily. It has advantages over UFH, including better bioavailability, longer plasma half-life, more predictable pharmacokinetics, and pharmacodynamics. LMWH is much more expensive than UFH. A recent review has found that LMWH has a reassuring profile, including reduced risk of antenatal bleeding, 0.43 (0.22-0.75); postpartum hemorrhage more than 500 ml, 0.94 (0.61-1.37); wound hematoma, 0.61 (0.36-0.98); thrombocytopenia, 0.11 (0.02-0.32); HIT, 0.00 (0.00-0.11); and osteoporosis, 0.04 (<0.01-0.20). Coumarins are vitamin-K antagonists that block the generation of vitamin KH2. The latter serves as a cofactor for the posttranslational carboxylation of glutamate residues to ι-carboxyglutamates on the N-terminal regions of prothrombin and factors VII, IX, and X as well as the anticlotting agents, PC and PS. The peak effect of warfarin, the most commonly used vitamin K antagonist, occurs 36 to 72 hours after initiating therapy and it has a half-life of 36 to 42 hours. Aspirin and other nonsteroidal antiinflammatory drugs and high doses of penicillins and moxalactam increase the risk of warfarin-associated bleeding by inhibiting platelet function. Because PC has a relatively shorter half-life compared with most of the vitamin K-dependent clotting factors, warfarin may initially create a relatively prothrombotic state. Indeed, it may take 6 days to achieve full antithrombotic effects, especially in pregnancy, given the elevated levels of factor VIII and often occurring APC resistance. In pregnancy, it is critical to maintain these women on therapeutic doses of UFH or LMWH for 5 days and until the international normalized ratio (INR) reaches the therapeutic range between 2.0 and 3.0 for 2 successive days.

Several other anticoagulants are now available that may have a role under limited circumstances in pregnancy. Danaparoid is another low-molecular-weight heparinoid and is especially useful in cases of HIT and in cases of heparin allergy. Fondaparinux is a synthetic heparin pentasaccharide that complexes with the antithrombin binding site for heparin to permit the selective inactivation of factor Xa but not thrombin. Given as a once-daily subcutaneous injection, fondaparinux is excreted in the kidney, has a half-life of 15 hours, and does not appear to induce HIT. Direct thrombin inhibitors represent another class of anticoagulants.

Hirudin is a 65-amino-acid protein derived from the medicinal leech (*Hirudo medicinalis*). It can be used in patients with HIT II and is readily available in a recombinant form, lepirudin. There is limited use of lepirudin in pregnancy. Argatroban (GlaxoSmithKline, Research Triangle Park, North Carolina) is a synthetic direct thrombin inhibitor that competitively binds to thrombin's active site, has a short half-life (45 minutes) and is cleared by the liver, making it the direct thrombin inhibitor of choice for patients with renal failure. Bivalirudin is a 20-amino-acid synthetic polypeptide analog of hirudin.

TREATMENT OF THROMBOEMBOLISM OR THROMBOPHILIA IN PREGNANCY

Before initiating anticoagulation therapy, a thrombophilia panel should be obtained as noted above. Functional clotting factor testing should be performed well after the cessation of anticoagulant therapy to diagnose a factor deficiency. Table 24-5 summarizes anticoagulant regimens for treatment

Table 24-5

Indication	Description	Antepartum		Postpartum	
		Therapeutic	Prophylactic	Therapeutic	Prophylactic
VTE current pregnancy		X		See (1)	
High-risk thrombophilia • Factor V Leiden (FVL) Homozygous	History of VTE or APO (2)	X			X
• Prothrombin G20210A mutation Homozygous • Antithrombin III deficiency	No history		X		X
Intermediate-risk thrombophilia • Compound Heterozygote (FVL/ Prothrombin G2010A)			X		X
Low-risk thrombophilia	Prior VTE		X		X
• Factor V Leiden Heterozygous • Prothrombin G20210A mutation Heterozygous	History of APO (2) but *not* VTE		±X (3)		X (4)
• Protein C deficiency	No history of VTE or APO (2)				X (4)
• Protein S deficiency • Hyperhomocysteinemia (refractory to folate therapy)					
No thrombophilia	Prior VTE				X
Hyperhomocysteinemia (5)	Prior VTE or APO (2)		X		X (4)

Continued

Table 24-5—cont'd

Indication	Description	Antepartum		Postpartum	
		Therapeutic	Prophylactic	Therapeutic	Prophylactic
Antiphospho-lipid antibody syndrome	(+)LAC or >20 gpl units IgG or IgM		X (+ASA)		X

APO, Adverse pregnancy outcome; VTE, venous thromboembolism.
VTE during current pregnancy should receive therapeutic anticoagulation for 20+ wks during pregnancy, followed by prophylactic therapy for up to 6 wks postpartum.
APO includes early onset severe preeclampsia, abruption, severe intrauterine growth restriction (IUGR), unexplained intrauterine fetal demise (IUFD) (>10 wks).
Patients with less thrombogenic thrombophilias and histories of APO should be treated prophy-lactically in the antepartum period if the clinical scenario suggests a high risk for recurrence or there are other thrombotic risk factors (e.g., obesity, immobilization).
If cesarean delivery or first-degree relative with history of VTE.
Cases of hyperhomocysteinemia unresponsive to folate, vitamin B6, and vitamin B12 therapy.

Unfractionated Heparin (UFH)
Initial dose of UFH for acute VTE to keep activated partial thromboplastin time (aPTT) 1.5-2.5 times control. Thereafter UFH may be given SQ q8-12hrs to keep aPTT 1.5-2 times control (when tested 6 hrs after injection) for therapeutic levels.
Prophylactic doses may range from 5000 to 10,000 units SQ q12h and can be titrated to achieve heparin levels (by protamine titration assay) of 0.1 to 0.2 U/ml.

Low Molecular Weight Heparin (LMWH)
Therapeutic doses of Lovenox (enoxaparin; Sanofi-Aventis, Bridgewater, New Jersey) may start at 1mg/kg SQ q12h. Therapeutic doses should be titrated to achieve anti-factor Xa levels of 0.6-1.0 U/ml (when tested 4-6 hrs after injection).
Prophylactic doses of Lovenox may start at 40 mg SQ q24h. Prophylactic doses should be titrated to achieve anti-factor Xa levels of 0.1 to 0.2 U/ml 4 hrs after injection
Regional anesthesia is contraindicated within 18-24 hours of LMWH and thus LMWH should be converted to UFH at 36 weeks or earlier if clinically indicated.
Postpartum
Heparin anticoagulation (LMWH or UFH) may be restarted 3-6 hours after vaginal delivery and 6-8 hours after cesarean.
Warfarin anticoagulation may be started postpartum day 1.
Therapeutic doses of LMWH or UFH must be continued for 5 days and until the INR reaches therapeutic range (2.0-3.0) for 2 successive days.
Maternal and Fetal Surveillance
Fetal growth should be monitored every 4-6 weeks beginning at 20 weeks in all patients on anticoagulation.
Nonstress tests and biophysical profiles may be appropriate at 36 weeks or earlier as clinically indicated.

and prophylactic settings. Women with new-onset VTE during a current pregnancy should receive therapeutic anticoagulation for at least 20 weeks during the pregnancy, followed by prophylactic therapy. After delivery, patients require a minimum of 6 weeks of anticoagulation. During pregnancy, UFH and LMWH are the anticoagulants of choice. Postpartum, oral anticoagulation with warfarin may be started and is considered safe in breast-feeding mothers. Because osteoporosis is more common with doses of heparin greater than 15,000 U/day used for more than 6 months, all patients treated with heparin should receive 1500 mg of calcium supplementation per day. Postpartum bone densitometry may be appropriate in such patients. In pregnancy, LMWH from multidose vials containing benzoyl alcohol, which is potentially toxic to the fetus and newborn, should be avoided.

The goals of therapy for an acute VTE in pregnancy are to maintain the activated partial thromboplastin time (aPTT) between 1.5 and 2.5 times the control when using UFH. The dose required may vary greatly between women secondary to interpatient differences in heparin-binding proteins in pregnancy. The aPTT should be evaluated every 4 to 6 hours during the initial phase of therapy and adjustments made in dosage as needed. Intravenous therapeutic UFH should be continued for at least 5 to 10 days or until clinical improvement is noted. Thereafter, therapeutic doses of UFH may then be administered subcutaneously every 8 to 12 hours to maintain the aPTT 1.5 to 2 times control 6 hours after the injection. These should be continued for 20 weeks followed by prophylactic dosages. Patients with highly thrombogenic thrombophilias such as AT deficiency or those homozygous for the FVL or prothrombin G20210A gene mutations should receive therapeutic anticoagulation throughout pregnancy.

If vaginal or cesarean delivery occurs more than 4 hours after a prophylactic dose of UFH, the patient is not at significant risk for hemorrhagic complications. Protamine sulfate may be administered to those patients with an elevated aPTT receiving prophylactic or therapeutic UFH who are about to deliver vaginally or by cesarean section.

Low-Molecular-Weight Heparin

For therapeutic dosing, the anti-factor Xa level should be maintained at 0.6 to 1.0 U/ml 4 to 6 hours after injection (e.g., starting with enoxaparin 1 mg/kg subcutaneously every 12 hours). Again treatment should continue for 20 weeks and then prophylactic dosages given (e.g., enoxaparin 40 mg subcutaneously every 12 or 24 hours), adjusted to maintain anti-factor Xa levels at 0.1 to 0.2 U/ml 4 hours after an injection. As noted, patients with highly thrombogenic thrombophilias require therapeutic anticoagulation throughout pregnancy. Because regional anesthesia is contraindicated within 18 to 24 hours of LMWH administration, we recommend switching to UFH at 36 weeks or earlier if preterm delivery is expected. If vaginal or cesarean delivery occurs more than 12 hours from prophylactic or 24 hours from therapeutic doses of LMWH, the patient should not experience anticoagulation-related problems with delivery. Protamine can partially reverse the anticoagulant effects of LMWH.

POSTPARTUM

Either UFH or LMWH can be restarted 3 to 6 hours after vaginal delivery or 6 to 8 hours after cesarean delivery. Warfarin should be started in the first post-delivery day. UFH or LMWH therapy is required for 5 days and until the INR reaches the therapeutic range between 2.0 and 3.0 for 2 successive days.

SURGERY AND THROMBOLYTIC THERAPY

Thrombolytic therapy is associated with a maternal mortality rate of 1.2%, fetal loss rate of 6%, and maternal hemorrhagic complication rate of 8%. Recombinant tissue plasminogen activator (rt-PA) poses significant hemorrhagic peripartum risks.

ANTICOAGULATION IN PREGNANCY: SPECIAL CONSIDERATIONS

1. **Recurrent VTE in women with prior VTE:** Antepartum heparin is not necessary in patients without thrombophilia and prior VTE associated with temporary risk factor, based on the study of Brill-Edwards et al. In a prospective evaluation of 125 women with a single previous episode of VTE, antepartum heparin was withheld. In the 95 patients who did not have a known thrombophilia and whose prior VTE was associated with a temporary risk factor, the recurrence of VTE was zero percent (CI 0-8.0). In patients with thrombophilia and/or idiopathic prior VTE, the RR of recurrent antepartum VTE was 5.9 (1.2%-16%). Antepartum prophylaxis is indicated in the latter group of patients. Postpartum anticoagulation is indicated in both groups.

2. **Antithrombin deficiency:** Patients with antithrombin deficiency represent the highest thrombogenic risk. Patients with antithrombin deficiency should receive antithrombin concentrate if they experience an acute arterial or venous thromboembolism. Human AT-III is available as Thrombate III (Bayer Healthcare, Montville, New Jersey), a sterile, preservative-free, nonpyrogenic, biologically stable lyophilized preparation of purified human AT-III. The baseline antithrombin level is expressed as the percent of the normal level based on the functional AT-III assay. The goal is to increase the antithrombin levels to those found in normal human plasma (around 100%).

SUMMARY

Thromboembolism remains a leading cause of maternal mortality. Prompt diagnosis and initiation of therapy are essential to optimize maternal and perinatal outcome. Doppler ultrasound is a valuable test in the evaluation of patients suspected of having a deep venous thrombosis, and ventilation perfusion scanning and spiral computed tomography (CT) scanning are key diagnostic tests in the evaluation of patients suspected of having a pulmonary embolus. Suitable candidates for thrombophilia screening include history of unexplained fetal loss at 10 or more weeks, history of severe preeclampsia/HELLP at less than 36 weeks, history of abruption, history of IUGR (5th percentile), personal history of thrombosis, and family history of thrombosis. UFH and LMWH are the mainstay of treatment and prevention strategies to reduce the risk of thrombotic complications. VTE should be treated with therapeutic anticoagulation for a minimum of 20 weeks, with prophylactic dosing extended to a minimum of 6 weeks' postpartum. Assessment of risk factors for thromboembolism will optimize treatment and prevention strategies and minimize hemorrhagic complications associated with anticoagulation.

KEY POINTS

- Venous thromboembolism is a leading cause of death in women and complicates at least 1 in 1000 pregnancies.
- Pregnancy is associated with significant elevations of a number of clotting factors. Fibrinogen concentration is doubled, there are 20% to 1000% increases in factors VII, VIII, IX, X, and XII, and von Willebrand factor increases 20% to 1000%. Normal pregnancy is associated with significantly decreased activity levels of protein S, typically one half the value of nonpregnancy.
- The high-risk thrombophilias include antithrombin III deficiency, homozygosity of Factor V Leiden or prothrombin gene mutation G20210A, and antiphospholipid antibody syndrome defined by the presence of thrombotic complications. Heterozygous Factor V Leiden is associated with a 0.2% risk of thromboembolism in pregnancy, whereas heterozygous PGM is associated with a 0.5% risk. Compound heterozygous FVL and PGM is associated with a 4.6% risk of thromboembolism.
- Suitable candidates for thrombophilia screening include: history of unexplained fetal loss at 10 weeks or more, history of severe preeclampsia/HELLP less than 36 weeks, history of abruption, history of IUGR ($\leq$ 5th percentile), personal history of thrombosis, and family history of thrombosis.
- Initial thrombophilia evaluation should include: PC (functional level); PS (functional level, free antigen); ATIII (functional level); FVL (PCR); prothrombin gene mutation 20210A (PCR); lupus anticoagulant; ACA IgG, IgM; platelet count; and fasting homocysteine levels. Other commonly ordered screens include ACA IgA; β-II glycoprotein I IgA; and MTHFR (not recommended).
- Heparin and aspirin administration is the best strategy for the treatment of recurrent pregnancy loss associated with antiphospholipid antibody syndrome.
- Therapeutic anticoagulation during the antepartum period should be reserved for VTE in the current pregnancy and high-risk thrombophilic conditions. Dosing of therapeutic anticoagulation should be titrated to keep the PTT between 1.5 to 2.5 times control for unfractionated heparin and anti-factor Xa levels between 0.6 and 1.0 U/ml for LMWH.
- Venous thromboembolism should be treated with therapeutic anticoagulation for a minimum of 20 weeks, with prophylactic dosing extended to a minimum of 6 weeks' postpartum.
- Heparin anticoagulation may be restarted 3 to 6 hours after vaginal delivery and 6 to 8 hours after cesarean delivery. Therapeutic doses of LMWH or unfractionated heparin must be continued for 5 days and until the INR reaches therapeutic range (2.0-3.0) for 2 successive days. Warfarin may be started postpartum day one.

SUGGESTED READINGS

Alfirevic Z: How strong is the association between maternal thrombophilia and adverse pregnancy outcome? A systematic review. *Eur J Obstet Gynecol Reprod Biol* 101:6, 2002.

Brill-Edwards P et al: Safety of withholding heparin in pregnant women with a history of venous thromboembolism. Recurrence of clot in this pregnancy study group. *N Engl J Med* 343:1439, 2000.

Dahlback B: Inherited resistance to activated protein C, a major cause of venous thrombosis, is due to a mutation in the factor V gene. *Haemostasis* 24:139, 1994.

Duhl AJ, Paidas MJ, Ural SH, Branch W, Casele H, Cox-Gill J, Hammersley SL, Hyers TM, Katz V, Kuhlman R, Nutecu EA, Thorp JA, Zender JL; Pregnancy and Thrombosis Working Group: Antithrombotic therapy and pregnancy: consenous report and recommendations for prevention and treatment of venous thromboembolism and adverse pregnancy outcomes. *Am J Obstet Gynecol* 197(5):457, 2007.

Gerhardt A et al: Prothrombin and factor V mutations in women with a history of thrombosis during pregnancy and the puerperium. *N Engl J Med* 342:374, 2000.

Gris JC: Case-control study of the frequency of thrombophilic disorders in couples with late foetal loss and no thrombotic antecedent—the Nimes Obstetricians and Haematologists Study5 (NOHA5). *Thromb Haemost* 81:891, 1999.

Gris JC et al: Low-molecular-weight heparin versus low-dose aspirin in women with one fetal loss and a constitutional thrombophilic disorder. *Blood* 103:3695, 2004.

Kupferminc MJ et al: Increased frequency of genetic thrombophilia in women with complications of pregnancy. *N Engl J Med* 340:9, 1999.

Paidas MJ et al: Protein Z, protein S levels are lower in patients with thrombophilia and subsequent pregnancy complications. *J Thromb Haemost* 3:497, 2005.

Rand JH et al: Pregnancy loss in the antiphospholipid-antibody syndrome—a possible thrombogenic mechanism. *N Engl J Med* 337:154, 1997.

Rey E, Kahn SR, David M, Shrier I: Thrombophilic disorders and fetal loss: a meta-analysis. *Lancet* 361:901, 2003.

25

HEMATOLOGIC DISORDERS IN PREGNANCY

Michael J. Paidas, De-Hui W. Ku, and Yale S. Arkel

HEMATOLOGIC CHANGES IN PREGNANCY

Pregnancy is associated with a variety of alternations in the hematologic system. Understanding the pregnancy-associated physiologic alternations is pivotal to correctly differentiating among normal physiology, diseases unique to pregnancy, and medical conditions affecting women during the antenatal and postnatal periods.

Red Blood Cell

A greater expansion of plasma volume relative to the increase in hemoglobin mass and erythrocyte volume is responsible for the modest fall in hemoglobin levels observed in healthy pregnant women. The greatest disproportion between the rates at which plasma and erythrocytes are added to the maternal circulation occurs during the second trimester. At the end of pregnancy, hemoglobin concentration increases because of the cessation of plasma expansion and continuing increase in hemoglobin mass. Given the pregnancy-associated changes in plasma volume and red cell mass, normal differences in hemoglobin concentrations between women and men, ethnic variation between white and black women, between women who are pregnant and those who are not, and the frequent use of iron supplementation in pregnancy, a precise definition of anemia in women is not straightforward. Table 25-1 lists the normal iron indices for pregnancy.

The Centers for Disease Control and Prevention has defined anemia as hemoglobin levels of less than 11 g/dl in the first and third trimesters and less than 10.5 g/dl in the second trimester. In general, women taking iron supplements have a mean hemoglobin concentration that is 1 g/dl greater than that of women not taking supplements. In a typical singleton gestation, the maternal iron requirement averages close to 1000 mg: approximately 300 mg for the fetus and placenta and approximately 500 mg, if available, for the expansion of maternal hemoglobin mass. Most women do not have adequate iron stores to handle the demands of pregnancy. Two hundred milligrams is shed through the gut, urine, and skin. Table 25-1 lists the normal iron indices for pregnancy. Of particular importance for

Table 25-1

Normal Iron Indices
during Pregnancy

Plasma iron	40-175 μg/dl
Plasma total iron-binding capacity	216-400 μg/dl
Transferrin saturation	16-60%
Serum ferritin	>10 μg/dl

pregnancy is the increased folic acid requirement. In nonpregnant women, the daily folic acid requirement is 50 to 100 μg/day. Because folate deficiency is associated with neural tube defects, all women of reproductive age are advised to consume 0.4 mg of folic acid daily.

Platelets

The most significant obstetrical consideration concerning platelet physiology in pregnancy is the frequent occurrence of a fall in the maternal platelet count. Platelet physiology in pregnancy is characterized by increased mean platelet volume and reduced lifespan. There are few and conflicting studies on platelet activation in pregnancy. Slightly lower mean platelet counts in pregnant women than in nonpregnant women is the most prominent change in platelets associated with pregnancy. Gestational thrombocytopenia occurs in 5% of pregnancies and is typically not associated with maternal, fetal, or neonatal sequelae. The lower limit of normal platelet counts in pregnancy has been reported to be 106 to 120×10^9/L. It is well recognized that platelet counts can drop much lower than this range, with a lower threshold of gestational thrombocytopenia being 70×10^9/L.

White Blood Cells

The most noticeable alteration of the white blood cell system is the increase in neutrophil count, which begins in the second month of pregnancy. This neutrophilia plateaus in the second or third trimester, where total white blood cell counts range from 9 and 15×10^9 cells per liter.

PREGNANCY-RELATED HEMOSTATIC ALTERATIONS IN COAGULATION FACTORS

It is well accepted that normal pregnancy is a prothrombotic state. Fibrinogen concentration is doubled. There are 20% to 1000% increases in factors VII, VIII, IX, X, and XII, and von Willebrand factor increases 20% to 1000%, with maximal levels reached at term. Prothrombin and factor V levels remain unchanged, and levels of factors XIII and XI decline modestly. Concomitantly, there is a decrease in the natural anticoagulant system, with impressive lower levels of protein S (PS) and increased resistance to activated protein C (APC). Impairment of the fibrinolytic process exists, as evidenced by increased levels of plasminogen activator inhibitor 1 and 2 (PAI-1 and PAI-2) along with increased levels of thrombin activatable fibrinolysis inhibitor (TAFI).

Protein S

PS is a vitamin K-dependent 69,000 molecular weight glycoprotein that has several anticoagulant functions, including its activity as a nonenzymatic cofactor to the anticoagulant serine protease APC. PS has a plasma half-life of 42 hours, considerably longer than protein C, whose half-life is approximately 6 to 8 hours. Circulating PS exists in both free (40%) and bound (60%) forms. Plasma PS is reversibly bound (60%) to (C4BP) C4b-binding protein, which serves as a carrier protein for PS. PS has also been shown to have an APC-independent anticoagulant function in the direct inhibition of the prothrombinase complex. PS also inhibits TAFI. The prevalence of PS deficiency is 0.03% to 1.3%, and inheritance is autosomal dominant.

Pregnancy is associated with decreased levels of PS activity and free PS antigen in the majority of patients. Most normal pregnancies acquire some degree of resistance to APC, when measured by the first-generation global assays and tests that measure endogenous thrombin potential. Factor X, its activation to FXa and participation in the activation of prothrombin, is a central element in the generation of thrombin. It is possible that derangements in the control of factor Xa contribute to adverse prothrombotic sequelae in pregnancy. In one study, PS levels were significantly lower in the second and third trimesters among patients with adverse pregnancy outcome, defined as intrauterine growth restriction, preeclampsia, preterm delivery, preterm rupture of membranes associated with preterm delivery, and bleeding in pregnancy, compared with patients with normal pregnancy outcome (second trimester $34.4 \pm 11.8\%$ vs. $38.9 \pm 10.3\%$, $p < .05$, respectively; and third trimester 27.5 ± 8.4 vs. 31.2 ± 7.4, $p < .025$, respectively). In a follow-up study, free PS antigen levels in the first trimester were found to be 39% (SD 10.5), compared with the reference range in nonpregnant women of 88% (SD 19), $p < .05$.

Protein Z

Protein Z (PZ) is a 62-kDa vitamin K-dependent plasma protein that serves as a cofactor for a PZ-dependent protease inhibitor (ZPI) of Factor Xa. PZ is critical for regulation of factor Xa activity in addition to tissue factor pathway inhibitor. PZ increases rapidly during the first months of life followed by slow increases during childhood, with adult levels reached during puberty. PZ deficiency influences the prothrombotic phenotype in factor V Leiden patients, and low plasma PZ levels have been reported in patients with antiphospholipid antibodies. There is also some evidence suggesting a role of PZ deficiency to a bleeding tendency. Although controversy exists surrounding the association between ischemic stroke and PZ deficiency (<1.0 μg/ml), there is a high prevalence of PZ deficiency in patients with unexplained early fetal loss (tenth to nineteenth weeks). Gris et al. found an increased risk of fetal loss associated with PZ deficiency (odds ratio of 6.7, 95% CI 3.1-14.8, $p < .001$), and noted that the patients with late fetal loss and recurrent miscarriages had lower PZ levels.

Paidas et al. found that there was a significant decrease in the PZ levels in patients ($n = 51$) with a variety of adverse pregnancy outcomes, including intrauterine growth restriction (IUGR), preeclampsia, preterm delivery, and bleeding in pregnancy compared with women ($n = 51$) with normal pregnancy outcomes (second trimester 1.5 ± 0.4 vs. 2.0 ± 0.5 μg/ml, $p < .0001$; and third trimester 1.6 ± 0.5 vs. 1.9 ± 0.5 μg/ml, $p < .0002$). PZ levels at the 20th percentile (1.30 μg/ml) were associated with an increased risk of adverse pregnancy outcome (odds ratio 4.25 [1.536-11.759], with a sensitivity of 93%, specificity 32%). Mean first trimester PZ level was significantly lower among patients with adverse pregnancy outcomes, compared with pregnant controls (1.81 ± 0.7 vs. 2.21± 0.8 µg/ml, respectively, $p < .001$). In patients with other known thrombophilic conditions, those with adverse pregnancy outcomes had a tendency for lower mean PZ levels compared with those thrombophilic women with normal pregnancy outcomes (1.5 ± 0.6 vs. 2.3 ± 0.9 µg/ml, respectively, $p < .0631$).

Gris et al. found an inverse correlation between anti-PZ immunoglobulin (Ig) M antibody levels and PZ concentrations ($p = -.43$) in patients with recurrent embryonic loss and PZ deficiency. The relationship between PZ antibodies and PZ levels is not straightforward. Anti-PZ IgG antibody and anti-PZ IgM antibody levels were not correlated with PZ levels in the entire cohort of patients with normal and abnormal outcomes. The immunologic response to coagulation factors in pregnancy requires further inquiry.

Gris et al. carried out a prospective randomized trial comparing the low molecular weight heparin (LMWH) enoxaparin (40 mg/day) with low-dose aspirin (100 mg/day) in 160 women with one unexplained fetal loss (≥ tenth week of gestation) and either factor V Leiden, prothrombin 20210, or PS deficiency. Birth weights were higher and there were fewer small-for-gestational-age infants in the enoxaparin group.

Activation Markers in Pregnancy

Bremme et al. found that normal pregnancy ($n = 26$ women) was associated with increased thrombin activity, increased soluble fibrin levels (9.2-13.4nmol/L), increased thrombin- antithrombin complexes (3.1-7.1 µg/L), and fibrinolysis, as evidenced by increased levels of fibrin D-dimer (91-198 µg/L). Considering only the first trimester, 50% of women had elevated TAT levels (11/22) and 36% of women had elevated levels of D-dimers (9/25). Only one patient, however, had a significantly elevated level of first-trimester soluble fibrin compared with the nonpregnant state. Soluble fibrin monomers have also been shown to be elevated in pregnancy. As can be seen from Table 25-2, activation markers are often increased in pregnancy.

Normal pregnancy is associated with a number of changes in the hemostatic system. The most significant results are the frequent occurrence of anemia in pregnancy; presence of neutrophilia, frequent occurrence of thrombocytopenia, increase in procoagulant factors, and diminished fibrinolysis, which overall contribute to a prothrombotic state.

RED BLOOD CELL DISORDERS

Anemia

The initial evaluation of a woman with moderate anemia includes hemoglobin electrophoresis and red cell indices to ensure adequate hemoglobin identification. It also should include hematocrit, examination of peripheral blood smear, and measurement of levels of serum iron, ferritin, or both. Any disorder that causes anemia in women of childbearing age may complicate pregnancy. A classification based primarily on etiology and including most of the common causes of anemia in pregnant women is shown in Box 25-1.

Table 25-2

Variables (mean $\pm$ SD)	First Tri*	Second Tri*	Third Tri*	Normal Range
Platelet ($\times 10^9$ L^{-1})	275 $\pm$ 64	256 $\pm$ 49	244 $\pm$ 52	150-400
Fibrinogen (g/L)	3.7 $\pm$ 0.6	4.4 $\pm$ 1.2	5.4 $\pm$ 0.8	2.1-4.2
Prothrombin complex (%)	120 $\pm$ 27	140 $\pm$ 27	130 $\pm$ 27	70-30
Antithrombin (U/ml)	1.02 $\pm$ 0.10	1.07 $\pm$ 0.14	1.07 $\pm$ 0.11	0.85-1.25
Protein C (U/ml)	0.92 $\pm$ 0.13	1.06 $\pm$ 0.17	.94 $\pm$ 0.2	0.68-1.25
Protein S, total (U/ml)	0.83 $\pm$ 0.11	0.73 $\pm$ 0.11	0.77 $\pm$ 0.10	0.70-1.70
Protein S, free (U/ml)	0.26 $\pm$ 0.07	0.17 $\pm$ 0.04	0.14 $\pm$ 0.04	0.20-0.50
Soluble fibrin (nmol/L)	9.2 $\pm$ 8.6	11.8 $\pm$ 7.7	13.4 $\pm$ 5.2	<15
Thrombin-antithrombin (μg/L)	3.1 $\pm$ 1.4	5.9 $\pm$ 2.6	7.1 $\pm$ 2.4	<2.7
D-dimers (μg/L)	91 $\pm$ 24	128 $\pm$ 49	198 $\pm$59	<80
Plasminogen activator inhibitor 1 (AU/ml)	7.4 $\pm$ 4.9	14.9 $\pm$ 5.2	37.8 $\pm$ 19.4	<15
Plasminogen activator inhibitor 2 (μg/L)	31 $\pm$ 14	84 $\pm$16	160 $\pm$ 31	<5
Cardiolipin antibodies positive	2/25	2/25	3/23	0
Protein Z (μg ml^{-1})†	2.01 $\pm$ 0.76	1.47 $\pm$ 0.45	1.55 $\pm$ 0.48	
Protein S (%)†		34.4 $\pm$ 11.8	27.5 $\pm$ 8.4	

*First Tri, wk 12-15, Second Tri, wk 24, Third Tri, wk 35.
†First trimester: 0-14 wk; second trimester: 14-27 wk; third trimester 27 wk.
Table modified from Bremme K: *Best Pract Res Clin Haematol* 16:153, 2003, Table 3, p. 157 Haemostatic changes in pregnancy; and Paidas MJ et al: Protein Z, protein S levels are lower in patients with thrombophilia and subsequent pregnancy complications. *J Thromb Haemost* 3:497, 2005.

Box 25-1 Causes of Anemia during Pregnancy

Acquired
- Iron deficiency
- Anemia caused by acute blood loss
- Megaloblastic anemia
- Acquired hemolytic anemia
- Anemia of inflammation or malignancy
- Aplastic or hypoplastic anemia

Hereditary
- α- and β-thalassemias
- Sickle cell hemoglobinopathies
- Other hemoglobinopathies
- Hereditary hemolytic anemias

Iron Deficiency Anemia

The two most common causes of anemia during pregnancy are the puerperium and iron deficiency and acute blood loss. Not infrequently, the two are related because excessive blood loss, with its concomitant loss of hemoglobin iron and depletion or iron stores, in one pregnancy is an important cause of iron deficiency anemia in a subsequent pregnancy.

The iron requirements of pregnancy are considerable, and most American women have small amounts of storage iron. In a typical gestation with a single fetus, the maternal need for iron induced by pregnancy averages close to 1000 mg: approximately 300 mg for the fetus and placenta and approximately 500 mg, if available, for the expansion of maternal hemoglobin mass. Another 200 mg is shed through the gut, urine, and skin. This total amount considerably exceeds the iron stores of most women.

With the rather rapid expansion of blood volume during the second trimester, a lack of iron often is manifested by an appreciable drop in hemoglobin concentration. Although the rate of expansion of blood volume is not as great in the third trimester, the need for iron is still increased because augmentation of maternal hemoglobin mass continues and considerable iron is now transported to the fetus. Thus iron deficiency anemia during pregnancy is the consequence primarily of expansion of plasma volume without normal expansion of maternal hemoglobin mass.

Moderate iron deficiency anemia during pregnancy—for example, a hemoglobin concentration of 9 g/dl—usually is not accompanied by obvious morphologic changes in erythrocytes. With this degree of anemia from iron deficiency, however, serum ferritin levels are lower than normal. In general, normal ferritin levels exclude iron deficiency, but decreased values do not confirm it. The serum iron-binding capacity is elevated, but by itself this is of little diagnostic value because it also is elevated during normal pregnancy in the absence of iron deficiency. Most clinicians consider a ratio of less than 15% for serum iron/iron-binding capacity to indicate iron deficiency anemia.

The objectives of treatment are correction of the deficit in hemoglobin mass and, eventually, restitution of iron stores. Taking into account the amount of iron absorption from the gastrointestinal tract, the clinician can accomplish both of these objectives with orally administered simple iron compounds—ferrous sulfate, fumarate, or gluconate—that provide a daily dose of about 200 mg of elemental iron (i.e., 325 mg of ferrous sulfate three times daily or iron compounds in combination with prenatal vitamins). (The Institute of Medicine recommends 20 mg/day for pregnant women, double the recommended dosage for nonpregnant women.) To replenish iron stores, oral therapy should be continued for 3 months or so after the anemia has been corrected. After 7 to 10 days of therapy with an iron compound, reticulocytosis can be seen and hemoglobin may increase by at least 1 g per week in patients with severe anemia.

In select cases—for example, patients with malabsorption syndromes, or those with severe anemia (hemoglobin <8.5g/dl) who will not take iron therapy—there is a role for parenteral iron therapy. There is a risk of anaphylaxis with iron dextran administration; therefore a test dose should be administered first. The maximal rate of the full dose is 1 ml/minute.

Subcutaneous erythropoietin has been administered successfully to correct iron deficiency anemia in pregnancy. In patients with significant anemia who had failed to correct anemia with oral iron therapy alone, the addition of erythropoietin to oral iron therapy resulted in correction of anemia within 2 weeks, in 73% of patients.

Despite the fact that iron deficiency anemia is the most common nutritional deficiency in the world, the maternal and perinatal complications associated with anemia had not been extensively studied. Severe anemia has been associated with increased low birthweight babies, induction rates, operative vaginal and cesarean deliveries, and prolonged labor.

Folic Acid Deficiency

In nonpregnant women, the daily folic acid requirement is 50 to 100 μg/day. Because folate deficiency is associated with neural tube defects, all women of reproductive age are advised to consume 0.4 mg of folic acid daily. Megaloblastic anemia during pregnancy is uncommon and almost always results from folic acid deficiency. This condition usually is found in women who do not consume fresh green leafy vegetables or foods with a high content of animal protein. Women with megaloblastic anemia may develop troublesome nausea, vomiting, and anorexia during pregnancy.

The sequence of changes that result from folate deficiency is unaltered by pregnancy. The earliest biochemical evidence is low plasma concentrations of folic acid. The earliest morphologic evidence is usually hypersegmentation of neutrophils. Macrocytes usually are seen on peripheral smear. As anemia becomes more intense, an occasional nucleated erythrocyte appears in the peripheral blood. As maternal folate deficiency and, in turn, the anemia become more severe, thrombocytopenia, leucopenia, or both may develop.

Treatment of pregnancy-induced megaloblastic anemia should include folic acid, a nutritious diet, and iron. As little as 1 mg of folic acid administered orally once daily produces a striking hematologic response. By 4 to 7 days after treatment is begun, the reticulocyte count is increased appreciably, and leukopenia and thrombocytopenia are promptly corrected. Severe megaloblastic anemia during pregnancy typically is accompanied by an appreciably smaller blood volume than that in a normal pregnancy, but soon after folic acid therapy has been started, the blood volume usually increases considerably and may intensify the anemia transiently. Folic acid requirements increase as gestation advances, and anemia may develop in the setting of folic acid deficiency. Pregnancies with multiple gestations should be supplemented with 1 mg of folic acid daily. Several drugs, including phenytoin, primidone, para-aminosalicylic acid, and sulfasalazine may decrease serum folate concentrations and cause deficiency.

Of note, oral contraceptives also may impair folate metabolism, and dihydrofolate reductase inhibitors (e.g., methotrexate, trimethoprim) can interfere with folic acid utilization.

Anemia Associated with Chronic Disease

Anemia may be associated with chronic disease states, such as inflammatory bowel disease, chronic renal failure, and systemic lupus erythematosus. The etiology of such anemia may result from both decreased production and increased destruction of erythrocytes. The treatment of chronic anemia in pregnancy may be difficult, and treatment response may vary. Besides iron and folic acid, human recombinant erythropoietin has been used for the treatment of these anemias in pregnant women, especially those associated with chronic renal failure. A potential worrisome side effect is hypertension.

Sickle Cell Hemoglobinopathies

Hemoglobin S results from a single β-chain substitution of glutamic acid by valine because of a substitution of A for T at codon 6 of the β-globin gene. Sickle cell anemia (SS disease), sickle cell hemoglobin C disease (SC disease), and sickle cell β-thalassemia disease (S-β-thalassemia disease) are the most common of the sickle hemoglobinopathies.

The inheritance of the gene for S hemoglobin from each parent results in sickle cell anemia (SS disease). Although pregnancy outcomes have been improving, complications from sickle hemoglobin diseases are still significant. This is especially true of women with hemoglobin SS disease, in whom anemia often becomes more intense, vasoocclusive episodes with severe pain—so-called sickle cell crises—usually become more frequent, and infections and pulmonary complications are more common. In addition to excessive maternal mortality, more than a third of pregnancies end in abortion, stillbirth, or neonatal death.

The management of pregnant women with sickle cell hemoglobinopathies includes close observation with careful evaluation of all symptoms, physical findings, and laboratory studies. One rather common danger is that the symptomatic women may categorically be considered to be suffering from sickle cell crisis. As a result, ectopic pregnancy, cholecystitis, or other serious obstetric or medical problems that cause pain, anemia, or both may be overlooked.

Intense sequestration of sickled erythrocytes with infarction in various organs may develop acutely, especially late in pregnancy, during labor and delivery, and early in the puerperium. Infarction usually is accompanied by severe pain, and because in many cases the bone marrow is involved, intense bone pain is common. Intravenous hydration is given, along with opioids administered parenterally for severe pain. A careful search for infection is warranted. Many of these women are dehydrated because of diminished oral intake secondary to pain, and they also often have fever, which exacerbates hypovolemia. Oxygen given via nasal cannula may increase oxygen tension and decrease the intensity of sickling at the capillary level. Although prophylactic red cell transfusions almost always eliminate pain episodes by preventing vasoocclusive episodes, their use is controversial because of the risks, such as transmission of disease, transfusion reactions, and iron overload. When partial exchange transfusion is used, the goal of therapy is to maintain hemoglobin A above 50% and the hematocrit above 25%.

Acute chest syndrome is characterized by pain, fever, cough, and pulmonary infiltrates. It also may result in significant illness and even death in women with sickle cell disease. The exact etiology of this syndrome is unclear, but it has been reported to be associated with infection, microvascular occlusion from sickle hemoglobin, and fat embolism. The treatment for this syndrome basically is supportive.

Special circumstances during pregnancy appreciably increase morbidity among these women. Bacteriuria is common, and urinary tract infections including acute pyelonephritis are increased substantially. Bacteriuria eradication is important to prevent most symptomatic infections. Pneumonia, especially caused by *Streptococcus pneumoniae*, is common, and polyvalent pneumococcal vaccine is recommended for these women. Because of substantial perinatal mortality and intrauterine growth restriction, careful fetal surveillance is mandatory, as is the use of other methods of antepartum assessment.

Sickle Cell Trait

About 8% of African Americans are heterozygous for the sickle cell gene. Sickle cell trait should not be considered a deterrent to pregnancy on the basis of increased risks to the mother. The risk of urinary tract infection is twice as high. Conflicting data exist regarding an association (increased or decreased) risk with pregnancy-induced hypertension. It appears that sickle cell trait does not unfavorably influence the frequency of abortion, perinatal mortality, or low birth weight.

The probability of a serious sickle cell hemoglobinopathy in offspring of women with sickle cell trait is one in four whenever the father carries a gene for an abnormal hemoglobin or for β-thalassemia. Prenatal diagnosis of sickle cell disease through amniocentesis or chorionic villus sampling is now available.

Thalassemias

Thalassemias are genetically determined hemoglobinopathies characterized by impaired production of one or more of the normal globin peptide chains. Hundreds of thalassemia syndromes have been described. Abnormal rates of hemoglobin synthesis may result in ineffective erythropoiesis, hemolysis, and various degrees of anemia. The different forms of thalassemia are classified according to the globin chain whose amount is deficient in relation to that of its partner chain.

Because there are two α-globin genes, the inheritance of α-thalassemia is more complicated than that of β-thalassemia. Four clinical syndromes that result from impaired synthesis of the α-globin chain have been identified. The normal genotype can be expressed as αα/αα. There are two major phenotypes of α-thalassemia. The deletion of all four α-globin chain genes (—/—) characterizes homozygous α-thalassemia. Because α-chains make fetal hemoglobin, the fetus is affected. Without α-globin chains, hemoglobin Bart (γ_4) and hemoglobin H (β_4) are formed as abnormal tetramers. Hemoglobin Bart has an appreciably increased affinity for oxygen. The fetus dies in utero or very soon after birth and demonstrates the typical clinical features of nonimmune hydrops fetalis. Alpha-thalassemia minor is caused by two gene deletions (-α/-α or αα/—) and hemoglobin H disease by three deletions (—/-α).

With β-thalassemia there is decreased β-chain production and excess α-chains precipitate to cause cell membrane damage. With heterozygous β-thalassemia minor, hypochromia, microcytosis, and slight to moderate anemia develop. The hemoglobin concentration typically is 8 to 10 g/dl late in the second trimester and increases to 9 to 11 g/dl near term; this compares with a hemoglobin level of 10 to 12 g/dl in the nonpregnant state. The hallmark of the common β-thalassemias is an elevated hemoglobin A_2 level.

In the typical case of β-thalassemia major, the neonate is healthy at birth, but as the hemoglobin F level falls, the infant becomes severely anemic and fails to thrive. If children are entered into an adequate transfusion program, they develop normally until the end of the first decade, when the effects of iron loading become apparent. Females surviving beyond childhood usually are sterile; life expectancy, even with transfusion therapy, is shortened. Although pregnancy is rare, successful outcomes have been reported. Over the past decades, bone marrow transplantation has been used with a high "cure" rate.

PLATELET DISORDERS

Gestational thrombocytopenia occurs in about 6% of pregnancies and is characterized by mild asymptomatic thrombocytopenia, occurring in a patient without any history of thrombocytopenia (other than in a prior pregnancy, recurrence risk 18%), typically occurring in the third trimester, without any fetal thrombocytopenia, and with spontaneous resolution. If a patient does not conform to these features, other etiologies for thrombocytopenia should be aggressively sought after. Routine obstetric management for the patient and fetus/neonate is recommended surrounding delivery.

Preeclampsia/ HELLP Syndrome

Preeclampsia is estimated to occur in 5% to 7% of all pregnancies and is commonly associated with a thrombocytopenia. Fifteen percent of all women with preeclampsia are estimated to have thrombocytopenia during the clinical course. In most cases, the platelet counts are above $50 \times 10^3/\mu l$; however, in an estimated 5% of cases the maternal thrombocytopenia may be severe, less than $50 \times 10^3/\mu l$. A platelet count less than $100 \times 10^3/\mu l$ is often considered a threshold for delivery in most research protocols. In more extreme cases, a patient may fit the criteria for HELLP syndrome (hemolysis, elevated liver function tests [LFTs], and low platelets), which is defined by the significant laboratory abnormalities. Rapid delivery of the fetus and placenta is indicated in these cases.

Idiopathic Thrombocytopenic Purpura

Idiopathic thrombocytopenic purpura (ITP), also called immune or autoimmune thrombocytopenic purpura, is an autoimmune disorder. Antiplatelet antibodies, usually IgG antibodies, initiate platelet destruction by macrophages in the reticuloendothelial system. The principal site of antibody production is the maternal spleen, followed by the bone marrow. Platelet destruction results in maternal thrombocytopenia. In addition, antiplatelet IgG antibodies can cross the placenta to cause fetal thrombocytopenia.

When new-onset thrombocytopenia is discovered in pregnancy, the diagnosis of ITP often is made as a diagnosis of exclusion, after other causes of thrombocytopenia are ruled out. Presently, the criteria for ITP includes thrombocytopenia, normal white and red blood cell counts, blood smear without microangiopathy, normal coagulation studies, and no other identifiable causes of thrombocytopenia. The platelets are usually large but not the size of lymphocytes as would be seen in congenital giant platelet syndromes. A bone marrow aspirate or biopsy is often performed and demonstrates an increased number of megakaryocytes and normal erythrocyte and leukocyte production.

The risk of significant fetal thrombocytopenia (platelet count $<50 \times 10^3/\mu l$) occurs in approximately 10% of cases. The risk of serious morbidity, namely intracranial hemorrhage, occurs in less than 1% of cases. An estimated rate of 2 per 100,000 births has been suggested for intracranial hemorrhage resulting from ITP. Currently, there are no adequate methods to predict severe fetal thrombocytopenia. The correlation between fetal and maternal platelet counts is not strong. Furthermore, there is poor correlation between maternal IgG circulating platelet antibody, platelet-associated antibody, and fetal platelet count. Given the rarity of sequelae from fetal thrombocytopenia resulting from ITP, routine obstetric management in most cases of either new-onset ITP or chronic ITP remains appropriate.

In select cases of ITP, a more aggressive approach to the management of labor and delivery may be indicated (i.e., prior affected sibling with severe thrombocytopenia or intracranial hemorrhage). Fetal blood sampling has been performed in these rare cases to measure the fetal platelet count to determine mode of delivery. If significant thrombocytopenia (platelet count $<50 \times 10^9/L$) is noted at fetal blood sampling, available options include cesarean delivery and treatment of the mother or neonate with intravenous gamma globulin (IVIG) or steroids.

Antenatal management of ITP depends on a number of factors, including the patient's experience with ITP, presence of other relevant medical conditions, the severity and setting of the thrombocytopenia, and gestational age at which it occurs. Early in pregnancy, treatment of thrombocytopenia is recommended if the maternal platelet count is less than the 30 to $50 \times 10^3/\mu l$ range, or if the patient is symptomatic. First-line treatment typically consists of steroid administration (1 mg/kg prednisone per day). Other options for severe thrombocytopenia include IVIG with regimens ranging from 400 mg/kg/day for 3 days to higher-dose IVIG (i.e., 1 g/kg/day for 2 days). Intravenous Rh immune globulin (anti-D or "WinRho") is also an option for ITP patients who are Rhesus positive. Mild anemia is a side effect of therapy. Splenectomy should be reserved for the most refractory cases because of the maternal and fetal surgical risks. Although splenectomy initially improves the maternal thrombocytopenia, thrombocytopenia can recur.

At delivery, the principal maternal risk is hemorrhage. A maternal platelet count of $50 \times 10^3/\mu l$ is considered safe for vaginal or cesarean delivery. For neuraxial anesthesia, a platelet count of $80 \times 10^9/L$ is considered adequate for catheter placement. For immediate treatment of thrombocytopenia for delivery, platelet transfusion is an option. Postpartum, medications associated with an increased risk of bleeding (e.g., nonsteroidal antiinflammatory agents) should be avoided.

Because thrombocytopenia can occur in neonates born of mothers with ITP, serial platelet counts in the newborn are required. Neonatal thrombocytopenia is correlated with prior maternal splenectomy, maternal platelet count less than 50×10^9/L, and neonatal thrombocytopenia in a sibling. Newborns with severe thrombocytopenia (typically in the range of $<20 \times 10^3/\mu$l) require immediate correction. Platelet transfusion may be given in cases of extreme thrombocytopenia or hemorrhage, although the transfused platelets typically have a shortened survival because of the presence of circulating antiplatelet antibodies.

Thrombotic Thrombocytopenic Purpura and Hemolytic Uremic Syndrome

Thrombotic thrombocytopenic purpura (TTP) and hemolytic uremic syndrome (HUS) are thrombotic microangiopathic diseases in which intravascular platelet activation causes transient ischemia that can mimic preeclampsia/HELLP syndrome during pregnancy. These diseases are characterized by thrombocytopenia and hemolytic anemia, often have multisystem organ failure, and occur with a frequency of 1 per 25,000 pregnancies. TTP has five distinguishing features: fever, hemolytic anemia, thrombocytopenia, neurologic symptoms, and renal abnormalities. Elevations in blood urea nitrogen (BUN) and creatinine are rarely greater than 100 mg/dl and 3 mg/dl, respectively. TTP is most common in women in the second and third decades of life. HUS typically has more significant renal impairment and hypertension and less neurologic involvement than TTP and is primarily a disease of children. Furthermore, HUS is commonly preceded by an antecedent gastrointestinal illness. Thrombocytopenia and bleeding are more severe in TTP.

The treatment for TTP and HUS is plasmapheresis. Patients with TTP have a progressively deteriorating course that is fatal (almost 90% cases) unless treated. Both TTP and HUS can occur following a normal pregnancy or occur following preeclampsia. Unlike preeclampsia, delivery is not associated with resolution.

Infection

Many viral and bacterial infections may result in maternal thrombocytopenia and may not be related to the pregnancy. Infections such as human immunodeficiency virus (HIV), cytomegalovirus (CMV), Epstein-Barr, and hepatitis B and C can all result in temporary thrombocytopenia. In 10% of HIV patients, thrombocytopenia may be the first clinical finding, although it can present at any time during the course of disease. The severity of the platelet deficiency varies, with 5% having platelet counts below $50 \times 10^3/\mu$l in one study. Testing for HIV virus should be routine in the newly diagnosed thrombocytopenic individual.

Pharmacologic

There are a countless number of therapies at our disposal that may result in thrombocytopenia. Drug-induced thrombocytopenia is immune mediated in most cases. Drugs such as heparin, acetaminophen, and trimethoprim-sulfamethoxazole are well-known drugs used during pregnancy.

Thrombocytopenia resulting from heparin therapy (HIT) is becoming more common in our field as the use of heparin during pregnancy becomes more widespread. It is a well-known entity and typically occurs 4 to 10 days after treatment is begun. There are two types. Type 1 is characterized by an early (within 2 days) mild thrombocytopenia that normalizes with continued use. It is thought to be a direct activation of platelets by the heparin molecule. Type 2 is far more severe and is thought to be an immune-mediated disorder resulting from the formation of heparin-platelet factor 4 complexes. Specific immunoglobulin binds to this complex and is thought to activate platelets resulting in aggregation and ultimately, premature removal from the peripheral circulation. Type 2 HIT can be confirmed by serotonin release assays, heparin-induced platelet aggregation assays, flow cytometry, or solid phase immunoassay. Despite the thrombocytopenia, arterial and venous thromboses have been associated with this condition. The etiology remains unknown. An estimated 10% to 20% of patients will have detectable drop in platelet count with heparin use; however, only 0.3% to 3% will have type 2. LMWHs are not as strongly associated with thrombocytopenia as unfractionated heparin. In most cases of type 2 disease, treatment is the cessation of heparin. However, consideration must be made for alternative anticoagulation resulting from the risks of thrombosis.

One good option for patients with HIT who require anticoagulation is fondaparinux, a synthetic heparin pentasaccharide that complexes with the antithrombin binding site for heparin to permit the selective inactivation of factor Xa but not thrombin. If the patient has no evidence of active thrombosis, prophylactic fondaparinux is recommended, whereas in the setting of active thrombosis, therapeutic fondaparinux is recommended. Fondaparinux does not cross the placenta and is considered a Class B medication but is not Food and Drug Administration (FDA) approved in pregnancy.

Direct thrombin inhibitors represent another class of anticoagulants for consideration in these special circumstances. Hirudin is a 65-amino-acid protein derived from the medicinal leech (*Hirudo medicinalis*) and is readily available in a recombinant form, lepirudin. It may be used in patients with HIT-type 2. Another option is argatroban, a synthetic direct thrombin inhibitor with a short half-life (45 minutes) that competitively binds to the active site of thrombin. Argatroban is cleared by the liver, making it the direct thrombin inhibitor of choice for patients with renal failure. One should be aware that there is limited use of lepirudin or argatroban in pregnancy.

The differential diagnosis for thrombocytopenia is extensive and the management varies tremendously with each etiology. Careful attention to a patient's history, physical examination, and laboratory studies is required to best manage these patients.

SUMMARY

Pronounced changes in the hematologic system accompany pregnancy and the puerperium. This chapter has reviewed the normal pregnancy alterations and common conditions affecting pregnancy.

KEY POINTS

- A greater expansion of plasma volume relative to the increase in hemoglobin mass and erythrocyte volume is responsible for the modest fall in hemoglobin levels observed in healthy pregnant women.

- The lower limit of normal platelet counts in pregnancy has been reported to be 106 to 120×10^9/L. It is well recognized that platelet counts can drop much lower than this range, with a lower threshold of gestational thrombocytopenia being 70×10^9/L.

- The circulating levels of several of the coagulation factors including fibrinogen, factors VII, VIII, X, and von Willebrand factor are increased.

- Pregnancy is associated with decreased levels of protein S (PS) activity and free PS antigen in the majority of patients.

- Normal pregnancy was associated with increased thrombin activity, increased soluble fibrin levels, and increased thrombin-antithrombin complexes, as well as fibrinolysis, evidenced by increased levels of fibrin D-dimer.

- After 7 to 10 days of therapy with an iron compound, reticulocytosis can be seen and hemoglobin may increase by at least 1 g per week in patients with severe anemia.

- Anemia may be associated with chronic disease states, such as inflammatory bowel disease, chronic renal failure, and systemic lupus erythematosus.

- Intense sequestration of sickled erythrocytes with infarction in various organs may develop acutely, especially late in pregnancy, during labor and delivery, and early in the puerperium.

- Sickle cell trait does not unfavorably influence the frequency of abortion, perinatal mortality, or low birth weight.

- With the thalassemias, abnormal rates of hemoglobin synthesis may result in ineffective erythropoiesis, hemolysis, and various degrees of anemia.

- Gestational thrombocytopenia is characterized by mild asymptomatic thrombocytopenia, occurring in a patient without any history of thrombocytopenia (other than in a prior pregnancy, recurrence risk 18%), typically occurring in the third trimester, without any fetal thrombocytopenia, and with spontaneous resolution.

- Given the rarity of sequelae from fetal thrombocytopenia resulting from ITP, routine obstetric management in most cases of either new-onset ITP or chronic ITP remains appropriate.

- Thrombotic thrombocytopenic purpura (TTP) and hemolytic uremic syndrome (HUS) are thrombotic microangiopathic diseases in which intravascular platelet activation causes transient ischemia that can mimic preeclampsia/HELLP syndrome during pregnancy.

SUGGESTED READINGS

Bremme, KA: Hemostatic changes in pregnancy. *Best Pract Res Clin Haematol* 16:153, 2003.

Burrows RF, Kelton JG: Fetal thrombocytopenia and its relation to maternal thrombocytopenia. *N Engl J Med* 329:1463, 1993.

Burrows RF, Kelton JG: Pregnancy in patients with idiopathic thrombocytopenic purpura: assessing the risks for the infant at delivery. *Obstet Gynecol Surv* 48:781, 1993.

Cines DB, Blanchette VS: Immune thrombocytopenic purpura. *N Engl J Med* 346:995, 2002.

George JN et al: Idiopathic thrombocytopenic purpura: a practice guideline developed by explicit methods for the American Society of Hematology. *Blood* 88:3, 1996.

Greer IA: Thrombosis in pregnancy: maternal and fetal issues. *Lancet* 353:1258, 1999.

Olivieri NF: The beta-thalassemias. *N Engl J Med* 341:99, 1999.

Payne SD et al: Maternal characteristics and risk of severe neonatal thrombocytopenia and intracranial hemorrhage in pregnancies complicated by autoimmune thrombocytopenia. *Am J Obstet Gynecol* 177:149, 1997.

Stuart MJ, Setty BN: Sickle cell acute chest syndrome: pathogenesis and rationale for treatment. *Blood* 94:1555, 1999.

Warkentin TE: Heparin-induced thrombocytopenia: diagnosis and management. *Circulation* 110:454, 2004.

26

COMMON AUTOIMMUNE DISORDERS IN PREGNANCY

Benjamin D. Hamar, Joshua A. Copel, and Jill P. Buyon

SYSTEMIC LUPUS ERYTHEMATOSUS

Definition

Systemic lupus erythematosus (SLE) is a chronic autoimmune disorder categorized by periods of disease flares and remissions. It is a heterogeneous disorder with a variety of clinical and laboratory manifestations. It can follow a relatively benign course affecting only the skin and musculoskeletal system or be more aggressive with life-threatening involvement of vital organs such as the kidney and brain.

Epidemiology

The prevalence of SLE varies with the population studied but is generally 0.5 to 12.5 per 10,000 and affects approximately 1 in 2000 to 3000 pregnancies. The lifetime risk of a woman developing SLE is 1 in 700. During the reproductive years (15-44 years) the disorder affects women 9 to 15 times more often than men although this falls to a threefold increase by menopause. Lupus affects black and Hispanic women two to four times more often than Caucasians.

Etiology

There is no known etiology for SLE. However, there is evidence to support a genetic predisposition or causal relationship because women with SLE are more likely to have certain human leukocyte antigen (HLA) types (HLA-B8, HLA-DR3, and HLA-DR2). Linkage studies suggest a genetic component: 5% to 12% of affected individuals have another affected relative, and 25% to 50% of monozygotic twins are concordant for the disease. Efforts to determine the specific genes responsible for development of SLE are underway in several laboratories across the country. It is clear that multiple genes are involved, many likely related to pathways of B- and T-cell biology and immune clearance mechanisms. Additionally, women with SLE have been found to be more likely to have persistence of fetal DNA (so-called microchimerism) compared with healthy controls. This suggests that the interaction between maternal and fetal DNA can play a role in the pathogenesis of SLE.[1]

Pathogenesis

Autoantibodies in SLE play a key role in mediating many of the disease effects. Lupus anticoagulant and other antiphospholipid antibodies (APAs) increase the risk for thrombosis. Renal damage is secondary to immune complex deposition, complement activation, and inflammation and subsequent fibrosis.

Placentas from women with SLE demonstrate characteristic changes: reduction in size, placental infarctions, intraplacental hemorrhage, deposition of immunoglobulin and complement, and thickening of the trophoblast basement membrane. These changes appear to be responsible for many of the effects of SLE on pregnancy outlined below (increased rates of preeclampsia, intrauterine growth restriction [IUGR], preterm delivery, etc.).

Clinical Presentation

The American Rheumatism Association (now called the American College of Rheumatology) set forth diagnostic criteria in 1982 that were formally revised in 1997 (Table 26-1). Patients must fulfill at least 4 of the 11 criteria at some point in the course of their disease although not necessarily at the same time. These criteria have been found to be 96% sensitive and 96% specific for the diagnosis of SLE.[2]

Lupus is characterized by the presence of a variety of autoantibodies with diagnostic and prognostic implications. Antinuclear antibody (ANA) is the most common antibody for screening for autoimmune syndromes. However, 10% of asymptomatic pregnant women without autoimmune disease have ANAs compared with 2% of nonpregnant controls. Because of the high prevalence in the general population, ANA is used primarily as a screening test for lupus. Antibodies to double-stranded DNA (dsDNA) and Smith (Sm) are more specific for lupus, and anti-dsDNA has been correlated with disease activity (generally renal involvement). Anti-SSA/Ro and anti-SSB/La are more often associated with Sjögren's syndrome but are also found in 40% and 15%, respectively, in women with SLE. Anti-SSA/Ro and anti-SSB/La are associated with the development of neonatal lupus, which is most often characterized by congenital heart block (CHB) or an annular rash.

Lupus flares are difficult to characterize because they represent worsening of a heterogeneous disease process. A variety of scoring systems have been developed to measure SLE disease status and to aid the diagnosis of a flare. Symptoms of flares include fatigue, fever, arthralgias/myalgias, weight loss, rash, renal deterioration, serositis, lymphadenopathy, and central nervous system symptoms. The titer of antibodies to Sm, RNP, SSA/Ro, or SSB/La may or may not fluctuate in parallel with disease flares. However, rising titers of antibodies to dsDNA (particularly in the setting of falling complement levels) may suggest an impending flare of disease and thus should trigger closer surveillance of the patient.

Table 26-1

Criterion	Definition
Malar rash	Fixed erythema, flat or raised, over the malar eminences, tending to spare the nasolabial folds
Discoid rash	Erythematous raised patches with adherent keratotic scaling and follicular plugging; atrophic scarring may occur in older lesions
Photosensitivity	Skin rash as a result of unusual reaction to sunlight, by patient history or physician observation
Oral ulcers	Oral or nasopharyngeal ulceration, usually painless, observed by a physician
Arthritis	Nonerosive arthritis involving 2 or more peripheral joints, characterized by tenderness, swelling, or effusion
Serositis	Pleuritis—convincing history of pleuritic pain or rub heard by a physician or evidence of pleural effusion OR Pericarditis—documented by ECG or rub or evidence of pericardial effusion
Renal disorder	Persistent proteinuria greater than 0.5 g/day or greater than 3+ proteinuria if quantitation is not performed OR Cellular casts—may be red cell, hemoglobin, granular, tubular, or mixed
Neurologic disorder	Seizures – in the absence of offending drugs or known metabolic derangements, e.g., uremia, ketoacidosis, or electrolyte imbalance OR Psychosis—in the absence of offending drugs or known metabolic derangements, e.g., uremia, ketoacidosis, or electrolyte imbalance
Hematologic disorder	Hemolytic anemia —with reticulocytosis OR Leukopenia—less than 4000/mm^3 on 2 or more occasions OR Lymphopenia—less than 1500/mm^3 on 2 or more occasions OR Thrombocytopenia—less than 100,000/mm^3 in the absence of offending drugs
Immunologic disorder	Anti-DNA antibody OR Anti-Sm antibody OR Positive findings of antiphospholipid antibodies based on: Abnormal serum level of IgG or IgM anticardiolipin antibodies OR Positive test result for lupus anticoagulant OR False-positive serologic test for syphilis known to be positive for at least 6 months and confirmed by *Treponema pallidum* immobilization or fluorescent treponemal antibody absorption test.

Continued

Table 26-1—cont'd

Criterion	Definition
Antinuclear antibody	An abnormal titer of antinuclear antibody by immunofluorescence or an equivalent assay at any point in time and in the absence of drugs known to be associated with "drug-induced lupus" syndrome

From Tan EM et al: The 1982 revised criteria for the classification of systemic lupus erythematosus. *Arth Rheum* 25:1271, 1982; Hochberg MC: Updating the American College of Rheumatology revised criteria for the classification of systemic lupus erythematosus (letter). *Arth Rheum* 40:1725, 1997.
A person is classified as having SLE if any 4 of the 11 criteria are present (serially or simultaneously) during any interval of the evaluation.
ECG, Electrocardiogram; *IgG*, immunoglobulin G; *IgM*, immunoglobulin M.

Differential Diagnosis

The main differential diagnosis for SLE is other rheumatologic/connective tissue disorders. Many of these autoimmune diseases share common diagnostic criteria and it may take time for the varied manifestations of these diseases to appear, permitting the ultimate diagnosis. Additionally, because of the varied nature of the criteria for diagnosis, patients presenting with several of the criteria could have other local or systemic disorders.

During pregnancy, differentiation of SLE from normal pregnancy symptoms or preeclampsia can be challenging. Lupus flares often feature inflammatory arthritis, significant leukopenia or thrombocytopenia, inflammatory rashes, pleuritis, and fevers. However, many of the manifestations of an SLE flare can be similar to preeclampsia (hypertension, proteinuria, thrombocytopenia, elevated hepatic transaminases, activation of the coagulation cascade), although the treatment for each is very different. The treatment for severe preeclampsia ultimately involves delivery, whereas lupus flares can be treated and the pregnancy often allowed to continue. A rising anti-dsDNA titer, active urinary sediment, and low complement levels (C3 and C4) suggest a lupus flare. In general, complement levels rise in pregnancy and are unaffected by uncomplicated preeclampsia. Conversely, rising uric acid levels or a greater degree of thrombocytopenia suggest severe preeclampsia and HELLP syndrome (hemolysis, elevated liver function tests [LFTs], and low platelets). As the pregnancy approaches term, efforts at discriminating between the two are not likely to be worthwhile: delivery will cure preeclampsia and if the symptoms do not improve, treatment of lupus flare can be initiated.

Morbidity

General Morbidity and Mortality

Because of the effect of SLE on multiple organ systems, patients with this disease have significantly increased morbidity and mortality. Women with SLE are more prone to cardiovascular disease, thromboembolic phenomena, infection, and renal disease. With better understanding of the disease process and potential complications, survival rates have improved with 5-, 10-, 15-, and 20-year survival rates of 93%, 85%, 79%, and 68%. Risk factors for mortality include renal damage, thrombocytopenia, lung involvement, high disease activity at diagnosis, and age 50 years or older at diagnosis. Fertility is not impaired in women with SLE unless they have a past history of prior cyclophosphamide treatment. A previous history of active lupus nephritis per se is not really associated with infertility unless there is renal failure. High-dose steroids can be associated with amenorrhea.

Effects of Pregnancy on Systemic Lupus Erythematosus

During pregnancy, there is a shift in cytokines from a type 1 helper T response (T_H1) to a type 2 helper T response (T_H2) pattern with predominance of the antiinflammatory and pro-B-cell cytokines interleukin (IL)-4 and IL-10. Because SLE is largely a humorally mediated autoimmune syndrome, one might expect that this cytokine shift may worsen the disease process or increase the rate of lupus flares in pregnancy.

Because of the heterogeneity of lupus patients and the variety of diagnostic criteria for lupus flares, there has been conflicting data regarding whether SLE exacerbations are more frequent in pregnancy. Some of the contributing factors to this controversy involve the variation in criteria for diagnosing lupus flares and the inherent heterogeneity of patients with lupus with different severity and activity of their lupus. Consequently, the reported incidence of lupus flares during pregnancy ranges from 13% to 74%. It is generally believed that the risk for flare in pregnancy is increased if women are not in remission before becoming pregnant. Approximately 35% of flares occur in the second trimester with another 35% occurring postpartum. The majority of flares are minor and do not require immunosuppressive therapy; however, serious manifestations can occur. Ruiz-Irastorza et al.[3] found flare rates were higher in pregnancy than in nonpregnant controls. When the pregnant women were followed throughout the first postpartum year, flares were noted to occur more often during pregnancy compared with the year following their deliveries. However, flares during pregnancy were no more severe than those experienced by the nonpregnant controls or postpartum. Other authors have found equivalent rates of flares in pregnancy compared with nonpregnant controls.

Lupus nephropathy is the end result of autoimmune-mediated inflammation and renal damage. Pregnancy causes a worsening in renal function in approximately 20% of women with nephropathy but is reversible 95% of the time. The risk of renal deterioration is directly correlated with prepregnant renal status. Additionally, poor renal function is correlated with poor pregnancy outcome with higher loss rates seen in women with nephrotic proteinuria or baseline creatinine above 1.5 mg/dl. Women with renal disease are also more likely to have pregnancies complicated by gestational hypertension, preeclampsia, IUGR, and premature birth.

Effects of Systemic Lupus Erythematosus on Pregnancy

Pregnancy outcome and risk of stillbirth are related to the baseline disease status prior to pregnancy and do not appear to be affected by the presence or absence of flares in pregnancy. Stillbirth rates in women with SLE have been found to be 150 per 1000 births, 25 times the national average. When pregnancies in women with SLE are compared with control women and to women more than 5 years before the diagnosis of SLE, complication and loss rates are greater in women with SLE in pregnancy. Additionally, if SLE is diagnosed during pregnancy, complication rates and fetal loss rates are increased.

The predominant mediator of fetal loss among SLE patents is the presence of concomitant antiphospholipid antibody syndrome (APS) that is present in approximately 30% of women with SLE. In women with active renal disease, pregnancy loss rates are as high as 30%, and for women with more advanced renal disease fetal loss rates approach 60%. Women with stable lupus nephritis marked by plasma creatinine values less than 1.5 mg/dl, proteinuria less than 2 g/24 hours, and no hypertension have lower risks of adverse pregnancy outcome.

Preeclampsia occurs in 20% to 30% of women with SLE with higher rates seen in women with underlying hypertension, renal disease, and APS. IUGR has been reported in 12% to 32% of lupus pregnancies, which was found to be higher than control populations. Preterm birth is increased in SLE pregnancies with rates as high as 50% to 60% because of preeclampsia, IUGR, abnormal fetal testing, and preterm premature rupture of membranes (PPROM). Rupture of membranes in women with SLE is more common in preterm and term pregnancies when compared with controls and appears to be unrelated to disease status or serology but may be confounded by steroid use (a known risk factor for rupture of membranes).

Neonatal lupus erythematosus (NLE) occurs in 1% to 2% of the infants of mothers with anti-SSA/Ro or anti-SSB/La antibodies regardless of whether or not the mother has SLE. The disease is thought to be due to immune-mediated damage of the fetus by transplacental autoantibodies with resulting inflammation. The syndrome is most commonly characterized by fetal and neonatal CHB, skin lesions, and occasionally thrombocytopenia, anemia, and hepatitis. Although the other manifestations are transient humorally mediated effects with resolution in the first few months of life, CHB is a permanent condition. The anti-SSA/Ro and anti-SSB/La maternal antibodies cross the placenta and can damage the atrioventricular conducting system, which results in varying degrees of heart block and, less often, a myocarditis. Fetal CHB is most commonly diagnosed between 18 and 24 weeks' gestation. These autoantibodies may act via apoptosis or by direct interference with cardiac conduction through calcium channels. The risk of CHB in women with anti-SSA/Ro antibodies and no prior affected infants is approximately 2% but increases to 18% in women with anti-SSA/Ro antibodies and a history of previous infant with CHB or a skin rash. The majority of women whose fetuses or infants have CHB are asymptomatic but are subsequently found to be anti-SSA/Ro or anti-SSB/La positive. About half of these women will develop symptoms of a rheumatic disease; most often these are dry eyes and mouth consistent with Sjögren syndrome. These women should be reassured that they do not have SLE in the absence of other features and they are less than 50% likely to develop SLE in the future. Although third-degree or "complete" CHB is permanent, there is some uncontrolled evidence that first- or second-degree can be reversed with antenatal fluorinated steroid therapy and that progression to more severe forms of heart block may be prevented. Additionally, steroid therapy has shown some reversal of hydropic features in fetuses with CHB and evidence of cardiac failure. At present, there is no evidence supporting the routine use of prophylactic steroid therapy in women with anti-SSA/Ro or anti-SSB-La antibodies to prevent the onset of CHB.

**Management
During
Pregnancy**

Management of SLE during pregnancy begins with preconceptional counseling. At this time, maternal disease status can be assessed and risks of pregnancy discussed. Evaluation for any preexisting renal disease is performed with a 24-hour urine collection and serum creatinine to measure proteinuria and creatinine clearance. Remission for 6 months before pregnancy reduces adverse outcomes.

Early pregnancy assessment should include assessment of maternal disease status including 24-hour urine collection, plasma creatinine, complete blood count, anti-SSA/Ro antibody, anti-SSB/La antibody, anti-dsDNA antibody, lupus anticoagulant, anticardiolipin antibody, C3, and C4 levels. Repeat anti-dsDNA, 24-hour urine, plasma creatinine, C3, and C4 levels to monitor disease status should be performed each trimester. Lupus anticoagulant and anticardiolipin antibodies can be repeated in the second trimester to screen for development of APS. Early genetic risk assessment is important because lupus pregnancies carry increased maternal risk and early diagnosis of genetic abnormalities gives patients the option of termination of a nonviable pregnancy. Because of the increased risk of premature delivery, establishment of reliable dating is important.

Prepregnant drug regimens, if safe in pregnancy, should be continued in pregnancy to maintain remission. A summary of some of the therapeutic agents and their reproductive risks can be found in Table 26-2. If APS is also present, anticoagulation can reduce the associated complications. Nonsteroidal antiinflammatory agents are contraindicated after 28 weeks because of risk of closure of the fetal ductus arteriosus. Hydroxychloroquine, an antimalarial medication helpful in reducing disease flares, is

427

Table 26-2

Systemic Lupus
Erythematosus
Therapeutic Agents

Drug	Safety in Pregnancy	Comments
Glucocorticoids	Safe	Association with growth restriction at high dose, need stress-dose steroids at delivery or for medical illnesses if chronic use through pregnancy. Increased risk of preterm rupture of membranes, preterm delivery
Hydroxychloroquine	Generally considered safe	Antimalarial. Reduces disease flares
Nonsteroidal antiinflammatory agents	See comments	Association with oligohydraminos, and ductus arteriosus closure. Avoid after 28 weeks
Azathioprine (6-mercaptopurine)	See comments	Risk of fetal growth restriction and immune suppression. Use as second-line agent
Cyclophosphamide	Unsafe	Alkylating agent. Skeletal and palate defects, also defects in eyes and limbs
Methotrexate	Unsafe	Folic acid antagonist. Abortifacient and teratogen.

often maintained during pregnancy. Glucocorticoids are also "safe" in pregnancy, although if patients are on chronic steroids, stress-dose steroids should be given at delivery. Azathioprine is an immunosuppressive agent that is metabolized to 6-mercaptopurine and is a cytotoxic purine analog. Most investigators have found azathioprine to be "safe" in pregnancy although there is a risk of growth restriction and fetal immune suppression. Other cytotoxic agents such as cyclophosphamide and methotrexate are contraindicated in pregnancy and are to be avoided.

Making the diagnosis of lupus flare in pregnancy requires excluding the other diagnoses as outlined previously. Flares can be managed conservatively with adjustment of medication regimen as outlined previously or addition of analgesics such as acetaminophen. Glucocorticoid therapy can be initiated for more severe flares. The exact treatment of the flare will vary with the nature and severity of the flare.

Fetal surveillance includes genetic risk assessment and measures of fetal well-being. Fetal growth is assessed in 4-week intervals in the second and third trimester with more frequent assessment if growth restriction is suspected. Doppler evaluation is reserved for assessment of fetal well-being if estimated fetal weight is less than the 10th percentile. Weekly nonstress testing with assessment of amniotic fluid can begin at 30 weeks.

When women are followed in an intense, multidisciplinary clinic with pregnancies initiated during disease quiescence and treatment of underlying disease, fetal outcomes appear to be improved. Diagnosis and treatment of APS improves fetal loss rates.

ANTIPHOSPHOLIPID ANTIBODY SYNDROME

Definition

APS is characterized by antibodies to phospholipid-binding proteins resulting in thrombosis, adverse pregnancy outcome, or recurrent pregnancy loss.

Epidemiology

APAs are found in 1% to 5% of asymptomatic pregnant women. However, APAs are present in 8% to 20% of women with recurrent pregnancy loss, 20% of women with stillbirth, and 30% of women with unexplained thrombosis.

Etiology

It is unknown why women develop APS. There is a high prevalence of women with APAs without the clinical manifestation of the syndrome. These women are at increased risk of developing thromboses and other clinical manifestations but the magnitude and risk factors are unknown for development of the syndrome itself. Some have postulated the requirement of a "second hit" to trigger APS (i.e., endothelial damage or other disruptive vascular event), but the inciting events are unknown.

Pathogenesis

APAs are a class of self-recognition immunoglobulins directed against proteins adhering anionic phospholipids that can be detected by screening for antibodies directly binding these protein targets (e.g., beta-2-glycoprotein-1, prothrombin, or annexin V) or by indirectly assessing antibodies reacting to proteins present in a phospholipid matrix (e.g., cardiolipin and phosphatidylserine) or by assessing the effects of these antibodies on clotting reactions in a phospholipid environment (i.e., lupus anticoagulants).[4]

There are several hypotheses to explain the mechanism by which APAs exert their procoagulant effect. First, APAs activate endothelial cells to upregulate cell adhesion molecules and enhance secretion of targeting cytokines. Second, anticardiolipin antibodies (ACAs) have been shown to bind to oxidized cardiolipin, suggesting that they play a role in oxidative injury to the endothelium. Third, APAs have been theorized to interfere with the function of phospholipid bound coagulation cascade modulators (e.g., annexin V, beta-2-glyocprotein-1, thrombomodulin). Fourth, APA-mediated activation of the complement cascade can lead to damage of the placental vasculature, leading to growth restriction and demise. Finally, a "second hit" vascular injury hypothesis has been advanced because APAs bind to charged phospholipids, which are usually expressed only in perturbed cellular membranes seen in cellular injury or apoptosis.

It is thought that APA-mediated injury to the placental vasculature is responsible for the growth restriction and fetal loss seen in APS. Localized placental thrombosis can lead to decreased placental perfusion and subsequent placental insufficiency, which would explain the increased losses after 10 weeks' gestational age. This theory has been supported by a murine model, in which the addition of human APAs induces murine fetal loss. The addition of APAs in this model leads to immunoglobulin deposition at the placental bed and fetal wastage. These phenomena are not seen in mice with complement deficiencies or who are given complement cascade inhibitors, suggesting that the complement cascade is an important common pathogenic pathway. Additionally, APAs may impair trophoblastic invasion of the spiral arteries and hormone production, which would explain the increased embryonic abortion and early pregnancy losses. Whether or not those women with recurrent early pregnancy loss and those with losses after 10 weeks' gestation represent different populations requiring different treatments is unclear at this time.

Clinical Presentation

APS is diagnosed by the presence of thrombotic or obstetric features and the presence of APAs as outlined by the 1999 International Consensus Statement and are summarized in Box 26-1. Laboratory evaluation (outlined below) for lupus anticoagulant or ACA is used to confirm the syndrome. Thromboses can be either venous or arterial and are often recurrent. Thromboses can lead to stroke or other dysfunction. Prospective evaluation of women with APS without treatment have shown fetal loss rates as high as 50% to 90%. Other clinical features include thrombocytopenia, hemolytic anemia, livedo reticularis, other cutaneous manifestations, and end-organ damage (i.e., renal) from chronic thrombotic microangiopathy. Cardiac valve abnormalities are found in 35% to 75% of women with APS; the majority are asymptomatic and benign.

Lupus anticoagulants (LACs) are detected by the prolongation of various phospholipid-dependent clotting assays and are reported as present or

> **Box 26-1** Criteria for the Classification of Antiphospholipid Antibody Syndrome
>
> **Clinical Criteria**
> 1. Vascular thrombosis
> 2. Pregnancy morbidity
>   a. Unexplained intrauterine fetal demise at ≥10 weeks of a morphologically normal fetus
>   b. Severe preeclampsia/eclampsia or severe placental insufficiency before 34 weeks
>   c. Three or more unexplained spontaneous abortions at <10 weeks
>
> **Laboratory Criteria**
> 1. Anticardiolipin antibody (IgG or IgM) at moderate or high titer,* on 2 or more occasions at least 6 weeks apart
> 2. Lupus anticoagulant present on 2 or more occasions at least 6 weeks apart
> Presence of at least one clinical criterion and one laboratory criterion is necessary for the diagnosis of antiphospholipid antibody syndrome.

Wilson WA et al: International consensus statement on preliminary classification criteria for definite antiphospholipid antibody syndrome. *Arth Rheum* 42:1309, 1999. Copyright © 2001 Wiley-Liss, Inc. Reprinted with permission of Wiley-Liss, Inc., a subsidiary of John Wiley & Sons, Inc.
*Test results for anticardiolipin antibody titers according to standards established by Harris et al: *Br J Haematol* 74:1, 1990. Negative 0-10 MPL or GPL, Low-positive >10-20 MPL or GPL, Moderate >20-80 MPL or GPL, High positive >80 MPL or GPL.

absent. Confirmatory testing includes failure of the addition of platelet-poor plasma to correct the prolongation, which excludes factor deficiency as an explanation for the test result. The presence of a lupus inhibitor detected by various lupus anticoagulant assays is more specific than ACA for APS.

Anticardiolipin antibodies are detected by indirect β_2-glycoprotein I dependent immunoassays and are reported by antibody class and low or high titer. It appears that the clinically relevant classes are immunoglobulin (Ig) G and IgM at high titer. Although LAC and ACA are often concordant and sometimes share epitope specificity, they are distinct entities.

Other antibodies have been evaluated including direct detection of anti-β_2-glycoprotein I antibodies and other phospholipid-associated antibody classes (e.g., anti-phosphatidylserine), but their clinical utility is unclear. These antibodies are thus not included in the diagnostic criteria. Although β_2-glycoprotein I antibodies are not included in the diagnostic criteria, it appears that there is an association with some of the clinical features of APS.

Differential Diagnosis

There are many conditions that lead to thrombosis (coagulopathy, vasculitis, etc.) and adverse pregnancy outcome (coagulopathy, preeclampsia, genetic abnormalities, etc.). Establishment of the clinical diagnosis of APS includes exclusion of these conditions.

Other conditions are associated with APAs, including cancer, infection, and drug use, although these are usually low titer and not persistent. Other syndromes such as SLE have a high prevalence of APAs and the presence of APAs should prompt an evaluation to exclude these conditions.

Treatment and Expected Outcome

Treatment goals include improvement of fetal outcomes and reduction in risk for maternal thrombosis. Historic treatment consisted of aspirin or glucocorticoids. However, heparin was shown to be as effective as steroids with a lower risk of premature delivery and gestational diabetes, and has become the standard therapy. Either unfractionated or low molecular weight heparin (LMWH) may be used but because of the lower risk of heparin-induced thrombocytopenia with LMWH, it is becoming the agent of choice. A recent meta-analysis showed that the live-birth rate was improved by 54% with heparin therapy. One cautionary note is that despite anticoagulation, 20% to 30% of women with APS have fetal losses. Intravenous IgG (IVIG) has been shown to be effective, although it is unclear whether it is superior to heparin therapy. The cost and side effects of IVIG currently limit it to women with severe APS or those who have been refractory to heparin therapy.

Preconceptional counseling is an important component of the management of APS in pregnancy. This allows patients the opportunity to discuss the magnitude of risk in pregnancy. Patients who are on maintenance anticoagulation with warfarin can be switched to regular heparin or LMWH in anticipation of pregnancy. Patients can begin aspirin therapy at their first positive pregnancy test and heparin therapy at or after 7 weeks. Because there is no maternal blood flow through the placenta before 9 weeks, it is unclear whether heparin is beneficial before this point and may potentiate implantation bleeding.

Women with definite diagnosis of APS should be treated during pregnancy. Those women with a history of prior venous or arterial thrombosis have a high rate of recurrence and should receive life-long anticoagulation. Women with lower-titer ACA (<20 glycerophospholipids [GPL] or monophosphoryl lipids [MPL] units) and those without LAC but with higher-titer ACA (20-50 GPL or MPL units) who have no history of thrombosis or recurrent adverse pregnancy outcomes are not at increased risk and do not appear to require treatment. However, women with high-titer ACA (>20 MPL or GPL units) and no history of thrombosis but no prior pregnancy may be at an increased risk of fetal loss, but it is unclear whether anticoagulation will improve their outcomes. It is similarly unclear whether women with APAs other than IgM or IgG (i.e., IgA) will benefit from anticoagulation.

In women who meet criteria for treatment outlined previously, our practice is to give LMWH and daily low-dose aspirin (81 mg) from diagnosis of fetal cardiac activity until at least 6 weeks postpartum. Women with a history of prior thromboembolism or prior stillbirth should have therapeutic anticoagulation consisting of 1 mg/kg enoxaparin every 12 hours or 1.5 mg/kg daily. Those women with a history of recurrent miscarriage without history of prior thrombosis may be maintained on a prophylactic regimen of 40 mg of enoxaparin daily. Aspirin monotherapy may be considered for women with positive serologies but without any history of clots or recurrent miscarriage. Because of the interference of some APAs with traditional measures of coagulation, antifactor-Xa levels are followed with

431

therapeutic goals of 0.5 to 1.0 unit/ml. Because of the 1% to 2% risk of heparin-induced osteoporosis and fracture, we recommend daily calcium and vitamin D supplementation and daily weight-bearing exercise as tolerated. At 36 weeks, LMWH can be switched to unfractionated heparin to facilitate epidural placement in labor and/or anticoagulation management at delivery. Aspirin should also be discontinued at this time, although some recommend continuing aspirin throughout pregnancy, even though there may be a slight increase risk of abruption in this latter setting and there is a theoretic risk of inhibition of fetal and neonatal platelet function. Post-partum anticoagulation with either warfarin or LMWH is mandated in all APS patients for at least 6 weeks.

Fetal surveillance involves serial fetal biometry every 4 weeks beginning in the second trimester to evaluate fetal growth for evidence of placental insufficiency. If fetal growth begins to decline, more frequent assessment of fetal weight and Doppler studies for assessment of uteroplacental blood flow can be considered. Screening for preeclampsia is important given the association of APS with severe, early preeclampsia. Weekly non-stress test (NST) and amniotic fluid assessment can begin at 28 weeks or earlier if clinically indicated.

Treatment of APS during pregnancy with active fetal surveillance has shown improved outcomes, with live birth rates as high as 70% to 80%. Nonetheless, antepartum complications remain common: 18% of women develop preeclampsia and 31% of infants are small for gestational age. Additionally, there is a high rate of premature delivery (40%-50%), with the majority of these premature births occurring around 34 weeks.

RHEUMATOID ARTHRITIS

Definition

Rheumatoid arthritis (RA) is a chronic systemic inflammatory disease characterized by symmetrical polyarthritis of the small joints of the hands and feet and knees and elbows. The disease may be remitting but if not controlled can lead to deformity and destruction of joints.

Epidemiology

RA affects 1% to 2% of the population with an overall annual incidence of 7.5 per 10,000. RA affects three times as many women as men.

Etiology

There is no known etiology for RA although a number of theories have been proposed, including infection-triggered autoimmunity, immune interactions, and synoviocyte transformation. Evidence exists for a genetic susceptibility because women with RA are more likely to have HLA-DR4. Research to determine the basis of this association is ongoing.

Pathogenesis

The exact inciting events that cause the pathologic effects of RA are unknown. However, it seems that both B-cell and T-cell mediated effects lead to activation of an immune response directed against the joint synovium. As mentioned previously, pregnancy is associated with a shift from T_H1 to T_H2 cytokines with increased production of the antiinflammatory cytokines IL-4 and IL-10 and decreased production of the proinflammatory cytokines tumor necrosis factor (TNF) -α, interferon (IFN) -γ, and IL-2. Proinflammatory cytokines (particularly TNF-α) mediate the increase in activity of synoviocytes, which increase the production of matrix-metalloproteinases, serine proteinases, and other extracellular matrix degradation agents. The action of these proteinases and the synoviocytes act to break down the synovium and erode the joint spaces, which leads to the clinical syndrome.

There is evidence that sex hormones play a role in the development and disease activity of RA: female predominance, increased incidence with menopause, relationship of activity with the menstrual cycle, and improvement during pregnancy. Nulliparity is a risk factor for development of RA, but oral contraceptive use does not appear to provide a protective effect. Estrogen is known to downregulate proinflammatory cytokines such as TNF-α, which provides a potential mechanism for this effect.

Clinical Presentation

The American College of Rheumatology set forth guidelines for the diagnosis of RA in 1988, including morning stiffness, soft-tissue swelling of three or more joint areas, arthritis involving the small bones of the hand, symmetrical arthritis, rheumatoid nodules, the presence of rheumatoid factor

Table 26-3

The 1987 Revised American Rheumatism Association Criteria for Diagnosis of Rheumatoid Arthritis

Criterion	Definition
1. Morning stiffness	Morning stiffness in and around the joints, lasting at least 1 hour before maximal improvement
2. Arthritis of 3 or more joint areas	At least 3 joint areas simultaneously with soft tissue swelling or fluid (not bony overgrowth alone). Possible areas: right or left proximal interphalangeal (PIP), metacarpophalangeal (MCP), wrist, elbow, knee, ankle, and metatarsophalangeal (MTP)
3. Arthritis of hand joints	At least 1 area swollen (as defined above) in a wrist, MCP, or PIP joint
4. Symmetric arthritis	Simultaneous involvement of the same joint area (as defined in 2) on both sides of the body
5. Rheumatoid nodules	Subcutaneous nodules, over bony prominences, or extensor surfaces, or in juxtaarticular regions
6. Serum rheumatoid factor	Demonstration of abnormal amounts of serum rheumatoid factor with appropriate controls
7. Radiographic changes	Erosions or unequivocal bony decalcifications localized in or most marked adjacent to the involved joints (osteoarthritis changes alone do not qualify)

From Arnett FC et al: The American Rheumatism Association 1987 revised criteria for the classification of rheumatoid arthritis. *Arth Rheum* 31:315-24, 1988. Copyright © 2001 Wiley-Liss, Inc. Reprinted with permission of Wiley-Liss, Inc., a subsidiary of John Wiley & Sons, Inc.
Patients are classified as having rheumatoid arthritis if they have 4 of 7 of these criteria. Criteria 1 through 4 must be present for at least 6 weeks. Patients with 2 clinical diagnoses are not excluded.

(RF), and radiographic erosions (Table 26-3). Patients must demonstrate four of the seven criteria, which have 91% to 94% sensitivity and 89% specificity for diagnosis of RA. RF, an IgM antibody to the Fc receptor of IgG antibodies, has 54% sensitivity and 91% specificity for diagnosis of RA if used alone. RA has no effect on fertility rates.

Differential Diagnosis

The main diseases in the differential include osteoarthritis, other arthritides, and other autoimmune phenomena characterized by arthralgias including SLE. RA is characterized by a symmetrical arthritis, which can help narrow the differential.

Treatment and Expected Outcome

RA improves during pregnancy in 70% to 90% of women, and this is usually evident in the first trimester. The disease relapses in 90% of women to prepregnancy severity by 6 months postpartum. Breast feeding increases relapse rates. The improvement was initially thought to be due to the increased cortisol levels in pregnancy, but this does not appear to be the only mechanism. Reduction in TNF-α resulting from the cytokine shift outlined previously has been suggested as the main reason for improvement during pregnancy.

Interaction with the fetal genotype appears to play a role in the likelihood of remission in pregnancy. Fetal-maternal disparity in HLA-DR and DQ antigens is more often characterized by remission or improvement in disease. The mechanism for this improvement is unknown.

Therapy involves treatment with antiinflammatory agents and disease-modifying antirheumatic drugs (DMARDs). A summary of agents used in the management of RA and their reproductive risks can be found in Table 26-4. Classic antiinflammatory agents include nonsteroidal antiinflammatory drugs (NSAIDs) and glucocorticoids. As mentioned previously, NSAIDs are contraindicated after 28 weeks' gestation. Glucocorticoids are felt to be safe if the benefits outweigh the risks. Synthetic DMARDs include methotrexate, leflunomide, minocycline, gold salts, penicillamine, and hydroxychloroquine. Methotrexate is one of the mainstays of DMARD therapy but is contraindicated in pregnancy. Similarly, leflunomide, minocycline, gold salts, and penicillamine are contraindicated in pregnancy. Recent biomolecular advances include the development of so-called biologic DMARDs including TNF-α inhibitors and IL-1 inhibition. The immunomodulatory drug leflunomide has shown great promise but is suspected to be teratogenic (Pregnancy Category X). It has an extremely long half-life, taking up to 2 years to reach undetectable levels. As a result, it should be avoided by women of childbearing age. TNF antagonists such as etanercept, adalimumab, and infliximab show great promise and appear to be safe in pregnancy (Pregnancy Category B). The interleukin-1 antagonist anakinra has similar promise as the latter drugs and similar limitations.

RA does not appear to have any effects on the pregnancy itself. There is no increase in fetal loss or pregnancy complications that have been related to RA. Consequently, there is no need for increased fetal surveillance or testing during pregnancies complicated by RA.

Table 26-4

Rheumatoid
Arthritis Drugs
and Mechanism
of Action

Drug	Pregnancy Safety	Comments
Glucocorticoids	Safe	Association with growth restriction at high dose, need stress-dose steroids at delivery or for medical illnesses if chronic use through pregnancy. Increased risk of preterm rupture of membranes, preterm delivery.
Nonsteroidal antiinflammatory agents	See comments	Association with oligohydraminos and ductus arteriosus closure. Avoid after 28 weeks.
Hydroxychloroquine	Generally felt to be safe	Antimalarial, doses in malaria and rheumatic diseases not associated with malformations or adverse outcomes.
Gold salts	See comments	Transplacental passage occurs, teratogenic in animal models, inadequate data in humans. Most recommend discontinuing before pregnancy.
D-penicillamine	Unsafe	Chelating agent. Association with congenital connective tissue disorders.
Methotrexate	Unsafe	Folate antagonist. Abortifacient and teratogen.
Minocycline	Unsafe	Antibiotic in tetracycline family. Exposure in pregnancy leads to tooth discoloration and osteotoxicity.
Leflunomide (Arava; Sanofi-Aventis US, Bridgewater, N.J.)	Unsafe	Inhibitor of pyrimidine synthesis. Evidence of multiple anomalies in animal models. Extremely long half-life.
Etanercept (Enbrel; Amgen, Thousand Oaks, CA)	Unknown	Fusion protein consisting of TNF receptor and portion of human immunoglobulin 1.
Adalimumab (Humira; Abbott Laboratories, Abbott Park, IL)	Unknown	Recombinant TNF-α antibody. Insufficient human data.
Infliximab (Remicade; Centocor Pharmaceuticals, Horsham, PA)	Unknown	Chimeric TNF-α antibody with mouse variable region and human constant region. Insufficient human data.
Anakinra (Kineret; Amgen)	Unknown	Synthetic IL-1 receptor antagonist. Insufficient human data.

IL, Interleukin; *TNF,* tumor necrosis factor.

MYASTHENIA GRAVIS

Definition

Myasthenia gravis (MG) is an autoimmune disorder characterized by antibodies to the acetylcholine receptor at the neuromuscular junction leading to variably expressed striated muscle weakness.

Epidemiology

The prevalence of MG is estimated at 1 in 10,000 and is more often seen in women than men. Women tend to develop MG during their reproductive years, whereas men develop it later in life. The prevalence in pregnancy is approximately 6.4 per 100,000 deliveries.

Etiology and Pathogenesis

Antibodies to the acetylcholine receptor at the neuromuscular junction impair neuromuscular conduction and lead to muscle fatigue in striated muscles. This is both a B- and T-cell mediated phenomenon. Consequently, women with MG are sensitive to neuromuscular blocking agents and treatment with acetylcholinesterase inhibitors improves symptoms. Smooth muscle activity does not appear to be affected.

Clinical Presentation

Women present with muscle fatigue in a variety of patterns. The weakness may be localized to the external ocular muscles and levator palpebrae, facial and bulbar muscles, or proximal limb muscles. Weakness may be more generalized and even life-threatening if the swallowing or respiratory muscles are affected.

Diagnosis can be made by history, response to neuromuscular stimulation, and serology. Administration of edrophonium can transiently restore muscular function in women with MG and helps to make the diagnosis. Additionally, repetitive neuromuscular stimulation in women with MG leads to muscular weakness. The presence of acetylcholine receptor antibodies helps to support the diagnosis of MG.

Disease activity has been associated with thymus function, and a thymectomy may improve symptoms in women with MG. There is an association with thymoma and women with new-onset disease should be evaluated for this.

Differential Diagnosis

Other disorders characterized by muscle weakness may be considered such as congenital myasthenic syndromes, drug-induced myasthenia, hyperthyroidism, Graves' disease, Lambert-Eaton myasthenic syndrome, botulism, progressive external ophthalmoplegia, and intracranial mass lesions. As mentioned previously, women should be evaluated for thymomas as well.

Morbidity

The risk of mortality during pregnancy inversely correlates with disease duration with the lowest risk seen about 7 years from onset of disease. One review found that maternal mortality was 4% during pregnancy in women with MG.

MG does not appear to have a significant effect on pregnancy outcome. Population data from Norway found no difference in mean birthweight, prematurity, and neonatal mortality in pregnancies complicated by MG. There was an increase in delivery complications and intervention in women with MG.

A transient neonatal syndrome is seen in 10% to 20% of infants born to mothers with MG because of maternal transfer of antibodies. Although it often correlates with maternal disease severity and antibody levels, exceptions are possible. Symptoms of weakness, hypotonia, and respiratory distress can develop in the first 12 to 48 hours after birth. Symptoms improve as antibody titers decrease and tend to resolve within the first 4 weeks of life.

Management During Pregnancy

The effect of pregnancy on MG is unpredictable and inconsistent with subsequent pregnancies. In women in remission at the onset of pregnancy, 17% will relapse during the pregnancy and postpartum period. In women on therapy, symptoms improved in 39%, remained unchanged in 42%, and worsened in 19%. Improvement was seen primarily in the second and third trimester and worsening primarily occurred in the first trimester and postpartum period.

Acetylcholinesterase inhibitors are one of the mainstays of treatment, and pyridostigmine bromide may be used safely during pregnancy at the recommended doses of less than 600 mg/day. Women with severe MG may require steroid or immunosuppressive therapy and the risk-to-benefit ratio of these medications should be considered during pregnancy.

Myasthenia crisis is characterized by severe weakness and respiratory compromise. These exacerbations can be managed with immunosuppression or if severe, with IVIG or plasmapheresis. Patients with respiratory compromise may require assisted ventilation.

Magnesium sulfate should never be given to women with MG. Magnesium sulfate diminishes the depolarizing action of acetylcholine, reduces transmitters at the motor end-plate, and depresses muscle membrane excitability. Reports of severe exacerbations and even maternal mortality have been described in women with MG who received magnesium sulfate for seizure prophylaxis in preeclampsia. Narcotics can potentiate respiratory depression and lead to compromise. Beta-adrenergic agents can potentiate latent myocardiopathy in MG patients and lead to complications. Other agents that have been found to increase myasthenic weakness include: barbiturates, lithium, aminoglycosides, tetracycline, and chloroquine.

Anesthesia is a concern in women with MG. Because of the sensitivity to neuromuscular blockade, nondepolarizing muscle relaxants agents should be avoided. Regional anesthesia is thus preferred in these patients. Local anesthetics are generally considered safe in pregnancy but amide-type local anesthetics such as lidocaine are better choices in MG because of their metabolism by mechanisms other than cholinesterase enzymes.

437

SCLERODERMA

Definition

Scleroderma is an autoimmune disease characterized by either localized or systemic fibrosis. The symptoms can be localized (linear scleroderma or morphea), limited, or systemic. Limited scleroderma tends to involve the hands and (to a lesser degree) the face and neck, often associated with the CREST syndrome (Calcinosis, Raynaud phenomenon, Esophageal dysmotility, Sclerodactyly, and Telangiectasias).

Epidemiology

Scleroderma has an incidence of 10 to 20 per million with a prevalence of 240 per million. It affects women three to five times more often than men with a mean onset of symptoms in the early 40s. Fertility is not impaired in scleroderma and with more women having children later, there is an increase in the number of pregnancies complicated by scleroderma.

Etiology

The precise etiology of scleroderma is not known but many mechanisms have been postulated. Viral triggering of autoimmune phenomena in a genetically susceptible individual is one etiologic theory. Other noninfectious environmental exposures have been postulated including organic solvents such as vinyl chloride, L-tryptophan supplementation, and petroleum distillates. Medications such as bleomycin can cause a scleroderma-like syndrome with fibrosis and Raynaud phenomenon.

Recent work has shown that there is in utero fetal-maternal cell traffic that can persist for decades after delivery. The persistence of fetal cell lines years after delivery has been termed "microchimerism" and is found more often in women with scleroderma than controls. The exact etiologic mechanism is unknown but creation of new antigens, cell-cell dysregulation, or other triggering of an autoimmune response are all possibilities.

Pathogenesis

Scleroderma is characterized by immune activation, vascular damage, and excessive synthesis of extracellular matrix and collagen deposition. These processes lead to the sclerosis, fibrosis, and vascular injury that are seen in scleroderma. Sclerosis of the skin leads to the characteristic hand and face appearance. Scleroderma can involve the distal esophagus and sphincter leading to esophageal hypomotility and sphincter incompetence. Autoimmune vascular injury and endothelin-mediated vasoconstriction and fibrosis lead to the vascular effects of scleroderma.

Clinical Presentation

Patients present with variable amounts of sclerosis of the skin of the hands, face, and body. Patients can also present with evidence of vascular disease and Raynaud phenomenon. Evidence of end-organ fibrotic damage involving the kidneys, esophagus, lungs, and heart can be seen as well.

Serologic tests can reveal characteristic antibodies including anti-centromere, anti-topoisomerase-I (Scl-80), anti-RNA polymerase, or U3-RNP antibodies. An ANA antibody preparation can be positive as well. Anti-centromere antibodies are more often associated with CREST syndrome. Anti-topoisomerase-I (Scl-70) is not very sensitive but is specific for systemic sclerosis. Anti-RNA polymerase antibodies are also associated with systemic sclerosis.

Morbidity

Scleroderma does not appear to have much affect on pregnancy. Early case reports suggested an increase in adverse maternal and fetal outcomes. However, later case-control series suggest that these adverse outcomes are not increased in patients with scleroderma. Specifically, miscarriage, prematurity, and fetal loss rates were similar between cases and controls. These studies do show an increase in small full-term infants though the risk for IUGR is unclear. A prospective study showed an increase in prematurity but no evidence of growth restriction or other maternal or fetal complications.[5]

The effect of pregnancy on scleroderma is similarly mild. The consensus of case reports and case-control studies is that there is no change in disease status during pregnancy. There are some reports of increased exacerbations of Raynaud phenomenon, arthritis, and skin thickening in up to a third of patients. In the previously mentioned prospective study by Steen, 20% experienced worsening of symptoms (arthralgias and reflux), 20% experienced improvement (Raynaud), and 60% had no change in their disease symptoms. The 10-year survival rate for women with scleroderma is unchanged when pregnancy history is considered. Cardiopulmonary problems do not appear to be affected by pregnancy.

Renal crisis was seen in 11% of the patients followed prospectively by Steen. With the advent of angiotensin-converting enzyme (ACE) inhibitors, renal crisis is more easily managed and has been documented in case reports. ACE inhibitors have been associated with fetal cartilage and skeletal anomalies and renal agenesis. Given the morbidity of maternal renal disease, the benefits may outweigh the risks of therapy in women with scleroderma complicated by renal disease or crisis.

Management during Pregnancy

Women with scleroderma for less than 4 years, diffuse cutaneous scleroderma, or those who have an anti-topoisomerase-I antibody are at increased risk for aggressive disease during pregnancy. Additionally, disease status at the onset of pregnancy is correlated with disease activity in the pregnancy with more favorable outcomes seen in those women with quiescent disease. An assessment of the maternal disease, risk factors for severe disease, and end-organ (lung, renal, cardiovascular) effects is critical early in pregnancy.

Maternal symptoms can be managed through pharmacologic means. Arthralgias can be treated with acetaminophen. Corticosteroids should be avoided because they have been associated with the precipitation of renal crisis. Reflux can be managed with antacids, histamine blockers, proton pump inhibitors, and promotility agents. Raynaud symptoms generally improve although some women require continuation of calcium channel blockers to control their symptoms. Systemic therapy for scleroderma (i.e., D-penicillamine, cytotoxic agents, colchicines, or cyclosporine) should be weaned before pregnancy as they have been associated with adverse fetal effects (see Table 26-4).

Women with scleroderma present an obstetrical and anesthetic challenge during labor and delivery and this should be discussed well in advance of labor. Owing to the difficulty of intubation because of strictures and aspiration risks, general anesthesia should be avoided. Skin thickening makes venous access difficult and increases vaginal constriction and obstruction. As mentioned previously, antepartum echocardiogram for assessment of cardiac function, pulmonary function tests, and assessment of renal function is essential for peripartum management.

SJÖGREN'S SYNDROME

Definition

Sjögren's syndrome is an autoimmune disease characterized by lymphocytic infiltration of the exocrine glands and a characteristic autoantibody profile. Sjögren's syndrome can be primary or secondary (associated with another autoimmune syndrome).

Epidemiology

Sjögren's syndrome has an annual incidence of 4 per 100,000. Women are nine times more often affected than men. Peak incidence is between 40 and 60 years, although the latency between initial symptoms and diagnosis averages 10 years.

Etiology

No definite etiology has been found although there are several interesting hypotheses. Because of the disproportionate number of women affected, sex hormones are thought to have a causal role. Because of the similarity of Sjögren's syndrome with graft-versus-host disease, several researchers have proposed that fetal microchimerism in the mother following a pregnancy can induce a fetal graft-versus-host-like syndrome resulting in Sjögren's syndrome. Evidence of fetal microchimerism is more common in women with Sjögren's syndrome than controls, which lends support to this theory. Additionally, symptoms similar to Sjögren's syndrome develop in patients receiving allograft bone marrow transplant but not in patients receiving autologous bone marrow transplants.

Pathogenesis

The pathogenesis of Sjögren's syndrome is multifactorial with autoimmune, genetic, and neuroendocrine components. Lymphocytes target the exocrine glands and in particular the parotid and salivary glands. Altered cytokine production and other signaling pathways are also responsible for altering glandular function.

Clinical Presentation

Women with Sjögren's syndrome present with symptoms of dryness of the eyes, mouth, or other mucous membranes, such as the vagina. The parotid gland is enlarged in one third of patients. ANA is present in many women with Sjögren's syndrome but SSA/Ro and SSB/La antibodies are more specific. The gold standard for diagnosis is a labial salivary gland biopsy showing lympho-cytic collections but is usually not necessary for diagnosis. Additional diagnostic tests include quantitative assessment of salivary or tear production.

Differential Diagnosis

The clinical findings of Sjögren's syndrome are often minor and sufficiently nonspecific that the differential diagnosis is broad. Viral illnesses including hepatitis C can mimic the clinical signs of Sjögren's syndrome.

Treatment and Expected Outcome

Treatment is symptomatic with artificial tears and topical treatment for dry mucous membranes. Recent advances have made muscarinic agonists available that increase salivary excretion but these are not well-studied in pregnancy and are generally avoided. Women with Sjögren's syndrome are at increased risk for lymphoproliferative disorders with approximately 5% developing malignant lymphomas. This is thought to be a multistep process from polyclonal lymphoproliferation to monoclonal lymphoproliferation, to mucosal-associated lymphoid tissue (MALT) lymphoma, and finally to high-grade malignant lymphoma. Women with Sjögren's syndrome thus require careful clinical examination and follow-up to evaluate for lymphoproliferative disease.

If anti-SSA/Ro or anti-SSB/La antibodies are present, surveillance for fetal heart block should be undertaken as outlined previously. With the exception of the risk for neonatal lupus (CHB, skin manifestations, etc.), Sjögren's syndrome has little effect on pregnancy outcome.

KEY POINTS

Systemic Lupus Erythematosus (SLE)

- SLE is an autoimmune mediated syndrome characterized by flares of disease activity and remissions.
- Flares may increase in pregnancy and the postpartum period.
- Autoantibodies are a frequent component including lupus anticoagulant and antiphospholipid antibodies.
- Differentiating lupus flares from preeclampsia can be difficult and is important for the management of gravidas with SLE.
- Women with SLE are at increased risk for adverse pregnancy outcomes including preeclampsia, stillbirth, preterm birth, and growth restriction.
- Neonatal lupus syndrome occurs in 1% to 2% of women with anti-SSA/Ro or anti-SSB/La antibodies.
- Prepregnant drug regimens (if safe in pregnancy) should be continued.

Antiphospholipid Antibody Syndrome (APS)

- APS is a humoral mediated autoimmune phenomenon characterized by vascular thrombosis and other adverse perinatal outcomes.
- Antiphospholipid antibodies (APAs) are found in 1% to 5% of asymptomatic gravidas.
- APAs exert a procoagulant effect.
- Treatment with anticoagulation can reduce the rate of complications.

Rheumatoid Arthritis (RA)

- RA is a cell-mediated autoimmune phenomenon that leads to damage of the joint synovium.
- Symptoms improve in 70% to 90% of women during pregnancy but relapse in 90% postpartum.

Myasthenia Gravis (MG)

- MG is an autoimmune disorder leading to striated muscle weakness.
- Antibodies are directed against the acetylcholine receptor.
- A transient neonatal syndrome is seen in 10% to 20% of women with MG.

Scleroderma

- Scleroderma is associated with localized or systemic fibrosis.
- CREST syndrome is a variant of scleroderma.
- Pregnancy has little effect on scleroderma.

KEY POINTS—cont'd

Sjögren's syndrome (SS)

- SS is characterized by lymphocytic infiltration of the exocrine glands and autoantibodies.
- Anti-SSA/Ro and anti-SSB/La antibodies are found in many women with SS.

REFERENCES

1. Abbud Filho M, Pavario-Bertelli EC, Alvarenga MP, Fernandez IM, Toledo RA, Tajara EH, Savoldi-Barbosa M, Goldmann GH, Goloni-Bertollo EM: Systemic lupus erythematosus and microchimerism in autoimmunity. *Transplantation Proc* 34:2951, 2002.
2. Tan EM, Cohen AS, Fries JF, Masi AT, McShane DJ, Rothfield NF, Schaller JG, Talal N, Winchester RJ: The 1982 revised criteria for the classification of systemic lupus erythematosus. *Arth Rheum* 25:1271, 1982.
3. Ruiz-Irastorza G et al: Increased rate of lupus flare during pregnancy and the puerperium: a prospective study of 78 pregnancies. *Br J Rheum* 35:133, 1996.
4. Galli M, Luciani D, Bertolini G, Barbui T: Anti-beta 2-glycoprotein I, antiprothrombin antibodies, and the risk of thrombosis in the antiphospholipid syndrome. *Blood* 102:2717, 2003.
5. Steen VD: Scleroderma and pregnancy. *Rheum Dis Clin North Am* 23:133, 1997.

SUGGESTED READINGS

Backos M et al: Pregnancy complications in women with recurrent miscarriage associated with antiphospholipid antibodies treated with low dose aspirin and heparin. *Br J Obstet Gynecol* 106:102, 1999.

Batocchi AP et al: Course and treatment of myasthenia gravis during pregnancy. *Neurology* 52:447, 1999.

Bianchi DW: Fetomaternal cell trafficking: a new cause of disease? *Am J Med Genetics* 91:22, 2000.

Buyon JP, Clancy RM: Maternal autoantibodies and congenital heart block: mediators, markers, and therapeutic approach. *Semin Arth Rheum* 33:140, 2003.

Buyon JP: Neonatal lupus syndrome. In Lahita R, editor: *Systemic Lupus Erythematosus*, ed 4. San Diego, 2004, Elsevier Academic Press, pp 449-484.

Choy EHS, Panayi GS: Cytokine pathways and joint inflammation in rheumatoid arthritis. *N Engl J Med* 344:907, 2001.

Ciafaloni E, Massey JM: The management of myasthenia gravis in pregnancy. *Semin Neurol* 24:95, 2004.

Derksen RHWM, Khamashta MA, Branch DW: Management of the obstetric antiphospholipid syndrome. *Arth Rheum* 50:1028, 2004.

Drachman DB: Myasthenia gravis. *N Engl J Med* 330:1797, 1994.

Empson M, Lassere M, Craig JC: Recurrent pregnancy loss with antiphospholipid antibody: a systemic review of therapeutic trials. *Obstet Gynecol* 99:135, 2002.

Endo Y, Negishi I, Ishikawa O: Possible contribution of microchimerism to the pathogenesis of Sjögren syndrome. *Rheumatology* 41:490, 2002.

Fausett MB, Branch DW: Autoimmunity and pregnancy loss. *Semin Reprod Med* 18:379, 2000.

Fox RI, Stern M, Michelson P: Update in Sjögren syndrome. *Curr Opin Rheumatol* 12:391, 2000.

Hoff JM, Daltveit AK, Gilhus NE: Myasthenia gravis: consequences for pregnancy, delivery, and the newborn. *Neurology* 61:1362, 2003.

Julkunen H: Pregnancy and lupus nephritis. *Scand J Urol Nephrol* 35:319, 2001.

Lambert N, Nelson JL: Microchimerism in autoimmune disease: more questions than answers? *Autoimmun Rev* 2:133, 2003.

Lee LA: Neonatal lupus erythematosus. *J Invest Dermatol* 100:9, 1993.

Levine JS, Branch DW, Rauch J: The antiphospholipid syndrome. *N Engl J Med* 346:752, 2002.

Lockshin MD, Sammaritano LR: Lupus pregnancy. *Autoimmunity* 36:33, 2003.

Mahoney EJ, Spiegel JH: Sjögren's disease. *Otolaryngology Clin North Am* 36:733, 2003.

Masaki Y, Sugai S: Lymphoproliferative disorders in Sjögren's syndrome. *Autoimmun Rev* 3:175, 2004.

Nelson JL, Østensoen M: Pregnancy and rheumatoid arthritis. *Rheum Dis Clin North Am* 23:195, 1997.

O'Dell JR: Therapeutic strategies for rheumatoid arthritis. *N Engl J Med* 350:2591, 2004.

Olsen NJ, Stein CM: New drugs for rheumatoid arthritis. *N Engl J Med* 350:2167, 2004.

Rand JH et al: Pregnancy loss in the antiphospholipid-antibody syndrome—a possible thrombogenic mechanism. *N Engl J Med* 337:154, 1997.

Ruiz-Irastorza G et al: Systemic lupus erythematosus. *Lancet* 357:1027, 2000.

Saleeb S et al: Comparison of treatment with fluorinated glucocorticoids to natural history of autoantibody-associated congenital heart block: retrospective review of the research registry for neonatal lupus. *Arth Rheum* 42:2335, 1999.

Salmon JE, Girardi G, Holers VM: Activation of complement mediates antiphospholipid antibody-mediated pregnancy loss. *Lupus* 12:535, 2003.

Shehata HA, Nelson-Piercy C, Khamashata MA: Management of pregnancy in antiphospholipid syndrome. *Rheum Dis Clin North Am* 27:643, 2001.

Smith JB, Haynes MK: Rheumatoid arthritis—a molecular understanding. *Ann Intern Med* 136:908, 2002.

Steen VD: Pregnancy in women with systemic sclerosis. *Obstet Gynecol* 94:15, 1999.

Steen VD: Fertility and pregnancy outcome in women with systemic sclerosis. *Arth Rheum* 42:763, 1999.

Warren JB, Silver RM: Autoimmune disease in pregnancy: systemic lupus erythematosus and antiphospholipid syndrome. *Obstet Gynecol Clin North Am* 31:345, 2004.

27

NEUROLOGIC DISORDERS IN PREGNANCY

Nikki Koklanaris and Men-Jean Lee

EPILEPSY

Definition

Epilepsy, also known as a seizure disorder, is a chronic neurological condition that is characterized by recurrent seizures or sudden recurring attacks of motor, sensory, or psychic malfunction with or without loss of consciousness or convulsions. Women with a preexisting diagnosis of epilepsy have normal fertility and pregnancy, and normal women can also develop a new-onset seizure disorder during pregnancy that requires investigation and management. These patients deserve special attention during the prenatal period.

The different types of seizures are generally classified as partial or generalized, with subcategories dependent on the symptoms occurring with the seizure (Table 27-1). These should be distinguished from the generalized, self-limited seizures known as eclampsia that occur only in association with pregnancy and that are associated with new-onset hypertension and proteinuria. Furthermore, about 20% of patients referred for evaluation of seizures have been found to have psychogenic seizures or pseudoseizures that are somatization disorders. Pseudoseizures resemble epileptic seizures but are not associated with abnormal electrical activity in the brain.

Epidemiology

There are approximately 1.1 million women of childbearing age with epilepsy in the United States who give birth to more than 20,000 infants each year. Women in underdeveloped parts of the world and women of low socioeconomic status within the United States have a higher prevalence of seizure disorder. Approximately 45% of women with epilepsy before pregnancy have increased frequency of seizures during pregnancy, 5% note a decrease, and 50% remain unchanged. Most of the increase in seizure frequency during pregnancy can be attributed to noncompliance with antiepileptic drugs (AEDs) and/or sleep deprivation.

Etiology

Seizures are a result of paroxysmal brain dysfunction resulting from excess neuronal discharge. Primary generalized seizures begin with widespread electrical discharge throughout both hemispheres of the brain. Although

Table 27-1

1981 International
Classification
of Seizures*

Partial Seizures Beginning Locally	Generalized Seizures
Simple (consciousness not impaired)	Absence seizures
With motor symptoms	(petit mal)
With somatosensory or special sensory symptoms	Typical
With autonomic symptoms	Atypical
With psychic symptoms	
Complex (with impairment of consciousness)	Myoclonic seizures
Beginning as simple partial seizure (progressing to	Clonic seizures
complex seizure)	Tonic seizures
Impairment of consciousness at onset	Tonic-clonic seizures
a. Impairment of consciousness only	(grand-mal)
b. With automatism	Atonic seizures
Partial seizures becoming secondarily generalized	

*Commission on Classification, International League Against Epilepsy: Proposed provisions of clinical and electroencephalographical classification of epileptic seizures. *Epilepsia* 22(4):489-501, 1981. © 1981 Blackwell Publishing, Ltd.

most are idiopathic, generalized seizures can have a genetic basis. Partial seizures begin with an electrical discharge in one limited area of the brain. Although partial seizures can be attributed to head injury, brain infection, stroke, or tumor, the cause is unknown in most cases. Some people may have only a single seizure during their lives; for instance, a case of febrile seizure in childhood or a hypoglycemic seizure in a diabetic. However, one seizure does not constitute a diagnosis of epilepsy. Patients with epilepsy have repeatedly witnessed seizures.

Pathogenesis

Seizure disorders fall into two general categories. In *primary* or *idiopathic epilepsy*, the cellular/molecular cause of the disorder remains largely or entirely unknown. In *secondary* or *symptomatic* epilepsy, seizures result from a known structural or metabolic disease of the brain. Women with secondary seizures must be counseled on the basis of the specific underlying etiology of their disease. Those with idiopathic epilepsy should be counseled regarding an increased risk of seizure disorder in their offspring of 2.0% to 4.0%. Paternal epilepsy has not been implicated in an increased rate of epilepsy among offspring. Pregnancy is associated with changes in two important hormones that have effects on seizure activity. Estrogen increases the electrical activity of the brain, and progesterone has the reverse effect.

Clinical Presentation

History

When evaluating a woman with epilepsy who is requesting preconceptional counseling or one who is already pregnant and seeking prenatal care, it is important to determine the type of seizure, etiology of seizure, seizure frequency, the current AED and dosage, if she is under the care of a neurologist, and if her seizures are witnessed. In addition, if the woman is already pregnant, it is essential to ascertain the gestational age of the pregnancy, compliance with AED, and the number of seizures she has had since conception, if any. If the patient denies having any more seizures, one should determine the length of time she has been seizure free. Ideally, a woman with epilepsy should receive preconceptional counseling on the effect of seizure disorder and AEDs on pregnancy and recommendations for supplementation with folic acid. The teratogenicity of AEDs are discussed in detail later (see "Treatment and Expected Outcome").

Symptoms

Seizures can cause brief changes in a person's body movements, consciousness, emotions, and senses, such as taste, smell, vision, or hearing. Absence or petit mal seizures are generalized seizures associated with brief episodes of staring in which awareness and responsiveness are impaired. Grand mal seizure is an older term for a tonic-clonic generalized seizure in which the patient experiences a loss of consciousness and presents with jerking motions of the arms and legs. These seizures are often associated with tongue biting, loss of bowel or bladder function, and/or cyanosis if breathing is affected. During pregnancy, the frequency of these seizures may increase.

Generalized seizures associated with a loss of consciousness present a particular concern during pregnancy because of abdominal trauma secondary to falls and fetal exposure to hypoxia because of inhibition of maternal respiration. After the mid-trimester, fetal bradycardias can be noted following a generalized seizure, which often normalizes within a few minutes following the seizure episode. If a seizure lasts more than 30 minutes, or a patient experiences three seizures without a normal period in between, a dangerous condition called convulsive status epilepticus requires emergency treatment.

Laboratory Findings

Most patients with epilepsy are diagnosed before pregnancy. The diagnosis is usually made by confirmation of the description of the seizure and by electroencephalography (EEG). Other imaging tests such as computed tomography (CT) scan or magnetic resonance imaging (MRI) of the brain may be required to investigate potential causes of new-onset seizures.

The increased seizure rate in pregnancy may be attributed to the changes in anticonvulsant pharmacokinetics. Increased systemic clearance and volume of distribution during pregnancy can result in decreased drug concentration in the serum. However, relative decreases in protein binding sites resulting from decreased plasma albumin may also increase free levels of AED. When following medication levels in the blood, the *free* fraction (a nonprotein bound [free] level) should be measured. AED levels should be checked during the preconceptional visit to establish a baseline norm. If a woman is taking an AED during pregnancy, medication levels should be checked at least once a trimester and during the final month of pregnancy. More frequent monitoring of drug levels should be performed if the patient is still suffering from seizures and AED dosages are being adjusted. AED dosage will likely need further adjustment in the postpartum period. In general, if there is an adjustment of AED that is made during pregnancy, the free drug level is usually checked 1 week or more after the change in therapy to allow the serum levels to reach steady state.

Differential Diagnosis

When seizures first present after 20 weeks of gestation or in the postpartum period, the generalized convulsion unique to pregnancy must be considered: eclampsia. In a known preeclamptic patient, intravenous magnesium sulfate has been shown to be superior to phenytoin, a standard AED, for seizure prophylaxis. It is important to differentiate eclamptic seizures that are treated with magnesium sulfate from epileptic seizures that respond better to benzodiazepines such as intravenous diazepam or lorazepam, which are considered the agents of choice for new-onset epileptic seizures that develop during pregnancy. In a patient with a known—or previously undiagnosed—seizure disorder, additional findings suggestive of eclampsia over epilepsy must be sought to clarify the diagnosis. Preeclampsia is defined by a new-onset hypertension with proteinuria and possible liver function test abnormalities, thrombocytopenia, and elevated creatinine and uric acid that may predate the development of an eclamptic seizure. Pseudoseizures must also be considered in the differential diagnosis of seizures that occur during pregnancy in a patient in whom the diagnosis of preeclampsia/eclampsia is excluded by gestational age of the pregnancy and laboratory data. Pseudoseizures are three times as likely to be found in female than in male patients, are more commonly observed in young adults, and may occur in patients who have previously experienced true epileptic seizures.

Pseudoseizures may be suspected when the patient continues to complain of convulsions despite the fact that serum AED levels are therapeutic, the seizures are unwitnessed, and the patient does not experience symptoms found in the typical post-ictal recovery period (e.g., shame, embarrassment, confusion, bruising, injuries, difficulty talking, bowel/bladder incontinence, and tongue-biting). Video-EEG monitoring or a witnessed seizure by an experienced neurologist are effective ways of diagnosing nonepileptic seizures. These symptoms are difficult to treat, especially if there is an underlying psychologic disorder. However, pseudoseizures should be correctly identified to avoid AED toxicities resulting from unnecessary overdosing, particularly during pregnancy.

Treatment and Expected Outcome

Preconceptional Counseling

Ideally, all women with epilepsy should receive preconceptional counseling on the effect of seizure disorder and AED on pregnancy and information on supplementation with folic acid to prevent birth defects associated with AED. Because teratogenicity from AED is a major concern for both the physician and patient, many women want to stop taking their medication. If a woman has been seizure free for 2 to 5 years, it is possible to attempt to wean her off all AEDs in collaboration with her neurologist before attempting conception. She must be counseled that this may precipitate a recurrence of seizures and necessitate resumption of the AED. In addition, if the woman is on multiple AEDs with rare seizures, the preconceptional visit should include a consultation with the neurologist to determine whether her seizures could be adequately controlled by weaning to monotherapy before attempting conception.

There is no safe AED to take during pregnancy. All AEDs have the potential to be teratogenic. The constellation of major malformations, growth restriction, and hypoplasia of the midface and fingers is known as *anticonvulsant embryopathy* or *fetal anticonvulsant syndrome* (FAS). However, for years it was widely believed that epilepsy itself—not the anticonvulsants used to treat the disorder—was teratogenic. More recent studies suggest that it is the use of AEDs not the presence of epilepsy per se that leads to the greater incidence of congenital anomalies in the offspring of women who take these medications (Table 27-2).

The frequency of anticonvulsant embryopathy has been reported to be 20.6% in pregnant women treated with monotherapy when compared with 8.5% in women without epilepsy. Infants exposed to two or more AEDs had a birth defect rate of 28.0%. The rate of major malformations has been reported to be as high as 25% in infants of women receiving four or more AEDs. The risk for congenital malformations in the offspring of women with untreated epilepsy has not been found to be higher than among nonepileptic controls. Not all fetuses exposed to AED during pregnancy develop a birth defect. Exposure to AEDs in a genetically susceptible fetus may be the critical combination that creates anticonvulsant embryopathy. One theory that accounts for increased susceptibility targets a deficiency of the detoxifying enzyme epoxide hydrolase. Another possible etiology is the increase in free radicals formed by the drugs.

The single AED responsible for the greatest number of major malformations has not been identified. A large retrospective study of more than 1400 children confirmed that most AED regimens were associated with an increased risk of major anomalies in the offspring, noting the following as having the greatest risk: valproate and carbamazepine monotherapy, caffeine in combination with phenobarbital, and benzodiazepines in polytherapy.

Table 27-2

Fetal and Neonatal Anomalies Associated with Anticonvulsant Embryopathy

Minor Anomalies	Major Anomalies
6%-20% of neonates born to women with epilepsy	4%-6% of neonates born to women with epilepsy

Craniofacial anomalies:
  Broad nasal bridge
  Ocular hypertelorism
  Short upturned nose
  Epicanthal folds
  Abnormal ears
  Low hairline
	Congenital heart disease*
	  Atrial septal defect
	  Ventricular septal defect
	  Tetralogy of Fallot
	  Coarctation of the aorta
	  Patent ductus arteriosis
	  Pulmonary stenosis

Distal digital and nail hypoplasia	Neural tube defects†
	  Typically spina bifida
	Cleft lip and palate
	Urogenital defects
	  Hypospadias

From Rosa F: Spina bifida in infants of women treated with carbamazepine during pregnancy. *N Engl J Med* 324:674, 1991; Lindhout D, Schmidt D: In-utero exposure to valproate and neural tube defects. *Lancet* 2:1392, 1986.
*Rates of congenital heart disease are 0.5% in the general population and 1.5%-2% in women with epilepsy.
†Rates of neural tube defects are especially high with carbamazepine and valproate use, at a rate of 10 and 20 times that of the general population, respectively.

Regarding valproate, 1% to 2% of fetuses exposed in utero will develop neural tube defects (NTDs), underscoring the need for early, targeted ultrasonography in these pregnancies. Additionally, the rate of cardiovascular disorders is increased in the fetuses of women taking valproate, and fetal echocardiogram (ECHO) is often advised. The Antiepileptic Drug Pregnancy Registry followed 123 valproate-exposed pregnancies and found the prevalence of major birth defects in offspring of women taking valproate monotherapy to be 8.9% as compared with 2.8% in offspring of women receiving other AEDs and 1.6% in unexposed controls.

Fetuses exposed to phenytoin are at increased risk of orofacial clefts, cardiac malformations, and genitourinary defects. Also, there have been case reports linking in utero exposure to phenytoin with the subsequent development of neuroblastoma.

Carbamazepine use in pregnancy is also associated with an increased rate of major malformations. Around 1% of fetuses exposed in utero to carbamazepine have spina bifida aperta.

Prenatal vitamins and folic acid (4 mg per day) may decrease the risk of birth defects. The MRC Vitamin study (which excluded women with epilepsy) demonstrated that folic acid supplementation starting in the months before conception and continued through the first trimester was associated with a 72% reduction in the incidence of NTDs. However, low serum folate levels in women with epilepsy are independently associated with an increased risk of major fetal malformations. There is a concern regarding supplementation of epileptic women with folic acid, which has been found to decrease the efficacy of phenytoin during pregnancy. Because of the increased incidence of NTDs associated with valproate and carbamazepine, high-dose folic acid supplementation during the periconceptional period is now widely accepted. The American College of Obstetrics and Gynecology recommends 4.0 mg/day of folic acid for women with epilepsy who are being treated with AEDs—the dose typically recommended for women with a previously affected child. The woman should also be advised that uncontrolled seizures and the associated hypoxic episodes during pregnancy also pose harm to the fetus. Therefore noncompliance with AED or self-discontinuing AED without the supervision of her neurologist may also be detrimental to her health and that of her unborn child.

Prenatal Care

Ideally, women with epilepsy who desire pregnancy should present for preconceptional counseling. Whether a woman presents for such counseling or presents for prenatal care already pregnant, the visit should include a detailed discussion of the risk of teratogenicity from AEDs versus the benefits of remaining seizure-free during pregnancy.

Despite these valid fears over teratogenic effects of AEDs, the patients should be reminded about the concerns about the direct effect of maternal seizures on the fetus. Fetal hypoxia may occur as a result of decreased uteroplacental flow during a seizure, but it is not known what threshold must be crossed in terms of seizure number or duration to jeopardize the fetus. Fetal heart rate deceleration for greater than 20 minutes following a maternal generalized tonic-clonic seizure has been reported. Cases of fetal intracranial hemorrhage and fetal demise after a single generalized tonic-clonic seizure have also been described. Status epilepticus is a rare but grave complication that can occur in pregnancy and can result in both maternal and fetal deaths. Of note, seizures may lead to trauma, which can directly or indirectly injure the fetus secondary to abruption or preterm rupture of the membranes. Patients should be counseled of these risks, particularly regarding driving or climbing heights.

Furthermore, by the time most patients realize that they are pregnant and present for prenatal care (typically after 8-10 weeks following their last menstrual period), fetal heart formation and neural tube closure is already completed. Those women who are already pregnant and are reluctant to take the AED while pregnant should be counseled that discontinuing AED after embryogenesis is completed will not prevent structural fetal anomalies and it would behoove the woman to continue with her medications to prevent convulsions and their physical complications. If a patient has self-discontinued her AED before pregnancy and presents to the obstetrician already pregnant, the neurologist should be consulted as to whether or not the patient should resume her medication.

Finally, the health care provider should reinforce general recommendations for the woman to receive adequate sleep and stress reduction during pregnancy to increase the threshold to precipitating a seizure. Extra precautions should be made in the patient's home and workplace to ensure a safe environment to protect the patient, the fetus, and others who might be harmed by seizure-related accidents. Seizures during driving or cigarette smoking can cause injury to the woman with epilepsy but also to other people. The support of family, friends, and health care providers in discussing safety precautions and activity restrictions for these patients will help to prevent serious accidents before, during, and after pregnancy.

Screening for Malformations

Given the increased frequency of malformations, genetic counseling and prenatal screening should be offered to all women with epilepsy. NTDs can be screened for using maternal serum α-fetoprotein (MSAFP). The sensitivity of MSAFP for detecting an open NTD is 85%; therefore 15% will be missed when it is the only screening tool used. A targeted ultrasound should also be performed between 18 and 20 weeks to screen for neural tube and other defects.

The accuracy of ultrasound diagnosis of NTD depends heavily on the experience of the operator, the quality of the equipment, and the amount of time dedicated to the scan. In the RADIUS trial, an 80% sensitivity of ultrasound *plus* MSAFP in detecting NTDs was reported, whereas the sensitivity of ultrasound alone was 85% in a recent retrospective multicenter trial. The sensitivity in detecting NTD is increased by including cranial signs of NTDs—the "banana sign" and the "lemon sign"—in their screen. If abnormal serum screening and/or abnormal ultrasound findings are detected, amniocentesis should be offered for karyotyping, amniotic fluid α-fetoprotein (AFP) levels, and amniotic fluid acetylcholinesterase testing. Additionally, given the increased risk for cardiac malformations in these pregnancies, fetal echocardiography is also recommended.

Obstetric Outcomes and Labor/Delivery

There is an increased rate of nonproteinuric hypertension and inducted labor among women with epilepsy; however, the rates of other antenatal, intrapartum, and neonatal complications are similar to those of the general population. Epilepsy itself is not an indication for induction of labor; however, semielective inductions have been undertaken because of the distance the patient has to travel and/or in an attempt to minimize the stress that is known to precipitate seizures.

Patients should be aware that most women with epilepsy have uncomplicated vaginal deliveries. There is a 1% to 2% chance of a seizure occurring during labor and another 1% to 2% chance of a seizure within the first 24 hours postpartum. Because sleep deprivation may provoke seizures, regional obstetric anesthesia may be used to allow the patient to rest during labor.

During a prolonged labor oral absorption of scheduled AEDs may be limited by emesis. Phenobarbital, (fos)phenytoin, and valproic acid can be given intravenously at the same maintenance dosage in labor. Seizures during labor should be treated with parenteral benzodiapines such as lorazepam 4 mg given slowly over 2 to 5 minutes. This dose may be repeated in 10 to 15 minutes, with a maximal dose of 8 mg. Of note, lorazepam does cross the placenta and the newborn may experience respiratory depression or hypotonia if the drug is administered near the time of delivery. The pediatric staff should be informed if these medications were used in labor so that appropriate reversal agents are available for neonatal resuscitation. The patient should be placed on her left side to minimize the risk of aspiration. Consideration must be given to the fact that the woman may also be experiencing an eclamptic seizure, and additional signs and symptoms should be evaluated.

It has been noted that AED use in pregnancy is associated with early-onset neonatal hemorrhage, particularly with enzyme-inducing AEDs (carbamazepine, phenytoin, phenobarbital, primidone, and oxcarbazepine). Although there have been no randomized clinical trials to prove the efficacy of maternal administration of vitamin K in the prenatal period to prevent neonatal bleeding in the postnatal period, oral vitamin K is a relatively inexpensive prophylactic therapy that can be considered. If vitamin K is given antenatally, most clinicians use a dose of 10 to 20 mg orally per day beginning at 36 weeks of gestation. In addition, the American Academy of Pediatrics recommends that all newborns routinely receive 0.5 to 1 mg of vitamin K intramuscularly immediately after delivery.

Anticonvulsant Therapy

Older AEDs, particularly valproate, phenytoin, phenobarbital, and carbamazepine, are associated with an increased rate of malformations. For specific details on the defects characteristic of fetuses exposed to these drugs, please see Table 27-3.

Table 27-3

Valproate (Depakene, Depakote; Abbott Laboratories, Abbott Park, Illinois)*	Phenytoin (Dilantin; Pfizer, New York, New York)[†]	Carbamazepine (Tegretol; Novartis, East Hanover, New Jersey)	Phenobarbital (Luminal; Abbott Laboratories)[†]
1%-2% develop neural tube defects Meningomyelocele Cardiovascular Urogenital	Orofacial clefts Cardiac malformations Genitourinary defects Case reports of neuroblastoma development after in utero exposure to phenytoin[‡]	Approximately 0.9% rate of spina bifida[§]	Cardiac defects Orofacial defects Urogenital defects

*Of 123 pregnancies followed by the Antiepileptic Drug Pregnancy Registry, the rate of major malformations in women on valproate monotherapy was 8.9% vs. 2.8% in offspring of women on other antiepileptic drugs (AEDs) and 1.6% in controls not taking any AED.[§]
[†]Holmes LB: The teratogenicity of anticonvulsant drugs: a progress report. *J Med Genetics* 39: 245-7, 2002.
[‡]Satge D, Sasco AJ, Little J: Antenatal therapeutic drug exposure and fetal/neonatal tumours: review of 89 cases. *Paediatr Perinat Epidemiol* 12:84, 1998.
[§]Rosa FW: Spina bifida in infants of women treated with carbamazepine during pregnancy. *N Engl J Med* 324:674, 1991.

In recent years a number of new AEDs have come into clinical use for partial seizures and as secondary agents for generalized seizures (Table 27-4). Obstetricians should become familiar with the new AEDs because they are associated with different features that make them more suitable for pregnant women. However, their teratogenic profiles are not yet known. Animal reproductive toxicology studies appear to be favorable for some of the newer AEDs, particularly compared with the older ones. However, these encouraging findings from animal tests are not necessarily predictive of the safety of the newer AEDs in humans. Positive aspects of the newer AEDs include a low potential for interaction with other drugs, which reduces the risk of toxic metabolite production. Also, most newer AEDs do not have antifolate properties. Further long-term studies will be needed for a final consensus on the safety and efficacy of these drugs.

Postpartum Care and Breast Feeding

During the postpartum period, women should have monitoring of serum AED levels, receive care to ensure regular sleeping habits, and receive precautions to ensure maternal and neonatal safety during daily activities. Breast feeding is safe for women who are being treated with any of the AEDs. If excessive infant sedation is noted, particularly with phenobarbital or primidone, infant levels of AED can be checked to determine whether too much medication is being passed through breast milk. If so, the infants can be weaned slowly and monitored for any signs of withdrawal. In general, because the immunologic and nutritional benefits of breast feeding outweigh

Table 27-4

Commonly Encountered Newer Antiepileptic Drugs (Brand Names in Parentheses)

Drug	Common Dosage	Presumed Action	Indications	Side Effects
Gabapentin (Neurontin; Pfizer, New York, New York)	1200-2400 mg qd	Enhances GABA activity	Partial seizures and secondarily generalized seizures	Somnolence, improved mood, increased irritability
Lamotrigine (Lamictal; Glaxo SmithKline, Research Triangle Park, North Carolina)	700 mg qd	Inhibits sodium current (similar to phenytoin and carbamazepine)	Partial seizures and secondarily generalized seizures	Tremor, improved mood, Stevens-Johnson syndrome
Felbamate (Felbatol; Medpointe Pharmaceuticals, Somerset, New Jersey)	400-600 mg bid or tid	Inhibits sodium current and enhances GABA activity	Partial seizures and secondarily generalized seizures	Irritability, anxiety, aplastic anemia, liver failure
Levetiracetam (Keppra; UCB, Smyrna, Georgia)	500-1500 mg bid	Unknown	Partial seizures	Somnolence, anxiety, irritability, depression
Oxcarbazepine (Trileptal; Novartis, East Hanover, New Jersey)	300-600 mg bid	Metabolized to carbamazepine	Partial seizures	Fatigue, dizziness, hyponatremia
Topiramate (Topamax; McNeil Consumer & Specialty Pharmaceuticals, Fort Washington, Pennsylvania)	200 mg bid	Inhibits sodium current and enhances GABA activity	Partial seizures and secondarily generalized seizures	Improved mood, tremor, renal calculi
Tiagabine (Gabitril; Cephalon, Fraxer, Pennsylvania)	4-12 mg bid or qid	Enhances GABA activity	Partial seizures and generalized seizures	Depression, confusion

From Pschirrer ER: Seizure disorders in pregnancy. *Obstet Gynecol Clin North Am* 31:373, vii, 2004; Dichter MA, Brodie MJ: New antiepileptic drugs. *N Engl J Med* 334:1583, 1996.
bid, Twice daily; *GABA,* γ-aminobutyric acid; *qd,* once a day; *qid,* four times a day; *tid,* three times a day.

the risks of rare neonatal complications from AED exposure in breast milk, there are no contraindications to breast feeding in women with epilepsy.

OTHER NEUROLOGIC DISORDERS

Spinal Cord Injury

More than 7% of spinal cord injuries occur in women of reproductive age, and these patients have unique management considerations. Fertility is not compromised and there are generally no contraindications to vaginal delivery. Several issues should be considered in treating these patients: the high risk of autonomic hyperreflexia in labor, the risk of bladder distention, and the lack of pain from contractions if the lesion is from T5-T10.

Autonomic hyperreflexia is a potentially life-threatening disorder that can be precipitated by distention or irritation of the cervix, vagina, bowel, or bladder. The manifestations result from sympathetic hyperactivity below the level of the lesion—the portion of the cord isolated from hypothalamic control. When autonomic hyperreflexia develops in labor, cardiac arrhythmias and malignant hypertension can result, and uteroplacental vasoconstriction can occur. The symptoms are exacerbated by contractions and improve between contractions.

Antepartum consultation with an anesthesiologist is strongly suggested to discuss the prevention of this complication in labor by providing adequate epidural anesthesia and extending regional anesthetic to a T10 level. In addition to blood pressure and cardiac rhythm monitoring, an indwelling Foley catheter should be placed prophylactically to avoid bladder distention during labor.

As noted previously, these patients may not be able to perceive their contractions depending on the level of their lesion. Weekly cervical examinations in the late third trimester to assess favorability of the cervix and instruction of the patient to palpate for uterine contractions are useful tools to promptly make the diagnosis of labor.

Myasthenia Gravis

Myasthenia gravis (MG) is an autoimmune disorder resulting from abnormal T-cell regulation and the production of antibodies against the acetylcholine receptor (AChR) on the neuromuscular end plate of skeletal muscle. The hallmarks are variable muscle weakness and fatigability.

The effect of pregnancy on MG is variable. Seventeen percent of asymptomatic patients who were not on treatment before the pregnancy relapse during pregnancy. Of symptomatic patients requiring medication to manage their disease, 39% improve, 42% are unchanged, and 19% worsen during pregnancy. A maternal thymectomy may need to be considered in refractory cases of MG during pregnancy.

Patients who are taking pyridostigmine (Mestinon; Valeant Pharmaceuticals, Aliso Viejo, California) should remain on their medication to control symptoms, keeping in mind that the dose may need to be adjusted given the increased renal clearance and maternal blood volume of pregnancy. When adjusting pyridostigmine dosage during pregnancy, one should increase the frequency of dosing (decrease the interval between dosing) before increasing

455

the amount of drug being taken at each time point. Two medications are to be avoided in the pregnant patient with MG: aminoglycosides, because of their effect on the motor end plate, and magnesium sulfate, which can precipitate a severe myasthenic crisis.

As in patients with spinal cord injury, antepartum consultation with an anesthesiologist is recommended. Myasthenic crisis—respiratory and pharyngeal muscle paresis—can be lethal without prompt intubation. Also, patients with MG who require general anesthesia are at increased risk for requiring prolonged mechanical ventilation. Regarding drug interactions, anticholinesterases in combination with succinylcholine can cause respiratory collapse.

Cesarean is reserved for the usual obstetric indications. Skeletal muscle fatigue may impair pushing during the second stage, although the uterus—a smooth muscle organ—contracts as in patients without the disease. An instrumented delivery can be safely performed in the fatigued MG patient.

Pediatricians should be present at the time of delivery to evaluate the neonate. Approximately 9% of offspring of women with MG have transplacental passage of anti-AChR antibodies that render them at risk for neonatal MG and require respiratory support. Immunosuppressive therapy, plasmapheresis, and intravenous human immunoglobulins can be administered to the infant safely if needed However, the diagnosis of MS should be considered in patients presenting with perinantal optic neuritis.

Multiple Sclerosis

Multiple sclerosis (MS) is a demyelinating disease that affects men and women equally. It commonly develops in the 20- to 40-year age range and is more common in those who live in colder climates. The onset can be subtle, with symptoms of muscle weakness, visual disturbances, and loss of coordination. The disease is characterized by periods of exacerbation and remission, and the life expectancy and the rate of progression are difficult to predict.

Older studies suggest that there is no change in fertility in patients with MS and no apparent increase in perinatal morbidity and mortality. The effect of pregnancy on MS exacerbation is controversial. Postpartum exacerbations increase threefold from the 9 months during pregnancy. Twenty percent to 40% of women with stable MS during pregnancy will experience a postpartum exacerbation. The rate is highest in the first 3 months postpartum and stabilizes after the sixth postpartum month. These flares do not appear to contribute to long-term disability. Breast feeding does not increase the risk of MS exacerbation. However, the diagnosis of MS should be considered in patients presenting with perinatal opic neuritis.

There are data to suggest that pregnancy itself is protective in patients with MS and may delay the onset of wheelchair dependence. Patients with at least one pregnancy after the onset of disease had a mean time to wheelchair dependence of 18.6 years versus 12.5 years in those without a pregnancy after diagnosis of MS.

Pregnancy does affect treatment of the disease because some of the agents used to treat MS are known teratogens, including methotrexate and Cytoxan (Bristol-Myers Squibb, Princeton, New Jersey). Traditional therapy for MS includes glucocorticoids and adrenocorticotrophin (ACTH), both of which are safe to use during pregnancy in consultation with a perinatologist. Women who are taking any of the disease-modifying drugs—interferon beta-1a (Avonex; Biogen Idec, Research Triangle Park, North Carolina), interferon beta-1b (Betaseron; Bayer HealthCare Pharmaceuticals, Montville, New Jersey), interferon beta-1a (Rebif; Biogen Idec), glatiramer acetate (Copaxone; Teva Pharmaceuticals, North Wales, Pennsylvania), or mitoxantrone (Novantrone; Wyeth Consumer Healthcare, Richmond, Virginia)—should discuss their plan to become pregnant with their prescribing physician. The disease-modifying drugs are not recommended during breast feeding because it is not known whether they are excreted in breast milk. A woman should also review any other medications she is taking with her neurologist and obstetrician to identify those that are safe during pregnancy and breast feeding. Interferon beta-1a and interferon beta-1b are both category C for use in pregnancy, and glatiramer acetate is a category B medication. Patients must be counseled on the risks and benefits of using these medications in pregnancy. One option is to discontinue the immune-modulating therapy during pregnancy with resumption after the patient has completed breast feeding if her disease is stable. Women who use steroids for acute MS exacerbations may continue to use them throughout the pregnancy. Patients on chronic steroids should receive stress doses of steroids in labor and the postpartum period.

Women who have gait problems may experience difficulty walking during late pregnancy as they become heavier and their center of gravity shifts. Increased use of assistive devices to walk or use of a wheelchair may be considered. Bladder and bowel problems, which can occur in all pregnant women, may be aggravated in women with MS who have preexisting urinary or bowel dysfunction. Women with MS have a higher rate of urinary tract infection and should be screened monthly with urine cultures during the pregnancy. MS patients may also be more subject to fatigue. Also, those with deficits that impair pushing may require an assisted second stage. There are no contraindications to general or regional anesthesia. Mothers with weakness and lack of coordination may need extra help in caring for a newborn.

Carpal Tunnel Syndrome

The median nerve and flexor tendons pass through the carpal tunnel of wrist bones and the flexor retinaculum. In pregnancy, weight gain and edema can result in compression of the median nerve as it passes through this tunnel. While many pregnant women complain of palmar pain, less than 1% actually have true carpal tunnel syndrome, which consists of pain, numbness, and/or tingling in the distribution of the median nerve in the hand and wrist. Compressing the median nerve and percussing the wrist and forearm with a reflex hammer—the Tinel maneuver—can exacerbate the pain. These symptoms appear to be more common in primigravidas with generalized edema.

For most patients, supportive and conservative therapy is adequate. This includes splinting of the wrist until the symptoms subside in postpartum as the edema of pregnancy resolves. Local steroid injection can be considered in patients who do not improve with wrist splints. However, surgery should not be delayed in patients with deteriorating muscle tone and motor function. Decompression surgery can be performed under local anesthesia or an axillary block. Surgery is recommended for women with sensory loss or when neurologic testing demonstrates motor latency that is more than 5 msec.

Bell's Palsy

Bell's palsy is a facial nerve paralysis that typically involves all three peripheral branches, leading to asymmetric facial drooping and difficulty closing the eye of the affected side. The risk in pregnancy is more than three times that of nonpregnant women, and approximately 85% of cases appear in the third trimester or postpartum. Treatment in pregnancy is controversial because most patients recover without therapy.

Bell's palsy can be confused with the facial nerve palsy that is commonly associated with Lyme disease. Facial palsy occurs in 50% to 63% of patients with Lyme disease in the United States and Europe. However, patients with Lyme disease and facial nerve palsy can be differentiated from patients with Bell's palsy by the presence of other clinical features of Lyme disease. When patients with facial nerve palsy were compared with a retrospective cohort of nine women with facial palsy and serologic evidence of Lyme disease, all of the patients with serologic evidence of *Borrelia burgdorferi* had other clinical manifestations of Lyme disease.

Recently the combination of steroids (usually prednisone 60-80 mg/day) plus an antiviral agent such as valacyclovir (1 g three times daily) has become standard treatment because it is thought that Bell's palsy may be due to herpes simplex virus. Although the combination of corticosteroids and acyclovir has not been definitively proven, the available evidence suggests that it may be useful in improving outcomes. Of note, the combination of these medications has not been specifically tested in pregnancy. Symptomatic treatment with an eye patch and artificial tears may also be a useful adjunctive therapy.

VENTRICULOPERITONEAL SHUNT

Gravidas with cerebrospinal fluid shunts pose several unique management issues. Ventriculoperitoneal (VP) shunt malfunction can occur in 25% to 50% of these women in pregnancy. Occlusion of the shunt most often occurs in the third trimester—when the enlarging uterus may occlude the intraperitoneal portion of the catheter. Symptoms of shunt occlusion include confusion, lethargy, nausea and vomiting, headache, and nerve palsies.

Patients with a shunt should be managed in consultation with a neurologist. A baseline MRI should be performed to assess ventricular size in the patient who presents for preconceptional counseling. There are no controlled studies on the best method of delivery for these women, but the general agreement is that vaginal delivery can be attempted to avoid exposure of the VP shunt during a cesarean delivery. Shortening the second stage has been recommended to avoid increasing intracranial pressure with pushing. Intrapartum intravenous antibiotic prophylaxis to prevent shunt infection may be considered.

CEREBROVASCULAR DISEASE

Infarction or Thrombotic Stroke

Cerebral infarction may occur during pregnancy because of hypercoagulable states such as preeclampsia, infection, or thrombophilias. Rare etiologies of arterial occlusion include amniotic fluid embolus and a paradoxical embolization from the pelvic vein to the cranium via a patent foramen ovale. Antiphospholipid antibody syndrome is also associated with maternal thrombosis, although the risk is highly variable and exacerbated by coexistent coagulopathies. Sagittal sinus thrombosis is a common location of intracranial thrombosis in women with thrombophilia.

The relative risk of a cerebral infarction is 0.7 during pregnancy and increases 8.7 times the in the postpartum period. Risk factors for stroke related to pregnancy include cesarean delivery and pregnancy-related hypertension.

Transient ischemic attacks may precede occlusion of one of the major arteries, and the clinician should be sensitive to subtle neurologic cues. When a patient presents with neurologic signs during pregnancy, the symptoms must be investigated and treated as in nonpregnant patients. An imaging study of the brain is an essential component of the evaluation. A noncontrast head CT is typically the first diagnostic study in patients with suspected stroke. CT has the benefits of widespread access and speed of acquisition, but MRI may be more sensitive for the diagnosis of early infarction. Whenever possible, radiographic diagnostic procedures performed during pregnancy should be undertaken with shielding of the maternal abdomen. Small subarachnoid hemorrhages can be missed by both CT and MRI and require lumbar puncture to make a diagnosis.

Pregnant patients can undergo neurosurgery, but care must be taken to avoid deep hypotension, which compromises uteroplacental flow. Anticoagulation for stroke in pregnancy has not been well studied. Warfarin use carries with it teratogenic risk in the first trimester and potential for fetal intraventricular hemorrhage when used later in the pregnancy. Although heparin does not cross the placenta it can be difficult to obtain therapeutic dosing in pregnancy. Low molecular weight heparin (LMWH) can be dosed twice daily and has the advantages of better bioavailability and less heparin-induced thrombocytopenia. However, it is considerably more expensive than unfractionated heparin.

Hemorrhagic Stroke

Women of reproductive age may have asymptomatic cerebral aneurysms or arteriovenous malformations (AVMs). These vascular lesions can rupture during pregnancy, leading to hemorrhagic stroke. The adjusted risk of intracerebral hemorrhage is 2.5 in pregnancy and increases to 28.3 in the postpartum period. AVMs tend to bleed in the second trimester, whereas aneurysms lead to subarachnoid hemorrhages in the third trimester.

Small AVMs (less than 2 cm^3) have an average annual risk of rupture of 3.4%. Medium AVMs (2 to 5 cm^3) have an average annual risk of rupture of 3.7%. Pregnancy does not increase the risk rate of first cerebral hemorrhage from an AVM. A 3.5% risk of first bleed during pregnancy has been reported. This risk is evenly distributed across gestation, without any apparent increased likelihood of hemorrhage during labor and delivery. Women with a previous cerebral hemorrhage will be at a greater risk of rebleed in pregnancy (5.8%) if left untreated.

Women with chronic hypertension are at higher risk for developing intracerebral aneurysms. Saccular aneurysms often rupture into the subarachnoid space, accounting for 70% to 80% of spontaneous subarachnoid hemorrhages (SAHs). They are associated with a very high mortality, accounting for 10% of all deaths from stroke. The risk of rebleeding is greatest in the first

48 hours and is associated with a high mortality rate. Surgical clipping of the involved aneurysm is of proven benefit, although the timing of surgery remains the subject of some controversy.

Both ruptured AVMs and aneurysms can present with a sudden onset of severe headache with or without nausea. There can be meningeal signs on physical examination. CT or MRI should be performed expeditiously. There are no contraindications to lumbar puncture in the pregnant woman. To more precisely identify the anatomic features and location of the lesion, intracranial angiography with shielding may also be necessary.

Surgical treatment may involve embolization of AVMs or clipping of aneurysms. Hypertension and hypotension should be avoided. Pregnant patients with subarachnoid hemorrhage resulting from ruptured aneurysms can also be successfully treated via an endoscopic approach, avoiding craniotomy. Up to 60% of patients die in the first 30 days as the result of SAH. About 10% die immediately without any warning; an additional 25% die or become disabled as a result of the initial hemorrhage. For women with uncorrected intracranial vascular lesions, a planned cesarean delivery is warranted to avoid increased intracranial vascular pressure that might lead to intracranial bleed. General anesthesia should be avoided for cesarean delivery because intubation may cause hypertension. Operative vaginal delivery with shortening of the second stage of labor to avoid unnecessary increases in intracranial pressure can be considered in women who have undergone surgical treatment of the vascular malformations or aneurysms.

KEY POINTS

Epilepsy

- Attempts should be made to control seizures with monotherapy to minimize risk of AED embryopathy.
- Folic acid (4 mg per day) supplementation should begin preconceptionally to prevent NTD.
- Sleep deprivation may increase seizure frequency.
- Patients may discontinue AED if seizure free for 2 years.
- Genetic counseling and prenatal screening for congenital anomalies should be offered after pregnancy is confirmed.

Spinal Cord Injury

- Autonomic hyperreflexia should be avoided while the patient with a T5-10 injury is in labor.
- Bladder distention can be avoided with indwelling Foley catheter to prevent autonomic hyperreflexia.
- Obstetrical anesthesiologists should be consulted in early labor to provide continuous lumbar epidural anesthesia to the T10 level to prevent autonomic hyperreflexia.
- Women with spinal cord injuries may not be able to feel contractions, so labor should be diagnosed early by cervical examination and abdominal palpation for contractions.

KEY POINTS—cont'd

Myasthenia Gravis

- The pyridostigmine often must be increased during pregnancy and this should be accomplished by increasing the frequency of the medication first before increasing the dosage amount.
- Gentamicin antibiotic is contraindicated in patients with MG.
- Magnesium sulfate tocolysis for preterm labor or seizure prophylaxis for preeclampsia should be avoided in women with MG.
- General anesthesia should be avoided if cesarean delivery is needed.
- Neonates are at risk for self-limited congenital MG.

Multiple Sclerosis

- A consultation with a neurologist should be made preconceptionally or early in pregnancy to determine whether immune modulator therapy must be continued throughout the pregnancy.
- Corticosteroids can be taken safely throughout pregnancy if necessary.
- Patient is at increased risk for flares in the postpartum period.
- Monthly urine cultures can be performed to screen for urinary tract infection in MS patients with bladder dysfunction.

Carpal Tunnel Syndrome

- Wrist splints are the initial therapy for symptomatic relief of carpal tunnel syndrome complaints.
- Neurology and orthopedics consultation may be needed if patient is experiencing motor weakness and requires more invasive therapy.

Bell's Palsy

- An eye patch and artificial tears provide supportive care for the pregnant patient.
- A short course of corticosteroids and acyclovir can be considered to shorten the course of disease.

Ventriculoperitoneal Shunt

- Symptoms of shunt occlusion include confusion, nausea, vomiting, and headache, which can develop particularly in the third trimester.
- The second stage of labor can be shortened to avoid increased intracranial pressure.
- Intravenous antibiotic prophylaxis can be considered.

Cerebral Vascular Disease

- Low molecular weight heparin can be safely be used for thrombotic strokes in pregnancy.
- The patient should undergo a thrombophilia workup for thrombotic stroke.
- Women with known AVMs or cerebral aneurysms should have surgical correction before attempting pregnancy.
- If intracranial vascular lesions are not corrected, cesarean delivery is indicated.
- If the vascular lesions are surgically corrected, vaginal delivery with shortening of second stage can be offered.

SUGGESTED READINGS

Holmes LB et al: The teratogenicity of anticonvulsant drugs. *N Engl J Med* 344:1132, 2001.

Palmieri C, Canger R: Teratogenic potential of the newer antiepileptic drugs. What is known and how should this influence prescribing? *CNS Drugs* 16:755, 2002.

Pennell PB: Pregnancy in the woman with epilepsy: maternal and fetal outcomes. *Semin Neurol* 22:299, 2002.

Pschirrer ER: Seizure disorders in pregnancy. *Obstet Gynecol Clin North Am* 31:373, 2004.

http://www.epilepsy.com.

28

DERMATOSIS OF PREGNANCY

Miriam Keltz Pomeranz and Olympia Kovich

The physiologic changes associated with pregnancy may lead to a variety of cutaneous manifestations. Changes in hormonal levels during this period may also induce or exacerbate a wide variety of common dermatoses. The focus of this chapter, however, is on those dermatoses specific to pregnancy, namely, those that occur only in pregnant and puerperal women.

Relatively few dermatoses are confined solely to pregnant and puerperal women, thus limiting the scope of our discussion to several disease entities. This chapter covers pemphigoid gestationis, pruritic urticarial papules and plaques of pregnancy (PUPPP), prurigo of pregnancy, and pustular psoriasis of pregnancy. Additionally, this chapter includes a discussion of cholestasis of pregnancy, which is not considered a true dermatosis of pregnancy.

PEMPHIGOID GESTATIONIS

This entity has also been variably referred to as herpes gestationis or gestational pemphigoid. The names pemphigoid gestationis or gestational pemphigoid are most accurate. It is clinically a pemphigoid-like disease. The antigen targeted in this dermatitis belongs to the pemphigoid group. The misleading name herpes gestationis implies an infectious disease associated with herpes, which is untrue (Box 28-1).

Epidemiology

Pemphigoid gestationis is an autoimmune bullous disease with an estimated incidence ranging between 1 in 10,000 and 1 in 60,000 pregnancies. This rare disorder is more common in Caucasian patients, particularly those with HLA-DR3 and HLA-DR4 haplotypes. It has been reported in pregnant patients and those with trophoblastic tumors and molar pregnancies.

Clinical Features

Pemphigoid gestationis most commonly begins during the second or third trimester. Intense pruritus, often preceding cutaneous lesions, is a key feature of this disorder. The classic presentation of disease, occurring in approximately 50% of patients, begins with urticarial plaques or papules surrounding the umbilicus but not necessarily localized to striae (Figure 28-1). These initial lesions then form tense bullae, with new lesions extending to involve the trunk

Box 28-1 Pemphigoid Gestationis at a Glance

- Nomenclature: pemphigoid gestationis, herpes gestationis, gestational pemphigoid
- Etiology: autoimmune, not infectious, disorder
- Clinical features
  - Onset during second or third trimester
  - Periumbilical urticarial papules/plaques progress to tense blisters
- Differential diagnosis: PUPPP, erythema multiforme, contact dermatitis, drug eruption
- Diagnosis: skin biopsy and direct immunofluorescence studies establish diagnosis
- Treatment: systemic corticosteroids
- Prognosis
  - Maternal: risk of recurrence with subsequent pregnancies, use of OCPs, menses; increased lifetime risk of Grave's disease
  - Fetal: at risk for growth retardation and prematurity; low incidence of neonatal disease, with mild course

OCP, Oral contraceptive pills; *PUPPP,* pruritic urticarial papules and plaques of pregnancy.

and extremities. Rare involvement of the face or mucous membranes has been reported.

Etiology

Although the target antigen of pemphigoid gestationis has been identified, the mechanism of initiating autoimmunity has not been proven. It is postulated that the expression of paternal major histocompatibility complex (MHC) class II antigens in the placenta triggers an autoimmune response

Figure 28-1

Pemphigoid gestationis. Note the periumbilical localization of the urticarial papules and plaques.

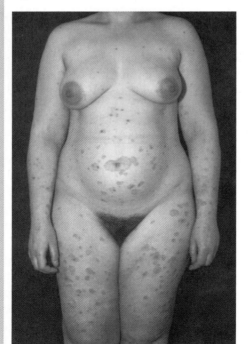

against a placental antigen. This antigen is present in both the skin and amnion and has been identified as BP antigen 2, also known as type XVII collagen, a 180-kDa epidermal protein. Once antibodies have been formed in the placenta, they can cross-react with skin and cause maternal disease.

This hypothesis is supported by the fact that this antigen may be found in the placenta beginning in the second trimester, coincident with the onset of disease. However, the inconsistent association between a change in partner and the occurrence of pemphigoid gestationis undermines this hypothesis. Thus the pathogenesis of this disease is not entirely understood.

Differential Diagnosis

Pemphigoid gestationis should be differentiated from PUPPP. The predilection of PUPPP for striae as opposed to the truly periumbilical initial localization in pemphigoid gestationis is a useful clinical clue. Other entities in the differential diagnosis include erythema multiforme, contact dermatitis, and drug eruptions. Therefore a careful history, specifically with regard to possible environmental exposures and medication use, is warranted.

465

Natural History

Pemphigoid gestationis usually remits before delivery but three quarters of patients experience a flare at delivery or in the immediate postpartum period. Nevertheless the majority of cases will spontaneously resolve within weeks to months after delivery. Only six cases of long-lasting postpartum pemphigoid gestationis have been reported, with two of these patients meeting criteria for an evolution of their disease into bullous pemphigoid. Interestingly, a hormonal component in the pathogenesis of this disease is supported by the occurrence of flares with the use of oral contraceptives in 25% of patients and during the premenstrual period. Pemphigoid gestationis may present during any pregnancy, with a high frequency of recurrence with subsequent pregnancies. In 5% of patients, pemphigoid gestationis may skip pregnancies.

Laboratory

Routine laboratory tests, including complement levels, are normal; there are no diagnostic laboratory tests. Histopathologic examination of a skin biopsy reveals a subepidermal vesicle with a perivascular infiltrate of lymphocytes, histiocytes, and eosinophils. The presence of eosinophils is the most constant and conspicuous feature.

Direct immunofluorescence of perilesional skin reveals the linear deposition of C3 along the dermoepidermal junction. This finding is pathognomonic for pemphigoid gestationis in a pregnant patient. Complement-added indirect immunofluorescence microscopy reveals the presence of anti-basement membrane zone antibodies in 93% of cases. Older methods of indirect immunofluorescence were not nearly as sensitive. In addition, enzyme-linked immunosorbent assay (ELISA) is another sensitive technique for detecting autoantibodies (86.3% of cases) and titers have been demonstrated to correlate with disease activity.

Treatment

Although antihistamines and topical corticosteroids have been used to alleviate pruritus, systemic corticosteroids (0.5-1.0 mg/kg/day) are needed to control most cases. Because of the high incidence of postpartum flares, therapy may need to be continued through delivery or reinstituted in the postpartum period.

Prognosis

As mentioned previously, mothers with pemphigoid gestationis are at risk for recurrence of disease in the postpartum period, during menstrual cycles, with use of oral contraceptives, and with subsequent pregnancies. An increased incidence of antithyroid antibodies has been reported and patients with pemphigoid gestationis are at an increased lifetime risk of Graves' disease.

Mild placental insufficiency resulting from the autoimmune response increases the risk of small-for-gestational age births and premature delivery (16% before 36 weeks and 32% before 38 weeks' gestation). The incidence of a neonatal eruption is low (2.8%-10%) and usually follows a mild course, resolving within weeks.

466

PRURITIC URTICARIAL PAPULES AND PLAQUES OF PREGNANCY

The entity called pruritic urticarial papules and plaques of pregnancy is known by the acronym PUPPP in the United States. Some authors have renamed it polymorphic eruption of pregnancy (PEP), which is the favored name in the United Kingdom (Box 28-2).

Epidemiology

Of the dermatoses specific to pregnancy, PUPPP is the most common, with an estimated incidence of 1 in 160 to 1 in 300 pregnancies. Although usually diagnosed in primigravidas in the third trimester, PUPPP is also seen in multiparous women, especially with multiple gestations. For this reason, elevated hormone levels and excessive weight gain have been postulated as potential etiologic factors.

Clinical Features

As its name indicates, PUPPP is a polymorphous eruption. PUPPP usually begins at the end of the third-trimester gestation with urticarial wheals, but the morphology of lesions may change during its mean duration of 6 weeks (Figure 28-2). Urticarial plaques may develop overlying vesicles (40% of

---

Box 28-2 Pruritic Urticarial Papules and Plaques of Pregnancy at a Glance

- Nomenclature: pruritic urticarial papules and plaques of pregnancy (PUPPP), polymorphic eruption of pregnancy (PEP), toxic erythema of pregnancy, Bourne's "toxemic rash of pregnancy," Nurse's "late onset prurigo" of pregnancy
- Etiology: unknown
- Clinical features
  - Onset in third trimester of nulliparous women or multiple gestation pregnancies
  - Pruritic urticarial lesions begin in abdominal striae
- Differential diagnosis: pemphigoid gestationis, erythema multiforme, contact dermatitis, drug reactions, viral infections, infestations
- Diagnosis: clinical
- Treatment: topical corticosteroids, antihistamines and rarely oral corticosteroids
- Prognosis: No maternal or fetal morbidity

Figure 28-2

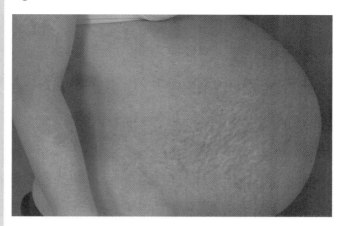

cases); later lesions may be annular or polycyclic (18% of cases) or targetoid (20% of cases). Up to 70% of patients with PUPPP may develop widespread erythema.

A distinguishing feature is the location of the lesions, which have a predilection for the abdominal striae; this is the site of initial involvement in two thirds of cases. In contrast to pemphigoid gestationis, PUPPP spares the periumbilical region. Other common sites of involvement include the thighs, buttocks, and extremities, with sparing of the palms, soles, and mucous membranes. Pruritus is a universal feature, but the most debilitating pruritus usually lasts about 1 week.

Etiology

The pathogenesis of PUPPP has not been elucidated, but certain clinical features and studies suggest various mechanisms. One theory is that increased abdominal distention alters vascular permeability, enabling the migration of fetal cells into maternal skin. This theory, supported by the discovery of fetal DNA in the cutaneous lesions of PUPPP, purports that an immune reaction may be elicited either by fetal cells against maternal antigens or that the fetal cells may be targeted. A second hypothesis is also based on abdominal distention; damage to connective tissue may cause normal proteins to be processed as antigens, with a resultant inflammatory reaction. Yet a third theory of pathogenesis considers the potential role of hormones. Various studies have demonstrated increased immunoreactivity of progesterone receptors in PUPPP lesions and decreased serum cortisol levels in women with PUPPP.

Differential Diagnosis

As mentioned previously, the location of PUPPP lesions in the abdominal striae and the absence of true vesicles/bullae help differentiate this entity from pemphigoid gestationis. Direct immunofluorescence (DIF) studies on a biopsy specimen will also distinguish PUPPP (negative or nonspecific findings on DIF) from pemphigoid gestationis (linear C3 deposition on DIF). PUPPP may also be confused with erythema multiforme when the morphology of lesions is targetoid (three distinct rings); sparing of the palms, soles, and mucous membranes is an important distinguishing feature. Other entities to consider in the differential diagnosis include contact dermatitis, drug reactions, viral syndromes, and infestations (scabies).

Natural History

PUPPP is a self-limited condition that usually begins late in the third trimester. Although it lasts for a mean duration of 6 weeks, the worst pruritus typically subsides after 1 week. It generally resolves early in the postpartum period and does not routinely recur with subsequent pregnancies.

Laboratory

No specific abnormalities are associated with PUPPP, but liver function tests may be performed to investigate other possible causes of pruritus. Biopsy results are nonspecific, variably demonstrating spongiosis, parakeratosis, and a perivascular dermal lymphocytic infiltrate, which may contain eosinophils and dermal edema. DIF fails to demonstrate linear deposition of C3 at the dermoepidermal junction, which is the hallmark of pemphigoid gestationis. Indirect immunofluorescence is invariably negative.

Treatment

Control of maternal pruritus directs treatment, typically with topical steroids and oral antihistamines. The use of oral corticosteroids is rarely required. Early delivery is generally not indicated.

Prognosis

PUPPP does not affect maternal or fetal outcomes, other than the discomfort of pruritus. Recurrence with subsequent pregnancies appears uncommon.

PRURIGO OF PREGNANCY

Prurigo of pregnancy, also referred to as prurigo gestationis, is a less well-defined dermatosis. Pruritic folliculitis, considered a separate entity by some authorities, may be included under this heading with certain distinct features (Box 28-3).

Box 28-3   Prurigo of Pregnancy at a Glance

- Nomenclature: prurigo of pregnancy, prurigo gestationis, Besnier's "prurigo gestationis," Nurse's "early onset" form of prurigo, Spangler's "papular dermatitis of pregnancy," linear IgM disease of pregnancy, pruritic folliculitis
- Etiology: unknown
- Clinical features
  - Excoriated, crusted papules on extensor surfaces of extremities and trunk
  - Associated pruritus
- Differential diagnosis: PUPPP, drug reactions, scabies, cholestasis of pregnancy, bacterial folliculitis, other dermatoses
- Treatment: symptomatic (topical steroids, antihistamines)
- Prognosis: No fetal or maternal risk

PUPPP, Pruritic urticarial papules and plaques of pregnancy.

468

Epidemiology

Prurigo of pregnancy is a diagnosis of exclusion, established only after other potential etiologies of pruritus such as cholestasis or atopic dermatitis have been ruled out. Prurigo of pregnancy occurs more commonly in the second and third trimesters, with an estimated incidence of 1 in 300 to 1 in 450 pregnancies.

Clinical Features

Patients with prurigo of pregnancy present with flesh-colored or erythematous papules, which are often excoriated or crusted because of the associated scratching. The lesions are often grouped on the extensor surfaces of the extremities and the trunk. In the subset of pruritic folliculitis, papules and occasional pustules are centered around hair follicles, most commonly on the upper trunk.

Etiology

Although the etiology of this entity is unknown, a potential association with atopy has been suggested by the finding of elevated serum IgE and positive history of atopy in affected women.

469

Differential Diagnosis

Other dermatoses unrelated to pregnancy, such as drug reactions and scabies, may present with pruritus but should be distinguished by clinical features. Cholestasis of pregnancy should be excluded by laboratory tests. If these laboratory tests are abnormal, then, by definition, the condition is not prurigo of pregnancy. If confirmed by elevated levels of serum bile acids, the diagnosis is then cholestasis of pregnancy, which is referred to as prurigo gravidarum in the older literature. Bacterial folliculitis should be investigated by culture of a pustule, if present.

Natural History

Prurigo of pregnancy usually resolves spontaneously in the postpartum period, although it rarely persists for several months after delivery. Recurrences with subsequent pregnancies may occur.

Laboratory

There are no specific laboratory abnormalities and liver function tests must be normal (to exclude cholestasis of pregnancy) to establish the diagnosis. Histopathology reveals nonspecific findings of a dermal perivascular infiltrate lacking eosinophils and variable acanthosis, hyperkeratosis, or parakeratosis of the epidermis. Both direct and indirect immunofluorescence studies are negative. Biopsy of a lesion of pruritic folliculitis may demonstrate intrafollicular neutrophils.

Treatment

Treatment is aimed at symptomatic relief of pruritus with topical steroids and antihistamines. Pruritic folliculitis has been treated similarly; the use of benzoyl peroxide or ultraviolet B phototherapy has also been effective in anecdotal reports.

Prognosis

No evidence demonstrates risk to the fetus or mother, other than one study that showed reduced birth weight in fetuses of mothers with pruritic folliculitis. There are variable data on recurrence with subsequent pregnancies.

PUSTULAR PSORIASIS OF PREGNANCY

Pustular psoriasis of pregnancy was previously referred to as impetigo herpetiformis. Some now consider this entity to represent a flare of psoriasis during pregnancy and not a distinct dermatosis of pregnancy (Box 28-4).

Epidemiology

Although 50% of women with chronic psoriasis may report improvement in the peripartum period, the occurrence of pustular psoriasis of pregnancy generally occurs in women without a past history of psoriasis and remits permanently postpartum. This exceedingly rare disorder has only 350 reported cases in the literature as of 2000.

Clinical Features

Pustular psoriasis may develop during any trimester but onset occurs most commonly in the third trimester. Lesions often first appear in intertriginous regions, as erythematous plaques studded with rings of pustules. As the lesions evolve, the center becomes eroded and crusted as the plaque enlarges. Subsequent lesions develop on the trunk and extremities; oral and esophageal erosions may occur. Additional cutaneous features include onycholysis of the nails (lifting of the nail plate from the nail bed) and nail pitting.

Systemic features include malaise, anorexia, nausea, vomiting, diarrhea, fever, and chills. An associated hypocalcemia may lead to tetany, delirium, and seizures. Notably, there is often a lack of pruritus.

Etiology

There is no clear understanding of this disorder, although it may be related to hormonal changes of pregnancy. Hypocalcemia and hypoparathyroidism may be inciting factors or secondary phenomena. In contrast to the implications of the name impetigo herpetiformis, this disorder is not infectious.

Differential Diagnosis

Infectious etiologies of pustules, including candidiasis and impetigo, should be investigated through appropriate cultures. Pustular drug eruptions, notably acute generalized exanthematous pustulosis, may be excluded through history. Other pregnancy-related dermatoses, including pruritic folliculitis and pemphigoid gestationis, may be differentiated on the basis of

---

Box 28-4   Pustular Psoriasis of Pregnancy at a Glance

- Nomenclature: pustular psoriasis of pregnancy, impetigo herpetiformis
- Etiology: unknown, not infectious
- Clinical features
  - Erythematous plaques with rings of pustules begin in intertriginous areas
  - Associated systemic symptoms, notably hypocalcemia
- Differential diagnosis: candidiasis, impetigo, pustular drug eruptions, other pustular dermatoses
- Treatment: systemic corticosteroids, correction of hypocalcemia (if present)
- Prognosis: increased risk of stillbirth and neonatal death resulting from placental insufficiency
  - Recurrence with subsequent pregnancies is common

morphology and location of lesions. Finally, other pustular dermatoses, such as subcorneal pustular dermatosis and dermatitis herpetiformis should be considered.

Natural History

The eruption usually persists until delivery but generally resolves in the postpartum period. Recurrence with subsequent pregnancies is common, with a trend toward earlier onset and increased severity of presentation after the initial episode. Rarely the disease may reappear with menses or use of oral contraceptive pills.

Laboratory

Leukocytosis and elevated erythrocyte sedimentation rate are common laboratory findings associated with pustular psoriasis of pregnancy. Importantly, hypocalcemia may be present, which may be related to hypoparathyroidism and lead to significant clinical features. Additional findings include albuminuria, pyuria, and hematuria. Pustules are sterile.

471

Histopathology reveals spongiform pustules with neutrophils in the epidermis, parakeratosis and psoriasiform hyperplasia, identical to findings in nonpregnant patients with pustular psoriasis.

Treatment

Systemic corticosteroids are the mainstay of treatment, with high doses often needed to control disease. It is of absolute necessity to correct hypocalcemia, if present, and monitor electrolytes. In severe cases, early delivery may be warranted.

Prognosis

An association with placental insufficiency has been reported, leading to a risk of stillbirth and neonatal death. As stated previously, recurrence with increased severity is common with subsequent pregnancies.

CHOLESTASIS OF PREGNANCY

Cholestasis of pregnancy, often referred to as prurigo gravidarum in older literature, does not have primary skin lesions; it therefore might not be considered a true "dermatosis" of pregnancy. However, because it causes the patient to present with pruritus as the chief complaint, it belongs in a discussion of pregnancy and skin disease (Box 28-5).

Box 28-5   Cholestasis of Pregnancy at a Glance

- Nomenclature: cholestasis of pregnancy, obstetric cholestasis, intrahepatic cholestasis of pregnancy, cholestatic jaundice of pregnancy, prurigo gravidarum
- Etiology: unknown
- Clinical features
  - Pruritus and excoriations in the absence of primary cutaneous lesions
  - Jaundice in 20% of patients
- Differential diagnosis: viral hepatitis, primary biliary cirrhosis
- Treatment: antihistamines, cholestyramine, ursodeoxycholic acid
- Prognosis: increased risk of prematurity, fetal distress, and intrauterine death

Epidemiology

The incidence of this disorder is estimated at 70 in 10,000 pregnancies in the United States. It has previously been reported with an increased prevalence in Scandinavia, Chile, and Bolivia, which may be attributed to dietary or genetic factors. Cholestasis of pregnancy is seen more often with multiple-gestation pregnancies. In 50% of cases, a family history is reported, with a purported dominant inheritance pattern. Studies have confirmed that the incidence of cholestasis of pregnancy is higher in women with hepatitis C.

Clinical Features

The clinical hallmark of cholestasis of pregnancy is excoriations in the absence of primary lesions. The associated pruritus is severe, often worse at night, and involves the palms and soles. Onset is most frequent in the third trimester, associated with a concomitant urinary tract infection in up to 50% of patients. Earlier onset of symptoms may be observed in patients with hepatitis C and may herald the complication of spontaneous prematurity.

Although viral hepatitis is the most common cause of obstetric jaundice, a minority of patients with cholestasis of pregnancy will develop jaundice, with associated dark urine and light-colored stools, typically within 2 to 4 weeks of onset of symptoms. Jaundice may be accompanied by subclinical steatorrhea, resulting in deficiency of vitamin K, which leads to prolonged prothrombin time and a risk of hemorrhage.

Etiology

Various theories have been proposed to explain the phenomenon of cholestasis of pregnancy. Decreased hepatic blood flow or hormonal factors during pregnancy may play a role. Additionally, clustering within families and the finding of mutations at various genetic loci suggest a polygenetic basis of disease.

Differential Diagnosis

Appropriate screening to rule out viral hepatitis is warranted. If primary cutaneous lesions are noted on physical exam, then a primary dermatosis should be considered.

Natural History

Pruritus persists until delivery, but resolves in the immediate postpartum period (24-48 hours). Jaundice typically resolves in the first weeks after delivery. In 60% to 70% of cases, recurrence during subsequent pregnancies occurs. The use of oral contraceptives may also lead to recurrence in the postpartum period. Patients with cholestasis of pregnancy are at increased risk for developing cholelithiasis or gallbladder disease.

Laboratory

The most sensitive marker of cholestasis of pregnancy is elevation of serum bile acids (cholic acid, deoxycholic acid, chenodeoxycholic acid), which may be from 3 to 100 times above the normal range. Total serum bile acid levels greater than 10 to 11 μmol/L are considered to be diagnostic. A ratio of cholic to chenodeoxycholic acid is usually 4:1 in women with cholestasis of pregnancy, as opposed to a ratio of less than 1.5 in unaffected pregnant and nonpregnant women. Additional findings include a mild elevation in direct bilirubin and mild liver function abnormalities. Hepatitis serologies should be evaluated.

Skin biopsy is not warranted and nonspecific. Though not indicated, liver biopsy will demonstrate centrilobular cholestasis with bile thrombi within dilated canaliculi. Ultrasound of the liver is normal.

Treatment

Various modalities have been reported in the treatment of cholestasis of pregnancy, beginning with topical emollients, antipruritics, and antihistamines to control pruritus. Other treatments include cholestyramine and phenobarbital, ultraviolet B (UVB) phototherapy, and ursodeoxycholic acid (UDCA). UDCA has been reported to be effective both in control of symptoms and reducing adverse fetal events; it is classified as pregnancy category B. Because of concerns regarding efficacy and side effects of cholestyramine and phenobarbital, most clinicians will initially treat cholestasis with a combination of topical emollients and antihistamines, followed by UDCA if symptoms worsen.

Monitoring prothrombin time is crucial to minimizing potential fetal intracranial hemorrhage; intramuscular vitamin K should be administered as needed.

Prognosis

Reported complications associated with cholestasis of pregnancy include increased incidence of stillbirth, premature delivery, postpartum hemorrhage, and fetal intracranial hemorrhage. One prospective study demonstrated an increased risk of complications in women with higher bile acid levels (≥ 40 µmol/L). Other data demonstrate that intrauterine death occurs most often after 37 weeks of gestation in single gestation pregnancies. The additional finding of hepatitis C infection has not been shown to impart any additional risk for fetal outcome. These risks may be reduced by treatment.

Many authorities support delivery at 36 to 38 weeks gestation or sooner, if fetal lung maturity is documented. Most concerning is that adverse fetal outcomes, such as demise and abruptio, seem not to be well predicted by antenatal testing. Regardless, twice-weekly fetal testing should be instituted when the diagnosis of cholestasis is made, as well as an evaluation of fetal growth.

KEY POINTS

- Pemphigoid gestationis (herpes gestationis), a blistering disorder during pregnancy, is associated with increased risk of in utero growth retardation and premature labor; it often recurs with subsequent pregnancies.
- Pemphigoid gestationis often requires treatment with systemic steroids through delivery.
- PUPPP is not associated with significant risks to the mother or the fetus. Early delivery is not necessary.
- Pustular psoriasis of pregnancy (impetigo herpetiformis) can result in fetal demise and early delivery may be necessary.
- Pustular psoriasis of pregnancy often recurs with subsequent pregnancies.
- Cholestasis of pregnancy can be diagnosed in a pruritic pregnant patient with elevated serum bile acids. It can cause premature labor and fetal demise. It may recur in subsequent pregnancies.
- Cholestasis of pregnancy can be treated with ursodeoxycholic acid, but one should consider delivery at 36 to 38 weeks' gestation.

SUGGESTED READINGS

Al-Fares S, Jones SV, Black MM: The specific dermatoses of pregnancy: a re-appraisal. *J Eur Acad Dermatol Venereol* 15:197, 2001.

Glantz A, Marschall H-U, Mattsson L-A: Intrahepatic cholestasis of pregnancy: relationships between bile acid levels and fetal complication rates. *Hepatology* 40:467, 2004.

Kroumpouzos G, Cohen LM: Specific dermatoses of pregnancy: an evidence-based systematic review. *Am J Obstet Gynecol* 188:1083, 2003.

Paternoster DM et al: Intra-hepatic cholestasis of pregnancy in hepatitis C infection. *Acta Obstet Gynecol Scand* 81:99, 2002.

Paus TC et al: Diagnosis and therapy of intrahepatic cholestasis of pregnancy. *Z Gastroenterol* 42:623, 2004.

Shornick JK: Pregnancy dermatoses. In Bolognia JL, Jorizzo JL, Rapini RP, editors: *Dermatology*. London, 2003, Mosby, pp 425-432.

Sitaru C et al: Immunoblotting and enzyme-linked immunsorbent assay for the diagnosis of pemphigoid gestationis. *Obstet Gynecol* 103:757, 2004.

Williamson C et al: Clinical outcome in a series of cases of obstetric cholestasis identified via a patient support group. *Br J Obstet Gynaecol* 111:676, 2004.

INDEX

Note: Page numbers followed by f refer to figures; page numbers followed by t refer to tables; page numbers followed by b refer to boxes.

477

481